Clinical Applications of Pharmacotherapy

Clinical Applications of Pharmacotherapy

Editor: Brendon Krauss

FOSTER ACADEMICS

www.fosteracademics.com

www.fosteracademics.com

FOSTER ACADEMICS

Cataloging-in-Publication Data

Clinical applications of pharmacotherapy / edited by Brendon Krauss.
p. cm.
Includes bibliographical references and index.
ISBN 978-1-63242-571-3
1. Chemotherapy. 2. Drugs. 3. Pharmacology. I. Krauss, Brendon.
RM263 .C55 2018
615.58--dc23

Foster Academics,
118-35 Queens Blvd., Suite 400,
Forest Hills, NY 11375, USA

ISBN 978-1-63242-571-3 (Hardback)

Contents

Preface

Over the recent decade, advancements and applications have progressed exponentially. This has led to the increased interest in this field and projects are being conducted to enhance knowledge. The main objective of this book is to present some of the critical challenges and provide insights into possible solutions. This book will answer the varied questions that arise in the field and also provide an increased scope for furthering studies.

Medical therapies can be divided into pharmacotherapy, surgery, radiation or physical therapy. The therapy used on patients which uses pharmaceutical drugs is known as pharmacotherapy. It uses drugs in a safe and appropriate manner to cure or treat diseases. This book outlines the processes and applications of pharmacotherapy in detail. There has been rapid progress in this field and its applications are finding their way across multiple areas of medicine. The book is meant for students who are looking for an elaborate reference text on pharmacotherapy.

I hope that this book, with its visionary approach, will be a valuable addition and will promote interest among readers. Each of the authors has provided their extraordinary competence in their specific fields by providing different perspectives as they come from diverse nations and regions. I thank them for their contributions.

Editor

1

Prognostic Parameters and Spinal Metastases: A Research Study

Jefferson W. Daniel*, José C. E. Veiga

Division of Neurosurgery, Santa Casa de São Paulo - Faculty of Medical Sciences, São Paulo, Brazil

Abstract

Object: To identify pre-operative prognostic parameters for survival in patients with spinal epidural neoplastic metastasis when the primary tumour is unknown.

Methods: This study was a retrospective chart review of patients who underwent surgery for spinal epidural neoplastic metastases between February 1997 and January 2011. The inclusion criteria were as follows: known post-operative survival period, a Karnofsky Performance Score equal to or greater than 30 points and a post-operative neoplastic metastasis histological type. The Kaplan-Meier method was used to estimate post-operative survival, and the Log-Rank test was used for statistical inference.

Results: A total of 52 patients who underwent 52 surgical procedures were identified. The mean age at the time of spinal surgery was 53.92 years (std. deviation, 19.09). The median survival after surgery was 70 days (95% CI 49.97–90.02), and post-operative mortality occurred within 6 months in 38 (73.07%) patients. Lung cancer, prostate cancer, myeloma and lymphoma, the 4 most common primary tumour types, affected 32 (61.53%) patients. The three identified prognostic parameters were the following: pre-operative walking incapacity (American Spinal Injury Association, A and B), present in 86.53% of the patients (p-value = 0.107); special care dependency (Karnofsky Performance Score, 10–40 points), present in 90.38% of the patients (p-value = 0.322); and vertebral epidural neoplastic metastases that were in contact with the thecal sac (Weinstein-Boriani-Biagini, sector D), present in 94.23% of the patients (p-value = 0.643). When the three secondary prognostic parameters were combined, the mean post-operative survival was 45 days; when at least one was present, the survival was 82 days (p-value = 0.175).

Conclusions: Walking incapacity, special care dependency and contact between the neoplastic metastases and the thecal sac can help determine the ultimate survival of this patient population and, potentially, which patients would benefit from surgery versus palliation alone. A 2- to 3-month post-operative survival period justified surgical treatment.

Editor: Anthony W.I. Lo, Queen Mary Hospital, Hong Kong

Funding: The authors received no specific funding for this work. The authors report no conflicts of interest concerning the materials or methods used in this study or the findings described in this paper.

Competing Interests: The authors have declared that no competing interests exist.

* Email: jefferson.w.daniel@gmail.com

Introduction

The vertebral column is the most common site of skeletal metastases and is involved in approximately 40% of the patients who die of cancer [1–4]. Spinal epidural metastases as the initial manifestation of cancer comprise 20% of all spinal epidural metastases [5,6], and the cumulative probability of spinal cord compression caused by malignant disease in the 5 years preceding death from cancer is 2.5% [6,7]. Surgical treatment is required in 5–10% [8] of the patients, and the incidence of patients with unknown primary tumours ranges from 0.4–38% [9–14]. Prognostic indicators are used to select candidates for surgery and to estimate their survival [4,5,8–10,15–36]. In patients who harbour spinal epidural neoplastic metastasis, surgery is indicated for the diagnosis of the histological type of the tumour, segmental vertebrae instability and neurological deficit, particularly muscular force motor deficit [1,5,18,22,23].

In 2012, the estimated incidence of new primary cancers in Brazil was 518,510 (2.6%) in a population of 193,946,886. The overall cancer survival period statistics were imprecise because of discrepancies in death notifications [37]. There are no official government statistics for the prevalence of spinal metastases and unknown primary tumours [37]. Accessible pre-operative secondary prognostic parameters tailored for developing countries is a gap in the literature and could supplement the lack of cancer outcome data, specifically for patients with spinal epidural neoplastic metastases.

In the clinical setting with patients with unknown primary tumours and indications for surgery, secondary parameters that estimate the post-operative survival period are helpful for selecting the correct surgical procedure [10,15]. Indices, scales and algorithms constitute evidence-based tools for survival prognostication that can contribute to decisions regarding the best therapeutic options [4,18,24,29–33,38,39].

The primary prognostic parameters for survival in spinal epidural neoplastic metastases are the primary tumour and the histological tumour type [8–10,15,16,18,22,23,30,34,36]. When these parameters are unknown, secondary parameters are used to estimate patient survival [8–10,15,16,18,22,23,30,36,38]. An estimated three-month post-operative survival period seems reasonable for the decision-making process regarding whether surgery should be performed [23]. The critical judgment and clinical experience of physicians are the criteria for this decision. The surgical risks and benefits are evaluated for these patients, and the aim of treatment is the best possible quality of life during the patients' abbreviated survival periods [5,25–27,35].

Clinically, the origin sites of histologically documented carcinomas cannot be identified in approximately 3–13% of patients, even after complete neoplasm staging [10–13]. In autopsy studies, 15–25% of primary neoplasms remain unidentified [11]. In 13% of spinal epidural neoplastic metastases, the primary tumour is unknown [12].

The unknown primary tumour prognostication hiatus between imaging diagnosis and definitive histological type diagnosis was the rationale for this study. Walking incapacity, special care dependency and contact between the spinal epidural neoplastic metastases and the thecal sac within the spinal canal can be used to estimate survival and can act as secondary prognostic parameter of survival for patients with spinal epidural neoplastic metastases, regardless of whether the primary neoplasm is known. The present hypothesis is that these three accessible pre-operative prognostic factors might assist in calculating a survival estimate. With accurate post-operative survival estimations, patient care might improve, allowing patients to spend more quality time with family/friends and on end-of-life planning. The authors describe these three indicators as useful survival estimation tools. In this model, no other factors were explored regarding their predictive value.

Methods

Data review

This research involved a retrospective review of data collected from patients who underwent surgery for spinal epidural neoplastic metastases in the Division of Neurosurgery at the Santa Casa of São Paulo Faculty of Medical Sciences between January 1997 and February 2011. The sources of the health records were written data and a chart review limited to the prognosis, diagnosis and surgical treatment. The main author collected the data.

Patients of all ages and both genders who met the following criteria were included in the study: a known survival period after surgery, spinal epidural neoplastic metastases, a Karnofsky Performance Score (KPS) [40] equal to or greater than 30 points and neoplastic metastases with a known histological type. Patients who received surgery at other institutions, with primary spine tumours and with primary spinal cord tumours were excluded. Of the 74 (100%) patients who received surgery, 52 (70%) met the inclusion criteria, and 22 (30%) were excluded from the study. A lack of post-operative hospital discharge follow-up and loss of contact with the patients or their legal guardians resulted in the exclusion of 21 patients whose home addresses and telephone numbers were unknown. The only living patient was excluded because a known post-operative survival period was a patient inclusion criterion.

The recorded data included the following information: the dates of surgery and death; registry of the surgical regime type (urgent and elective surgeries); surgical procedure data; known and unknown histological type diagnoses in the pre-operative period; walking capacity according to the American Spinal Injury Association Impairment Scale (ASIA) [41]; clinical functional performance according to the KPS [40]; anatomical relationship between the spinal epidural neoplastic metastasis and the thecal sac according to the Weinstein-Boriani-Biagini Surgical Tumour Staging System (WBB Surgical Tumour Staging System) [42]; Revised Tokuhashi Scoring System of Metastatic Spine Tumour Prognosis [31], which was calculated in the post-operative period; histological type of the spinal epidural neoplastic metastasis according to the World Health Organization Tumour Classification System; knowledge of the primary tumour site; adjuvant chemotherapy and/or radiation therapy; hospitalisation period and length of follow-up. Pathologists from the institution's Pathology Department reviewed the post-operative tumour histological diagnoses.

In this study, survival was defined as the period from the day of surgery to the day of death, which was confirmed by documents from the hospital registry or by the testimony of family members for all 52 (100%) patients. Ambulation was defined as the capacity for independent walking with or without an aid (cane or walker). An unknown primary neoplasm was defined as a metastasis for which the tissue of origin is unknown [11,13]. The surgical regime was established as urgent when performed within 24 hours of hospitalisation and as elective when performed after 24 hours. Neoplastic disease staging was performed in accord with the criteria established in the literature, including patient physical exams, imaging studies, laboratory tests, tumour pathology analysis and surgical reports [8,18,43,44].

Parameter contextualisation

The aim of this study was to identify accessible prognostic parameters with statistical validity for indicating post-operative survival, other than the primary tumour and the neoplasm histological type. Discrepancies in the collected data concerning prognostic parameters, such as tumour sensitivity to adjuvant chemotherapy and/or radiation therapy, visceral metastases and skeletal metastases, were incomplete in the pre-operative urgent surgery regime and inaccessible for survival prognostication; thus, these factors were not analysed statistically. Walking incapacity, special care dependency of the patient and contact between the spinal epidural neoplasms were accessible and hypothesised to be statistically significant as prognostic parameters to estimate post-operative survival in the pre-operative period. In addition to the hypothesised statistical validity, these three prognostic parameters and measurement methods were selected because they are validated measurement and classification methods in Brazilian Portuguese. They are in the public domain, familiar to medical residents and the medical staff and reproducible. In addition, they possess internal institutional validity. Our institution is a philanthropic, private, high-volume quaternary care centre that includes a teaching hospital. It was founded in 1883, and patients are referred from throughout the country and from other countries in South America. The Brazilian Basic Legislation of the Unified Health System (*Sistema Único de Saúde*) treats all patients free of charge, and hospital reimbursement is the responsibility of the federal government. All patients in this study received treatment at no charge.

The classification item *palsy* on the Revised Tokuhashi Scoring System of Metastatic Spine Tumor Prognosis [31] was modified. The ASIA Scale [41] was substituted for the Frankel Score [45]. Prof. Dr. Yasuaki Tokuhashi authorised this modification (Tokuhashi Y., personal communication, 2012). Walking incapacity and limb muscle strength were measured during the neurological exam and were expressed on the ASIA Scale [41] as A and B, with walking capacity expressed as ASIA [41] C, D and E. Pre-operative Tokuhashi Index [31] calculations were not feasible because information on the primary and secondary tumours was insufficient for 36 (69.23%) patients in this study.

The KPS [40] was used to indicate the functional performance of the patients and to infer the clinical compromise secondary to the neoplastic process. The KPS [40] allows for the classification and stratification of patients with complex clinical conditions [46].

The WBB Surgical Tumour Staging System [42] is designed for vertebral primary tumour staging and surgical strategic planning. The system is reproducible for research studies and was applied to classify the anatomical relationship between the primary or secondary neoplasm and the tissues, organs and spinal canal [42]. Magnetic resonance and computerised tomography spinal imaging situated the neoplastic metastases in the vertebrae and indicated their relationship to the thecal sac. Control post-operative spinal imaging was performed during the hospitalisation period. Vertebral segment instability was inferred in the presence of spinal epidural neoplastic metastases secondary to the vertebral segment lytic destructive process of the neoplasm. Although a specific evaluation of spinal segment instability was not within the scope of this study, we agreed with the instability criteria of the Spine Instability Neoplastic Score [19] for neoplastic metastases of the spine.

Parameters of prognosis

Survival was individually compared with each of the following prognostic parameters: the primary tumour and its histological type (primary parameter), walking incapacity, clinical functional performance and contact between the spinal epidural neoplastic metastasis and the thecal sac (secondary parameters). Additionally, survival was compared with the combination of the three mentioned secondary parameters. The six primary tumour sites that affected only one patient each were collected in a group labelled *other*, which was included in the statistical analysis (Kaplan-Meier Method) with the seven other primary tumour sites.

Surgical methods and indications

The authors and neurosurgeons of the Division of Neurosurgery at the Santa Casa of São Paulo Faculty of Medical Sciences performed 52 surgeries in 52 patients. Five neurosurgeons assisted by neurosurgical residents used standardised surgical methods in the patients. Spinal canal neural tissue decompression was accomplished using a dorsal or ventral spinal surgical approach. In all of the patients, spinal column stabilisation was accomplished with the use of autologous bone and/or supplementary surgical instrumentation.

The three secondary prognostic parameters offered surgical indications for spinal epidural neoplastic metastases. When the primary tumour and/or other metastatic tumours were known in the pre-operative period, the Tokuhashi Index Score [31] was calculated by summing the four following criteria:

1. The clinical state measured by the KPS [40] (equal to or greater than 30 points);
2. The neurological state measured by a fixed or progressive neurological deficit, classified as grades A, B, C or D on the ASIA Impairment Scale [41];
3. The presence of spinal epidural neoplastic metastases within the spinal canal causing nervous tissue compression, as classified by the WBB Surgical Tumour Staging System [42];
4. The survival prognosis estimated by the Tokuhashi Index [31] (equal to or greater than three points).

Ethical considerations

The research project was approved on August 27, 2010, by the Ethics Committee on Human Research in the Santa Casa of São Paulo Faculty of Medical Sciences (protocol number 281/10). Informed oral consent was obtained from the patients' legal guardians and conformed to the standards of the Declaration of Helsinki. The 52 (100%) research subjects included had died before the study cut-off date of February 28, 2011; thus, written consent was not obtained. The Ethics Committee on Human Research in the Santa Casa of São Paulo Faculty of Medical Sciences approved the use of oral consent.

Statistical analysis

The Kaplan-Meier method was used to estimate the post-operative survival in the bivariate analyses of the three prognostic parameters and the histological types. The Log-Rank test was used for statistical inference. The level of statistical significance was 5% for the chi-squared distribution tests (one-tailed hypothesis). The statistical software used was the IBM *Statistical Package for the Social Sciences* (SPSS, Inc., Chicago, IL, USA), version 13.0.

Results

Patient demographic data

A total of 52 research subjects underwent 52 operations. There were no reoperations. The average age of the 52 patients was 53.92 years, with a range of 6–83 years (std. deviation 19.09). There were 32 (61.53%) male and 20 (38.46%) female patients. The time from the initial symptoms to the main neurological symptoms at hospital admission was 103 days on average and varied from 1 to 730 days (std. deviation 145.66). Back pain and/ or pain in the limbs were the initial spinal neoplasm symptoms in 27 (51.9%) of the patients, and motor impairment was the main symptom prior to surgery in 51 (98.07%) of the patients. Hospitalisation lasted for 30.29 days on average (std. deviation 23.00). The average follow-up period after surgery was 179 days (minimum 1, maximum 993 days).

Surgical data

The surgical procedures were performed in an urgent or elective regime for 31 (59.61%) and 21 (40.39%) patients, respectively. A stand-alone dorsal-lateral spinal column surgical access was performed in 48 (92.30%) patients, a ventral surgical access in 2 (3.85%) patients, and fluoroscopy-guided percutaneous biopsy in another 2 (3.85%) patients. Thoracic segmental tumour involvement was present in 42 (80.76%) of the 52 patients who underwent surgery. The anatomical topographic spinal neoplastic metastasis distribution was as follows: thoracic, 33 (63.46%); lumbar, 6 (11.53%); cervical/thoracic, 6 (11.53%); cervical, 3 (5.76%); thoracic/lumbar, 2 (3.84%); thoracic/lumbar/sacral, 1 (1.92%); and sacral, 1 (1.92%).

Survival data

The average survival period was 179.38 days (95% CI 107.49–251.27), and the median survival period was 70 days (95% CI 49.97–90.02) after surgery. Tokuhashi's [31] criterion of predicted prognosis classified post-operative survival into the following three time periods: mortality within 6 months after surgery in 38 (73.07%) patients, with 16 (30.76%) deaths occurring within the first post-operative month; between six and eleven months in 3

(5.76%) patients; and twelve months or longer after surgery in 11 (21.15%) patients. The median of the Tokuhashi Scoring System [31] was 7 points, ranging from 2–14 points (95% CI 6.46–7.66), which indicated that the expected post-operative survival after palliative surgery was less than 6 months. The post-operative median survival periods were 97 days (95% CI 69.56–124.44) for the 16 (30.77%) patients who received adjuvant chemotherapy and/or radiation therapy and 45 days (95% CI 0–92.04) for the 36 (69.23%) that did not. The adjuvant chemotherapy and/or radiation therapy cycles were incomplete for 7 (43.75%) patients and complete for 9 (56.25%) patients in this 16-patient group. The post-operative survival of the 7 patients with incomplete adjuvant therapy was less than 90 days. Because of the discrepancies of these results, the adjuvant therapy data were not statistically analysed as prognostic parameters with regard to the survival period.

Parameters for prognosis

Histological data. The primary neoplasm site and histological type were unknown in 36 (69.23%) patients in the pre-operative period. The following primary tumour types were identified after surgery: myeloma (8 patients), lung carcinoma (6), sarcoma (5), prostate carcinoma (5), lymphoma (4), undifferentiated carcinoma (4), thyroid carcinoma (1), pineal germinoma (1), gastric adenoma (1) and kidney blastoma (1). The tumour prevalence is listed in Table 1.

For the overall comparisons, the Log-Rank was used to test the equality of the survival distributions for the tumour types, with a p-value of 0.023.

Walking incapacity. Walking incapacity was present in 45 (86.53%) patients in the pre-operative period and in 47 (90.38%) patients after surgery. The median survival periods (measured in days) for the patients who were able to walk (ASIA [41] C, D and E) or unable to walk (ASIA [41] A and B) in the pre-operative period were 502 days (95% CI 0–1579.82) and 59 days (95% CI 12.99–105), respectively (p-value = 0.107).

Functional performance. The functional performance evaluation (measured with the KPS [40]) did not change between the pre-operative and post-operative periods. The scores were in the 10- to 40-point range in 47 (90.38%) patients. The scores of the other 5 (9.61%) patients varied between 50 and 70 points, and none of the patients had scores in the 80- to 100-point KPS [40] range.

The median survival periods (measured in days) in the post-operative period for the patients who were partially dependent on special care (50–70 points on the KPS [40]) and patients who were completely dependent on special care (0–40 points) were 82 days (95% CI 39–124.9) and 70 days (95% CI 33.7–106.2), respectively (p-value = 0.322).

Contact between a neoplastic metastasis and the thecal sac. In the pre-operative period, the neoplastic metastases were within the spinal canal and in contact with the thecal sac in 49 (94.23%) patients. They were restricted to the vertebrae in 3 (5.76%) of the 52 patients. These metastases were classified as WBB Surgical Tumour Staging System [42] anatomic sectors D and C, respectively. The control post-operative spinal imaging confirmed that there was no contact between the spinal epidural neoplastic metastases and the thecal sac.

The median post-operative survival periods (measured in days) for the patients harbouring vertebral metastases, without or with thecal sac contact, as measured with the WBB Surgical Tumour Staging System [42], were 72 days for WBB [42] sector C (95% CI 68.7–75.2) and 67 days for WBB [42] sector D (95% CI 24.4–109.5); (p-value = 0.643), respectively.

Combined secondary prognostic parameters. The patients who harboured the three secondary prognostic parameters (in combination) were compared with the patients who did not (no combination) to determine the post-operative survival of these two subgroups. In the 43 (82.69%) patients with walking incapacity, special care dependency and contact between the neoplastic metastasis and thecal sac, the median survival time was 45 days (95% CI 9.66–80.33). In the other subgroup, 9 patients (17.31%) had at least one, but not all three, of the secondary parameters of prognosis, resulting in a median survival time of 82 days (95% CI 76.15–87.84; p-value = 0.175) (Fig. 1).

Discussion

Knowledge of the cancer type, tumour sensitivity to adjuvant chemotherapy and/or radiation therapy, visceral metastases and skeletal metastases are the main prognostic parameters for survival in patients undergoing a neoplastic process [4,5,8–10,15–36,38]. The rationale for this study was to identify accessible secondary prognostic parameters for use when the primary tumour is unknown. During the time interval between a spinal epidural neoplastic metastasis diagnosis by imaging and a definitive histological type diagnosis, an estimate of the period of survival

Table 1. Primary sites, histological types, post-operative survival, prevalence and reliability estimates of neoplastic metastases in 52 patients.

Histological type	Median survival/days	Prevalence	CI*
Lung carcinoma	19	9 (17.30%)	14.6–23.3
Undifferentiated carcinoma	28	5 (9.61%)	6.5–49.4
Lymphoma	35	8 (15.38%)	0–26.4
Breast carcinoma	43	4 (7.69%)	0–412.4
Prostate carcinoma	45	6 (11.53%)	0–102.6
Sarcoma	72	5 (9.61%)	67.7–76.2
Myeloma	100	9 (17.30%)	41.5–158.4
Other**	502	6 (11.53%)	0–1, 004.9

*Confidence interval.

**Other: thyroid carcinoma, 506 days; pineal gland germinoma, 606 days; nephroblastoma, 877 days; suprarenal gland carcinoma, 502 days; kidney carcinoma, 87 days; and gastric adenoma, 72 days.

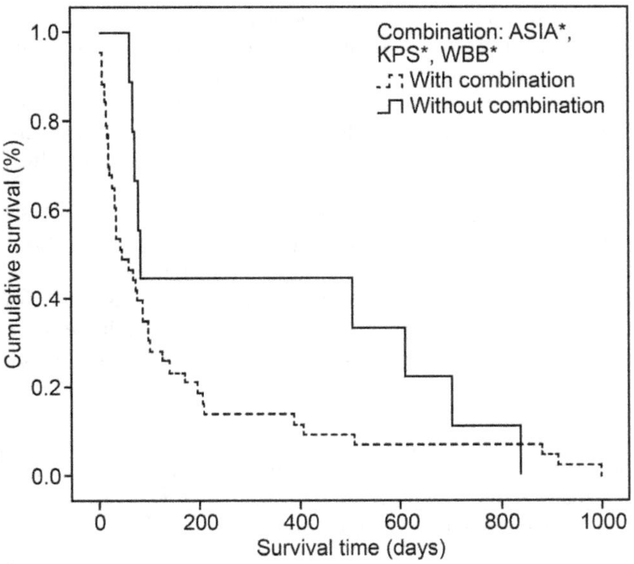

Figure 1. Kaplan-Meier survival curve demonstrating the survival profiles (multiple comparisons procedure). ASIA Scale [41]*: American Spinal Injury Association Impairment Scale; KPS [40]*: Karnofsky Performance Score; WBB Classification [42]*: Weinstein-Boriani-Biagini Surgical Tumour Staging System.

allows physicians to select the best treatment, whether it is surgical or another treatment. This study differs from the published literature because of the three selected secondary parameters of prognosis and the proposal to estimate post-operative survival in the pre-operative period when the primary tumour is unknown. This study is confirmatory.

Demographic characteristics

Compared with the populations in other studies, our patients were younger, with an average age of 54 years. The predominance of males in the sample was similar to that in other studies [13,15,20,21,28,29,39]. The average 3-month interval of time between the initial neurological symptoms and hospital admission was greater than the time interval in other studies [17]. The predominance of axial and/or appendicular pain as the initial symptom and motor impairment as the primary symptom agreed with the literature [8,13,17,20,29]. The average 30-day hospitalisation period was similar to the 27-day average reported by Putz et al. [29]; it was longer than the 6-day period reported by Arrigo et al. [15].

Survival

In this series, the patients had a shorter average survival compared with that in other studies. Within the first 6 months after surgery, 38 (73.07%) of the treated patients had died. Because of delays in patient referral, the neoplastic process was frequently advanced at the time of hospitalisation, which might explain the abbreviated post-operative survival period. The following authors reported varying results for the average survival time: Yang et al. [36], 6 to 9 months; Aizenberg et al. [9], 8 months; Lau et al. [23], 10 months; Arrigo et al. [15], 8 months; Gasbarrini et al. [39], 41 months; and Holman et al. [21], 15 months.

The average post-operative Tokuhashi Index Score [31] utilised for prognostication was 7 points, in accord with the expected post-operative survival of up to 6 months. The Tokuhashi Index Score Point Interpretation [31] ranged from 1–8 points for this group of 41 (78.84%) patients. The Tokuhashi Index Scoring [31] was low and compatible with the advanced neoplastic process in most of the 52 studied patients. These findings are in accord with the literature [29,32,34]. The Tokuhashi Index Scores [31] we obtained confirmed their predictive capacity in this study when compared with the overall post-operative survival of our patients, which was 6 months. We agree with Oliveira et al. [3] that the Tokuhashi Index Score [31] for pre-operative prognostication was not useful in guiding the treatment type because in the majority of patients with vertebral metastases, their pre-operative prognostication variables were incomplete.

All 52 (100%) of the research subjects died. Death occurred in 41 (78.84%) of the 52 patients between 0 and 12 months, which might explain the shorter period of post-operative follow-up compared with those in other series. Follow-up was conducted for more than 11 months in 11 (21.15%) of the patients. A post-operative patient follow-up period of approximately 10 months has been reported in the literature [17]. Lau et al. [23] reported the results of a 2-year retrospective post-operative follow-up of 99 patients from 2005 to 2011.

Sixteen (30.76%) patients received adjuvant chemotherapy and/or radiation therapy in 9 complete and 7 incomplete cycles. This small number of patients submitted to adjuvant therapy likely resulted because 38 (73.07%) of the patients had advanced neoplastic processes and survived less than 6 months after surgery. The median post-operative survival period was longer for the 9 patients who completed the adjuvant chemotherapy and/or radiation therapy cycles than those who completed the surgical series, 97 days (95% CI 69.56–124.44) and 70 days (95% CI 49.97–90.02), respectively. This small difference suggests a tendency for a longer post-operative survival period when surgery and adjuvant therapy are associated in the treatment plan. The literature supports this point of view [4,18,22,23,37,39]. Hirabayashi et al. [20] stated that 75 (70%) of the 107 patients they studied from 1985 to 2001 were subjected to adjuvant therapy and underwent surgery for spinal epidural neoplastic metastases, and these patients had a 10-month survival period.

Histological data

Cancer type was the strongest survival indicator in this study (p-value = 0.023). The tumours were analysed as a group for overall survival and compared with the secondary prognostic parameters. As expected, the primary tumour site and histological type of the neoplasm were significant as primary prognostic parameters because of the biological characteristics of each neoplasm, which were specific to each patient.

The primary tumour was unknown before surgery in 36 (69.23%) of the patients because of incomplete neoplasm staging prior to elective surgery or urgent surgery. A definitive histological type diagnosis was obtained in the post-operative period in all 52 (100%) patients using a multidisciplinary neoplasm staging work-up.

When the median survival period after surgery was compared between the shortest and the longest life spans, the patients with lung carcinomas survived for 19 days on average (95% CI 14.6–23.3), whereas those with myelomas survived for 100 days (95% CI 41.5–158.4). Lung carcinoma exhibited the most aggressive biological behaviour in our series. These findings are in accord with the existing literature [20,34].

Waking incapacity

Walking incapacity was the strongest secondary parameter of prognosis in this series (p-value = 0.107). The capacity to walk implies a capacity for self-care. The authors observed that the 47 (90.38%) post-operative patients who could not walk were dependent on institutional care for personal hygiene, feeding and locomotion and had aggravated neoplastic disease. These patients fared worse than those who could walk.

Walking capacity has been used as a secondary parameter of prognosis in the post-operative period in the literature [8,20,30,31,35], and in this study, pre-operative walking incapacity was used. The ASIA Scale [41] was used instead of the Frankel Index [45] to ensure accuracy and precision in the results, which were reproduced throughout the study. The ASIA Scale [41] measures the motor and sensitive functions (accuracy) and the motor and sensitive S4 and S5 sacral segment functions (precision) [41]. Putz et al. [29] measured motor deficiencies using a modified ASIA Scale [41]. Other authors have used the Frankel Index [9,12,15,20–22,28,31,45] or have omitted motor deficiency measurements [10,23,33,38].

Functional performance

Patient special care dependency (KPS [40]: 0–40 points) was the second most relevant of the three secondary prognostic parameters (p-value = 0.322). This study indicated that the lower the point sum was, the higher the grade of clinical need caused by the neoplastic process was. In this series, all of the patients were hospitalised, disabled and reliant on active vital support for life. As such, walking incapacity might have contributed to their limited survival. None of the 47 (90.38%) patients improved in their functional status in the post-operative period.

The KPS [40] is used as a prognostic factor in patient assessment to measure and compare the functional statuses of individual patients [46]. In the literature, the KPS [40] is inserted in the Revised Tokuhashi Scoring System of Metastatic Spine Tumour Prognosis [24,29,31] or is used as an independent method of quantifying functional performance [12,16,34].

Contact between the neoplastic metastases and the thecal sac

Contact between the neoplastic metastasis and the thecal sac was the weakest of the three secondary prognostic parameters in this study (p-value = 0.643). This parameter has not been previously reported in the literature as a prognostic parameter. The vertebral neoplastic commitment is itself a prognostic factor, and the neoplastic thecal sac contact might not be as relevant as hypothesised in this study.

Primary versus secondary prognostic parameters

When the primary parameter of prognosis is unknown, we propose the use of secondary parameters of prognosis. The secondary parameters of prognosis, in decreasing order of statistical relevance for post-operative survival, were as follows: impaired walking (ASIA [41] A and B), 59 days (95% CI 12.99–105); special care dependency (KPS [40] 0–40 points), 70 days (95% CI 33.7–106.2); and contact between the spinal epidural neoplastic metastasis and thecal sac within the spinal canal (WBB Surgical Tumour Staging System [42] sector D), 67 days (95% CI 24.4–109.5).

When these three parameters were combined, the mean post-operative survival was 45 days (95% CI 9.66–80.33); when at least one parameter was present, the survival was 82 days (95% CI 76.15–87.84). The reason for this difference of 37 days between the two subgroups was not identified; however, the biological behaviour of the primary tumour is presumed to be the most important prognostic factor. The combined secondary parameters of prognosis (p-value = 0.175) indicated the probability that the observed statistics occurred only by chance in at least 17% of the cases, in contrast to 2% for the primary parameter of prognosis. These secondary prognostic parameters reflect a trend towards predicting survival in this model; however, these parameters might only reach significance upon testing a larger sample size, which should be addressed in future studies.

The median post-operative survival for the 16 (30.77%) patients with known pre-operative primary tumours was 59 days (95% CI 11.96–106.04), and it was 72 days (95% CI 51.45–92.54) for the 36 (69.23%) patients with unknown tumours. The reason for this difference was not identified, and the 52 research subjects were statically analysed as a whole, thus validating the use of the aforementioned 3 prognostic parameters for known and unknown primary tumours (p-value of 0.023).

There is no sense of prejudice or subjectivity for deviation from the truth, and the prognostication results are incidental because of the small sample groups; however, these parameters are considered a useful prognostication tool.

Surgical data and indications

A 2- to 3-month post-operative survival period justified surgical treatment in our series of 52 patients, although this time period is clearly an abbreviated post-operative period of survival. Surgical treatment was tailored to the dying patient and aimed to improve the quality of their last days. Post-operative nursing care for a surgically stabilised spinal segment facilitated patient bed mobilisation, personal hygiene and transportation between hospital facilities and home.

These authors agree with the following criteria for surgical indications developed by Lau et al. [23]: life expectancy of at least 3 months when the primary tumour is known, imaging evidence of spinal neoplastic metastasis, neurological deficit and intractable pain and/or concern for instability.

Installed paraplegia within 24 hours and rapid progressive paraparesis were the indications for urgent surgery performed within 24 hours of hospitalisation in 31 (59.61%) of our patients. None of the patients regained walking capacity within the first post-operative week. These patients might have experienced improvements in walking impairment if their survival had been longer than the median 70 days; for this reason, surgery was performed. Other indications for surgery in this series, in accord with the literature, were as follows: spinal segmental instability, intractable pain and diagnosis of the histological type of neoplastic metastasis [1,4,8,18,22].

The limitations of this study, including its retrospective nature, small sample size and long time interval (14 years), are outweighed by its internal institutional validity and the beneficial use of the 3 proposed prognostic parameters in a series with 69.23% unknown primary tumour pre-operative patients. The results are not statistically significant, and the three identified prognostic parameters are known in the literature [8,18,24,31,32,35,42]. Treatment was not withheld from the research subjects that had the surgical indications listed in the methods section. Comparisons between operated versus non-operated patients were not the focus of this study. As the study continues, the authors' aim is to compare the two groups, and the authors are aware that predictive factors are statistically worthy when they are compared to a control group. Larger prospective studies are needed to address these limitations.

Conclusions

The results of this study allow an accurate estimate of survival for patients with spinal epidural neoplastic metastases with unknown primary tumours in a pre-operative urgent regime. The intended implications of this study were to predict the survival and criteria for surgical indications. In addition to knowledge of the cancer type, the following three identified prognostic factors were useful in predicting survival: walking incapacity, special care dependency and contact between the neoplastic metastasis and the thecal sac. These factors could facilitate the determination of the ultimate survival of this patient population and the identification those who would benefit from surgery versus palliation. For a patient with an advanced neoplastic process and an unknown primary tumour, forecasting an abbreviated 2- to 3-month survival estimate indicates surgery and could increase the quality time that patients have to spend with family and friends and on end-of-life planning. With respect to the surgeon facing this critical clinical situation, he or she might be more comfortable performing a suitable palliative surgery that aims to stabilise the committed spinal segment and obtain a histological tumour type diagnosis with the aforementioned statistical indications. This study could be included in future cohort studies for meta-analysis. Multicentre trials are necessary to determine the future guidelines and standards for survival prognostication.

Acknowledgments

The authors extend their gratitude to the medical staff and residents in the Department of Surgery and the Division of Neurosurgery, Santa Casa de São Paulo - Faculty of Medical Sciences, São Paulo, SP, Brazil, for their collaboration and for making this manuscript possible.

Portions of this work were presented in abstract form under the title "Three survival prognostic indicators for spinal column epidural neoplasm metastasis when the primary neoplasm is unknown" at the Global Spine Congress, Hong Kong Exhibition Centre; Hong Kong, China, April 4–6, 2013.

Author Contributions

Conceived and designed the experiments: JWD. Performed the experiments: JWD. Analyzed the data: JCEV. Contributed reagents/materials/analysis tools: JWD JCEV. Contributed to the writing of the manuscript: JWD JCEV.

References

1. Araujo JLV, Veiga JCE, Figueredo EG, Barboza VR, Daniel JW, et al. (2013) Management of metastatic spinal column neoplasms - an update. Rev Col Bras Cir 40: 508–513.
2. Bryne TN (1992) Spinal cord compression from epidural metastases. New Engl J Med 327: 614–619.
3. Oliveira MF, Barros BA, Rotta JM, Botelho RV (2013) Tokuhashi Scoring System has limited applicability in the majority of patients with spinal cord compression secondary to vertebral metastasis. Arq Neuropsiquiatr 71: 798–801.
4. Quraishi NA, Gokaslan ZL, Boriani S (2010) The surgical management of metastatic epidural compression of the spinal cord. J Bone Joint Surg Br 92: 1054–1060.
5. Choi D, Crockard A, Bunger C, Harms J, Kawahara N, et al. (2010) Review of metastatic spine tumour classification and indications for surgery: the consensus statement of the Global Spine Tumour Study Group. Eur Spine J 19: 215–222.
6. Mut M, Shiff D, Shaffrey ME (2005) Metastases to the nervous system: spinal epidural and intramedullary metastases. J Neuro-Oncol 75: 43–56.
7. Loblaw DA, Perry J, Chambers A, Laperriere NJ (2005) Systematic review of the diagnosis and management of malignant extrdural spinal cord compression: the cancer care Ontario practice guidelines initiative's neuro-oncology disease site group. J Clin Oncol 23: 2028–2037.
8. Sciubba DM, Petteys RJ, Dekutoski MB, Fisher CG, Fehlings MG, et al. (2010) Diagnosis and management of metastatic spine disease. J Neurosurg Spine 13: 94–108.
9. Aizenberg MR, Fox BD, Suki D, McCutcheon IE, Rao G, et al. (2012) Surgical management of unknown primary tumors metastatic to the spine: clinical article. J Neurosurg Spine 16: 86–92.
10. Douglas S, Huttenlocher S, Bajrovic A, Rudat V, Schild SE, et al. (2012) Prognostic factors for different outcomes in patients with metastatic spinal cord compression from cancer of unknown primary. BMC Cancer 12: 261.
11. National Cancer Institute (2012) General information about carcinoma of unknown primary. Bethesda, MD: NIH. Available at: http://www.cancer.gov/cancertopics/pdq/treatment/unknownprimary/HealthPr ofessional. Accessed 24 January 2013.
12. Paholpak P, Sirichativapee W, Wisanuyotin T, Kosuwon W, Jeeravipoolvarn P (2012) Prevalence of known and unknown primary tumor sites in spinal metastasis patients. Open Orthop J 6: 440–444.
13. Pavlidis N, Briasoulis E, Hainsworth J, Greco FA (2003) Diagnostic and therapeutic management of cancer of an unknown primary. Eur J Cancer 39: 1990–2005.
14. Varadhachary GR (2007) Carcinoma of unknown primary origin. Gastrointest Cancer Res 1: 229–235.
15. Arrigo RT, Kalanithi P, Cheng I, Alamin T, Carragee EJ, et al. (2011) Predictors of survival after surgical treatment of spinal metastasis. Neurosurgery 68: 674–681.
16. Bartels RH, Feuth T, van der Maazen R, Verbeek AL, Kappelle AC, et al. (2007) Development of a model with which to predict the life expectancy of patients with spinal epidural metastasis. Cancer 110: 2042–2049.
17. Chaichana KL, Pendleton C, Wolinsky JP, Gokaslan ZL, Sciubba DM (2009) Vertebral compression fractures in patients presenting with metastatic epidural spinal cord compression. Neurosurgery 65: 267–274.
18. Daniel JW, Veiga JCE (2007) Guidelines for treatment of epidural spinal metastases [in Portuguese]. Arq Bras Neurocir 26: 93–110.
19. Fisher CG, DiPaola CP, Ryken TC, Bilsky MH, Shaffrey CI, et al. (2010) A novel classification system for spinal instability in neoplastic disease: an evidence-based approach and expert consensus from the Spine Oncology Study Group. Spine (Phila Pa 1976) 35: E1221–E1229.
20. Hirabayashi H, Ebara S, Kinoshita T, Yuzawa Y, Nakamura I, et al. (2003) Clinical outcome and survival after palliative surgery for spinal metastases: palliative surgery in spinal metastases. Cancer 97: 476–484.
21. Holman PJ, Suki D, Mccutcheon I, Wolinsky JP, Rhines LD, et al. (2005) Surgical management of metastatic disease of the lumbar spine: experience with 139 patients. J Neurosurg Spine 2: 550–563.
22. Kataoka M, Kunisada T, Tanaka M, Takeda K, Itani S, et al. (2012) Statistical analysis of prognostic factors for survival in patients with spinal metastasis. Acta Med Okayama 66: 213–219.
23. Lau D, Leach MR, La Marca F, Park P (2012) Independent predictors of survival and the impact of repeat surgery in patients undergoing surgical treatment of spinal metastasis. J Neurosurg Spine 17: 565–576.
24. Leithner A, Radl R, Gruber G, Hochegger M, Leithner K, et al. (2008) Predictive value of seven preoperative prognostic scoring systems for spinal metastases. Eur Spine J 17: 1488–1495.
25. L'Espérance S, Vincent F, Gaudreault M, Ouellet JA, Li M, et al. (2012) Treatment of metastatic spinal cord compression: cepo review and clinical recommendations. Curr Oncol 19: e478–e490.
26. Mannion RJ, Wilby M, Goodward S, Lyratzopoulos G, Lang RJC (2007) The surgical management of metastatic spinal disease: prospective assessment and long-term follow-up. Br J Neurosurg 21: 593–598.
27. Meyer SA, Singh H, Jenkins AL (2010) Surgical treatment of metastatic spinal tumors. Mt Sinai J Med 77: 124–129.
28. North RB, LaRocca VR, Schwartz J, North CA, Zahurak M, et al. (2005) Surgical management of spinal metastases: analysis of prognostic factors during a 10-year experience. J Neurosurg Spine 2: 564–573.
29. Putz C, Wiedenhöfer B, Gerner HJ, Fürstenberg CH (2008) Tokuhashi prognosis score: an important tool in prediction of the neurological outcome in metastatic spinal cord compression: A retrospective clinical study. Spine (Phila Pa 1976) 33: 2669–2674.
30. Sioutos PJ, Arbit E, Meshulam CF, Galicich JH (1995) Spinal metastases from solid tumors. Analysis of factors affecting survival. Cancer 76: 1453–1459.
31. Tokuhashi Y, Matsuzaki H, Oda H, Oshima M, Ryu J (2005) A revised scoring system for preoperative evaluation of metastatic spine tumor prognosis. Spine (Phila Pa 1976) 30: 2186–2191.
32. Tokuhashi Y, Ajiro Y, Umezawa N (2009) Outcome of treatment for spinal metastases using scoring system for preoperative evaluation of prognosis. Spine (Phila Pa 1976) 34: 69–73.
33. Tomita K, Kawahara N, Kobayashi T, Yoshida A, Murakami H, et al. (2001) Surgical strategy for spinal metastases. Spine (Phila Pa 1976) 26: 298–306.
34. Wibmer C, Leithner A, Hofmann G, Clar H, Kapitan M, et al. (2011) Survival analysis of 254 patients after manifestation of spinal metastases: evaluation of seven preoperative scoring systems. Spine (Phila Pa 1976) 36: 1977–1986.
35. Yamashita T, Siemionow KB, Mroz TE, Podichetty V, Lieberman IH (2011) A prospective analysis of prognostic factors in patients with spinal metastases: use of the revised Tokuhashi score. Spine (Phila Pa 1976) 36: 910–917.
36. Yang SB, Cho W, Chang UK (2012) Analysis of prognostic factors relating to postoperative survival in spinal metastases. J Korean Neurosurg Soc 51: 127–134.
37. Instituto Nacional de Câncer, Coordenação Geral de Ações Estratégicas (2011) Estimate 2012: cancer incidence in Brazil [in Portuguese]. Available at: http://www.inca.gov.br/estimativa/2012/. Accessed 20 August 2013.
38. Fourney DR, Gokaslan ZL (2006) Use of "MAPs" for determining the optimal surgical approach to metastatic disease of the thoracolumbar spine: anterior, posterior, or combined. J Neurosurg Spine 2: 40–49.

39. Gasbarrini A, Li H, Cappuccio M, Mirabile L, Paderni S, et al. (2010) Efficacy evaluation of a new treatment algorithm for spinal metastases. Spine (Phila Pa 1976) 35: 1466–1470.
40. Karnofsky DA, Burchenal JH (1949) The clinical evaluation of chemotherapeutic agents in cancer. In: MacLeod CM, editor. Evaluation of chemotherapeutic agents. New York: Columbia University Press. 191–205.
41. Marino RJ, Barros T, Biering-Sorensen F, Burns SP, Donovan WH, et al. (2003) International standards for neurological classification of spinal cord injury. J Spinal Cord Med 26: S50–S56.
42. Boriani S, Biagini R, De Lure F, Bertoni F, Malagu-Ti M, et al. (1996) En bloc resections of bone tumors of the thoracolumbar spine: a preliminary report on 29 patients. Spine (Phila Pa 1976) 21: 1927–1931.
43. Iizuka Y, Iizuka H, Tsutsmi S, Nakagawa Y, Nakajima T, et al. (2009) Diagnosis of a previously unidentified primary site in patients with spinal metastasis: diagnostic usefulness of laboratory analysis, CT scanning and CT- guided biopsy. Eur Spine J 18: 1431–1435.
44. National Cancer Institute (2012) Cancer staging. Bethesda, MD: NIH. Available at: http://www.cancer.gov/cancertopics/factsheet/detection/staging. Accessed 3 July 2013.
45. Frankel HL, Hancock DO, Hyslop G, Melzak J, Michaelis LS, et al. (1969) The value of postural reduction in the initial management of closed injuries of the spine with paraplegia and tetraplegia. Paraplegia 7: 179–192.
46. Péus D, Newcomb N, Hofer S (2013) Appraisal of the Karnofsky Performance Status and proposal of a simple algorithmic system for its evaluation. BMC Med Inform Decis Mak 13: 72.

2

Statin Use and Breast Cancer Survival: A Nationwide Cohort Study from Finland

Teemu J. Murtola[1,2]*, Kala Visvanathan[3,4], Miia Artama[5], Harri Vainio[6], Eero Pukkala[7,8]

1 University of Tampere, School of Medicine, Tampere, Finland, **2** Tampere University Hospital, Department of Urology, Tampere, Finland, **3** Johns Hopkins Bloomberg School of Public Health, Department of Epidemiology, Baltimore, Maryland, United States of America, **4** Sidney Kimmel Comprehensive Cancer Center, Johns Hopkins School of Medicine, Baltimore Maryland, United States of America, **5** University of Helsinki, Helsinki, Finland, **6** Finnish Institute of Occupational Health, Helsinki, Finland, **7** University of Tampere, School of Health Sciences, Tampere, Finland, **8** The Finnish Cancer Registry, Institute for Statistical and Epidemiological Cancer Research, Helsinki, Finland

Abstract

Recent studies have suggested that statins, an established drug group in the prevention of cardiovascular mortality, could delay or prevent breast cancer recurrence but the effect on disease-specific mortality remains unclear. We evaluated risk of breast cancer death among statin users in a population-based cohort of breast cancer patients. The study cohort included all newly diagnosed breast cancer patients in Finland during 1995–2003 (31,236 cases), identified from the Finnish Cancer Registry. Information on statin use before and after the diagnosis was obtained from a national prescription database. We used the Cox proportional hazards regression method to estimate mortality among statin users with statin use as time-dependent variable. A total of 4,151 participants had used statins. During the median follow-up of 3.25 years after the diagnosis (range 0.08–9.0 years) 6,011 participants died, of which 3,619 (60.2%) was due to breast cancer. After adjustment for age, tumor characteristics, and treatment selection, both post-diagnostic and pre-diagnostic statin use were associated with lowered risk of breast cancer death (HR 0.46, 95% CI 0.38–0.55 and HR 0.54, 95% CI 0.44–0.67, respectively). The risk decrease by post-diagnostic statin use was likely affected by healthy adherer bias; that is, the greater likelihood of dying cancer patients to discontinue statin use as the association was not clearly dose-dependent and observed already at low-dose/short-term use. The dose- and time-dependence of the survival benefit among pre-diagnostic statin users suggests a possible causal effect that should be evaluated further in a clinical trial testing statins' effect on survival in breast cancer patients.

Editor: James M. Wright, University of British Columbia, Canada

Funding: This work was supported by a post-doctoral research grant from the Finnish Cultural Foundation (http://www.skr.fi/en), a traveling grant from the Finnish Surgical Society (http://www.kirurgiyhdistys.fi/), and a working grant from the Finnish Medical Association (http://www.laaketieteensaatio.fi/fin/in_english/). The funders had no role in study design, data collection and analysis, decision to publish, or preparation of the manuscript.

Competing Interests: TJM has received lecture fees from Janssen Cilag and has attended medical meetings at the expense of Janssen-Cilag and GlaxoSmithKline. The other authors have declared that no competing interests exist.

* Email: teemu.murtola@uta.fi

Introduction

Breast cancer is the leading cause of cancer death among women globally. [1] Experimental studies suggest that statins, a well-established group of cholesterol-lowering drugs, may have antitumor properties against this common cancer. [2–4].

Statins reduce cholesterol biosynthesis in the liver by inhibiting 3-hydroxy-3-methylglutaryl-coenzyme-A reductase (HMGCR), the rate-limiting enzyme in the mevalonate pathway. In addition to cholesterol, this pathway produces isoprenoids that are critical for regulation of cell growth. [5] The pathway is also essential for tumor promoting effects of oncogene p53. [6] Further, cholesterol is a critical component of intracellular lipid-rafts, which are crucial for intracellular signaling. [7] Thus statins' anticancer effects have a biologically plausible background.

Despite promising preclinical results, there is no clear association between statin use and breast cancer incidence. [8] However, some recent studies have reported lowered overall cancer mortality among statin users, [9–13] including one study that reported decreased breast cancer mortality among pre-diagnostic statin users, [13] and other studies have suggested that statin use is associated with improved recurrence-free survival among breast cancer patients. [14–17] Therefore statins may exert a greater effect on cancer progression versus initiation.

We studied the association between statin use and breast cancer mortality among breast cancer patients in a nationwide population-based cohort.

Materials and Methods

Data sources

We used the Finnish cancer registry to obtain information on all breast cancer cases diagnosed in Finland from 1995 to 2003. Due to mandatory reporting of all cancer diagnoses made in the

Finnish health care units, the Finnish Cancer Registry has good national coverage, including over 99% of cancer cases in Finland. [18] The information on breast cancer cases included the date of diagnosis, tumor stage (local vs. metastatic, available for 92% of cases in our cohort), tumor morphology (available for all cases), initial treatment selection (surgery, radiation therapy, chemotherapy, hormonal therapy or other) and date and cause of death (cancer death vs. death due to other causes). Information on tumor hormone receptor status or screening history was not available. However, the screening participation rate for breast cancer screening in Finland has been reported to be up to 90% [19].

Detailed, individual-level information on usage of cholesterol-lowering drugs between Jan. 1,1995 and Dec. 31, 2003 was obtained from the national prescription database managed by Social Insurance Institution of Finland (SII). Cancer cases were linked to the prescription database using a unique personal identification number.

SII is a governmental agency providing reimbursements to each Finnish citizen for the cost of medicines prescribed by a physician and purchased in outpatient setting. All reimbursed purchases of drugs approved by the SII (most prescription drugs in clinical use) are recorded in the database. [20] The prescription database includes information on date, dosage, package size and number of packages obtained for each reimbursed purchase.

The cholesterol-lowering drugs in clinical use during the study period and recorded by the prescription database were statins (atorvastatin, cerivastatin, fluvastatin, lovastatin, pravastatin, rosuvastatin and simvastatin), fibrates (bezafibrate, clofibrate, fenofibrate and gemfibrozil) and bile-acid binding resins (cholestyramin and cholestipol).

Identification of the study cohort

All histologically confirmed invasive breast cancer cases diagnosed in Finnish health care units from 1995 to 2003 and recorded in the Finnish Cancer Registry were included in our

Table 1. Baseline population characteristics of all breast cancer cases diagnosed in Finland during 1995–2003.

	Non-users of any cholesterol-lowering drugs	Statin users[a]	Fibrate or resin users[a]
n (%)	26,941 (86.2%)	4,151 (13.3%)	313 (1%)
Median age at diagnosis (yrs)	58	64	65
P-value	Reference	<0.001	<0.001
Age-group[b]			
>=55 years	15,919 (59.3%)	3,383 (81.5%)	249 (79.6%)
<55 years	10,918 (40.7%)	768 (18.5%)	64 (20.4%)
P-value	Reference	<0.001	<0.001
Deaths; n (% of the subgroup)	5,658 (21.0%)	318 (7.6%)	50 (16.0%)
Breast cancer deaths; n (% of all deaths)	3,434 (60.7%)	166 (52.2%)	27 (54%)
Years of follow-up (median; 95% range)	3.17 (0.08–8.50)	3.83 (0.08–8.67)	3.50 (0.25–8.51)
Stage at diagnosis:			
Local; n (%)	22,747 (84.8%)	3,696 (89.0%)	277 (88.5%)
Metastatic; n (%)	1,899 (7.1%)	152 (3.7%)	11 (3.5%)
Unknown	2,191 (8.2%)	303 (7.3%)	25 (8.0%)
P-value	Reference	<0.001	0.036
Tumor morphology:			
Ductal ca	20,524 (76.2%)	3,252 (78%)	263 (84%)
Lobular ca	4,278 (15.9%)	643 (15.4%)	32 (10.2%)
Other	2,139 (7.9%)	274 (6.6%)	18 (5.8%)
P-value	Reference	0·005	0.002
Treatment selection:			
Any surgery; n (%)	24,908 (92.5%)	3,989 (95.7%)	297 (94.9%)
P-value	Reference	0.003	NS
Any radiation therapy; n (%)	14,474 (53.7%)	2,291 (55.0%)	170 (54.3%)
Chemotherapy	6,367 (23.6%)	628 (15.1%)	51 (16.3%)
P-value	Reference	<0·001	0.012
Hormonal therapy	6,787 (25.2%)	849 (20.4%)	73 (23.3%)
P-value	Reference	<0·001	NS
Other therapy	220 (0.8%)	17 (0.4%)	1 (0.3%)
P-value	Reference	<0.001	NS

[a]Any pre-diagnostic or post-diagnostic use.

[b]Age cutoffs selected to reflect menopausal status of the majority of women at breast cancer diagnosis.

Table 2. Risk of breast cancer death by amount, duration and intensity of post-diagnostic statin use compared to non-users in a cohort of all breast cancer cases diagnosed in Finland during 1995–2003.

	Breast cancer mortality									
	Localized					Metastatic				
Statin use	n of cases (non-users/users)	n of deaths (non-users/users)	person-years of follow-up (non-users/users)	HR (95% CI)$_{age\text{-}adjusted}$	HR (95% CI)$_{multivar.\ adjusted}$[a]	n of cases (non-users/users)	n of deaths (non-users/users)	person-years of follow-up (non-users/users)	HR (95% CI)$_{age\text{-}adjusted}$	HR (95% CI)$_{multivar.\ adjusted}$[a]
Never	23,098/3,455	2,129/105	86,491/14,831	Reference	Reference	1,930/130	1,011/29	3,323/260	Reference	Reference
Current				0.34 (0.27–0.44)	0.35 (0.28–0.45)				0.48 (0.33–0.72)	0.49 (0.33–0.73)
Previous				1.36 (0.97–1.91)	1.44 (1.02–2.02)				1.78 (0.66–4.78)	1.04 (0.38–2.80)
Amount of statin use										
1st tertile (10–322 DDD)	1,138	47	4,361	0.51 (0.38–0.69)	0.54 (0.40–0.72)	60	21	86	0.70 (0.45–1.08)	0.66 (0.42–1.01)
2nd tertile (333–800 DDD)	1,152	32	4,386	0.43 (0.30–0.60)	0.43 (0.31–0.61)	49	6	93	0.36 (0.17–0.76)	0.37 (0.18–0.79)
3rd tertile (801 DDD or more)	1,165	26	6,075	0.41 (0.27–0.61)	0.42 (0.28–0.62)	21	2	82	0.21 (0.03–1.52)	0.24 (0.03–1.74)
Duration of statin use										
1 year	1,126	39	3,810	0.49 (0.35–0.67)	0.51 (0.37–0.70)	80	20	82	0.56 (0.36–0.86)	0.57 (0.37–0.89)
2–3 years	1,382	39	5,513	0.41 (0.30–0.55)	0.42 (0.31–0.57)	39	7	123	0.42 (0.19–0.94)	0.38 (0.17–0.86)
4 years or longer	947	27	5,508	0.52 (0.34–0.77)	0.52 (0.35–0.78)	11	2	55	0.90 (0.22–3.66)	0.73 (0.18–2.98)
Intensity of statin use (DDDs/year)										
14–183	1,143	54	4,847	0.59 (0.44–0.78)	0.61 (0.45–0.81)	56	17	114	0.87 (0.53–1.43)	0.66 (0.40–1.09)
184–300	1,208	29	4,985	0.36 (0.25–0.52)	0.36 (0.25–0.53)	35	11	71	0.41 (0.19–0.85)	0.43 (0.20–0.90)
301 or more	1,104	22	4,999	0.42 (0.29–0.60)	0.43 (0.30–0.62)	39	1	75	0.33 (0.15–0.73)	0.42 (0.19–0.94)

[a]Calculated with Cox regression model adjusted for age, tumor stage and morphology, treatment selection and pre-diagnostic statin use.
DDD = Defined Daily Dose.

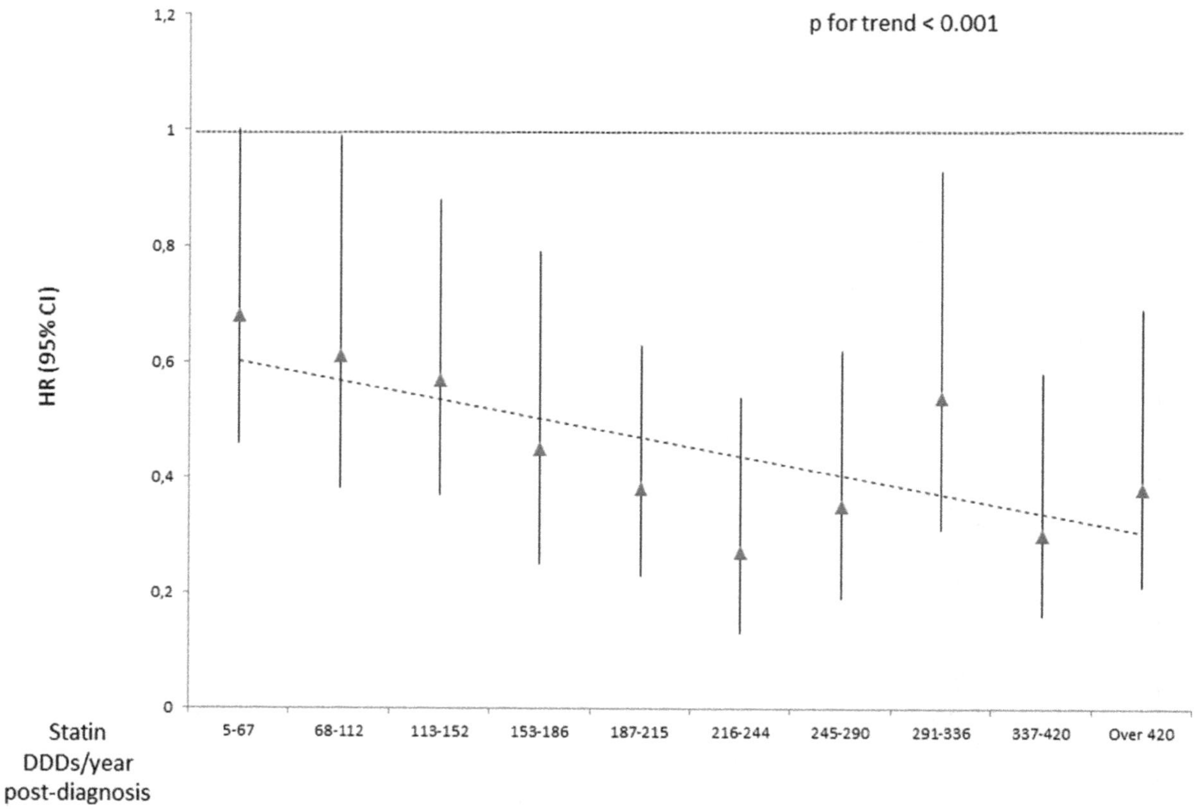

Figure 1. Trend in breast cancer mortality by intensity (doses/year) of post-diagnostic statin use. Nationwide cohort of all female breast cancer patients in Finland during 1995–2003.

study cohort, a total of 31,236 cases (31,114 women, 122 men). Men were excluded from this analysis.

Lipid-lowering drug usage

The status on post-diagnostic statin use was updated prospectively for each year of follow-up since breast cancer diagnosis. The study participant was categorized as statin user only for the years with recorded statin purchases, regardless of the amount. Persons who discontinued prior post-diagnostic statin use were categorized separately as previous users. Cumulative amount (daily doses), duration (years) and intensity (doses/year of usage) of post-diagnostic use were analyzed as prospective time-dependent continuous variables. At discontinuation the cumulative amount/duration/intensity of statin use stayed at the level reached before the usage was stopped.

For prediagnostic use women who were using statins at the year of diagnosis were categorized as current pre-diagnostic users; those who had use the drugs before but had stopped prior to the diagnosis were categorized as previous pre-diagnostic users. Total cumulative amount, duration and intensity of pre-diagnostic statin use were calculated since 1995 up to the year of diagnosis.

The amount of usage was standardized for different statins using the defined daily doses (DDDs) recommended by the World Health Organization (WHO ATC/DDD index database). [21] The DDD is the assumed average maintenance dose per day for a drug used for its main indication in adults. For each year of follow-up, the total milligram amount for each drug was calculated based on all purchases reimbursed that year. Yearly mg amount was divided by the amount corresponding to 1 DDD to obtain the yearly DDDs. Duration of medication use was calculated as the cumulative number of years of follow-up with recorded statin purchases. The total cumulative amount and duration of usage were obtained by adding together yearly DDDs or years with statin purchases from the entire follow-up. Intensity of statin use, i.e. the number of statin doses used per year was calculated by dividing the yearly number of DDDs with years of usage (DDDs/year). The study population was stratified into tertiles (post-diagnostic use) or by median (pre-diagnostic use) of amount, duration and intensity of usage in order to compare long-term/high-dose/high-intensity use with short-term/low-dose/low-intensity usage.

Statistical analysis

We used Chi-square test (for categorical variables) and Mann-Whitney-U test (for continuous variables) to evaluate statistical significance of the differences in baseline characteristics between medication users and non-users.

Hazard ratios (HRs) and 95% confidence intervals (CIs) for breast-cancer specific and all-cause mortality were estimated using Cox proportional hazards regression, with years since the date of breast cancer diagnosis as the time-metric. Each cohort member contributed person-time from the diagnosis until the date of death, emigration from the country or the end of study period (common closing date December 31st, 2003), whichever came first.

Tumor stage at diagnosis, morphology and treatment choice (surgery, radiation therapy, chemotherapy, hormone therapy or other) were included in the regression model as time-independent variables. The proportional hazards assumption was checked for each time-independent variable by including interaction term with follow-up time into the regression model. In each case, the

Table 3. Risk of breast cancer death by amount, duration and intensity of statin use pre-diagnosis compared to non-users in a cohort of all breast cancer cases diagnosed in Finland during 1995–2003, with information on medication use available since 1995.

	Breast cancer mortality								
	All cases			**Localized**			**Metastatic**		
Prediagnostic statin use[†]	**n of cases**	**n of deaths**	**HR (95% CI)** $_{multivar.\ adjusted}$*	**n of cases**	**n of deaths**	**HR (95% CI)** $_{multivar.\ adjusted}$*	**n of cases**	**n of deaths**	**HR (95% CI)** $_{multivar.\ adjusted}$*
None	28,871	3,486	Reference	24,599	2,159	Reference	1,932	1,003	Reference
Current	1,896	96	0.54 (0.44–0.67)	1,652	62	0.60 (0.46–0.77)	106	28	0.58 (0.40–0.84)
Previous	347	22	0.70 (0.46–1.07)	302	13	0.82 (0.48–1.42)	22	9	1.03 (0.53–2.00)
Amount of use[‡]									
1–495 DDD	1,123	82	0.69 (0.55–0.86)	978	54	0.76 (0.58–0.99)	61	22	0.79 (0.51–1.20)
496 DDD or more	1,120	36	0.40 (0.29–0.56)	976	21	0.44 (0.28–0.67)	67	15	0.51 (0.30–0.86)
P for trend[¶]			<0.001			<0.001			0.006
Years of use[‡]									
1–3 years	1,479	95	0.65 (0.53–0.80)	1,286	61	0.69 (0.53–0.89)	85	28	0.77 (0.53–1.12)
4 years or longer	764	23	0.37 (0.25–0.56)	668	14	0.45 (0.27–0.76)	43	9	0.43 (0.22–0.83)
P for trend[¶]			<0.001			<0.001			0.004
Intensity of use[‡]									
195 DDDs/year or less	1,122	78	0.66 (0.53–0.83)	981	48	0.71 (0.53–0.94)	69	24	0.70 (0.47–1.05)
over 196 DDDs/years	1,121	40	0.44 (0.32–0.60)	973	27	0.52 (0.36–0.76)	59	13	0.57 (0.33–0.98)
P for trend[¶]			<0.001			<0.001			0.010

*Calculated with Cox regression model adjusted for age, tumor morphology and treatment selection.
[†]Women with statin usage at the year of diagnosis categorized as current pre-diagnostic users; women with statin usage before the diagnosis but not at the year of diagnosis considered previous pre-diagnostic users.
[‡]Stratum cut-point set at median of amount, duration and intensity of usage.
[¶]Calculated by adding total cumulative number of pre-diagnostic DDDs, years of usage or intensity of use (DDDs/year) as a continuous variable into the Cox regression model.

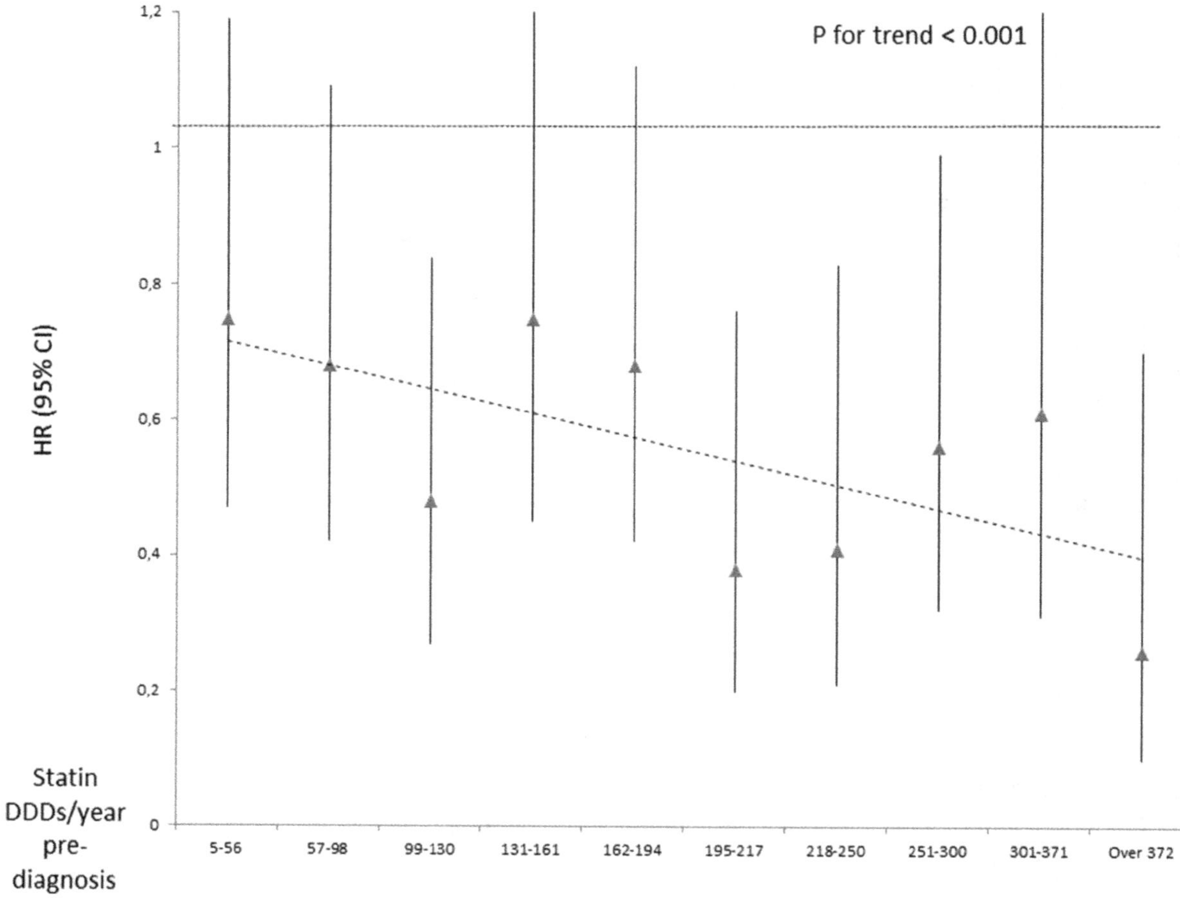

Figure 2. Trend in breast cancer mortality by intensity (doses/year) of pre-diagnostic statin use. Nationwide cohort of all female breast cancer patients in Finland during 1995–2003.

interaction term was not statistically significant, confirming the assumption.

All HRs are calculated using non-users of cholesterol-lowering drugs as the reference group. We performed the analyses separately with an age-adjusted model and a multivariable adjusted model (adjustment for age, tumor stage, morphology and treatment selection). Analyses on non-statin cholesterol-lowering drugs (fibrates and resins) were additionally adjusted for prior statin usage. We report multivariable-adjusted HRs unless otherwise stated.

Survival trends by increasing amount, duration or intensity of statin use were estimated by stratifying the analysis within tertiles of the amount/duration or deciles of intensity of statin usage. P values for trends by amount, duration or intensity of statin use were calculated by including these variables as continuous, time-dependent variables into Cox regression model.

The analyses were repeated separately for pre-diagnostic (statin use occurring before the years of diagnosis) and post-diagnostic statin use.

To address the potential for confounding by indication we evaluated and controlled for each person's likelihood of being a statin user post-diagnosis we calculated propensity score using logistic regression model with post-diagnostic statin use as the dependent variable and age, tumor stage, morphology, treatment selection and pre-diagnostic statin usage as categorical independent variables. [22] Of these, pre-diagnostic statin use was the strongest predictor of post-diagnostic use. The propensity from each variable was combined to form a total propensity score for statin use. The analysis was stratified by quartiles of the total propensity score to ensure comparable distribution of background characteristics between statin users and non-users.

We evaluated the impact of death due to non-cancer causes on observed breast cancer mortality with a competing risks regression as described by Fine and Gray, [23] using the same model adjustments as for the multivariable adjusted Cox regression model.

All reported p-values are two-sided. IBM SPSS statistics 20 statistical software (Chicago, Illinois, USA) was used for Cox regression analyses and STATA version 12 (StataCorp LP, College Station, Texas, USA) was used for competing risks regression.

Results

Population characteristics

Of the participants, 4,151 (13.3% of the cohort) had used statins between 1995 and 2003, while 313 (1% of the cohort) had used fibrates or resins (Table 1). Of the latter 187 (59.7%) had also used statins during the study period. The most commonly used statins were simvastatin (n = 2,031, 48.9% of statin users), atorvastatin (n = 1,507, 36.3%), and fluvastatin (n = 840, 20.2%).

In total, 1,801 women (5.8% of all) had used statins before breast cancer diagnosis, while 71 (0.2%) had used fibrates or

Table 4. Risk of breast cancer death by current pre-diagnostic and post-diagnostic statin use within a cohort of all breast cancer patients diagnosed in Finland during 1995–2003.

	Risk of breast cancer death	
	Pre-diagnostic statin use	**Post-diagnostic statin use**
	HR (95% CI) multivar. adjusted[a]	**HR (95% CI)** multivar. adjusted[a]
Propensity score[b]:		
1st quartile	1.23 (0.66–2.29)	0.42 (0.24–0.74)
2nd quartile	0.82 (0.39–1.73)	0.26 (0.12–0.59)
3rd quartile	0.79 (0.43–1.48)	0.51 (0.33–0.78)
4th quartile	0.84 (0.65–1.10)	0.50 (0.38–0.66)
Age		
>=55 years	0.73 (0.39–1.36)	0.44 (0.26–0.75)
<55 years	0.59 (0.47–0.72)	0.39 (0.31–0.48)
Pre-diagnostic statin use		
Yes	-	0.45 (0.27–0.75)
No Initial treatment choice	-	0.31 (0.22–0.44)
Surgery:		
Yes	0.63 (0.48–0.83)	0.39 (0.30–0.50)
No	0.63 (0.37–1.07)	0.49 (0.26–0.88)
Radiation therapy:		
Yes	0.68 (0.46–1.00)	0.30 (0.20–0.44)
No	0.45 (0.32–0.63)	0.38 (0.28–0.52)
Chemotherapy:		
Yes	0.75 (0.50–1.13)	0.45 (0.29–0.69)
No	0.48 (0.36–0.64)	0.38 (0.30–0.49)
Hormone therapy:		
Yes	0.70 (0.47–1.05)	0.53 (0.36–0.79)
No	0.47 (0.35–0.62)	0.33 (0.25–0.43)
Combination treatments:		
Surgery and radiation therapy	0.71 (0.54–0.93)	0.37 (0.28–0.49)
Surgery and chemotherapy	1.06 (0.76–1.47)	0.45 (0.31–0.64)
Surgery and hormone therapy	0.77 (0.54–1.09)	0.47 (0.33–0.67)
Radiation and chemotherapy	1.11 (0.78–1.57)	0.45 (0.31–0.66)
Radiation and hormone therapy	0.89 (0.63–1.28)	0.54 (0.37–0.78)

Analysis stratified by propensity for post-diagnostic statin use, population characteristics at baseline and primary treatment selection.
[a]Calculated with Cox regression model adjusted for age, tumor stage and morphology and treatment selection.
[b]Propensity for post-diagnostic statin usage as a function of age, tumor stage and morphology, initial treatment choice and pre-diagnostic statin use.

resins. The usage continued after the diagnosis in 85% and 38% of previous statin and fibrate/resin users, respectively.

A total of 2,350 new users started statin usage post-diagnosis. Of these 1,880 (80%) remained adherent users until the end of follow-up.

During the median follow-up of 3.25 years post-diagnosis 6,011 (19.2%) participants died, of which 3,619 (60.2%) due to breast cancer. The median follow-up did not differ significantly by medication usage. Compared to the non-users, medication users were older and more likely to have localized invasive ductal carcinoma than lobular carcinoma (Table 1). Surgical treatment was more common among statin users. Characteristics of fibrate and resin users were similar to statin users (Table 1).

Breast cancer survival by post-diagnostic statin use

Compared to the non-users, current post-diagnostic statin users had lowered risk of breast cancer death (multivariable adjusted HR 0.46, 95% CI 0.38–.055), whereas women who had stopped statin use post-diagnosis (previous users) had elevated risk compared to non-users (HR 1.67, 95% CI 1.22–2.27). The risk decrease among current statin users was observed both in localized and metastatic cases at diagnosis (Table 2).

In stratified analyses the risk decrease strengthened by increasing cumulative amount and intensity of post-diagnostic use, especially among participants with metastatic tumors (Table 2). No statistically significant trends were observed by increasing amount and duration of post-diagnostic statin use, but a significant decreasing trend in breast cancer mortality was observed with increasing intensity of statin usage (p for trend< 0.001) (Figure 1).

Table 5. Overall risk of death among post-diagnostic and pre-diagnostic statin users compared to non-users.

	Overall risk of death					
	Localized cases at diagnosis			Metastatic cases at diagnosis		
	n of cases	n of deaths	HR (95% CI) multivar. adjusted*	n of cases	n of deaths	HR (95% CI) multivar. adjusted*
Post-diagnostic statin use	**23,098/3,455 (non-users/users)**	**3,779/232 (non-users/users)**		**1,930/130 (non-users/users)**	**1,154/38 (non-users/users)**	
None			Ref			Ref
Current			0.39 (0.33–0.46)			0.55 (0.39–0.78)
Previous			1.27 (0.98–1.65)			1.16 (0.48–2.82)
Amount of statin use						
1st tertile (10–322 DDD)	1,138	91	0.56 (0.45–0.69)	60	26	0.73 (0.49–1.08)
2nd tertile (333–800 DDD)	1,152	73	0.48 (0.38–0.61)	49	9	0.41 (0.21–0.80)
3rd tertile (801 DDD or more)	1,165	44	0.37 (0.27–0.50)	21	3	0.38 (0.09–1.53)
Duration of statin use						
1 year	1,126	78	0.55 (0.44–0.69)	80	26	0.63 (0.43–0.93)
2–3 years	1,382	88	0.46 (0.37–0.57)	39	10	0.50 (0.26–0.96)
4 years or longer	947	42	0.41 (0.30–0.57)	11	2	0.58 (0.14–2.36)
Intensity of statin use (DDDs/year)						
14–183	1,143	102	0.59 (0.47–0.73)	56	23	0.79 (0.51–1.22)
184–300	1,208	66	0.41 (0.32–0.53)	35	12	0.42 (0.21–0.84)
301 or more	1,104	40	0.45 (0.34–0.58)	39	3	0.47 (0.23–0.94)
Pre-diagnostic statin use	**n of cases**	**n of deaths**	**HR (95% CI) multivar. adjusted***	**n of cases**	**n of deaths**	**HR (95% CI) multivar. adjusted***
None	24,599	3,841	Ref	1,932	1,144	Ref
Current	1,652	120	0.58 (0.49–0.70)	106	36	0.66 (0.47–0.92)
Previous	302	26	0.80 (0.54–1.17)	22	12	1.18 (0.67–2.10)
Amount of use						
1–495 DDD	978	94	0.69 (0.56–0.84)	61	29	0.91 (0.63–1.31)
496 DDD or more	976	52	0.51 (0.39–0.68)	67	19	0.58 (0.37–0.92)
Years of use						
1–3 years	1,286	114	0.66 (0.55–0.80)	85	35	0.84 (0.60–1.17)
4 years or longer	668	32	0.49 (0.34–0.69)	43	13	0.57 (0.33–0.99)
Intensity of use						
195 DDDs/year or less	981	89	0.68 (0.55–0.83)	69	32	0.82 (0.57–1.17)
Over 196 DDDs/years	973	57	0.54 (0.41–0.70)	59	16	0.63 (0.38–1.03)

Cohort of all breast cancer patients diagnosed in Finland during 1995–2003.
*Calculated with Cox regression model adjusted for age, tumor stage and morphology and treatment selection.
DDD = Defined Daily Dose.

Pre-diagnostic statin use and survival

Women who had used statins pre-diagnosis and were still users at the year of breast cancer diagnosis had lowered risk of breast cancer death compared to non-users (HR 0.54, 95% CI 0.44–0.67), whereas previous pre-diagnostic use (usage stopped before the year of diagnosis) was not associated with the risk (HR 0.70, 95% CI 0.46–1.07) (Table 3). A significant decreasing trend by increasing cumulative amount, duration and intensity of pre-diagnostic statin was observed (Table 3). This was observed both for localized and metastatic cases at diagnosis. Unlike for post-

Table 6. Breast cancer-specific and overall mortality by current pre-diagnostic and post-diagnostic use of specific statins.

Statin type*	Breast cancer mortality						All-cause mortality			
	Localized			Metastatic			Localized		Metastatic	
	n of cases	n of deaths	HR (95% CI) multivar. adjusted†	n of cases	n of deaths	HR (95% CI) multivar. adjusted†	n of deaths	HR (95% CI) multivar. adjusted†	n of deaths	HR (95% CI) multivar. adjusted†
No post-diagnostic statin use	23,098	2,129	Reference	1,930	1,011	Reference	3,779	Reference	1,154	Reference
Simvastatin										
Post-diagnostic use	1,612	45	0.40 (0.28–0.57)	50	8	0.31 (0.14–0.69)	94	0.43 (0.33–0.55)	13	0.46 (0.25–0.86)
Pre-diagnostic use	693	28	0.67 (0.46–0.98)	41	8	0.36 (0.18–0.73)	55	0.66 (0.51–0.87)	13	0.55 (0.32–0.95)
Atorvastatin										
Post-diagnostic use	1,241	20	0.23 (0.13–0.40)	47	9	0.68 (0.34–1.36)	46	0.35 (0.25–0.48)	11	0.66 (0.34–1.27)
Pre-diagnostic use	420	7	0.42 (0.20–0.87)	35	9	1.00 (0.12–8.61)	17	0.52 (0.32–0.83)	10	1.00 (0.14–6.95)
Fluvastatin										
Post-diagnostic use	548	22	0.33 (0.17–0.63)	17	5	0.53 (0.20–1.44)	39	0.31 (0.19–0.50)	5	0.45 (0.17–1.23)
Pre-diagnostic use	246	10	0.57 (0.30–1.05)	12	4	0.73 (0.27–1.99)	16	0.46 (0.28–0.75)	4	0.61 (0.22–1.66)
Pravastatin										
Post-diagnostic use	374	14	0.45 (0.21–0.94)	10	1	-	22	0.44 (0.25–0.76)	2	0.41 (0.10–1.63)
Pre-diagnostic use	121	9	1.20 (0.62–2.32)	6	0	-	13	0.92 (0.53–1.58)	1	0.35 (0.05–2.52)

Cohort of all breast cancer patients diagnosed in Finland during 1995–2003.
*Statin types are not mutually exclusive, i.e. person who has used two types of statins (e.g. atorvastatin and simvastatin) is counted as a user in both categories.
†Calculated with Cox regression model adjusted for age, tumor stage and morphology, treatment selection and pre-diagnostic statin use.

Table 7. Risk of breast cancer death by amount, years and intensity of post-diagnostic statin use as compared to non-users.

	Risk of breast cancer death		
Statin use	**n of cases**	**n of deaths**	**HR (95% CI)** multivar. adjusted[a]
Never	26,963/1,908 (users/non-users)	3,439/47 (users/non-users)	Reference
Current			0.31 (0.22–0.44)
Former			1.04 (0.60–1.80)
	Risk of breast cancer death by amount of post-Dx statin use		
Amount of statin use			
1st tertile (10–322 DDD)	755	25	0.41 (0.27–0.61)
2nd tertile (333–800 DDD)	600	13	0.32 (0.18–0.56)
3rd tertile (801 DDD or more)	553	9	0.45 (0.23–0.86)
	Risk of breast cancer death by years of post-Dx statin use		
Years of statin use			
1 year	687	23	0.41 (0.27–0.62)
2–3 years	760	16	0.35 (0.22–0.58)
4 years or longer	461	8	0.41 (0.19–0.86)
	Risk of breast cancer death by intensity of post-Dx statin use		
Intensity of statin use			
14–183 DDDs/year	773	25	0.44 (0.29–0.67)
184–300 DDDs/year	632	13	0.28 (0.15–0.52)
301 DDDs/year or more	503	9	0.42 (0.24–0.74)

Statin users limited to new post-diagnostic users only.
[a]Calculated with Cox regression model adjusted for age, tumor stage and morphology and treatment selection.
DDD = Defined Daily Dose.

diagnostic usage, no significant risk decrease was observed for low-intensity pre-diagnostic use, but only for high-intensity usage (Figure 2).

Stratified analyses

Stratification by quartiles of propensity score ensured similar propensity for post-diagnostic statin use between users and non-users in the first two quartiles (standardized mean difference 0.09 and 0.05, respectively). In the third and fourth quartiles the propensity score was not perfectly balanced between statin users and non-users (standardized mean difference 0.117 and 1.22, respectively), mainly because post-diagnostic statin users in these quartiles were mostly also pre-diagnostic users, which was the strongest predictor of post-diagnostic use causing high propensity scores.

For post-diagnostic statin use the risk of breast cancer death was similarly decreased in all quartiles of propensity score (Table 4). Further, stratification by pre-diagnostic statin use, age group or treatment selection did not clearly modify the risk decrease (Table 4).

The risk estimates for pre-diagnostic statin use were mostly non-significantly decreased in stratified analysis, with no clear effect modification (Table 4).

All-cause mortality

Similar to breast cancer-specific mortality also all-cause mortality was lowered in current, but not previous pre- and post-diagnostic statin users. Again, the association was clearer with continued and more intensive usage (Table 5).

Survival by statin type

All three most commonly used statins were associated with decreased risk of breast cancer death in participants with localized tumors both when used pre- or post-diagnosis (Table 6). Also post-diagnostic use of hydrophilic pravastatin was linked with lowered risk, whereas pre-diagnostic use was not. Among participants with metastatic disease at diagnosis, only simvastatin users had decreased risk of breast cancer death. However, the lack of significant associations for other statins may be due to small numbers. (Table 6).

Sensitivity analyses

Fibrates and bile-acid binding resins were not associated with all-cause mortality in patients with localized cancer (HR 1.06, 95% CI 0.47–2.37) but were linked to higher mortality in patients with metastatic disease (HR 1.85, 95% CI 1.07–3.20). The number of fibrate/resin users was too low to estimate breast cancer-specific mortality.

Decreased risk of breast cancer death among statin users was not explained by increased risk of death from other causes; the mortality decrease was observed also in multivariable adjusted competing risks regression, with non-cancer deaths as a competing cause of death (HR 0.27, 95% CI 0.22–0.32).

Women dying of breast cancer may have been more likely to drop statin use during the final months of life. However, the inverse association between post-diagnostic statin use and breast cancer mortality remained after exclusion of changes to statin usage status during the final year of follow-up (HR 0.33, 95% CI 0.24–0.45 and 0.63, 95% CI 0.39–1.02 for localized and metastatic cancer, respectively).

The impact of prevalent user bias was evaluated by limiting the analysis to new post-diagnostic statin users only. The risk decrease was observed also in this group of statin users, but with no dose-dependence by amount, duration or intensity of use (Table 7). However, after limiting the analysis to adherent new post-diagnostic users, a significant decreasing trend in breast cancer deaths was observed by years and intensity (p for trend = 0.018 and 0.006, respectively) but not by cumulative amount of post-diagnostic use.

Hazard of breast cancer death remained decreased among post-diagnostic statin users when the minimum follow-up was set to be 5 or 7 years (HR 0.23, 95% CI 0.13–0.39 and HR 0.42, 95% CI 0.19–0.95, respectively), suggesting that the risk decrease remains even in the long-term.

Discussion

We have demonstrated lowered risk of breast cancer death among statin users in a nationwide cohort of all breast cancer patients diagnosed in Finland during a period of nine years. The risk decrease was observed for both localized and metastatic disease at diagnosis, and both for pre-diagnostic and post-diagnostic statin use. The association was dose-dependent especially for pre-diagnostic usage. The risk decrease was not modified by differences in age, tumor characteristics and treatment selection between statin users and non-users. This association was not observed for other types of cholesterol-lowering drugs despite similar age, tumor and treatment characteristics, and was not explained by competing causes of death or decreased likelihood of statin usage at the end of life.

Our results could have been affected by healthy user bias, created by a tendency of healthier patients' greater likelihood to initiate and adhere to statin therapy, leading to decreased likelihood of outcomes not causally related to statin use, such as risk of accidents. [24] In case of cancer mortality this would mean that healthier cancer patients are more likely to initiate statin use, while less healthier would be less likely to initiate usage and more likely to stop previous use. Indeed, when analyzing current and previous post-diagnostic statin use the risk of death was elevated in women who had stopped previous statin use after the diagnosis. Thus post-diagnostic use was likely affected by the healthy adherer bias, i.e. by increased likelihood of fatally ill cancer patients to stop statin usage and lowered likelihood to start it which makes survival in statin users seem better than it really is. This is likely the reason for absence of clear dose-dependence for post-diagnostic statin use, the risk decrease being observed already at short-term and low-dose usage as well as with longer-term usage. However, for pre-diagnostic statin use the risk association was dependent on the amount, duration and intensity as well as timing of statin use, as would be expected in a causal association. As breast cancer could not have affected the patients' decisions on statin use before the diagnosis, the healthy adherer effect is unlikely to affect pre-diagnostic statin use.

A major strength of our study is the nationwide coverage of all incident breast cancer patients in Finland from 1995–2003, reducing the possibility of selection bias and allowing us several unique opportunities: the ability to evaluate the association by stage, perform analysis by statin type and compare mortality by the type of cholesterol-lowering drug being used. Another important strength is our detailed knowledge on timing, dosage and duration of statin use, allowing incorporation of the time varying nature of the medication use into analysis and reliable estimation of dose-dependence. Although our median follow-up was only 3.25 years post-diagnosis, the results were unchanged in sensitivity analysis with minimum follow-up set to seven years, showing that the mortality decrease remains also in the long-term.

Previous laboratory studies have demonstrated that statins inhibit breast cancer cell growth *in vitro*, [2–4] providing biological plausibility to statins' inhibitory effect on breast cancer progression. A pre-surgical clinical trial supported this by demonstrating decreased proliferation activity and increased apoptosis in high-grade, but not low-grade breast cancer tissue among patients randomized to receive either high-dose fluvastatin (80 mg/day) or low-dose fluvastatin (20 mg/day) for 3–6 weeks before mastectomy. [25] Another presurgical clinical study reported antiproliferative effect of atorvastatin on invasive breast cancer when given for two weeks before mastectomy at 80 mg/day dose. [26] This effect was observed only in tumors expressing HMGCR at baseline, suggesting that statins target this enzyme in breast cancer tissue. Another possible mechanism for the anti-cancer action is decreased estrone sulfate level. [27] Our results are consistent with previous studies reporting lowered overall cancer mortality in statin users. [9–13,17] Similar to our study, one study estimating effects of pre-diagnostic statin use reported lowered breast cancer mortality in a sub-analysis. [13] Another cohort study found no association between breast cancer mortality and self-reported lipid-lowering drug usage at diagnosis. [17] The results of this study could have been biased towards the null as it did not take into account post-diagnostic statin use. Our study is the largest study to examine this question with ability to analyze statin usage occurring both before and after breast cancer diagnosis.

Cardiovascular disease prevention trials have shown lowered overall mortality in statin users compared to the non-users. [28] A recent meta-analysis of such trials concluded that lowering LDL with statins did not affect cancer risk or mortality during median follow-up of 4.8 years. [29] However, due to the inclusion criteria of included trials most participants did not have cancer at the baseline. Because 5-year disease-specific survival in breast cancer is up to 89% [30] the risk of dying of breast cancer within the next 4.8 years in a cohort of cancer-free people at baseline is very low. Therefore the present clinical trials testing statins for prevention of cardiovascular outcomes have too short follow-up to study breast cancer mortality leading to underpowered analysis. In the meta-analysis 41 breast cancer deaths occurred among 85,683 women included in the trials, which translates to 0.96 deaths/10,000 women/year, which is lower than the average number of breast cancer deaths in the general population: 2.26 deaths/10,000 women/year. [30] This demonstrates how selected the participants of the cardiovascular disease prevention trials are in this regard, and the value of population-based studies such as ours. The final proof of statins' anticancer effects or the lack of such needs to come from clinical trials recruiting specifically cancer patients.

The significant mortality decrease in our study was evident already after short-term post-diagnostic statin use. Spontaneous decrease in serum cholesterol has been reported for years before cancer death. [31] Thus lower mortality observed already at the initiation of usage may have been because people dying of breast cancer had less hypercholesterolemia, i.e. indication for statin use. Nevertheless, statins may also have a direct short-term effect on cancer progression as recent clinical trials have demonstrated decreased breast cancer proliferation after just weeks of statin usage. [25,26] Whatever the reason for the initial mortality benefit between statin users and non-users, the dose-dependent decrease in breast cancer mortality by increasing intensity of usage supports a causal effect.

When analyzed separately the risk decrease was not clearly modified by statin potency, as similar risk decrease was observed for high-potent atorvastatin as for other statins. Also hydrophilic pravastatin was associated with a similar decrease as lipophilic statins. This suggests that statins' anticancer effects *in vivo* are due to a systemic effect common to all statins, such as cholesterol-lowering.

Our study has several limitations. We could not evaluate whether statins' effect on mortality was modified by tumor hormone receptor status as this information was unavailable. Neither did we have information on breast cancer screening history, which could have been more common among statin users, [32] possibly causing lead-time bias by earlier breast cancer diagnoses. However, the observed risk decrease even among metastatic cases at diagnosis indicates that lead-time bias may not affect our results to any great degree. Our data lacked information on life-style factors, such as obesity, and usage of medications apart from cholesterol-lowering drugs. It could be assumed that fibrate and resin users are in general similar to statin users regarding these unmeasured factors, yet lower mortality was observed only in statin users. Thus lifestyle factors may not have a great influence on our results. Finally, we did not have information on serum cholesterol levels in our cohort and could not assess the indications for statin usage.

In conclusion, statin users had lower risk of breast cancer death compared to non-users in a nationwide cohort of Finnish breast cancer patients. Combined with previous evidence from *in vitro* [2–4], epidemiological [14–17] and clinical studies [25,26] our study suggests that, apart from cardiovascular benefits, statins may have beneficial effect against breast cancer progression. However, because uncertainty remains due to biases related to differing likelihood for statin use in different patient groups our results need to be confirmed in a randomized clinical trial before statins can be recommended for breast cancer treatment.

Acknowledgments

We are thankful to Dr. Elizabeth Platz from the Johns Hopkins Bloomberg School of Public Health, Department of Epidemiology for her insightful comments and feedback on the present analysis and manuscript. TJ Murtola and E Pukkala had full access to all the data in the study and take responsibility for the integrity of the data and the accuracy of the data analysis.

Author Contributions

Conceived and designed the experiments: TJM KV EP. Performed the experiments: TJM KV. Analyzed the data: TJM KV EP. Contributed reagents/materials/analysis tools: MA HV EP. Contributed to the writing of the manuscript: TJM KV MA HV EP.

References

1. Ferlay J, Shin HR, Bray F, Forman D, Mathers C, et al. (2010) GLOBOCAN 2008 v2.0, Cancer Incidence and Mortality Worldwide: IARC CancerBase No. 10 [Internet]. Lyon, France: International Agency for Research on Cancer; 2010. Available: http://globocan.iarc.fr. Accessed 2014 Sep 30.
2. Demierre MF, Higgins PD, Gruber SB, Hawk E, Lippman SM (2005) Statins and cancer prevention. Nat Rev Cancer 5: 930–942.
3. Koyuturk M, Ersoz M, Altiok N (2007) Simvastatin induces apoptosis in human breast cancer cells: p53 and estrogen receptor independent pathway requiring signalling through JNK. Cancer Lett 250: 220–228.
4. Kubatka P, Zihlavnikova K, Kajo K, Péc M, Stollárová N, et al. (2011) Antineoplastic effects of simvastatin in experimental breast cancer. Klin Onkol 24: 41–45.
5. Garcia-Ruiz C, Morales A, Fernandez-Checa JC (2012) Statins and protein prenylation in cancer cell biology and therapy. Anticancer Agents Med Chem 12: 303–315.
6. Freed-Pastor WA, Mizuno H, Zhao X, Langerød A, Moon SH, et al. (2012) Mutant p53 disrupts mammary tissue architecture via the mevalonate pathway.Cell 148: 244–258.
7. Hilvo M, Denkert C, Lehtinen L, Müller B, Brockmöller S, et al. (2011) Novel theranostic opportunities offered by characterization of altered membrane lipid metabolism in breast cancer progression. Cancer Res. 71: 3236–3245.
8. Undela K, Srikanth V, Bansal D (2012) Statin use and risk of breast cancer: A meta-analysis of observational studies. Breast Cancer Res Treat 35: 261–269.
9. Berard E, Bongard V, Dallongeville J, Arveiler D, Ruidavets JB, et al. (2011) Cancer mortality according to lipid-lowering drugs and lipoproteins in a general population. Curr Med Res Opin 27: 1963–1971.
10. Eindhoven JA, Onuma Y, Oemrawsingh RM, Daemen J, van Nierop JW, et al. (2012) Long-term outcome after statin treatment in routine clinical practice: Results from a prospective PCI cohort study. EuroIntervention.7: 1420–1427.
11. Frohlich GM, Rufibach K, Enseleit F, Wolfrum M, von Babo M, et al. (2012) Statins and the risk of cancer after heart transplantation. Circulation 126: 440–447.
12. Haukka J, Niskanen L, Partonen T, Lönnqvist J, Tiihonen J (2012) Statin usage and all-cause and disease-specific mortality in a nationwide study. Pharmacoepidemiol Drug Saf 21: 61–69.
13. Nielsen SF, Nordestgaard BG, Bojesen SE (2012) Statin use and reduced cancer-related mortality. N Engl J Med 367: 1792–1802.
14. Ahern TP, Pedersen L, Tarp M, Cronin-Fenton DP, Garne JP, et al. (2011) Statin prescriptions and breast cancer recurrence risk: A Danish nationwide prospective cohort study. J Natl Cancer Inst 103: 1461–1468.
15. Chae YK, Valsecchi ME, Kim J, Bianchi AL, Khemasuwan D (2011) Reduced risk of breast cancer recurrence in patients using ACE inhibitors, ARBs, and/or statins. Cancer Invest 29: 585–593.
16. Kwan ML, Habel LA, Flick ED, Quesenberry CP, Caan B (2008) Post-diagnosis statin use and breast cancer recurrence in a prospective cohort study of early stage breast cancer survivors. Breast Cancer Res Treat 109: 573–579.
17. Nickels S, Vrieling A, Seibold P, Heinz J, Obi N, et al. (2013) Mortality and recurrence risk in relation to the use of lipid-lowering drugs in a prospective breast cancer patient cohort. PLoS One. 8: e75088.
18. Teppo L, Pukkala E, Lehtonen M (1994) Data quality and quality control of a population-based cancer registry. experience in finland. Acta Oncol [nro 7]. 33: 365–369.
19. Mäkelä M, Saalasti-Koskinen U, Saarenmaa I, Autti-Rämö I (2005) The impact of an extension of breast cancer screening. Update of Finohta's report 16/2000. Finohta's report 28, 2006. Finnish Office for Health Technology Assessment (Finohta)/National Research and Development Centre for Welfare and Health STAKES. Helsinki, Finland. Available: http://finohta.stakes.fi/NR/rdonlyres/54239E75-C9E1-4F85-81F2-81B68F93D2E0/0/r028f.pdf. Accessed 2014 Sep 30.
20. Martikainen J, Rajaniemi S (2002) Drug reimbursement systems in EU member states, Iceland and Norway. Helsinki: The Social Insurance Institution, Finland, Social security and health reports. 54: 130. Available: http://www.kela.fi/in/internet/liite.nsf/ABID/030303101726PN/$File/Drug_reimbursement.pdf?openElement. Accessed 2014 Sep 30.
21. World Health Organization. ATC/DDD index database. Available: http://www.whocc.no/atcddd/indexdatabase/index.php?query¼C10A. Accessed 2014 Sep 30.
22. Rosenbaum PR, Rubin DB (1984) Reducing bias in observational studies using subclassification on the propensity score. J Am Stat Assoc 516–524.
23. Fine JP, Gray RJ (1999) A Proportional Hazards Model for the Subdistribution of a Competing Risk. J Am Stat Assoc 94: 496–509.
24. Dormuth CR, Patrick AR, Shrank WH, Wright JM, Glynn RJ, et al. (2009) Statin adherence and risk of accidents: A cautionary tale. Circulation 119: 2051–2057.
25. Garwood ER, Kumar AS, Baehner FL, Moore DH, Au A, et al. (2010) Fluvastatin reduces proliferation and increases apoptosis in women with high grade breast cancer. Breast Cancer Res Treat 119: 137–144.
26. Bjarnadottir O, Romero Q, Bendahl PO, Jirström K, Rydén L, et al. (2013) Targeting HMG-CoA reductase with statins in a window-of-opportunity breast cancer trial. Breast Cancer Res Treat 138: 499–508.
27. Higgins MJ, Prowell TM, Blackford AL, Byrne C, Khouri NF, et al. (2012) A short-term biomarker modulation study of simvastatin in women at increased risk of a new breast cancer. Breast Cancer Res Treat 131: 915–924.
28. Cholesterol Treatment Trialists (CTT) Collaborators (2012) The effects of lowering LDL cholesterol with statin therapy in people at low risk of vascular disease: Meta-analysis of individual data from 27 randomised trials. Lancet 380: 581–590.
29. Cholesterol Treatment Trialists' (CTT) Collaboration (2012) Lack of Effect of Lowering LDL Cholesterol on Cancer: Meta-Analysis of Individual Data from 175,000 People in 27 Randomised Trials of Statin Therapy. PLoS ONE 7(1): e29849.

30. SEER Stat Fact Sheets: Breast Cancer. Available: http://seer.cancer.gov/statfacts/html/breast.html. Accessed 2014 Sep 30.
31. Eichholzer M, Stahelin HB, Gutzwiller Ludin FE, Bernasconi F (2000) Association of low plasma cholesterol with mortality for cancer at various sites in men: 17-y follow-up of the prospective Basel study, Am J Clin Nutr 71: 569–574.
32. Brookhart MA, Patrick AR, Dormuth C, Avorn J, Shrank W, et al. (2007) Adherence to lipid-lowering therapy and the use of preventive health services: An investigation of the healthy user effect. Am J Epidemiol 166: 348–354.

3

An Algorithm that Predicts the Viability and the Yield of Human Hepatocytes Isolated from Remnant Liver Pieces Obtained from Liver Resections

Serene M. L. Lee[1]❡, Celine Schelcher[2]❡, Rüdiger P. Laubender[3], Natalja Fröse[1], Reinhard M. K. Thasler[2], Tobias S. Schiergens[1], Ulrich Mansmann[3], Wolfgang E. Thasler[1]*

1 Department of General, Visceral, Transplantation, Vascular and Thoracic Surgery, Grosshadern Hospital, Ludwig Maximilians University, Munich, Germany, **2** Tissue Bank, Department of General, Visceral, Transplantation, Vascular and Thoracic Surgery, Grosshadern Hospital, Ludwig Maximilians University, Munich, Germany, **3** Institute for Medical Information Processing, Biometry and Epidemiology, Grosshadern Hospital, Ludwig Maximilians University, Munich, Germany

Abstract

Isolated human primary hepatocytes are an essential *in vitro* model for basic and clinical research. For successful application as a model, isolated hepatocytes need to have a good viability and be available in sufficient yield. Therefore, this study aims to identify donor characteristics, intra-operative factors, tissue processing and cell isolation parameters that affect the viability and yield of human hepatocytes. Remnant liver pieces from tissue designated as surgical waste were collected from 1034 donors with informed consent. Human hepatocytes were isolated by a two-step collagenase perfusion technique with modifications and hepatocyte yield and viability were subsequently determined. The accompanying patient data was collected and entered into a database. Univariate analyses found that the viability and the yield of hepatocytes were affected by many of the variables examined. Multivariate analyses were then carried out to confirm the factors that have a significant relationship with the viability and the yield. It was found that the viability of hepatocytes was significantly decreased by the presence of fibrosis, liver fat and with increasing gamma-glutamyltranspeptidase activity and bilirubin content. Yield was significantly decreased by the presence of liver fat, septal fibrosis, with increasing aspartate aminotransferase activity, cold ischemia times and weight of perfused liver. However, yield was significantly increased by chemotherapy treatment. In conclusion, this study determined the variables that have a significant effect on the viability and the yield of isolated human hepatocytes. These variables have been used to generate an algorithm that can calculate projected viability and yield of isolated human hepatocytes. In this way, projected viability can be determined even before isolation of hepatocytes, so that donors that result in high viability and yield can be identified. Further, if the viability and yield of the isolated hepatocytes is lower than expected, this will highlight a methodological problem that can be addressed.

Editor: Anna Alisi, Bambino Gesu' Children Hospital, Italy

Funding: WET received a grant from the Federal Ministry of Education and Research (grant name: Virtual Liver Network, grant number: 0315759) and a grant from Hepacult GmbH. The funders had no role in the study design, data collection and analysis, decision to publish or preparation of the manuscript.

Competing Interests: WET is one of the founders of Hepacult GmbH and remains one of the members of the board in this company. RMKT is a co-founder of Hepacult GmbH.

* Email: Wolfgang.Thasler@med.uni-muenchen.de

❡ These authors contributed equally to this work.

Introduction

The liver carries out a diverse range of necessary functions, such as homeostasis, metabolism and detoxification. As much of the research on the liver is human-centric, whether for the elucidation of mechanisms, translational research or cell-based therapy, isolated human liver cells remain an important *in vitro* model for basic and translational research.

One of the main uses of a human *in vitro* hepatocyte model is for the validation of studies done using animal models due to species differences. Olson *et al.*, [1] showed that when 150 drugs that cause human toxicity are tested, the concordance between toxicity found in animal studies and that observed in clinical practice is 70%. Similarly, Brambilla and Martelli found that when 42 compounds from various chemical families were tested for their toxicity in rat or human hepatocytes, 28 had similar toxicities, 10 were more toxic for rats, 3 were moderately more toxic for human hepatocytes and 1 was lethal for rat hepatocytes at a concentration 30-fold lower than that equally toxic for human hepatocytes [2]. In addition, animal models could also have less genetic variation than humans; Brambilla and Martell [2] found

Table 1. Summary of factors affecting the viability of isolated hepatocytes.

Variables	Decreased viability	No change in viability	Increased viability
Age	Increased age [12,38]	Different ages [15,39]	Decreased age* [16]
Gender		Male or female [12,13,39]	
Fibrosis	Fibrotic organs [39]		Organs that are not steatotic, fibrotic or cirrhotic [39]
Cirrhosis	Cirrhotic organs [39]		Organs that are not steatotic, fibrotic or cirrhotic [39]
Steatosis		Severely steatotic organs or organs that are not steatotic, fibrotic or cirrhotic [39]	Visually steatotic liver [12]
Disease	Malignant disease [15]	Colonic secondary, cholangiocarcinoma, carcinoid, hepatocellular tumour, unknown primary, hyatid cyst, lung secondary or multi-organ donors [12], primary biliary cirrhosis or primary sclerosing cholangitis [9]	Benign disease [15]
Chemotherapy		Treated or untreated [14]	
Serum enzymes	Increased pre-operative GGT levels [15]		
Operation type		Right hepatectomy, segmental resection, left hepatectomy, extended right, local excision or multi-organ donor [12]	
Warm ischemia	Increased time* [16]	Varying time [11], no pringle or varying Pringle times [12]	
Cold ischemia	>20 h [39]	Up to 4 h [12], varying times [38,39]	<10 h [39]

*Statistics done with multiple regression analysis. All other variables were analysed using univariate analyses.

Table 2. Summary of factors affecting the yield of isolated hepatocytes.

Variables	Decreased yield	No change in yield	Increased yield
Age	>50 years old [15]	Different ages [10,13,39,40]	
Gender		Male or female [12,13,39]	
Fibrosis	Fibrotic organs [39]		Organs that are not steatotic, fibrotic or cirrhotic [39]
Cirrhosis	Cirrhotic organs [39]		Organs that are not steatotic, fibrotic or cirrhotic [39]
Steatosis	Severely steatotic organs [39]	No steatosis, <10% steatosis or >10% steatosis [10], no steatosis or >10% steatosis [13]	Organs that are not steatotic, fibrotic or cirrhotic [39]
Disease	Malignant disease [15]	Benign hepatic diseases, metastases from colorectal cancer, hepatic primitive malignant tumours or metastases from non-colorectal cancer [10], colonic secondary, cholangiocarcinoma, carcinoid, hepatocellular tumour, unknown primary, hyatid cyst, lung secondary or multi-organ donors [12], benign hepatic disease, metastases from colorectal cancer, hepatic primitive malignant tumours or metastases from non-colorectal cancer [13], primary biliary cirrhosis or primary sclerosing cholangitis [9]	Benign disease [15]
Chemotherapy		Treated or untreated [10,14]	
Serum enzymes	Increased pre-operative GGT levels [10]	Increased pre-operative ALT or AST levels [10]	
Operation type		Right hepatectomy, segmental resection, left hepatectomy, extended right, local excision or multi-organ donor [12]	
Warm ischemia	Intermittent clamping [13]	Varying time [11],no pringle or varying Pringle times [12], no clamping, continuous or intermittent clamping [13]	No clamping [13]
Cold ischemia		Up to 4 h [12], up to 5 h [13], varying times [39]	
Perfused liver	100–200 g liver pieces [12], increased liver weight [16]	Varying weights [10,13]	

Table 3. Variables considered for statistical analyses.

Variables	Categories	Abbreviation	Unit
Donor characteristics			
Age		-	-
Gender	Male or female	-	-
Body mass index		BMI	-
Fibrosis	Yes or no	-	-
Cirrhosis	Yes or no	-	-
Diabetes	Yes or no	-	-
Obesity	Yes or no	-	-
Hypertension	Yes or no	-	-
Hypercholesterolemia	Yes or no	-	-
Hyperuricemia	Yes or no	-	-
Smoking	Yes, no or ex-smoker	-	-
Cigarettes per day		-	-
Liver fat	Yes or no	-	-
Liver fat		-	%
Tumour type	Benign or malignant	-	-
Surgical indication	Hepatocarcinoma (HCC), metastasis, focal nodular hyperplasia (FNH), klatskin, adenoma, cholangiocarcinoma (CCC) or others	-	-
Chemotherapy	Treated or untreated	-	-
ASA physical status classification system	1, 2, 3 or 6	ASA	-
Ludwig score	No or minimal fibrotic changes, periportal fibrosis, septal fibrosis or cirrhosis	-	-
Clinical chemistry results before operation			
Alkaline phosphatase activity		AP	U/L
Aspartate aminotransferase activity		GOT	U/L
Gamma-glutamyltranspeptidase activity		GGT	U/L
Alanine aminotransferase activity		GPT	U/L
Cholinesterase activity		CHE	U/L
Bilirubin		-	mg/dL
Partial thromboplastin time		PTT	s
Quick value		-	%
Operation parameters			
Operation type	Hemihepatectomy right (HR), Hemihepatectomy left (HL), segment resection (SR), atypical resection (AR) extended hepatectomy (EH), liver transplantation (LT) or lobectomy (L)	-	-
Warm ischemia *in vivo*		-	min
Warm ischemia *ex vivo*		-	min
Weight of resected liver		-	g
Tissue processing and cell isolation parameters			
Cold ischemia		-	min
Weight of perfused liver		-	g

that the inter-individual variability in hepatocyte responses to chemicals that cause cytotoxicity is greater for humans than for rats. This would make it harder to detect idiosyncratic drug-induced liver injury.

The usage of human hepatocytes comes with the additional advantage of following the 3R ethical framework [3] to replace the use of research animals when possible. This is as the liver tissue used in this study was obtained from human elective liver resections. After resection, the tissue was immediately brought to a pathologist, who would take what was required for histopathological evaluation. The rest of the tissue, which is not needed, was designated as surgical waste. If a patient had signed an informed

Table 4. The number of replicates (*N*) and the *P* values obtained after linear regression of the individual variables listed below to viability (%) or yield (million hepatocytes/g liver) of isolated human hepatocytes.

Variables	Viability[1]		Yield[2]	
	N	*P* value	*N*	*P* value
Donor characteristics				
Age	1030	0.027*	1026	0.00067*
Gender	1032	6.3×10^{-7}*	1028	1.6×10^{-6}*
Body mass index[3]	1006	0.022*	1002	0.026*
Fibrosis	910	0.0016*	905	0.074
Cirrhosis	907	0.76	902	1.1×10^{-5}*
Diabetes	1014	0.23	1009	0.022*
Obesity	1015	0.89	1010	0.44
Hypertension	1014	0.21	1009	0.052
Hypercholesterolemia	1012	0.32	1007	0.87
Hyperuricemia	1010	0.48	1005	0.037*
Smoking	573	0.93	569	0.091
Liver fat	886	0.00052*	881	0.021*
Liver fat (%)	522	0.47	517	3.6×10^{-8}*
Tumour type	995	0.51	991	0.063
Surgical indication	1017	0.053	1013	1.6×10^{-6}*
Chemotherapy	1027	0.31	1023	3.5×10^{-5}*
ASA physical status classification system	990	0.90	986	0.054
Ludwig score	813	0.0010*	809	7.5×10^{-5}*
Clinical chemistry results before operation				
Alkaline phosphatase activity (U/L)[3]	797	0.067	792	7.3×10^{-5}*
Aspartate aminotransferase activity (U/L)[3]	712	0.00012*	709	0.00016*
Gamma-glutamyltranspeptidase activity (U/L)[3]	690	0.0015*	687	4.2×10^{-7}*
Alanine aminotransferase activity (U/L)[3]	812	2.9×10^{-5}*	808	2.7×10^{-9}*
Cholinesterase activity (U/L)[3]	714	0.97	713	0.74
Bilirubin (mg/dL)[3]	810	0.0022*	805	0.00087*
Partial thromboplastin time (s)[3]	799	0.88	794	0.035*
Quick value (%)	803	0.027*	798	0.015*
Operation parameters				
Operation type	992	0.16	989	3.3×10^{-8}*
Warm ischemia *in vivo* (min)[3]	602	0.47	602	0.00068*
Warm ischemia *ex vivo* (min)[3]	888	3.9×10^{-5}*	887	0.00054*
Weight of resected liver (g)[3]	839	0.092	836	0.00066*
Tissue processing and cell isolation parameters				
Cold ischemia (min)[3]	913	0.027*	914	0.19
Weight of perfused liver (g)[3]	1030	0.68	1027	1.2×10^{-11}*

*Significant at $P<0.05$. Data are transformed to follow a normal distribution by logit[1], fourth root[2] or natural logarithm[3] transformation.

consent [4], this discarded tissue could then be collected for hepatocyte isolation.

In order to successfully use human hepatocytes as an *in vitro* model or for cell-based therapy, hepatocytes must be obtained with good viability and hence quality. Further, as the sources of human hepatocytes are limited and the cost of the entire process from informed consent to successfully obtaining hepatocytes is high, it is also important to understand the factors that can result in a compromised yield. Thus far, the literature on factors that affect viability and yield is contradictory (Tables 1 and 2). Further, the previously done studies had a small sample size ranging from 10 to 149 donors. Therefore, this study aimed to determine, with a large number of donors and hepatocyte isolations carried out over 10 years, the donor characteristics, medical histories and

Table 5. The regression coefficients (β), P values and R^2 numbers of variables after multivariate analyses for the dependent variable of viability (%) of isolated human hepatocytes.

Variables	Viability[1]	
	β	P value
Donor characteristics		
Fibrosis	−0.18	0.040*
Liver fat	−0.22	0.0065*
Clinical chemistry results before operation		
Gamma-glutamyltranspeptidase activity (U/L)[2]	−0.088	0.017*
Bilirubin	−0.17	0.0095*
R^2 = 0.12, Intercept = 1.81		

Variables presented are chosen by backward elimination.
*Significant at $P<0.05$, with $N=218$. Data are transformed to follow a normal distribution by logit[1] or natural logarithm[2] transformation.

operation, tissue processing and cell isolation parameters that affect the viability and the yield of isolated human hepatocytes.

Material and Methods

Ethics Statement

The liver pieces used for hepatocyte isolation were collected from resected liver specimens designated as surgical waste after examination by a pathologist. In particular, the tissue used was dissected from the resection margin of tumours containing morphologically healthy tissue. All liver pieces were collected with their associated clinical data by the Tissue Bank under the Administration of the Human Tissue and Cell Research (HTCR) Foundation (http://www.htcr.de/english/contacts.html) [4]. The HTCR-process included written informed consent, was approved by the Ethics Committee of the Medical Faculty of Regensburg University Hospital (approval number 99/46) and Ethics Committee of the Medical Faculty of Ludwig Maximilians University (approval number 025-12) and complied with the Bavarian Data Protection Act.

Patients

In total, hepatocytes were isolated from remnant liver pieces from 1034 patients from Regensburg University Hospital (December 1997 to December 2002 and July 2010 to December 2011) and Grosshadern Hospital located in Munich (January 2003 to December 2013).

Corresponding data on the donor characteristics, medical histories and operation, tissue processing and cell isolation parameters were collected and entered into a database. The variables of interest for this study are listed on Table 3.

Isolation of Human Hepatocytes

Primary human hepatocytes were isolated using a two-step collagenase perfusion technique [5,6] with modifications [7]. In short, the larger blood vessels on a liver piece with one cut face were cannulated with irrigation cannulae with olive tips. The liver piece was then perfused first with 1 L of Solution 1, which contains 154 mM sodium chloride, 20 mM HEPES, 5.6 mM potassium chloride, 5 mM glucose and 25 mM sodium hydrogen carbonate. Next, it was perfused for 10 min with Solution 2 (152.5 mM sodium chloride, 19.8 mM HEPES, 5.5 mM potassium chloride, 5 mM glucose and 24.8 mM sodium hydrogen carbonate and 0.1 mM EGTA) followed by Solution 3 (152.5 mM sodium chloride, 19.8 mM HEPES, 5.5 mM potassium chloride, 5 mM glucose and 24.8 mM sodium hydrogen carbonate and 0.5 μM calcium chloride dihydrate) for 0.5 L. Finally, it was perfused with Solution 4 (120 mM sodium chloride, 10 mM HEPES, 0.9 mM calcium chloride dehydrate, 6.2 mM potassium chloride and 0.1% w/v albumin), which contains 0.1 to 0.15% w/v collagenase for 9 to 12 minutes or until the liver is sufficiently digested. The liver piece was then placed carefully in a crystallising dish for removal of the Glisson's capsule before gently shaking the cells loose. The cell suspension was then filtered through a 210 μm nylon mesh followed by a 70 μm nylon mesh before centrifuging at 72 g for 5 min at 4°C to pellet the hepatocytes. Hepatocytes were then washed 3 times before resuspending the cells in Cold Storage Solution (Hepacult GmbH, Germany).

A hemocytometer-based trypan blue dye exclusion assay was done to quantify the viability and total cells yielded by this isolation procedure.

Statistical Analyses

The data were summarised by adequate measures of location and spread. For modelling the outcomes of "viability" and "yield", linear regression modelling was used when the variables in Table 3 were considered.

To account for the possibility of non-linear relationships between the considered outcome and the continuous covariates (Table 3), fractional polynomials of first and second degree were applied. For this purpose, the multivariable fractional polynomials (MFP) algorithm [8] was used. This algorithm combines the selection of the functional forms of each continuous covariate using fractional polynomials with the selection of all continuous and non-continuous covariates via backward elimination. For the multiple regression models, only donors with a complete set of information for the variables of interest were used. Therefore, 218 donors were considered for viability and 128 donors were considered for yield. The selection level for potential predictors was set to 0.05.

In order to satisfy the assumption of normality, viabilities were transformed by applying the logit and yields by applying the fourth root. Graphical procedures were used to assess the fit of the model. All tests were performed two-sided and a p-value lower than 0.05

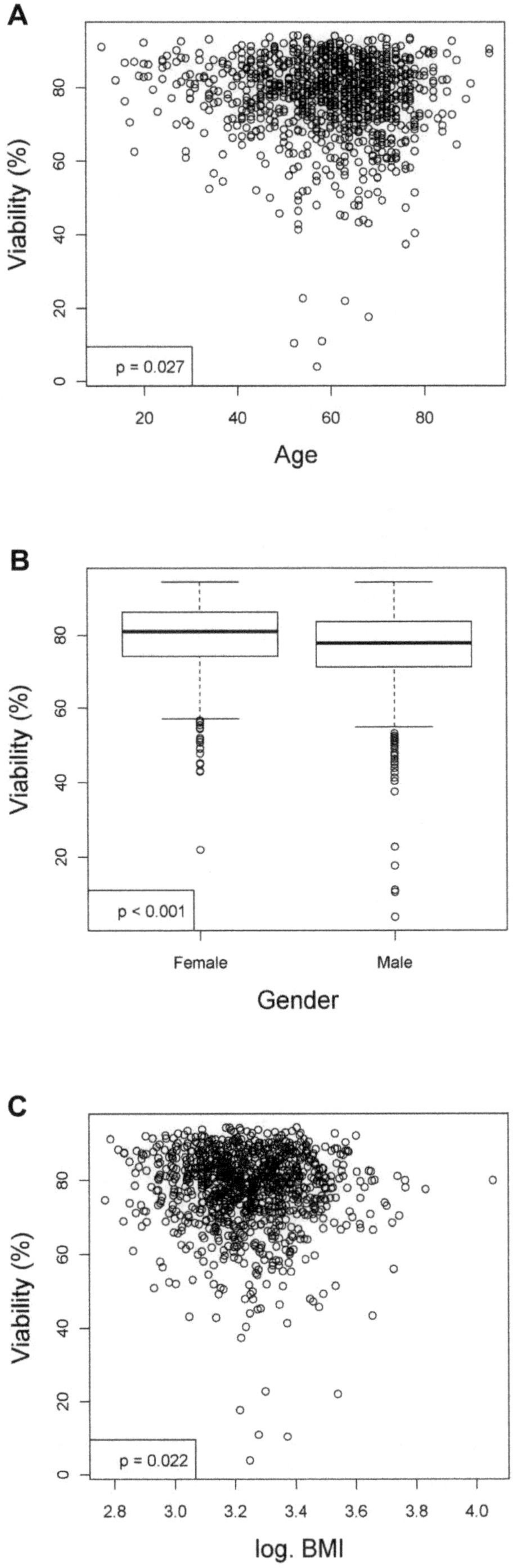

Figure 1. Donor characteristics that have significant relationships with the viability (%) of hepatocytes after linear regression analyses. Figures show relationships between viability and (**A**) age, (**B**) gender or (**C**) body mass index (BMI). Values were deemed significant when $P<0.05$.

was considered statistically significant. For all statistical analyses the software R (version 2.13.1) was used.

Results

A total of 1034 hepatocyte isolations were done with an average viability of 78±10% and average yield of 13±11 million viable hepatocytes per gram liver with the values represented in means ± standard deviation.

Univariate analyses to determine relationships of variables to viability and yield of hepatocytes

After linear regression analyses were carried out, variables with or without a significant relationship to the viability and the yield of hepatocytes were listed in Tables 4 and 5 respectively. In addition, figures were generated for the variables with significant relationships to the viability (Figures 1 to 4) and the yield (Figures 5 to 9) of hepatocytes.

It was found that the viability of hepatocytes was decreased by increases in age, body mass index (BMI), aspartate aminotransferase (GOT) activity, gamma-glutamyltranspeptidase (GGT) activity, alanine aminotransferase (GPT) activity, bilirubin content in the blood, quick value, warm ischemia time *in vivo* and cold ischemia time (Table S1). In addition, the viability of hepatocytes was also decreased for males and for donors with fibrosis, liver fat or Ludwig scores indicating periportal fibrosis or septal fibrosis (Table S1).

In the case of the yield of hepatocytes, it was found that the yield was decreased by increases in age, BMI, liver fat, alkaline phosphatase (AP) activity, GOT activity, GGT activity, GPT activity, bilirubin content in the blood, partial thromboplastin time (PTT), warm ischemia time *in vivo* and weight of resected or perfused liver (Table S2). Further, the yield of hepatocytes was also decreased for males and for donors with cirrhosis, diabetes, hyperuricemia or certain surgical indications, operation types or Ludwig scores (Table S2). However, the yield of hepatocytes can be increased by increases in warm ischemia time *ex vivo*, Quick value and in donors treated with chemotherapy (Table S2).

Multivariate analyses to determine the variables that affect the viability and the yield of hepatocytes

After multivariate analysis, the number of variables that have a significant effect on the viability of hepatocytes was reduced to 4 variables. It was found that the viability of hepatocytes was significantly decreased by the presence of fibrosis, liver fat and with increasing GGT activity and bilirubin content (Table 5).

For the yield of hepatocytes, it was found that yield was significantly decreased by the presence of liver fat and a Ludwig score indicating septal fibrosis. In addition, the yield of hepatocytes was decreased by increasing GOT activity, cold ischemia time and weight of perfused liver. However, the yield of hepatocytes was increased with chemotherapy treatment (Table 6).

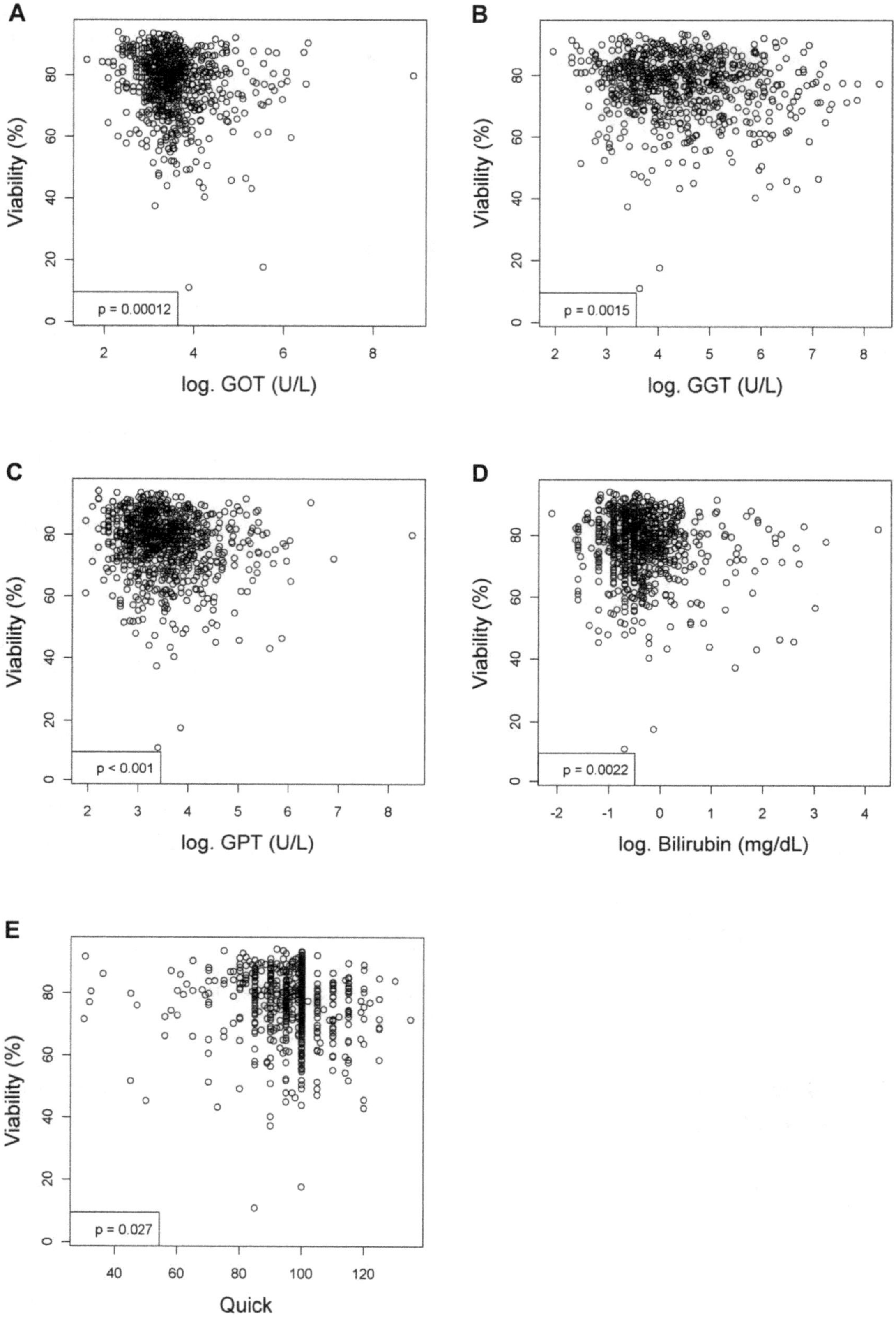

Figure 2. Variables measured in the blood or serum that have significant relationships with the viability (%) of hepatocytes after linear regression analyses. Figures show relationships between viability and (**A**) aspartate aminotransferase activity (GOT; U/L), (**B**) gamma-glutamyltranspeptidase activity (GGT; U/L), (**C**) alanine aminotransferase activity (GPT; U/L), (**D**) bilirubin (mg/dL) or (**E**) quick value (%). Values were deemed significant when $P<0.05$.

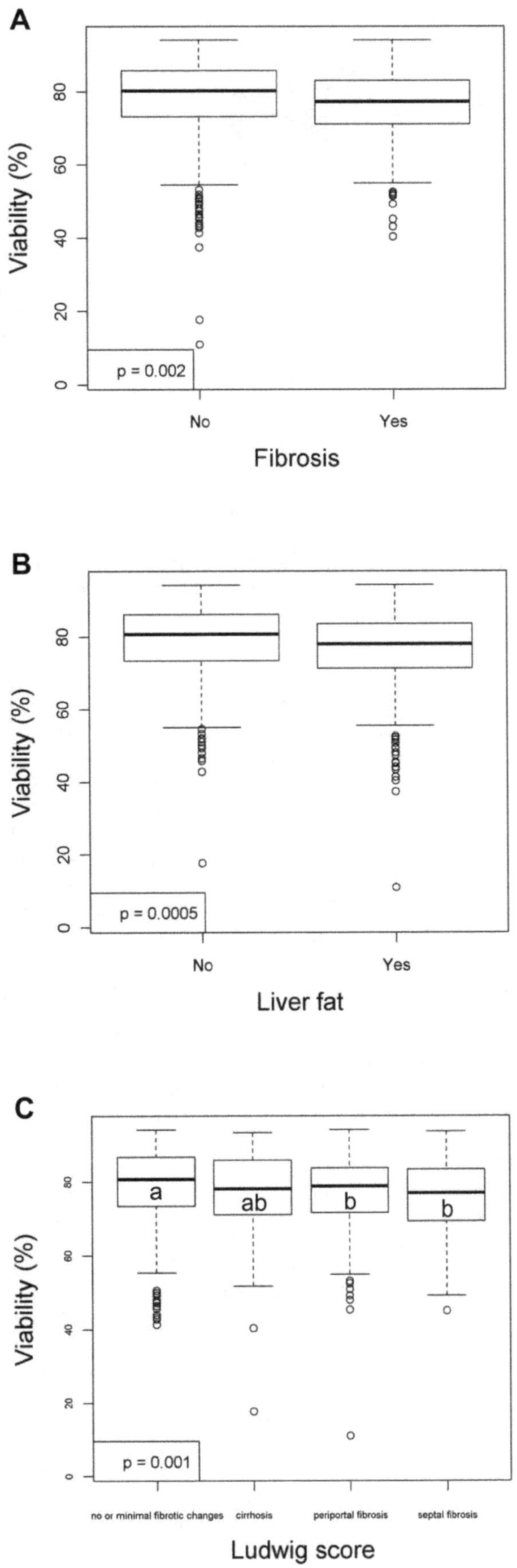

Figure 3. Liver variables that have significant relationships with the viability (%) of hepatocytes after linear regression analyses. Figures show relationships between viability and (**A**) fibrosis, (**B**) liver fat or (**C**) Ludwig score. Values were deemed significant when P<0.05. For the variable of Ludwig score, variables not sharing the same alphabet are significantly different, *P*<0.05.

Generation of a model that allows for the calculation of projected viability and yield of hepatocytes

The information obtained from the multivariate analyses allowed the generation of formulae for the calculation of projected viability and the yield of isolated human hepatocytes as shown below.

For the calculation of projected viability (%) of hepatocytes

Formula 1. Linear predictor of viability $= \beta_0 + \beta_1 \times \log_e(\text{bilirubin}) + \beta_2 \times \text{fibrosis} + \beta_3 \times \text{liver fat} + \beta_4 \times \log_e(\text{GGT}+1)$

The values of the various constants are as follows; $\beta_0 = 1.809$, $\beta_1 = -0.169$, $\beta_2 = -0.178$, $\beta_3 = -0.216$ and $\beta_4 = -0.088$. While the continuous variables can be directly substituted with the absolute values recorded for a patient, categorical variables have to be substituted with "0" or "1". For "fibrosis" – "0" for donors with no fibrosis and "1" for donors with fibrosis; for "liver fat" – "0" for donors with no liver fat and "1" for donors with liver fat.

Formula 2. Viability $(\%) = e^{(\text{linear predictor of viability})} \div (1 + e^{(\text{linear predictor of viability})}) \times 100$

For the calculation of projected yield (million hepatocytes/g liver)

Formula 3. Linear predictor of yield $= \beta_0 + \beta_1 \times \text{Chemotherapy} + \beta_2 \times \log_e(\text{Cold ischemia}+1) + \beta_3 \times \log_e(\text{Weight of perfused liver}+1) + \beta_4 \times \text{Liver fat }(\%) + \beta_5 \times (\text{Ludwig score})\text{ Cirrhosis} + \beta_6 \times (\text{Ludwig score})\text{ Periportal fibrosis} + \beta_7 \times (\text{Ludwig score})\text{ Septal fibrosis} + \beta_8 \times \log_e(\text{GOT activity}+1)$

The values of the various constants are as follows; $\beta_0 = 3.137$, $\beta_1 = 0.19$, $\beta_2 = -0.099$, $\beta_3 = -0.159$, $\beta_4 = -0.007$, $\beta_5 = -0.108$, $\beta_6 = 0.042$, $\beta_7 = -0.211$ and $\beta_8 = -0.114$. While the continuous variables can be directly substituted with the absolute values recorded for a patient, categorical variables have to be substituted with "0" or "1". For "chemotherapy" – "0" for donors with no chemotherapy and "1" for donors treated with chemotherapy; for the variable "Ludwig score", the Ludwig score category of the a donor should be set to "1" while all other not applicable Ludwig score categories should be set to "0" for calculation. For example, if the donor has "cirrhosis", this variable should be set to 1 at the same time as setting the variables "periportal fibrosis" and "septal fibrosis" to 0.

Formula 4. Yield (million hepatocytes/g liver) = linear predictor of yield^4

Validation of the models for calculating projected viability and yield of isolated hepatocytes

The appropriateness of the models for calculating the projected viability and yield of isolated hepatocytes are very similar and can be seen in Figures 10 and 11 respectively. Firstly, the residuals versus fitted plots (Figures 10A and 11A) show that there is no systematic relationship between the residuals and the predicted (or so-called fitted) values. These two figure panels (Figures 10A and

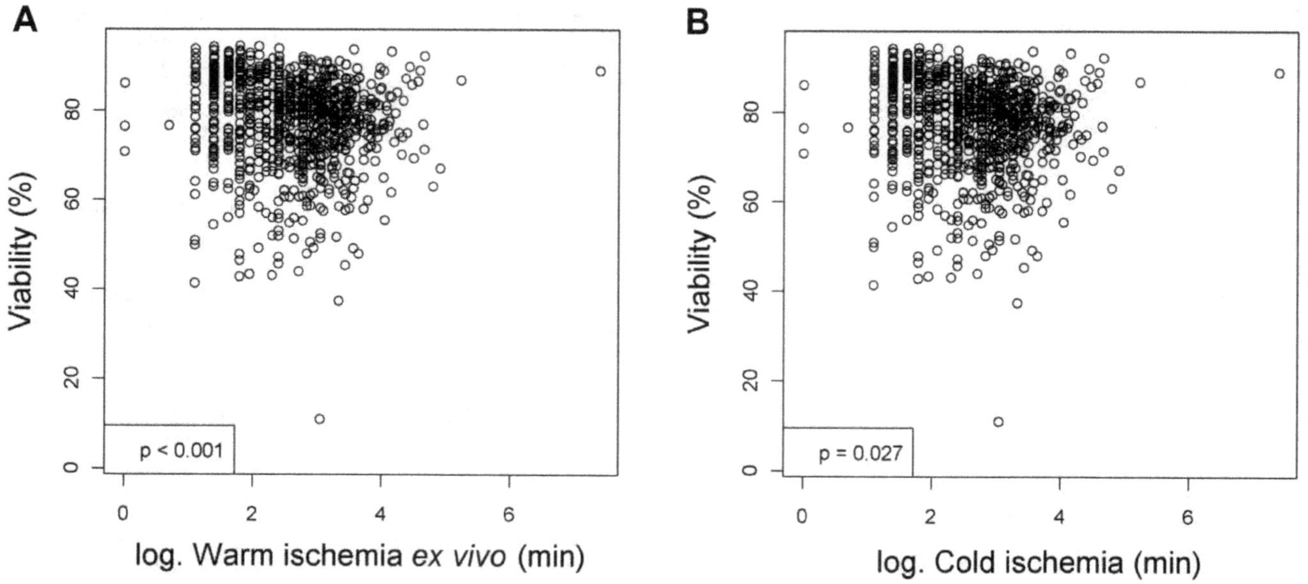

Figure 4. Tissue processing and cell isolation variables that have significant relationships with the viability (%) of hepatocytes after linear regression analyses. Figures show relationships between viability and (**A**) warm ischemia *ex vivo* (min) or (**B**) cold ischemia (min). Values were deemed significant when $P<0.05$.

11A) also show that there are no systematic tendencies in the errors, such as heteroscedasticity etc.

Secondly, the normal quintile plots (Figures 10B and 11B) show that the residuals are approximately normally distributed. This distribution is necessary in order to obtain valid test statistics and *P* values of the regression coefficient.

Thirdly, the square root of the standardised residuals versus fitted plots (Figures 10C and 11C) show that there is no systematic relationship between the residuals and the predicted (or fitted) values. As before, these graphs also do not show systematic tendencies in the errors such as heteroscedasticity. However, in contrast to the residuals versus fitted plot, the standardised residuals were normalised once again, so that the residuals to have unit variance, using an overall measure of the error variance.

Finally, the standardised residuals versus leverage plots (Figures 10D and 11D) show the influence of regression results when leaving out a single observation from the dataset. Leverage can be used to detect multivariate outliers in the data, but in this case, the leverage is so small that no limits indicating big leverage of a single or several observations appear in our data.

Discussion

This study aimed to determine donor characteristics, medical histories and operation, tissue processing and cell isolation parameters that affect the viability and the yield of isolated human hepatocytes. In order to do this, univariate analyses were first run to determine the variables that had a significant relationship to the viability or the yield of isolated human hepatocytes. Next, multiple regression analyses were run to determine the relative contributions of the various variables on the outcomes of viability and yield. From the results of the multiple regression analyses, a model was built to predict the viability and the yield of isolated hepatocytes (see Formulae 1–4 in results). Residual analyses were then done to check the regression assumptions in order to ensure that the model was appropriate.

This study has to the authors' knowledge, the largest number of donors examined for univariate analyses with 1034 donors and a sample size between 517 and 1032 for the individual variables. In contrast, other studies that carried out univariate analyses had sample sizes between 10 and 149 [9–15]. As a result, this study detects statistical significance in more variables than in the other studies (Tables 4, S1 and S2), probably due to an increase in statistical power. However, when multiple regression analyses were done, a reduced number of variables were found to be statistically significant. Typically, this is the case when multiple regression analyses are carried out, but it is important to consider that there is a loss of statistical power as the sample sizes were 218 for viability and 128 for yield of isolated hepatocytes as only cases with completed data on all the variables of interest were considered. However, as the other study that has conducted multiple regression analyses to the authors' knowledge has a sample size of 90 [16], this study still contributes useful information that will be discussed below.

When the absolute viability and yield numbers are considered, the hepatocytes isolated according to the authors' protocol [7] have a good balance of high viability (77 ± 0.3) and yield (13.4 ± 0.4) comparable to other groups with good results (Table 7). The comparison of variables found to have significant effects on the viability and yield of hepatocytes to what is known in the literature is challenging, as the results obtained by other groups are often contradictory (Tables 1 and 2). As such, the following paragraphs will instead focus on discussing the results of the multiple regression analyses.

After multiple regression analyses, this investigation has found that the viability of isolated human hepatocytes was significantly decreased by the presence of fibrosis, liver fat and with increasing GGT activity and bilirubin content (Formula 1). In the case of the

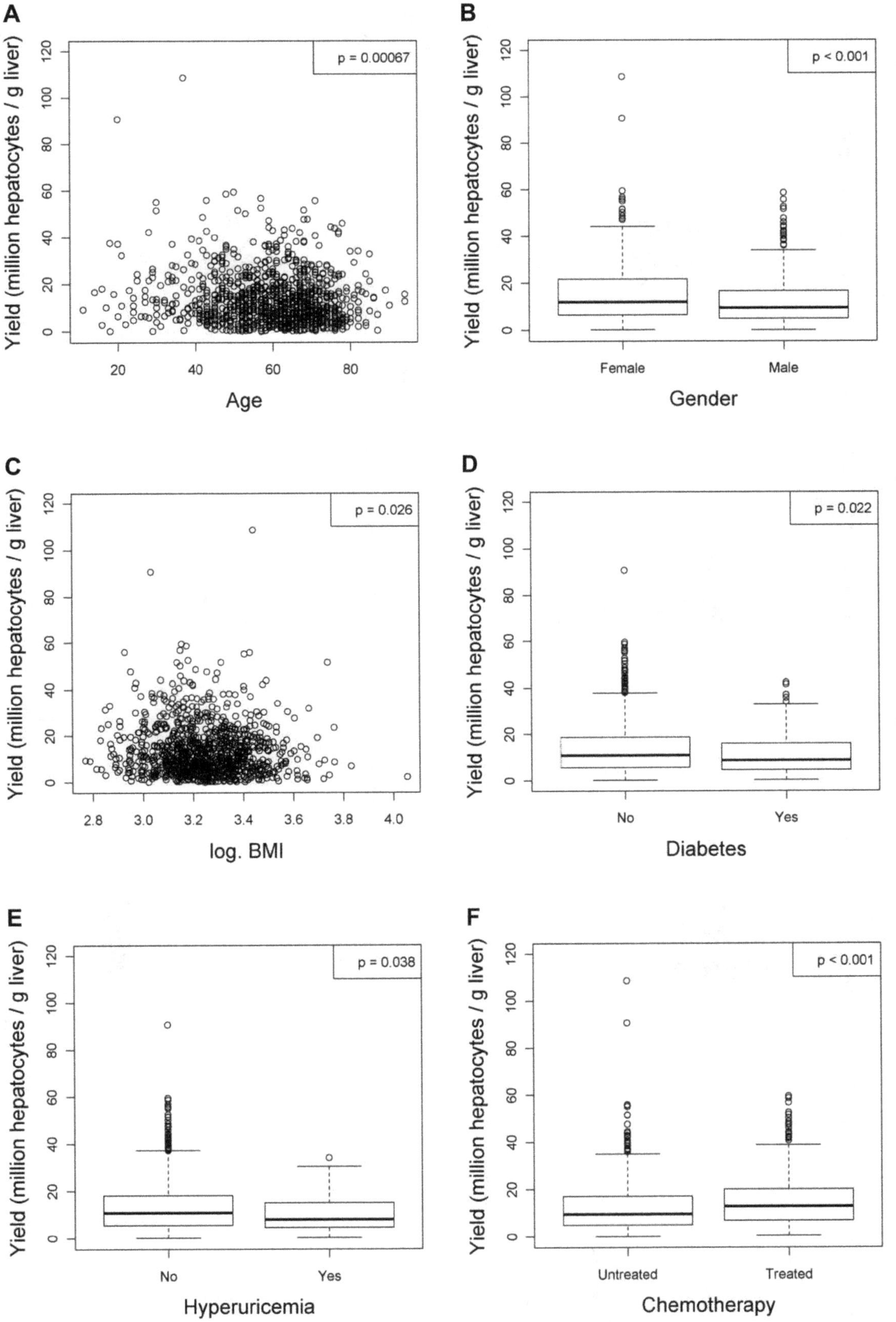

Figure 5. Donor characteristics that have significant relationships with the yield (million hepatocytes/gram liver) after linear regression analyses. Figures show relationships between yield and (**A**) age, (**B**) gender, (**C**) body mass index (BMI), (**D**) diabetes, (**E**) hyperuricemia or (**F**) chemotherapy. Values were deemed significant when $P<0.05$.

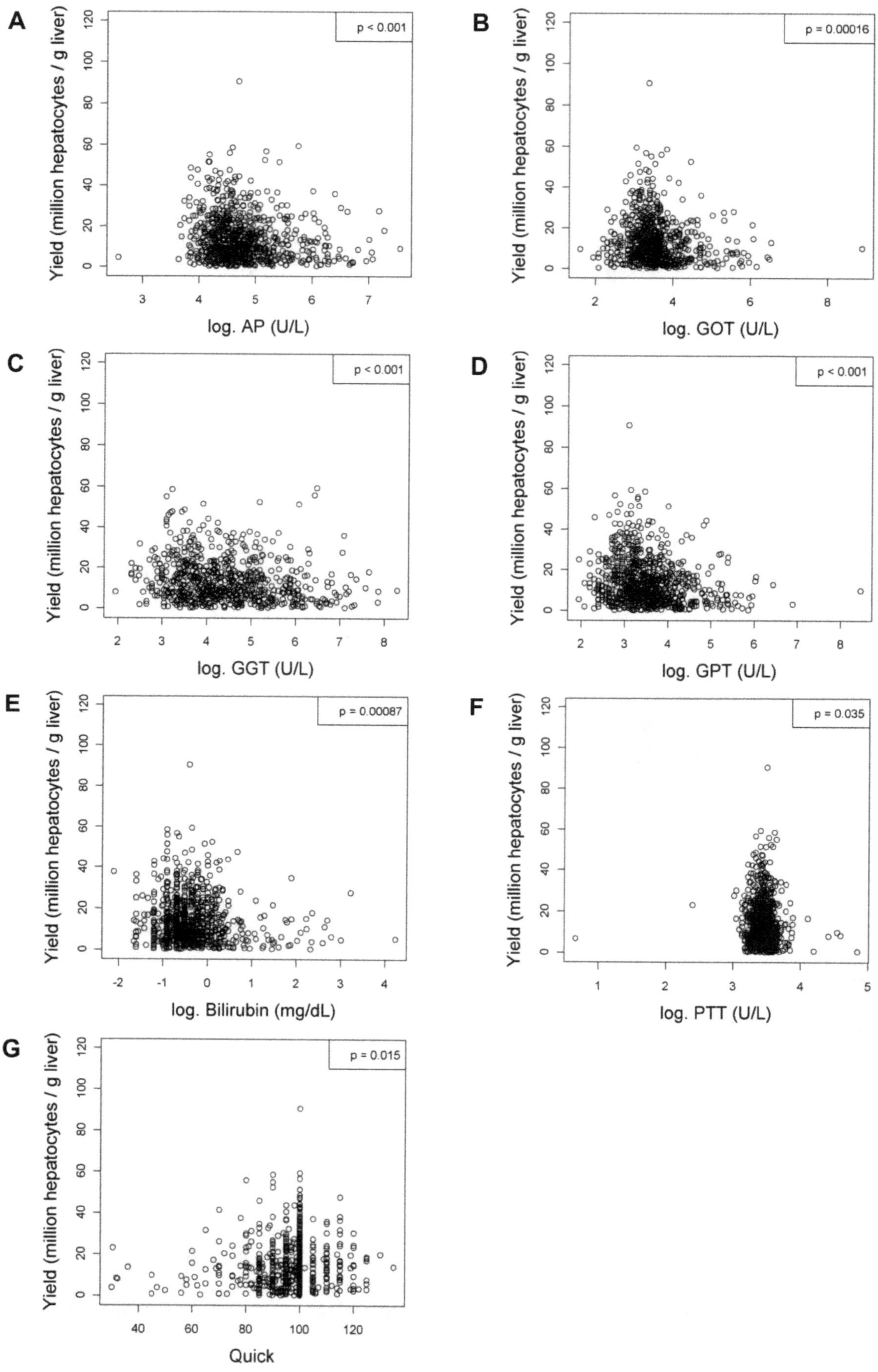
A
p < 0.001
Yield (million hepatocytes / g liver)
log. AP (U/L)
B
p = 0.00016
Yield (million hepatocytes / g liver)
log. GOT (U/L)
C
p < 0.001
Yield (million hepatocytes / g liver)
log. GGT (U/L)
D
p < 0.001
Yield (million hepatocytes / g liver)
log. GPT (U/L)
E
p = 0.00087
Yield (million hepatocytes / g liver)
log. Bilirubin (mg/dL)
F
p = 0.035
Yield (million hepatocytes / g liver)
log. PTT (U/L)
G
p = 0.015
Yield (million hepatocytes / g liver)
Quick

Figure 6. Variables measured in the blood or serum that have significant relationships with the yield (million hepatocytes/gram liver) after linear regression analyses. Figures show relationships between yield and (**A**) alkaline phosphatase activity (AP; U/L), (**B**) aspartate aminotransferase activity (GOT; U/L), (**C**) gamma-glutamyltranspeptidase activity (GGT; U/L), (**D**) alanine aminotransferase activity (GPT; U/L), (**E**) bilirubin (mg/dL), (**F**) partial thromboplastin time (PTT; s) or (**G**) quick value (%). Values were deemed significant when $P<0.05$.

yield of isolated human hepatocytes, it was found that the yield was significantly decreased by the presence of liver fat, a Ludwig score indicating septal fibrosis and by increasing GOT activity, cold ischemia time and weight of perfused liver. Further, the yield of hepatocytes was increased with chemotherapy treatment (Formula 3).

Increased cold ischemia time has been found to decrease the yield of isolated hepatocytes. In this study, the liver piece used for hepatocyte isolation was not perfused to remove the blood in the tissue before transport on ice to the laboratory. As a result, the formation of blood clots can occur in the tissue in the cases with longer transportation times even though the clotting process is slowed by low temperatures [17]. This could then affect the perfusion of the liver during the hepatocyte isolation process and decrease the yield. Yield is also decreased when the weight of the perfused liver is increased. Alexandre *et al.* [10] showed that the percentage of undigested tissue left after the isolation process is significantly increased in larger pieces of liver above 101 g. Also,

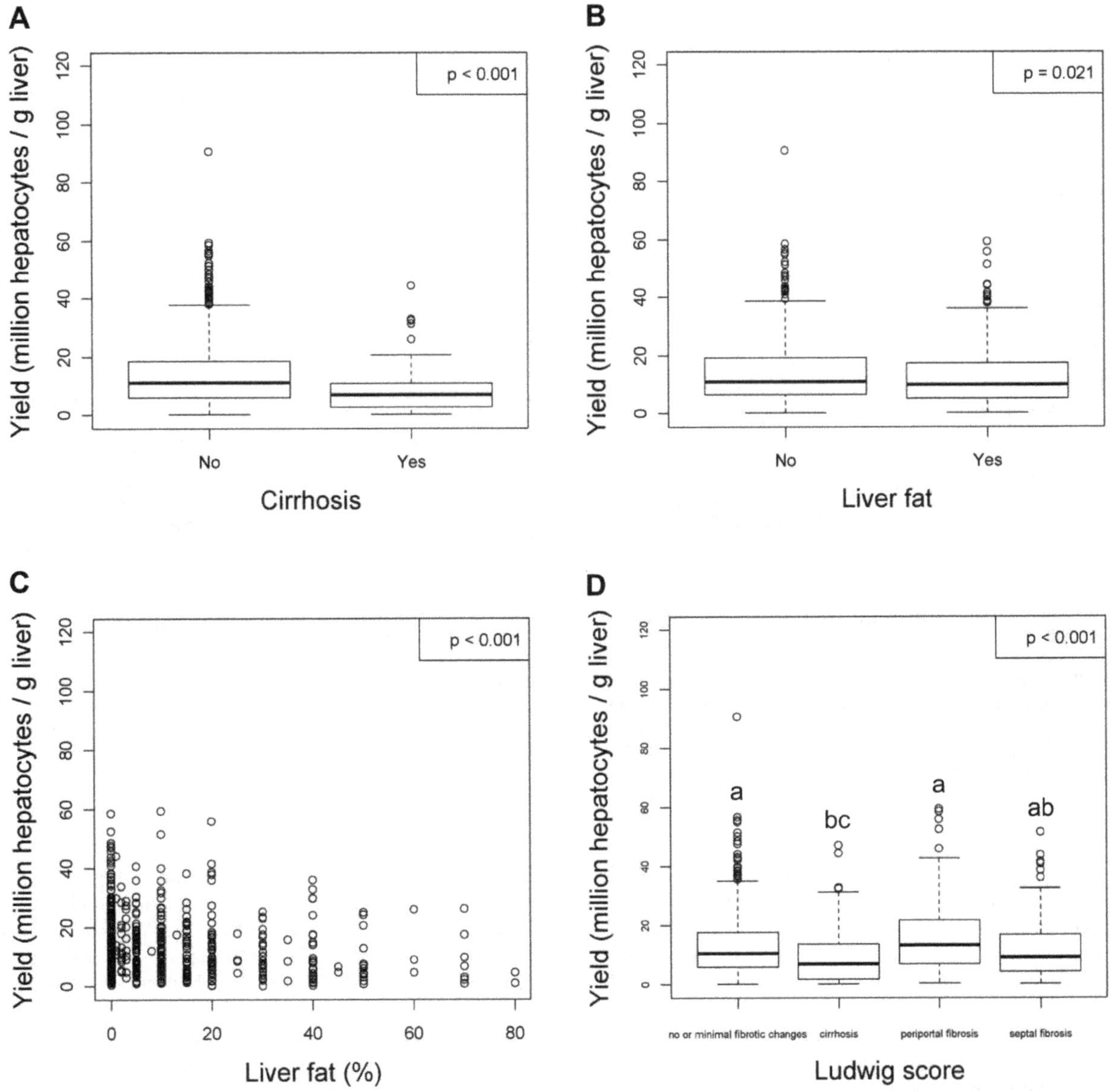

Figure 7. Liver variables that have significant relationships with the yield (million hepatocytes/gram liver) of hepatocytes after linear regression analyses. Figures show relationships between yield and (**A**) cirrhosis, (**B**) liver fat, (**C**) liver fat (%) or (**D**) Ludwig score. Values were deemed significant when $P<0.05$. For the variables of Ludwig score, operation type and surgical indication, variables not sharing the same alphabet are significantly different, $P<0.05$.

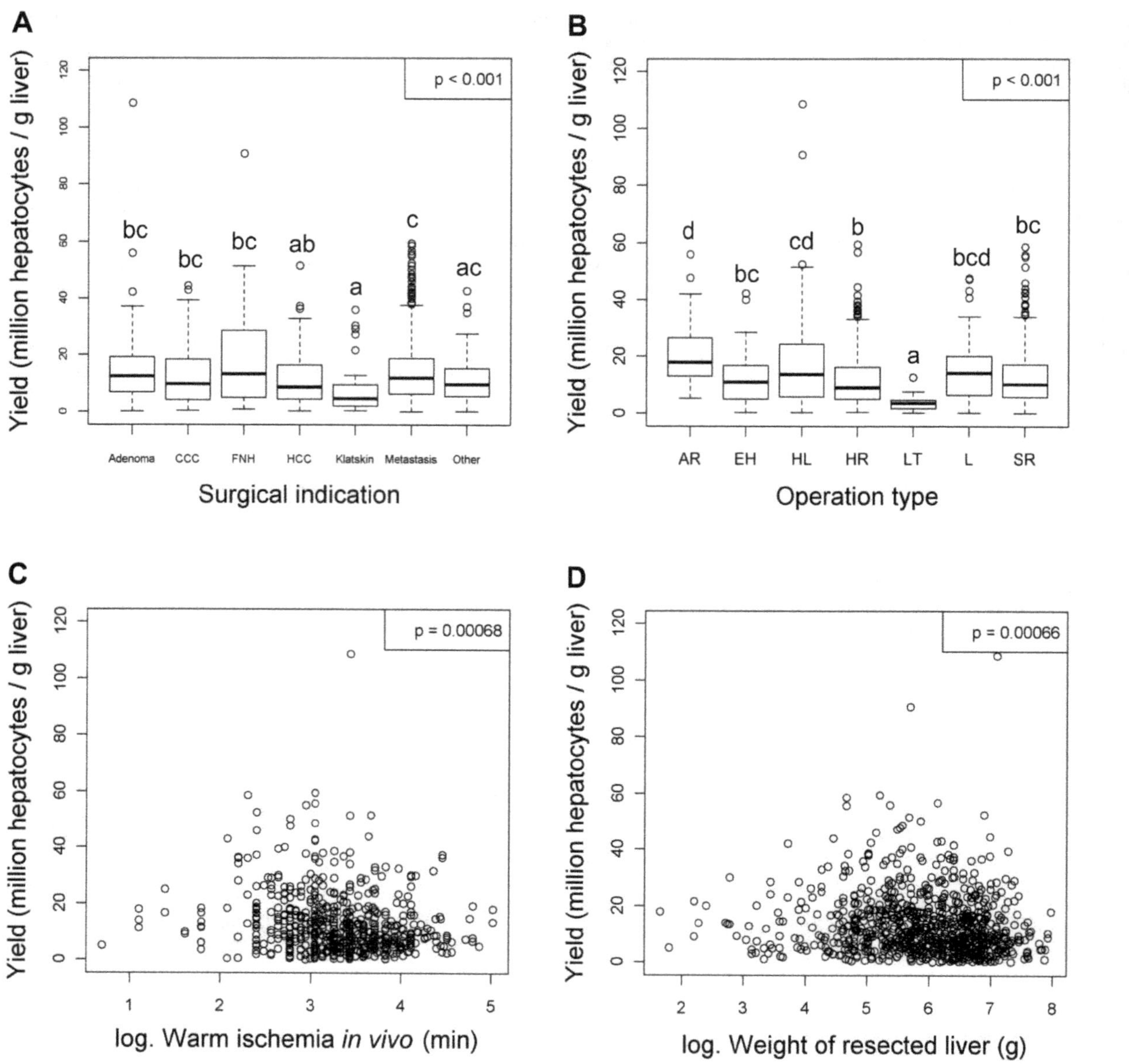

Figure 8. Operation variables that have significant relationships with the yield (million hepatocytes/gram liver) of hepatocytes after linear regression analyses. Figures show relationships between yield and (**A**) surgical indication, (**B**) operation type, (**C**) warm ischemia *in vivo* (min) or (**D**) weight of resected liver (g). Values were deemed significant when $P<0.05$. Abbreviations; hepatocarcinoma (HCC), focal nodular hyperplasia (FNH), cholangiocarcinoma (CCC), hemihepatectomy right (HR), hemihepatectomy left (HL), segment resection (SR), atypical resection (AR), extended hepatectomy (EH), lobectomy (L) and liver transplantation (LT).

the isolation set-up used in this study can provide a maximum of 8 cannulae for perfusing the liver piece [7]. Although the rate of perfusion per cannula is kept at similar levels independent of the size of the liver [7], it may be that portions of a larger liver are not perfused due to additionally available open blood vessels not being cannulated.

Fibrosis develops in response to many types of chronic liver diseases [18]. In such diseases, apoptosis plays a critical role both in liver injury and the subsequent fibrosis [18]. During the process of apoptosis, hepatocytes form apoptotic bodies that are phagocytosed by hepatic stellate cells resulting in an up-regulation of Transforming Growth Factor β (TGF-β) and procollagen α1, leading to subsequent inflammation and fibrogenesis [19–21]. Since fibrosis is closely linked with inflammation and cell death, it is not surprising that hepatocytes isolated from fibrotic livers have a significantly lower viability. In particular, this study found that septal fibrosis resulted in a significantly decreased yield of viable hepatocytes. The process of septal fibrosis begins with the extension of the septa between central veins through interhepatocellular space and the space of Disse on the sides of the sinusoids [22]. As fibrosis proceeds, capillarization and then venularization occurs [22,23]. During this process, the fenestrations in some hepatic sinusoids are lost and the development of basal laminae occur alongside the collagenization of the extravascular spaces of

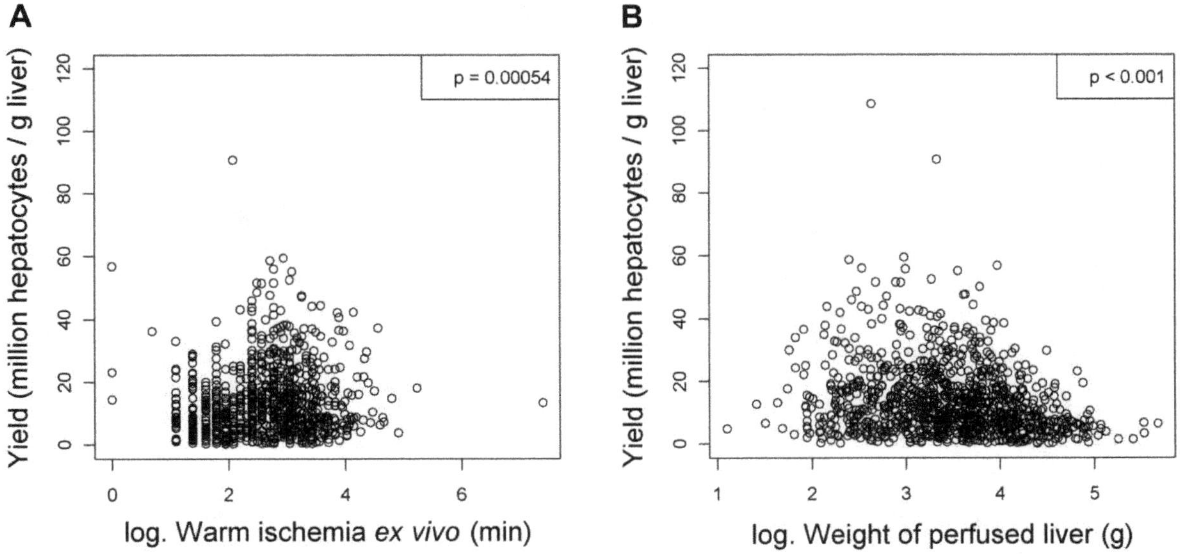

Figure 9. Tissue processing and cell isolation variables that have significant relationships with the yield (million hepatocytes/gram liver) of hepatocytes after linear regression analyses. Figures show relationships between yield and (**A**) warm ischemia *ex vivo* (min) or (**B**) weight of perfused liver (g). Values were deemed significant when P<0.05.

Disse [22,24]. This capillarization and fibrosis has been postulated to impair the leakage of macromolecules by creating a new barrier between the sinusoids and the hepatocytes [24]. This assertion has been supported by an approach utilising MRI, which shows that the extravascular distribution of high molecular weight contrast agents (6 or 52 kDa) is limited in a model of sinusoidal fibrosis [24]. These observations could explain the decreased yield obtained in this study due to septal fibrosis as collagenase that is 110 kDa will have limited access to the extracellular matrix in the direct vicinity of hepatocytes. Together with an increased amount of collagen surrounding capillaries that have to be digested, it is likely that the release of hepatocytes into a cell suspension is impaired and hence the reduced yield.

The presence of liver fat results in a significant decrease in the viability of hepatocytes. Hepatic steatosis, which is commonly found in obese or heavy alcohol drinkers, has been postulated to

Table 6. The regression coefficients (β), P values and R^2 numbers of variables after multivariate analyses for the dependent variable of yield (million hepatocytes/g liver) of isolated human hepatocytes.

Variables	Yield[1]	
	β	*P* value
Donor characteristics		
Liver fat (%)	−0.0069	0.0056*
Chemotherapy	0.19	0.0036*
Ludwig score		
-No or minimal fibrotic changes (reference)	-	-
-Periportal fibrosis	0.042	0.56
-Septal fibrosis	−0.21	0.047*
-Cirrhosis	−0.11	0.52
Clinical chemistry results before operation		
Aspartate aminotransferase activity (U/L)[2]	−0.11	0.016*
Tissue processing and cell isolation parameters		
Cold ischemia (min)[2]	−0.099	0.042*
Weight of perfused liver (g)	−0.16	0.0018*
R^2 = 0.32, Intercept = 3.14		

Variables presented are chosen by backward elimination.
*Significant at $P<0.05$, with $N=128$. Data are transformed to follow a normal distribution by fourth root[1] or natural logarithm[2] transformation.

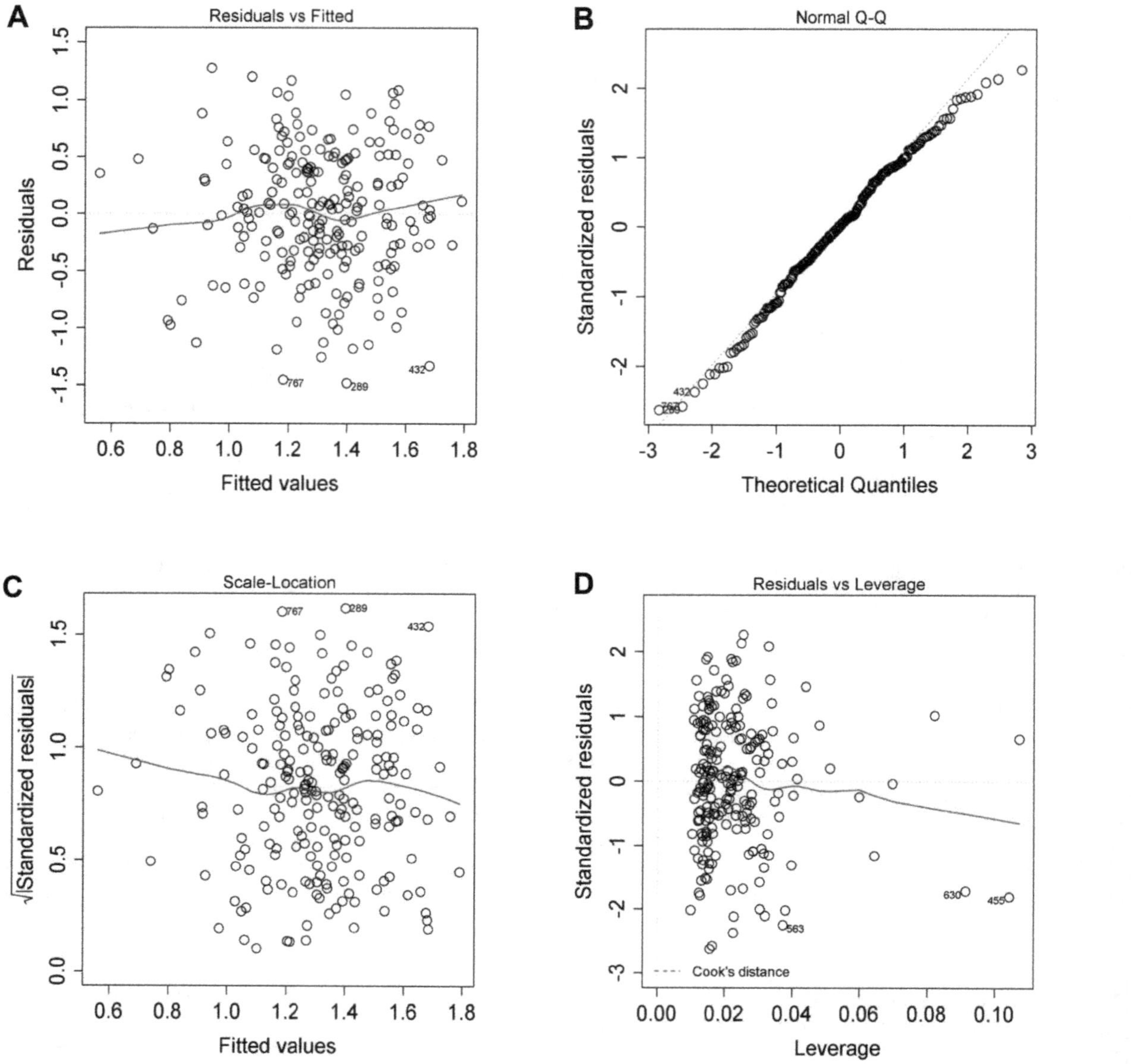

Figure 10. The model for calculating projected viability is appropriate. (**A**) Residuals versus fitted plot. (**B**) Normal quantile plot. (**C**) Square root of the standardised residuals versus fitted plot. (**D**) Standardised residuals versus leverage plot.

be a "first hit" that increases sensitivity to a "second hit" that could then trigger a cascade leading to steatohepatitis [25]. Steatohepatitis is characterised by inflammation and liver cell damage and could therefore lead to lower hepatocyte viability. Further, steatotic hepatocytes have been found to have increased sensitivity to hypoxic injury i.e. lower viability, due to the attenuation of Hypoxia Inducible Factor 1α expression and protein accumulation [26]. The presence of liver fat also results in a significant decrease in the yield of hepatocytes. It has been found that fat accumulation in hepatocytes results in microvascular alterations [27]. Various studies have demonstrated that lipid accumulation results in enlargement of hepatocytes, which widen the parenchymal cell plates, narrow and distort the lumens of the sinusoids and hence reduce the intrasinusoidal volume [27]. As a result, the sinusoids have impaired tissue perfusion and become poor conduits for conducting the collagenase-containing buffer used in the cell isolation process and possibly leading to a lower yield of hepatocytes. In addition, during centrifugation steps in the isolation process, steatotic hepatocytes tend to form a pellet less effectively, making it more likely that hepatocytes are lost when the supernatant is aspirated off (Authors' observation).

Levels of bilirubin and activities of GGT and GOT in the serum are standard assay parameters in liver function tests. Elevated levels of bilirubin and GGT, known indicators of hepatocyte injury [28,29], have been found here to lower viability of isolated hepatocytes. Increased activity of GOT significantly decreased the yield of hepatocytes. This could be because a high level of GOT has been found to be a diagnostic marker for a number of diseases that can affect microcirculation or have increased collagen deposition, such as advanced alcoholic disease [30] or non-alcoholic chronic liver diseases with significant fibrosis [31,32],

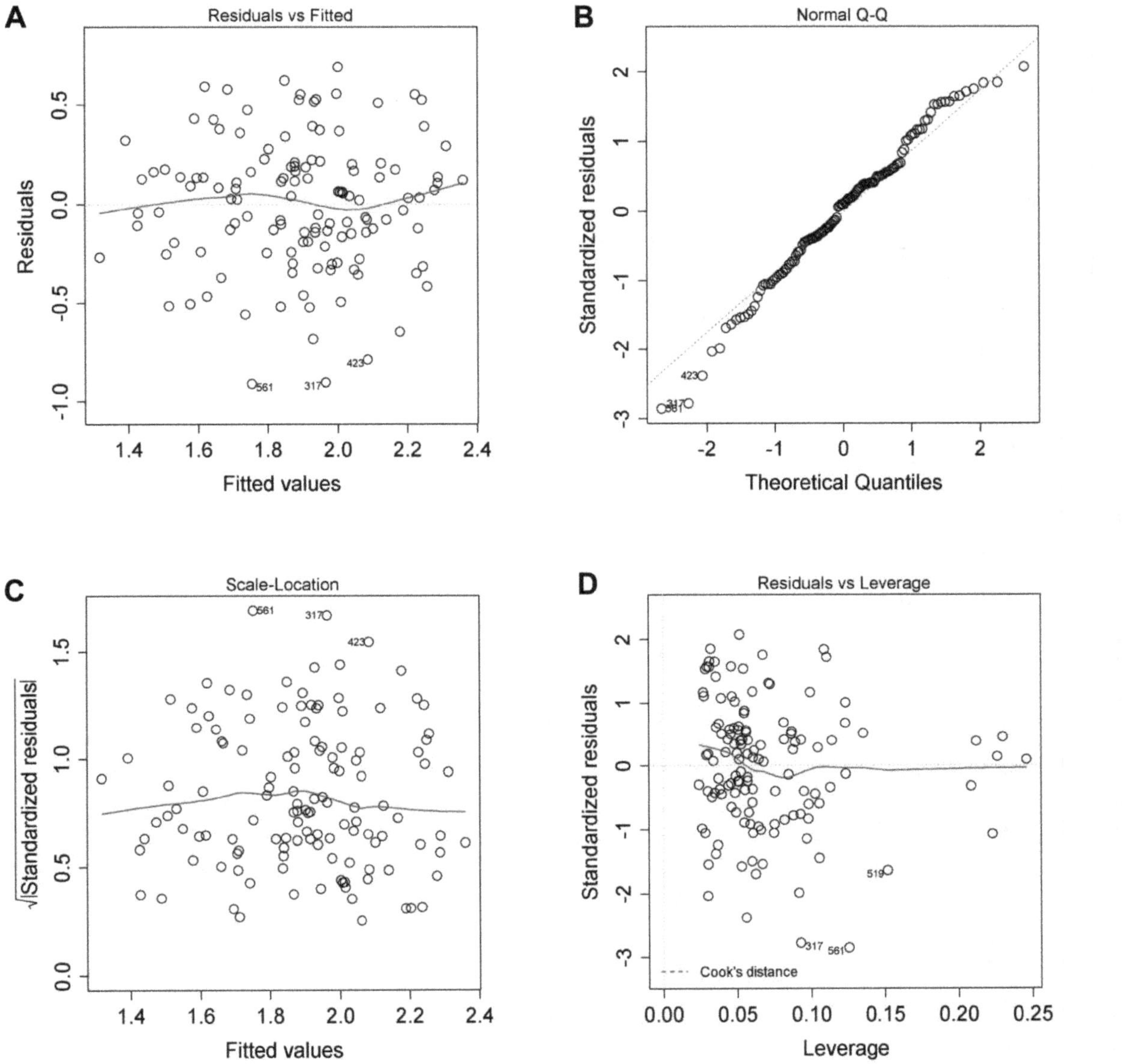

Figure 11. The model for calculating projected yield is appropriate. (**A**) Residuals versus fitted plot. (**B**) Normal quantile plot. (**C**) Square root of the standardised residuals versus fitted plot. (**D**) Standardised residuals versus leverage plot.

Hewes *et al.* [14] found that previous chemotherapy does not affect the median yield of isolated human hepatocytes (4.6 million viable cells per gram of liver). In contrast, this study found a significantly increased yield of hepatocytes from donors pre-treated with chemotherapy with median yields of 17 compared to 10 million viable cells per gram of liver from donors without chemotherapy. It could be possible that the analysis done here was able to pick up a significance due to an increased statistical power, as this study has 128 replicates compared to 47 replicates done in Hewes *et al.*'s study [14]. An additional support for this reasoning is that the univariate analysis done with 1027 replicates also indicated a statistical difference ($P = 3.5 \times 10^{-5}$). It is possible that chemotherapy has reduced extracellular matrix proteins, such as collagen, allowing for a more complete digestion of the liver piece with collagenase, which resulted in an increased yield of isolated hepatocytes. This is supported by the study of Drózdz and Kucharz [33], which found that a cytostatic drug, azathioprine caused a decrease in total collagen content in the liver. Further, Sorefenib, a drug that is approved for the treatment of hepatocarcinoma has been found to act as an antifibrotic agent that reduced collagen deposition in fibrosis models such as bile duct ligation, thioacetamide or dimethylnitrosamine administration in rats or carbon tetrachloride administration in mice [34–36]. Doxorubicin, another commonly used chemotherapeutic drug, also reduces collagen content in bile duct ligated rats by strongly inhibiting hepatic stellate cell proliferation [37].

In conclusion, this study has determined the variables that affect the viability and yield of isolated human hepatocytes. Further, this study has generated algorithms (Formulae 1–4) for the prediction of the viability or yield. A publicly accessible webpage (http://www.

Table 7. Viabilities (%) and yield (million hepatocytes per gram liver) of isolated human hepatocytes obtained by various groups.

Viability				Yield		*N*	Reference
Mean	Median	*N*	Reference	Mean	Median		
91±2	-	14	[11]	-	125	30	[41]
-	89	90	[16]	18.7±1.7	-	50	[15]
83±1	-	67	[12]	13.4±0.4	10.5	1028	Authors' own
83±1	-	72	[13]	10.6±7.8	-	41	[42]
80±8	-	41	[42]	8.2±5.7	-	42	[42]
78±0.3	-	10	[9]	7.9±1.2	-	14	[11]
77±0.3	79	1032	Authors' own	7.7±1.8	-	58	[13]
77±9	-	42	[42]	7.1±1.0	-	10	[9]
70±2	-	50	[15]	-	6.0	90	[16]
64±3	74	58	[39]	5.8±0.8	-	72	[13]
-	71	47	[14]	5.2±0.5	-	67	[12]
60±4	-	58	[13]	-	4.6	47	[14]
-	56	20	[38]	4.0±0.7	-	149	[10]
-	25	30	[41]	2.6±0.5	1.5	58	[39]

Values were expressed as means ± standard error of the mean.

klinikum.uni-muenchen.de/Chirurgische-Klinik-und-Poliklinik-Grosshadern/de/0700-forschung/ag-leberregeneration/core-facility/Qualitaetsrechner_Hepatozyten.html) where researchers can key in their variables for the automatic calculation of projected viability and yield using JavaScript, has been made available for ease of use. It is hoped that this resource will prove useful for the selection of suitable donors for hepatocyte isolation and also as a reference so that procedural problems can be spotted due to an unanticipated lower viability and yield obtained.

Supporting Information

Table S1 The number of replicates (*N*), *P* values, multiple R^2 values (R^2), intercepts, regression coefficients (β) obtained after linear regression of the individual variables to viability (%) of isolated human hepatocytes. *Significant relationship of the indicated variable to hepatocyte viability, $P<0.05$. For the variable of Ludwig score, variables not sharing the same superscript alphabet are significantly different, $P<0.05$. Viability values were transformed to follow a normal distribution by the logit[1].

Table S2 The number of replicates (*N*), *P* values, regression coefficients (β), intercepts and multiple R^2 values (R^2) obtained after linear regression of the individual variables to the yield (million/g liver) of isolated human hepatocytes. *Significant relationship of the indicated variable to hepatocyte yield, $P<0.05$. For the variables of Ludwig score, operation type and surgical indication, variables not sharing the same superscript alphabet are significantly different, $P<0.05$. Yield values were transformed to follow a normal distribution by the fourth root[1].

Acknowledgments

This work was made possible by the Human Tissue and Cell Research Foundation, which makes human tissues available for research. Our thanks also go to the technicians from the Grosshadern Hospital and the Regensburg University Hospital Tissue Banks for the collection of the liver samples and from the Cell Isolation Core Facility in Munich and Hepacult GmbH for carrying out the liver perfusion, hepatocyte isolation and data entry. Finally, special thanks go to Luke Bax for his help in creating the webpage, where investigators can enter their donor information to get a prediction of viability and yield of hepatocytes.

Author Contributions

Conceived and designed the experiments: WET SMLL CS. Performed the experiments: SMLL CS NF WET. Analyzed the data: SMLL CS RPL UM WET TSS. Contributed reagents/materials/analysis tools: WET RPL SMLL CS UM TSS RMKT. Wrote the paper: SMLL CS WET RMKT RPL UM TSS NF.

References

1. Olson H, Betton G, Robinson D, Thomas K, Monro A, et al. (2000) Concordance of the toxicity of pharmaceuticals in humans and in animals. Regul Toxicol Pharmacol 32: 56–67.
2. Brambilla G, Martelli A (1993) Human hepatocyte primary cultures in toxicity assessment. Cytotechnology 11 Suppl 1: S6–8.
3. Russell WMS, Burch RL (1959) The principles of humane experimental technique. London: Methuen.
4. Thasler WE, Weiss TS, Schillhorn K, Stoll PT, Irrgang B, et al. (2003) Charitable State-Controlled Foundation Human Tissue and Cell Research: Ethic and Legal Aspects in the Supply of Surgically Removed Human Tissue For Research in the Academic and Commercial Sector in Germany. Cell Tissue Bank 4: 49–56.
5. Berry MN, Friend DS (1969) High-yield preparation of isolated rat liver parenchymal cells: a biochemical and fine structural study. J Cell Biol 43: 506–520.
6. Seglen PO (1973) Preparation of rat liver cells. 3. Enzymatic requirements for tissue dispersion. Exp Cell Res 82: 391–398.
7. Lee SML SC, Demmel M, Hauner M, Thasler WE (2013) Isolation of human hepatocytes by a two-step collagenase perfusion procedure. J Vis Exp.
8. Sauerbrei W, Royston P (1999) Building multivariable prognostic and diagnostic models: transformation of the predictors by using fractional polynomials. Journal of the Royal Statistical Society Series a-Statistics in Society 162: 71–94.
9. Iqbal S, Elcombe CR, Elias E (1991) Maintenance of mixed-function oxidase and conjugation enzyme activities in hepatocyte cultures prepared from normal and diseased human liver. J Hepatol 12: 336–343.
10. Alexandre E, Cahn M, Abadie-Viollon C, Meyer N, Heyd B, et al. (2002) Influence of pre-, intra- and post-operative parameters of donor liver on the outcome of isolated human hepatocytes. Cell Tissue Bank 3: 223–233.
11. Serralta A, Donato MT, Orbis F, Castell JV, Mir J, et al. (2003) Functionality of cultured human hepatocytes from elective samples, cadaveric grafts and hepatectomies. Toxicol In Vitro 17: 769–774.
12. Lloyd TD, Orr S, Patel R, Crees G, Chavda S, et al. (2004) Effect of patient, operative and isolation factors on subsequent yield and viability of human hepatocytes for research use. Cell Tissue Bank 5: 81–87.
13. Richert L, Alexandre E, Lloyd T, Orr S, Viollon-Abadie C, et al. (2004) Tissue collection, transport and isolation procedures required to optimize human hepatocyte isolation from waste liver surgical resections. A multilaboratory study. Liver Int 24: 371–378.
14. Hewes JC, Riddy D, Morris RW, Woodrooffe AJ, Davidson BR, et al. (2006) A prospective study of isolated human hepatocyte function following liver resection for colorectal liver metastases: the effects of prior exposure to chemotherapy. J Hepatol 45: 263–270.
15. Vondran FW, Katenz E, Schwartlander R, Morgul MH, Raschzok N, et al. (2008) Isolation of primary human hepatocytes after partial hepatectomy: criteria for identification of the most promising liver specimen. Artif Organs 32: 205–213.
16. Kawahara T, Toso C, Douglas DN, Nourbakhsh M, Lewis JT, et al. (2010) Factors affecting hepatocyte isolation, engraftment, and replication in an in vivo model. Liver Transpl 16: 974–982.
17. Shionoya T (1927) Studies in Experimental Extracorporeal Thrombosis: Iv. Effects of Certain Physical and Mechanical Factors on Extracorporeal Thrombosis with and without the Use of Anticoagulants. J Exp Med 46: 957–961.
18. Yoon JH, Gores GJ (2002) Death receptor-mediated apoptosis and the liver. J Hepatol 37: 400–410.
19. Canbay A, Taimr P, Torok N, Higuchi H, Friedman S, et al. (2003) Apoptotic body engulfment by a human stellate cell line is profibrogenic. Lab Invest 83: 655–663.
20. Zhan SS, Jiang JX, Wu J, Halsted C, Friedman SL, et al. (2006) Phagocytosis of apoptotic bodies by hepatic stellate cells induces NADPH oxidase and is associated with liver fibrosis in vivo. Hepatology 43: 435–443.
21. Brenner C, Galluzzi L, Kepp O, Kroemer G (2013) Decoding cell death signals in liver inflammation. J Hepatol 59: 583–594.
22. Bhunchet E, Fujieda K (1993) Capillarization and venularization of hepatic sinusoids in porcine serum-induced rat liver fibrosis: a mechanism to maintain liver blood flow. Hepatology 18: 1450–1458.
23. Maria De Souza M, Tolentino M Jr, Assis BC, Cristina De Oliveira Gonzalez A, Maria Correia Silva T, et al. (2006) Pathogenesis of septal fibrosis of the liver. (An experimental study with a new model.). Pathol Res Pract 202: 883–889.
24. Van Beers BE, Materne R, Annet L, Hermoye L, Sempoux C, et al. (2003) Capillarization of the sinusoids in liver fibrosis: noninvasive assessment with contrast-enhanced MRI in the rabbit. Magn Reson Med 49: 692–699.
25. Day CP, James OF (1998) Steatohepatitis: a tale of two "hits"? Gastroenterology 114: 842–845.
26. Anavi S, Harmelin NB, Madar Z, Tirosh O (2012) Oxidative stress impairs HIF1alpha activation: a novel mechanism for increased vulnerability of steatotic hepatocytes to hypoxic stress. Free Radic Biol Med 52: 1531–1542.
27. Farrell GC, Teoh NC, McCuskey RS (2008) Hepatic microcirculation in fatty liver disease. Anat Rec (Hoboken) 291: 684–692.
28. Johnston DE (1999) Special considerations in interpreting liver function tests. Am Fam Physician 59: 2223–2230.
29. Ennulat D, Magid-Slav M, Rehm S, Tatsuoka KS (2010) Diagnostic performance of traditional hepatobiliary biomarkers of drug-induced liver injury in the rat. Toxicol Sci 116: 397–412.
30. Nyblom H, Berggren U, Balldin J, Olsson R (2004) High AST/ALT ratio may indicate advanced alcoholic liver disease rather than heavy drinking. Alcohol Alcohol 39: 336–339.
31. Shin WG, Park SH, Jun SY, Jung JO, Moon JH, et al. (2007) Simple tests to predict hepatic fibrosis in nonalcoholic chronic liver diseases. Gut Liver 1: 145–150.

32. Fotiadu A, Gagalis A, Akriviadis E, Kotoula V, Sinakos E, et al. (2010) Clinicopathological correlations in a series of adult patients with non-alcoholic fatty liver disease. Pathology International 60: 87–92.
33. Drozdz M, Kucharz E (1977) The effect of cytostatic drugs on collagen metabolism in guinea pigs. Arch Immunol Ther Exp (Warsz) 25: 773–778.
34. Wang Y, Gao J, Zhang D, Zhang J, Ma J, et al. (2010) New insights into the antifibrotic effects of sorafenib on hepatic stellate cells and liver fibrosis. J Hepatol 53: 132–144.
35. Deng YR, Ma HD, Tsuneyama K, Yang W, Wang YH, et al. (2013) STAT3-mediated attenuation of CCl-induced mouse liver fibrosis by the protein kinase inhibitor sorafenib. J Autoimmun.
36. Hong F, Chou H, Fiel MI, Friedman SL (2013) Antifibrotic activity of sorafenib in experimental hepatic fibrosis: refinement of inhibitory targets, dosing, and window of efficacy in vivo. Dig Dis Sci 58: 257–264.
37. Greupink R, Bakker HI, Bouma W, Reker-Smit C, Meijer DK, et al. (2006) The antiproliferative drug doxorubicin inhibits liver fibrosis in bile duct-ligated rats and can be selectively delivered to hepatic stellate cells in vivo. J Pharmacol Exp Ther 317: 514–521.
38. Mitry RR, Hughes RD, Aw MM, Terry C, Mieli-Vergani G, et al. (2003) Human hepatocyte isolation and relationship of cell viability to early graft function. Cell Transplant 12: 69–74.
39. Alexandrova K, Griesel C, Barthold M, Heuft HG, Ott M, et al. (2005) Large-scale isolation of human hepatocytes for therapeutic application. Cell Transplant 14: 845–853.
40. Gramignoli R, Tahan V, Dorko K, Skvorak KJ, Hansel MC, et al. (2013) New potential cell source for hepatocyte transplantation: discarded livers from metabolic disease liver transplants. Stem Cell Res 11: 563–573.
41. Bartlett DC, Hodson J, Bhogal RH, Youster J, Newsome PN (2014) Combined use of N-acetylcysteine and Liberase improves the viability and metabolic function of human hepatocytes isolated from human liver. Cytotherapy 16: 800–809.
42. Gramignoli R, Green ML, Tahan V, Dorko K, Skvorak KJ, et al. (2012) Development and application of purified tissue dissociation enzyme mixtures for human hepatocyte isolation. Cell Transplant 21: 1245–1260.

4

Cellular Intrinsic Mechanism Affecting the Outcome of AML Treated with Ara-C in a Syngeneic Mouse Model

Wenjun Zhao[1], Lirong Wei[1], Dongming Tan[1], Guangsong Su[1], Yanwen Zheng[1], Chao He[1], Zhengwei J. Mao[2], Timothy P. Singleton[3], Bin Yin[1,4,5]*

1 Cyrus Tang Hematology Center, Jiangsu Institute of Hematology, the First Affiliated Hospital, Soochow University, Suzhou, Jiangsu Province, PR China, **2** Division of Hematopathology, Department of Laboratory Medicine and Pathology, University of Minnesota Medical Center-Fairview, Minneapolis, Minnesota, United States of America, **3** Department of Laboratory of Medicine and Pathology, University of Minnesota, Minneapolis, Minnesota, United States of America, **4** Thrombosis and Hemostasis Key Lab of the Ministry of Health, Soochow University, Suzhou, Jiangsu Province, PR China, **5** Collaborative Innovation Center of Hematology, Soochow University, Suzhou, Jiangsu Province, PR China

Abstract

The mechanisms underlying acute myeloid leukemia (AML) treatment failure are not clear. Here, we established a mouse model of AML by syngeneic transplantation of BXH-2 derived myeloid leukemic cells and developed an efficacious Ara-C-based regimen for treatment of these mice. We proved that leukemic cell load was correlated with survival. We also demonstrated that the susceptibility of leukemia cells to Ara-C could significantly affect the survival. To examine the molecular alterations in cells with different sensitivity, genome-wide expression of the leukemic cells was profiled, revealing that overall 366 and 212 genes became upregulated or downregulated, respectively, in the resistant cells. Many of these genes are involved in the regulation of cell cycle, cellular proliferation, and apoptosis. Some of them were further validated by quantitative PCR. Interestingly, the Ara-C resistant cells retained the sensitivity to ABT-737, an inhibitor of anti-apoptosis proteins, and treatment with ABT-737 prolonged the life span of mice engrafted with resistant cells. These results suggest that leukemic load and intrinsic cellular resistance can affect the outcome of AML treated with Ara-C. Incorporation of apoptosis inhibitors, such as ABT-737, into traditional cytotoxic regimens merits consideration for the treatment of AML in a subset of patients with resistance to Ara-C. This work provided direct in vivo evidence that leukemic load and intrinsic cellular resistance can affect the outcome of AML treated with Ara-C, suggesting that incorporation of apoptosis inhibitors into traditional cytotoxic regimens merits consideration for the treatment of AML in a subset of patients with resistance to Ara-C.

Editor: Linda Bendall, University of Sydney, Australia

Funding: This study is supported by the National Key Scientific Project of China ("973 Program", No. 2011CB933501), the NSFC Project (No. 81070417), and the Priority Academic Program Development of Jiangsu Higher Education Institutions (PAPD program). The funders had no role in study design, data collection and analysis, decision to publish, or preparation of the manuscript.

Competing Interests: The authors have declared that no competing interests exist.

* Email: yinbin@hotmail.com

These authors contributed equally to this work.

Introduction

Acute myeloid leukemia (AML) is an aggressive hematologic malignancy characterized by a clonal expansion of myeloid blasts in the marrow and other sites. Despite the progresses made in AML therapy, such as hematopoietic stem cell transplantation, all-trans retinoic acid [1] and arsenic trioxide [2], the outcomes of most AML patients remain poor. In fact, the 5-year survival for patients with AML diagnosed from 2006 to 2010 was reported to be around 20% [3]. Failures in treatment of AML can be largely attributed to the refractoriness of leukemic cells to current therapies. However, the biological mechanisms underlying leukemic resistance to treatment are unclear.

Mouse models of leukemia have been attractive because of their close mimicking of human diseases in many aspects [4]. The past few years have witnessed a large amount of effort in the search for and the assessment of novel anti-leukemia treatment strategies in these mouse models. Recently, Mulloy's group evaluated standard cytosine-arabinoside (Ara-C) and doxorubicin regimens in AML xenografts using an immunodeficient mouse model, and showed that this system is useful for evaluation of novel chemotherapy in combination with standard induction treatment [5]. Because the microenvironment plays an important role in leukemic progression and response to therapy [6] and because immune cells are part of the tumor microenvironment [6], we investigated the effects of chemotherapy in immunocompetent mice and attempted to explore the mechanisms for differential drug responses.

Although enormous effort has been put into the exploration of targeted treatment of AML in the recent years, Ara-C remains one of the most effective drugs in the treatment of myeloid malignancies and demands more attentions [7,8]. It is specific to the S-phase of the cell cycle and therefore exhibits more toxicity to neoplastic cells that are in active synthesis of DNA. However, the outcomes of Ara-C-based treatment vary among patients. Genetic factors of leukemic cells have been associated with their response to treatment. MLL translocations predict poor outcome, whereas other chromosomal abnormalities such as AML1-ETO and inv(16), are associated with better prognosis [9,10]. Our earlier work demonstrated that Nf1 deficiency conferred Ara-C resistance to AML cells and that leukemic cells with loss-of-function mutation in p53 were selected for and grew out during the acquirement of resistance to Ara-C, indicating these genetic changes affected chemotherapeutic responses of leukemia [11,12]. Recently, p53 status has also been reported to significantly affect tumor response to targeted therapy [13]. Other factors contributing to the chemotherapeutic response need to be investigated.

To investigate the cellular mechanisms responsible for poor treatment response, we established a syngeneic mouse model of AML by transplanting BXH-2 derived myeloid leukemic cells to immunocompetent mice. The BXH-2 strain of mice spontaneously develops AML at a high incidence, mainly through retrovirally insertional mutagenesis arising from infection by a murine leukemia virus (MuLV) [14] Using this AML mouse model treated with an efficacious Ara-C-based regimen that we developed, we found that leukemic cell load, and the sensitivity of leukemic cells to Ara-C determined the survival. Gene expression profiling was performed to reveal the molecular changes in Ara-C resistant leukemic cells. Of interest, we demonstrated that the Ara-C resistant leukemic cells could be suppressed in vitro and in vivo by inhibition of anti-apoptosis proteins.

Materials and Methods

1. Ethics Statement

The cell line used in this study, B117, was originally established from primary AML cells developed in BXH-2 strain of mice, and published in independent studies thereafter [15]. This cell line is available upon request. All animal work was done in accordance with protocols approved by the Soochow University Institutional Animal Care and Use Committee.

2. Cell culture, drug and chemical

B117P and its derived cells were grown as described previously [15]. All culture media and supplements, except noted individually, were obtained from Invitrogen (Carlsbad, CA, USA). Ara-C was purchased from Pfizer Italia S.R.L (Neriviano, Italy). ABT-737 was obtained from Biochempartner Co. (Shanghai, China).

3. Animals

C57BL/6J and C3H/HeJ strains of mouse were obtained from Model Animal Research Center of Nanjing, and maintained in a Special Pathogen Free environment in our university animal facility. Six- to eight-week-old B6C3F1 mice generated by mating C57BL/6 and C3H/HeJ were used for leukemia transplantation and drug treatment. Moribund animals were euthanized as the end point in the survival experiments. Since this is an acute leukemia mouse model, these animals did not show obviously detectable sickness until a few hours prior to being moribund. To minimize suffering and difficulty of the mice, the husbandry conditions and health status of mice were monitored on a daily basis for any signs of sickness and maintained from fighting or tail clipping. During the late stage of the experiments, wet food was put on the floor of the cages. Moribund mice were euthanized using a CO_2 chamber. The criteria for humane euthanasia of mice involved in this study were determined by observation of signs of illness including lethargy, hunched posture, rough coat, and significant body weight loss. For collection of peripheral blood to count cells, mice were bled quickly followed by an immediate application of antibiotic analgesics.

4. Cytotoxicity assays

The MTS (3-(4,5-dimethylthiazol-2-yl)-5-(3-carboxymethoxyphenyl)-2-(4-sulfophenyl)- 2H-tetrazolium, Amresco, USA) tetrazolium assay was used to determine cytotoxic response of AML cell lines, as described before [12]. 1×10^5 cells were plated into flat-bottom 96-well plates (Corning Inc., Corning, NY, USA) in 200 μL of ASM media with various concentrations of Ara-C. After three days of incubation, 20 μL of MTS solution was added to each well and incubated at 37°C for 2 hours. The optical density at 650 nm was recorded as a reference, and subtracted from OD490 readings to eliminate nonspecific absorbance. Data from individual experiments are presented as the mean percentage of corrected OD490 of triplicate cultures ± SD.

5. Histopathology

The various mouse organ specimens were processed for histological analysis according to standard procedure [16]. Briefly, tissues were fixed in 4% paraformaldehyde, paraffin embedded, sectioned, and stained with hematoxylin and eosin. Morphological examination of leukemic cells and peripheral blood from leukemic recipient mice or normal mice used Wright-Giemsa staining method. Images were captured using an Olympus FSX100 at 20X for hematoxylin and eosin stained tissue sections, and 200X for hematoxylin and eosin or 600X for slides stained by Wright-Giemsa, respectively.

6. Flow cytometry

B117 cells and bone marrow cells flushed from mouse femurs and tibias were blocked prior to incubation with antibodies staining for Mac-1 and Gr-1 (BD Pharmingen, New Jersey, USA). To detect apoptosis, cells were stained with Annexin V-FITC apoptosis detection kit (Biouniquer, Nanjing, China) following the manufacturer's protocol. After staining, cells were washed and analyzed on a FACScan (BD Biosciences, Franklin Lakes, USA) using FlowJo software (Tree-Star Inc, Ashland, USA).

7. Measurement of B117P cell load using a specific proviral insertion tag

Genomic DNA was extracted from B117P and mouse white blood cells using the TIANamp Genomic DNA Kit (TianGen Co., China), according to the manufacturer's instructions. B117P specific proviral insertion tags were isolated using APE-PCR, as recently reported [17]. One of the tags was chosen as a molecular marker for B117P cells whose abundance can be reflected by measuring this tag using quantitative real-time polymerase chain reaction (See the following description of qPCR for details). The primers used for amplification of B117 tag were 5′ CTGAGATGAGGCGCAACAT 3′ (forward) and 5′ CCTGTGGTTCAAGTGAAGC 3′ (reverse), and β-actin gene as the internal reference 5′ GATCATTGCTCCTCCTGAGC 3′ (forward) and 5′ GACTCATCGTACTCCTGCTTG 3′ (reverse).

8. Gene expression profiling

Total RNA was extracted with TRIzol reagent according to the protocol (Molecular Research Center, Cincinnati, OH, USA), followed by DNase I treatment to eliminate potential genomic DNA contamination. Three samples of B117P and B117HS were analyzed by Super Biotek Co. Briefly, RNA was amplified and labeled using the OneArray Amino Allyl aRNA Amplification Kit

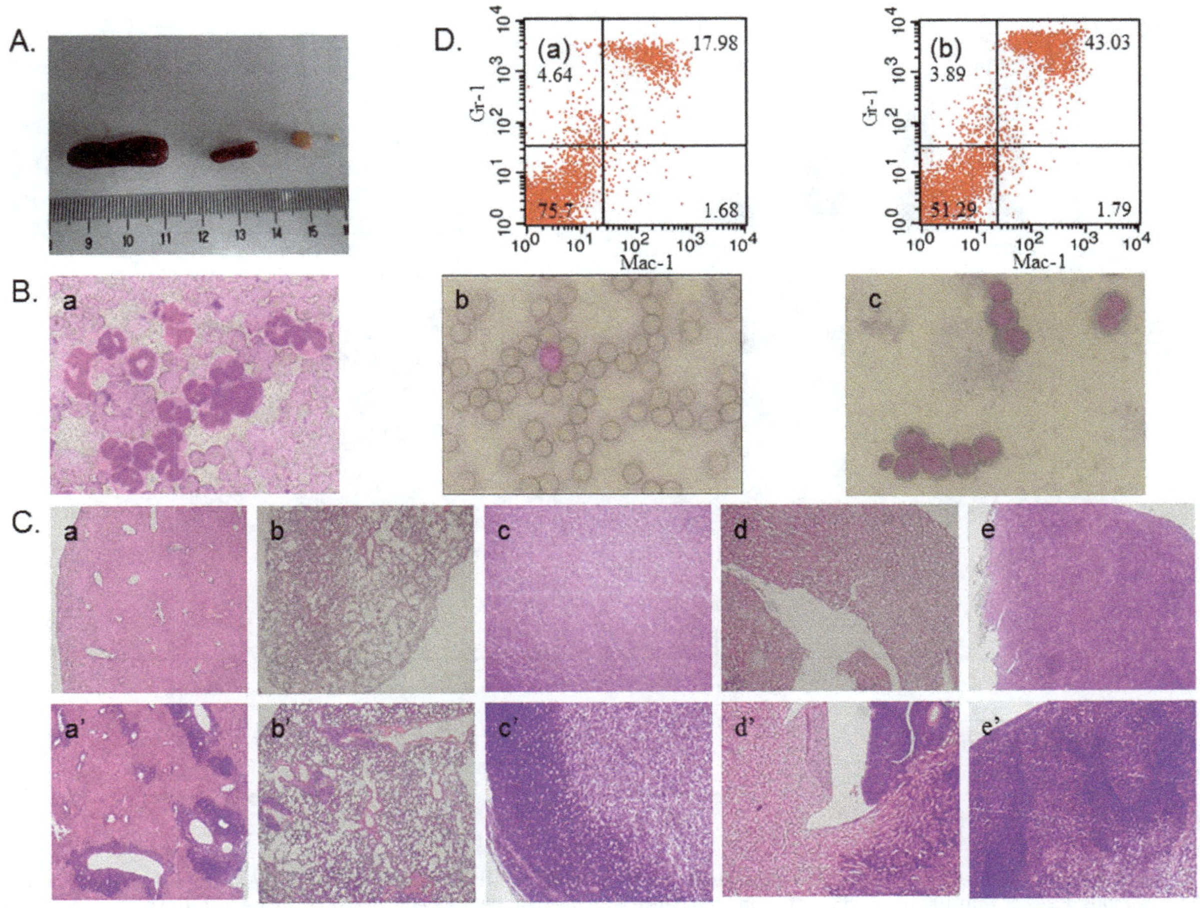

Figure 1. Establishment and characterization of an AML mouse model for evaluating treatment response by transplanting of BXH-2 derived myeloid leukemic cells into syngeneic mice (B6C3F1). Fig. 1A) Gross anatomic examination of spleen and lymph node collected from leukemic (left) or normal (right) mice. Fig. 1B) Morphological examination of peripheral blood smears from (a) recipient mice, (b) normal mice and (c) of B117 cells (Wright-Giemsa staining). Representative fields are shown here. Fig. 1C) Pathologic examination of organ sections, including liver (a & a'), lung (b & b'), lymph node (c & c'), kidney (d & d'), and spleen (e & e'), obtained from normal (a~e) versus leukemic (a'~e') mice (H & E staining). Fig. 1D) Immunophenotypic analysis of bone marrow cells recovered from normal (a) or leukemic (b) mice.

(Phalanx Biotech Group, Taiwan) and Cy5 dyes (Amersham Pharmacia, Piscataway, NJ, USA) and hybridized to Mouse Whole Genome OneArray with Phalanx hybridization buffer using Phalanx Hybridization System. Data was normalized using Rosetta Resolver System (Rosetta Biosoftware). A heat map of genes with $\log_2$ ratio ≥ 1 or $\log_2$ ratio ≤ -1 and p-value<0.05 was generated using Cluster 3.0 and TreeView and Gene set enrichment analysis was performed using ArrayTrack software (http://edkb.fda.gov/webstart/arraytrack/).

9. Quantitative real-time polymerase chain reaction (qPCR)

0.1 μg of total RNA was reverse transcribed with oligo(dT)n, using the SuperScript II First Strand cDNA Synthesis system (Invitrogen) according to the manual. qPCR was performed using SYBR Green method (Applied Biosystems, Foster city, CA, USA). Individual reaction contains diluted cDNA, 400 nM forward and reverse primers each, and 12.5 μL 2x PCR master mixes. PCR reaction was denatured at 95°C for 10 minutes, followed by 40 cycles of 95°C for 15 seconds and 60°C for 1 minute. The fold changes were calculated by the $2^{-\Delta\Delta Ct}$ method using ABI Prism 7500 SDS Software. The specific primers used for amplification of Dnmt3L were 5′ CTCTGGAAGAGCAATGGCTG 3′ (forward) and 5′ GACTTCGTACCTGATCATCTC 3′ (reverse), Plau 5′ GTGGCAGTGTACTTGGAGCT 3′ (forward) and 5′ GCATCTATCTCACAGTGCTC 3′ (reverse), CD72 5′ GAACAGCGCATCTAACCATCT 3′ (forward) and 5′ GTCGCAGTTGGTTGCTCTG 3′ (reverse), Uba7 5′ GAGTTATACTCCAGGCAGCT 3′ (forward) and 5′ CACTGAGCAGCCAAGTCAG 3′ (reverse), Pdrgl 5′ GAGTGTCTCTGAAGATGTGAT 3′ (forward) and 5′ GTTGACTCCGCAGCCTTTCT 3′ (reverse), and β-actin transcript levels for normalization 5′ CAAGCAGGAGTACGATGAGT 3′ (forward) and 5′ GCCATGCCAATGTTGTCTCT 3′ (reverse), respectively.

10. Statistical analysis

Two-tailed Student's t-tests were performed using Microsoft Excel. A p-value of <0.05 was considered statistically significant. Kaplan-Meier estimates were used to calculate survival, and log-rank was used to calculate the p-value. Survival was defined as from the day of injection of tumor cells.

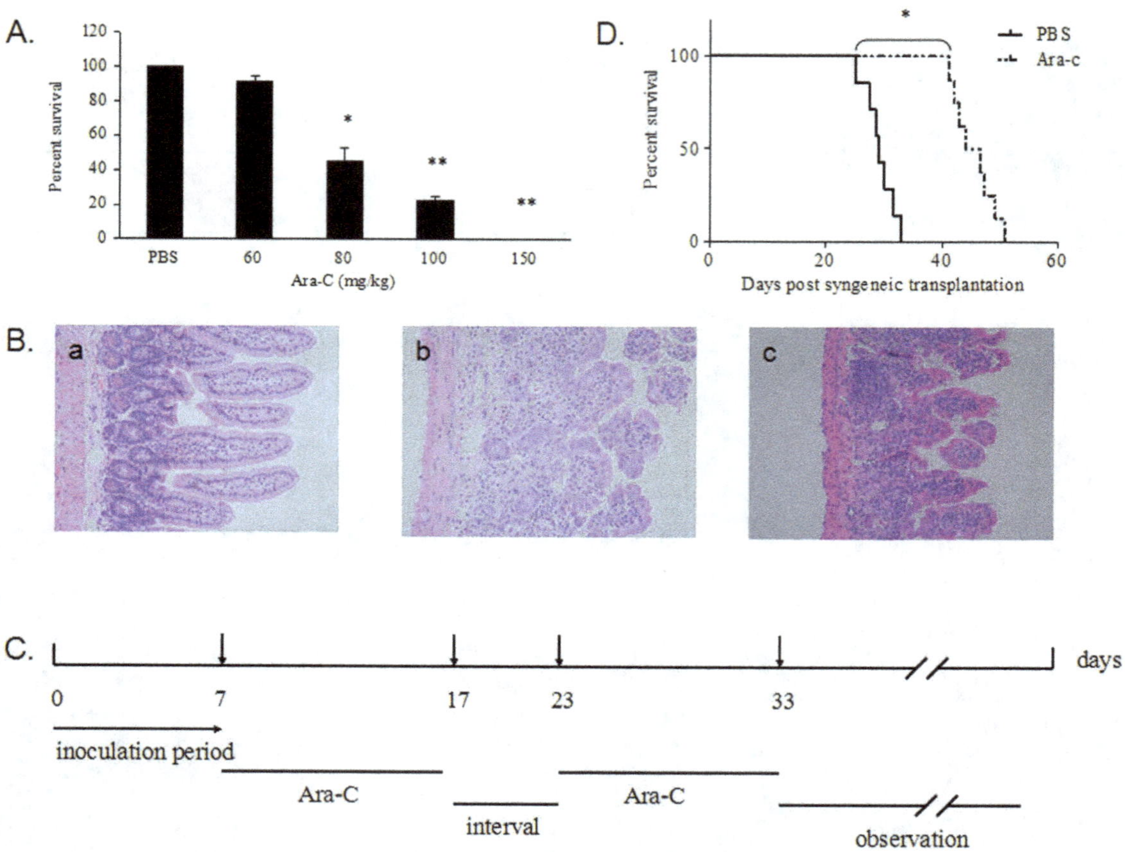

Figure 2. Development of an efficacious Ara-C-based regimen for the treatment of AML in mice. Fig. 2A) The survival rate of mice treated with Ara-C at various doses or with 100 μL of PBS control, in accordance with the treatment scheme described in the text. The mice were watched for a period of 50 days. The results shown here are representative of data obtained from 3 separate experiments. Fig. 2B) Histopathological examination of intestine affects Ara-C treatment. Fig. 2C) Treatment protocol for AML mice. The day of infusion of leukemic cells was considered as day 0. Fig. 2D) Suppression of leukemia using the treatment protocol. B6C3F1 mice transplanted with 2×10^5 B117P cells via tail vein were treated with either Ara-C (n = 12) or PBS (n = 12) as the control. *$p<0.05$.

Results

1. Establishment and characterization of a syngeneically transplanted AML mouse model for evaluation of treatment response

To establish an AML mouse model that is suitable for evaluation of chemotherapeutic response, we intravenously infused 2×10^5 B117 cells into a syngeneic B6C3F1 mouse. All recipient B6C3F1 mice (n = 12) reproducibly developed a hematologic disease resembling AML around a month following the transplantation, manifested by body weight loss, increased white blood cell counts, and being moribund. The necropsy showed enlarged spleen, lymph nodes and liver (Fig. 1A). Wright-Giemsa stained peripheral blood smears from diseased mice highlighted aggregates of heterogeneous blast cells with prominent nucleoli and nuclear indentations (Fig. 1B). Histopathological studies of liver, lung, lymph node, kidney and spleen revealed diffuse infiltration of the tissues with blast cells (Fig. 1C). Immunophenotypic staining of the bone marrow cells harvested from sick recipient mice showed an increased percentage of Mac-1^+Gr-1^+ cells (43%), compared with that for normal mice (18%) (Fig. 1D). These results indicated that an AML mouse model had been successfully created through a syngeneic transplantation of BXH-2 derived leukemia cells.

2. Development of an efficacious Ara-C based regimen for the treatment of AML in mice

One adverse effect of Ara-C treatment lies in its cause of damage to normal tissues. For the development of a protocol for Ara-C treatment of the mouse AML, it was important to determine the maximum tolerable dose (MTD) of Ara-C that could not only kill the tumor cells in vivo but also spare mice from the damage. To do so, we tested a range of doses of Ara-C on B6C3F1 mice that were intraperitoneally administered once a day for two courses of consecutive ten-day treatments with a five-day interval. We found that injection of 60 mg/kg of Ara-C gave rise to 5%~10% moribund animals which was further increased as the dose went up, till 100% reaching the end point mostly within the first course at 150 mg/kg (Fig. 2A). During the treatment, a significant body weight loss, a decrease in white blood cell counts, and frequent diarrhea were observed. Histopathological examination of intestine tissues of treated mice was indicative of a damage that became more severe with the increasing doses of Ara-C (Fig. 2B). These symptoms were consistent with the cytotoxicity of Ara-C. Therefore, the dose of 50 mg/kg of Ara-C was chosen for further studies.

Following several rounds of testings, we optimized the treatment scheme as illustrated in Fig. 2C. In order to examine its efficacy, AML mice created by intravenous infusion of 2×10^5 B117 cells were then treated with the protocol. Compared with the control

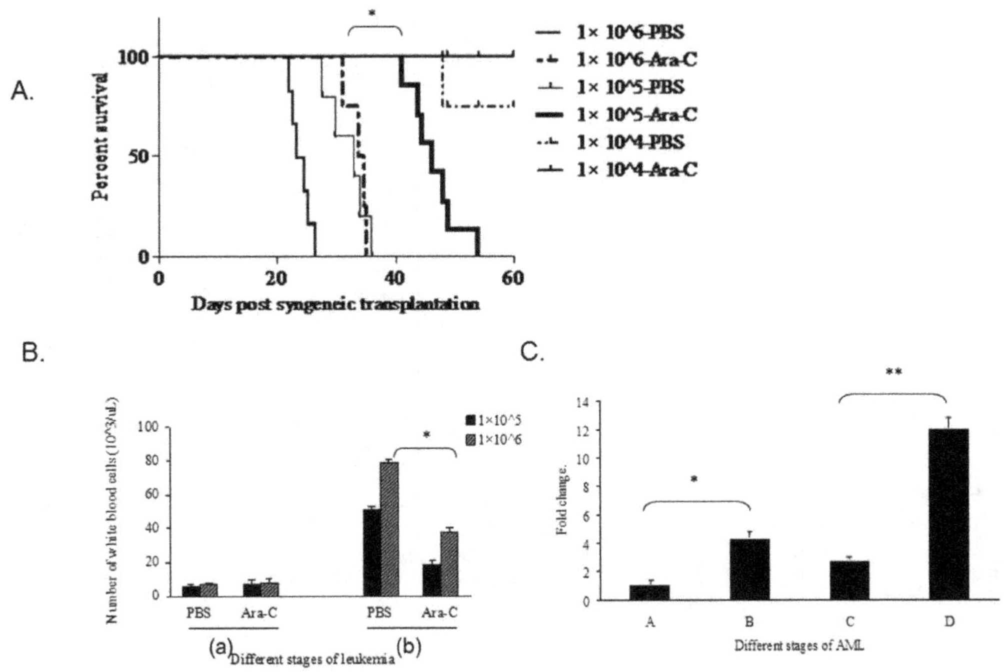

Figure 3. The effect of leukemic load on the survival of recipient mice. Fig. 3A) The survival of B6C3F1 mice receiving different dose of B117P cells and treated with either Ara-C or PBS. Each group included 12 mice. The mice were watched for 60 days. Fig. 3B) The white blood cell counts at different stages of transplanted leukemia in the mouse model. (a) before transplant, (b) after the first course of treatment. Fig. 3C) The abundance of B117 tag in the peripheral blood of recipient mice detected by q-PCR, taking β-actin as the reference, at different time points, (A) 2 days following the transplantation, (B) right before the treatment, (C) following the first course of treatment, (D) following the second course of treatment. $^*p<0.05$, $^{**}p<0.01$. The data were presented as mean +/− SD of triplicate.

(PBS) group, Ara-C treatment significantly prolonged the survival of mice for 12~14 days (Fig. 2D), suggesting that this Ara-C treatment protocol did not kill B6C3F1 mice but effectively suppressed leukemic cell growth in vivo.

3. The effect of leukemic load on the outcome of Ara-C treatment

To examine whether AML load had an impact on the treatment outcome, three different numbers of B117P cells were transplanted into B6C3F1 mice, followed by treatment either with PBS as control groups, or with Ara-C according to the above described protocol. As can be seen in Fig. 3A, infusion of 1×10^4 of B117P cells followed by Ara-C treatment did not cause moribund animal within the period of observation, whereas only 3 (25%) mice died in the PBS control group, indicative of an insufficient induction of reproducible leukemia at this cell dose. When the number of cells increased up to 1×10^5 and 1×10^6, the survival of recipient mice became shorter. Consistent with our previous observations, Ara-C treatment delayed the onset of disease, relative to the control groups. Notably, Ara-C treated mice infused with 1×10^5 B117P cells survived significantly longer than those with 1×10^6 cells, indicating that a higher level of blast cell load was associated with poor survival of Ara-C treated mice.

The recipient mice, when they became moribund, showed typical leukemic manifestations, with regard to their changed appearance and enlarged hematopoietic organs. The peripheral white blood cells of mice obtained at different stages of transplanted leukemia were counted, and the B117P tag quantified by qPCR. Following the first course of treatment, all four groups of mice displayed high counts of white blood cells, compared to normal B6C3F1 mice (Fig. 3B), consistent with moribund mice from transplanted leukemia and not from Ara-C toxicity. In PBS control groups, mice initially receiving 1×10^6 B117P cells died gradually, and had a greater increase in the numbers of white blood cells than mice injected with 1×10^5 cells which were still normal (Fig. 3C). Interestingly, Ara-C treated mice transplanted with either 1×10^5 or 1×10^6 cells had decreased cell counts in comparison with respective PBS control mice (Fig. 3B). This is consistent with our observation of the prolonged survival of Ara-C treated recipient mice, indicating, again, that this Ara-C treatment protocol could effectively reduce the number of blast cells. In addition, Ara-C treated mice infused with 1×10^6 cells exhibited an increased cell counts relative to mice receiving 1×10^5 cells (Fig. 3B). When they became sick after surviving the second course of treatment, mice showed markedly increased white blood cells (data not shown).

The abundance of B117P cells present in peripheral blood was also monitored by measuring the B117P-specific proviral insertion tag that has previously been identified by APE-PCR [17]. As shown in Fig. 3C, the B117P tag was detected as early as 2 days following the transplantation, and found to be increased later. The levels of B117P tag were decreased following the first course of Ara-C treatment, but became high again when animals were moribund after the second course of treatment. This indicated that changes of the number of B117P cells in the peripheral blood of mice followed a pattern similar to those of white blood cell counts.

The differential survival of mice receiving between 1×10^5 and 1×10^6 leukemic cells shown here suggested that leukemic load affected the survival of untreated recipient mice and the outcome of Ara-C therapy for AML.

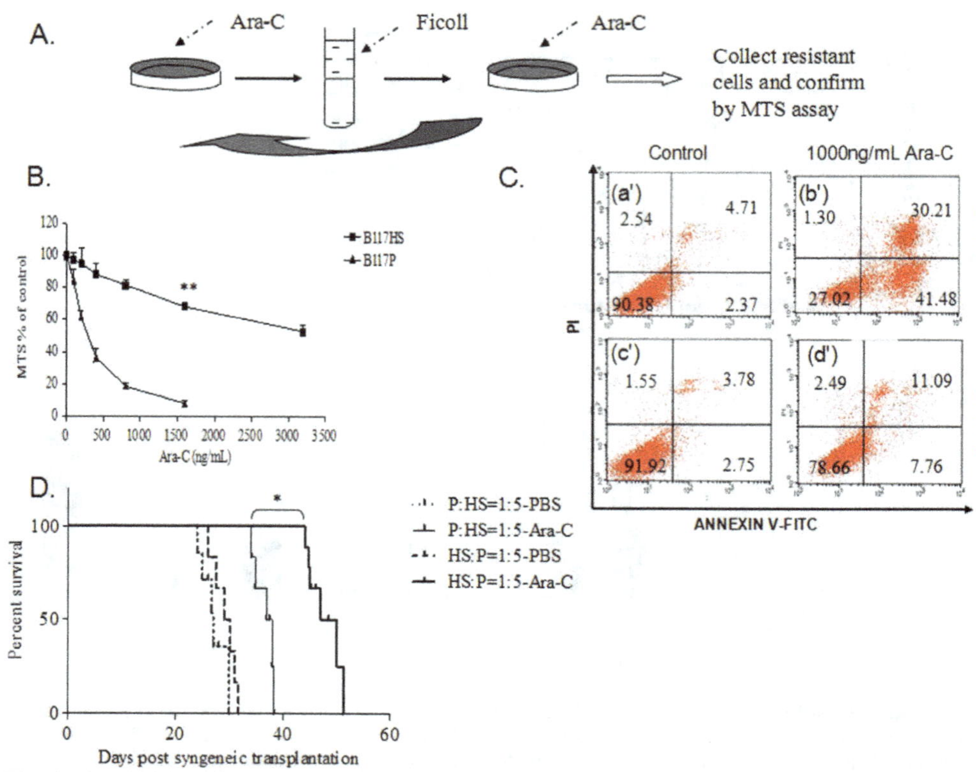

Figure 4. Sensitivity of leukemic cells to Ara-C determined the survival of treated AML mice. Fig. 4A) Selection scheme for generation of Ara-C resistant AML cells (B117HS). Fig. 4B) Comparision of B117P with B117HS in their sensitivities to Ara-C by MTS assay. **p<0.01. Fig. 4C) B117P or B117HS treated either with cell culture medium (a' and c') as control or with 1000 ng/mL Ara-C for 48 hours (b' and d') were subjected to flow cytometry analysis, according to the Methods. Fig. 4D) Survival of B6C3F1 mice transplanted with 2×10^5 leukemic cells containing different proportions of B117P and B117HS cells, followed by the treatment with Ara-C or PBS control. Each group included 12 B6C3F1 mice. *p<0.05.

4. Sensitivity of leukemia cells to Ara-C determined the survival of treated AML mice

We next asked whether the presence of drug-resistant cells in the leukemic population could impact the outcome of chemotherapy. Firstly, to generate isogenic leukemic cells with different drug sensitivity, we put B117P cells under selection against Ara-C at an initial concentration of 160 ng/mL. This concentration was chosen based on our previous observation that it could give rise to marked cytotoxicity but was no higher than the IC50 of B117P [12]. Thus, over 50% of treated cells could survive this initial treatment (data not shown). As depicted in Fig. 4A, a highly Ara-C resistant cell line, designated as B117HS, was derived from B117P by consecutive exposure to increasing concentrations of Ara-C, as described before [12]. It took about 10 weeks to produce B117HS. To verify the drug resistance of B117HS cells, we then performed MTS assay to determine their sensitivity to Ara-C. As shown in Fig. 4B, the IC50 of B117HS to Ara-C was about ten times higher than that of B117P. Flow cytometry analysis showed that treatment with 1000 ng/mL Ara-C induced apparent apoptosis of B117P and B117HS cells (Fig. 4C).

With the Ara-C resistant cells obtained, we next evaluated the effects of drug sensitivity of leukemic cells on the survival of transplanted animals. To better mimic the clinical context, we mixed B117P and B117HS at the ratio of 1:5 or 5:1, and transplanted the mixtures into B6C3F1 mice, prior to the drug treatment. All mice displayed similar signs of illness including lethargy, hunched posture, rough coat, and body weight loss, and eventually being moribund from AML. As shown in Fig. 4D, no obvious difference in the survival of mice between control groups B117P:B117HS (1:5) and B117P:B117HS (5:1) was detected. However, Kaplan-Meier analysis showed that, among Ara-C treated mice, B117P:B117HS (5:1) group survived significantly (p<0.05) longer than B117P:B117HS (1:5) group, indicating that an increased proportion of B117HS cells resulted in a poor outcome of chemotherapy. These data suggested that the existence of drug-resistant cells in leukemic population could affect the outcome of Ara-C treatment in vivo.

5. Gene expression profiling of leukemic cells sensitive or resistant to Ara-C

In order to further explore the intrinsic mechanism determining response to chemotherapy at a molecular level, a comparison of gene expression profiles between Ara-C resistant B117HS cells and their parental B117P-derived passage control cells was performed by Super Biotek using Mouse OneArray Microarray. Fluorescent aRNA targets were prepared from 1 or 2.5 μg total RNA samples using OneArray Amino Allyl aRNA Amplification Kit (Phalanx Biotech Group, Taiwan) and Cy5 dyes (Amersham Pharmacia, Piscataway, NJ, USA). Fluorescent targets were hybridized to the Mouse Whole Genome OneArray with Phalanx hybridization buffer using Phalanx Hybridization System. After 16 hrs hybridization at 50°C, non-specific binding targets were washed away by three different washing steps (Wash I 42°C 5 min; Wash II 42°C 5 min, 25°C 5 min; Wash III rinse 20 times), and the slides were dried by centrifugation and scanned by Axon 4000B scanner (Molecular Devices, Sunnyvale, CA, USA). The intensities of each probe were obtained by GenePix 4.1 software (Molecular Devices). Genechip hybridization data were collected,

Table 1. Genes upregulated or downregulated in B117HS compared with B117P.

Gene name	Super biotek probe set ID	Gene description	n-fold
Upregulated			
Thbs1	PH_mM_0014241	thrombospondin 1	99.99
CD63	PH_mM_0009050	CD63 antigen	99.99
Dnmt3L	PH_mM_0000812	DNA (cytosine-5-)-methyltransferase 3-like	70.09
Plau	mMC007080	plasminogen activator, urokinase	47.5
Tgfb3	mMC024423	transforming growth factor, beta 3	33.15
Rbpms	mMC016216	RNA binding protein gene with multiple splicing	19.03
Zmat3	mMC026312	zinc finger matrin type 3	18.95
ABCB9	mMR028795	ATP-binding cassette, sub-family B (MDR/TAP), member 9	16.46
Vopp1	mMC008041	vesicular, overexpressed in cancer, prosurvival protein 1	12.89
Gdf5	mMC004863	growth differentiation factor 5	11.9
Vegfa	PH_mM_0001624	vascular endothelial growth factor A	10.43
Kdr	PH_mM_0001297	kinase insert domain protein receptor	9.51
Stim1	PH_mM_0014218	stromal interaction molecule 1	8.05
Bcl2	mMR026887	B cell leukemia/lymphoma 2	5.26
Downregulated			
CD72	PH_mM_0008460	CD72 antigen	68.63
Psmb9	mMC008677	proteasome (prosome, macropain) subunit, beta type 9 (large multifunc- tional peptidase 2)	46.48
Parp8	mMC009866	poly (ADP-ribose) polymerase famil- y, member 8	33.08
Ripk3	PH_mM_0001581	receptor-interacting serine-threonine kinase 3	23.91
Traf3ip2	mMC006086	TRAF3 interacting protein 2	17.8
SOX4	mMR027907	SRY-box containing gene 4	16.22
Uba7	mMC023220	ubiquitin-like modifier activating enzyme 7	15.13
Pdrg1	mMC022475	p53 and DNA damage regulated 1	14.69
Cmpk2	mMC005508	cytidine monophosphate (UMP-CMP) kinase 2, mitochondrial	9.9
Lgals1	mMC003871	lectin, galactose binding, soluble 1	9.85
Ttc3	mMR026668	tetratricopeptide repeat domain 3	9.04

corrected, normalized, and statistically analyzed using programs including statistical Analysis of Microarray, GeneData Analyst, Principal Components Analysis and Cluster. As shown in Fig. 5A, a list of 578 genes with t-test ($p<0.01$) and fold-change (≥ 5.5) analysis was obtained, including 366 up-regulated and 266 down-regulated known genes in B117HS cells. Many of these genes were involved in resistance to chemotherapy or tumor formation and metastasis (Table 1). Expression changes for Dnmt3L, Plau, Bcl2, CD72, Uba7 and Pdrgl genes were confirmed by quantitative real-time PCR analysis using the ABI7500 (Fig. 5B). Our microarray study revealed extensive changes in gene expression levels of Ara-C resistant cells, and some of these may influence chemotherapy response and warrant further exploration.

6. Sensitivity of Ara-C resistant leukemic cells to an inhibitor of anti-apoptosis proteins (ABT-737)

Because of the result of gene expression profiling including up-regulated Bcl-2, we were curious whether Ara-C resistant cells were responsive to inhibition of anti-apoptotic proteins. Previous studies have shown that ABT-737, a BH3 mimetic, inhibited the pro-survival function of Bcl-2, Bcl-xL and Bcl-w, and induced apoptosis in a variety of cancer cell types [18–21]. We first examined the response of B117HS to ABT-737 in vitro. As shown in Fig. 6A, ABT-737 treated B117HS cells exhibited considerable apoptosis and/or necrosis compared to the control. To examine if B117P cells can be effectively treated by ABT-737, we performed MTS assay to measure the sensitivity of B117P to ABT-737. We found that B117P cells were sensitive to ABT-737 treatment, with an estimated IC50 of 2 μM (figure 6B(a)). Interestingly, B117HS exhibited a significantly lower IC50 compared with B117P ($p<0.05$; figure 6B(a)), indicating that B117HS became even more sensitive to ABT-737 than B117P cells. Then, we determined the sensitivity of cultured B117HS to the combined treatment with Ara-C plus ABT-737 by MTS assay, and found that combined use of 0.4 μM of ABT-737 and an escalation of concentrations of Ara-C ranging from 200 ng/mL to 3200 ng/mL significantly reduced the viability of B117HS cells relative to the treatment with Ara-C alone (Fig. 6B(b)). These data indicated that ABT-737 had a suppressive effect on Ara-C resistant cells, and encouraged us to further examine the in vivo activity of ABT-737. As we observed previously, single agent Ara-C was effective in delaying the progression of leukemia in recipient mice. Excitingly, the combined treatment with Ara-C and ABT-737 suppressed leukemia and prolonged the survival to an even greater extent than the group treated with Ara-C alone (Fig. 6C(a)). However, mice transplanted with B117P-dervied leukaemia had no significantly different survival following the treatment with ABT-737 plus Ara-C compared with Ara-C treatment alone (Fig. 6C(b)).

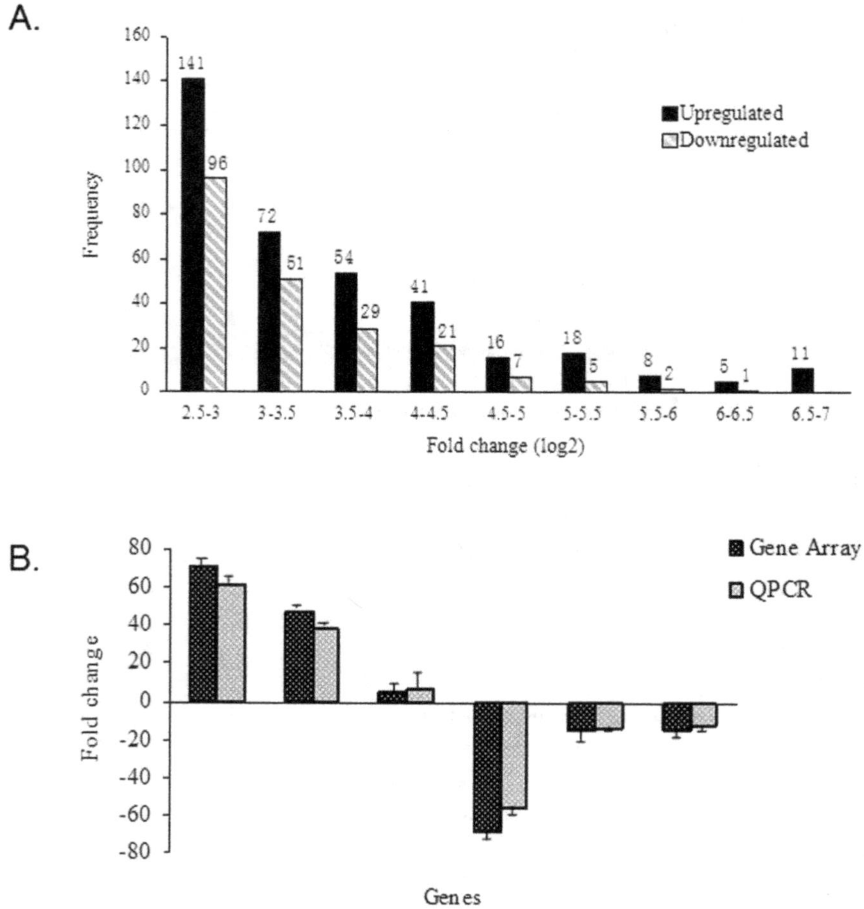

Figure 5. Gene expression profiling of leukemic cells sensitive or resistant to Ara-C. Fig. 5A) Histogram plot shows the distribution of genes with a fold change ($\log_2$) over 2.5. Fold changes were calculated by Rosetta Resolver 7.2 with error model adjusted by Amersham Pairwise Ration Builder for signal comparison of samples. Fig. 5B) Validation of the differences in expression of Dnmt3L, Plau, Bcl-2, CD72, Uba7 and Pdrg1 genes by quantitative PCR. In order to verify the direction and magnitude of the changes in gene expression induced by resistance of Ara-C in the gene microarrays, q-PCR was performed using primers to the selected genes whose expression levels were significantly altered in the array analysis.

Ara-C resistance of AML cells could be partially reversed by the treatment with ABT-737. These results suggest that inhibition of anti-apoptosis may improve the outcome of Ara-C treatment of AML with intrinsic resistance.

Discussion

The cure of AML represents a clinical challenge. Although a large body of work has focused on the responses of leukemic cells to a variety of chemotherapeutics, most patients die from relapse. In this report, we investigated the cellular factors contributing to poor prognosis. We found that leukemic cell load within a certain range and intrinsic cellular chemosensitivity are important factors determining the outcome of in vivo treatment of AML.

Targeted therapy of AML with small molecules has been intensely pursued over the past decade. The small compounds act on certain genes or their encoded products that are specifically or preferentially critical to malignant cell survival or proliferation, and can effectively kill tumor cells while having minor side effects. However, the array of molecules that have been developed so far have not proven efficacious in patients, in general [22]. On the other hand, since the standard first line of chemotherapy includes Ara-C we focused on the investigation of AML response to this classic drug.

A variety of mouse models have been developed to study the initiation, progression, and maintenance of AML including chromosome translocation-associated leukemia [23,24], and mutant gene-induced myeloid malignancy [25]. Recently, by crossing PML-RARA transgenic mice with BXH-2 mice, Kogan's group has identified a new cooperating pathway to leukemogenesis: Sox4 overexpression accelerated PML-RARα initiated acute promyelocytic leukemia with increased penetrance and reduced latency of disease [26]. Most of the AML mouse models that have been reported are xenografts of human leukemic cells. In contrast to ALL, AML xenotransplantation models are hampered by the problems of inadequate engraftment and a short life span of the animals [27]. Importantly, these systems are usually immunocompromised to facilitate successful engraftment. In this study, we developed an immunocompetent AML mouse model to complement xenotransplant models and mirror the pathology and response to chemotherapy in patients because it is known that the microenvironment can significantly affect tumor response to therapeutics. Based on this mouse model, we developed an Ara-C treatment protocol that has a minimum toxicity but this confirms that suppressed the growth of transplanted AML cells and prolonged the survival of recipient mice. In our study, we found that the two courses of 10-day consecutive treatment scheme with 50 mg/kg of Ara-C worked well.

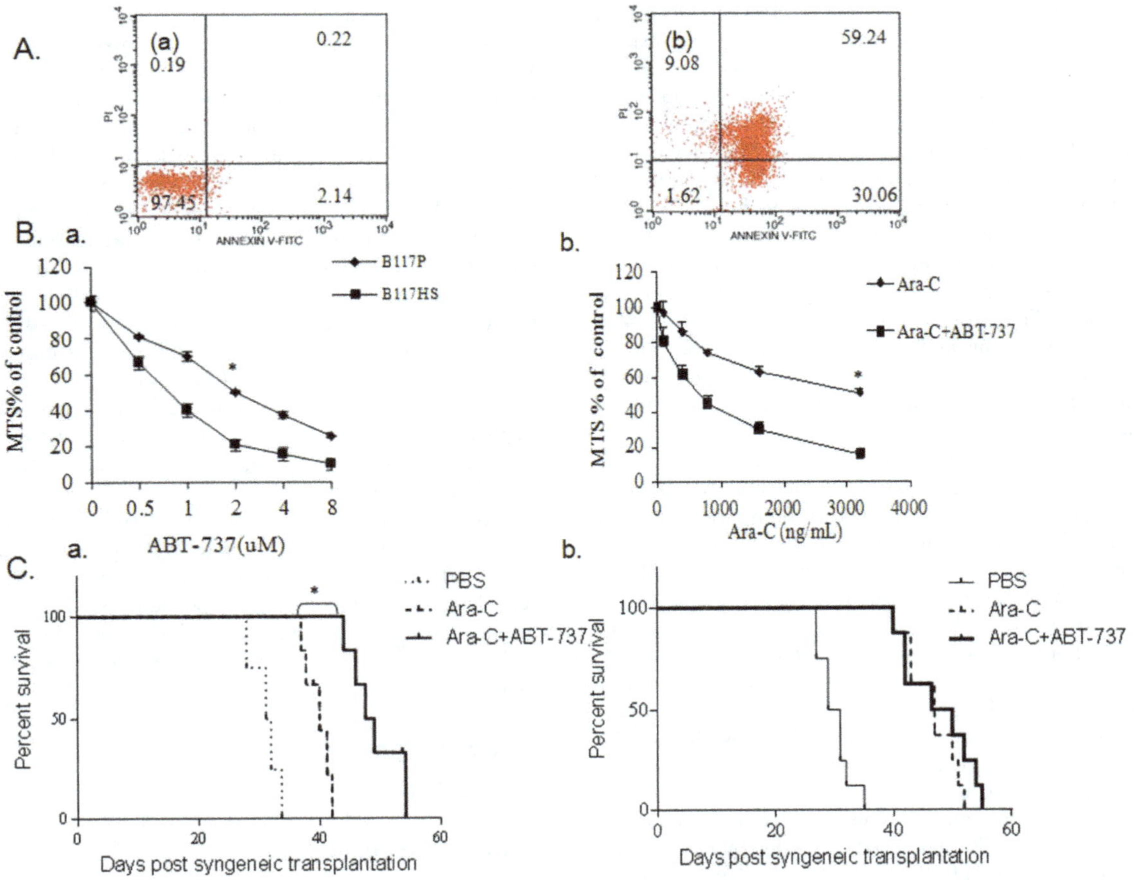

Figure 6. Sensitivity of Ara-C resistant leukemic cells to an inhibitor of anti-apoptosis proteins (ABT-737). Fig. 6A) In vitro induced apoptosis of B117HS cells by ABT-737. B117HS cells were treated with either DMEM medium as control (a) or with 2.0 μM of ABT-737 (b) for two days, followed by apoptosis analysis according to the Methods. Fig. 6B) Sensitivity of B117P and B117HS cells to ABT-737 (a). Cells were treated with 0.5 μM~8 μM of ABT-737 for three days prior to the MTS assay as described in the Methods. *$p<0.05$. Sensitivity of B117HS cells to Ara-C alone or in combination with ABT-737. (b). B117HS cells were treated with Ara-C alone or Ara-C combined with 0.4 μM of ABT-737 for three days prior to the MTS assay as described in the Methods. *$p<0.05$. Fig. 6C) Kaplan-Meier curves of recipient mice treated with Ara-C alone or in combination with ABT-737. B6C3F1 mice were infused with 2×10^5 B117HS cells (a) or B117P cells (b), followed by the treatment with PBS, Ara-C (50 mg/kg), or Ara-C (50 mg/kg) and ABT-737 (25 mg/kg), respectively. Each group contained 8 mice. *$p<0.05$.

In clinical practice, the number of leukemic blast cells is associated with the outcome of treatment. Measurement of leukemic load can be a useful tool in order to predict risk of relapse in patients [28]. Tumor load is also an important index for AML treatment by allogeneic bone marrow transplantation (BMT), and intermediate dose of Ara-C is suggested to be used to reduce leukemic load prior to allogeneic BMT [29]. In addition, it is helpful to monitor changes in tumor load following transplantation, since immunotherapy is known to be effective for low tumor burden. Some investigators have found an association between persistence of minimum residual disease and risk of relapse. Nevertheless, data from the literature remain contradictory and further correlations should be established [30]. Using a syngeneic transplantation mouse model, we showed that AML cell load of $1\times10^{5\sim6}$ were correlated with the survival of Ara-C treated recipient mice. In agreement, Mulloy observed that early treatment of transplanted AML cells before they expanded out could result in some cures, whereas mice with significant leukemic grafts were not cured using treatment by Ara-C plus doxorubicin [5]. Furthermore, Esteve et al. recently reported that patients with AML harboring a low burden of FLT3-ITD mutation and concomitant NPM1 mutation have a favorable outcome [31]. It appears that heavy leukemic load disrupts normal hematopoiesis more severely or more frequently results in leukemic infiltration of extramedullary organs which is commonly seen in patients with AML. Indeed, we noticed the marked infiltration of transplanted leukemia cells into organs, such as liver, lung, kidney, gastrointestinal tract (data not shown).

It is well established that tumor microenvironment and chronic inflammation play an important role in malignant transformation and progression [6]. Furthermore, it has been found that microenvironment can provide protection from cell death induced by treatment with chemotherapeutics or targeted small molecules for various types of tumors, including solid tumors, multiple myeloma, CLL, CML, AML as well [32–34]. Paradoxically, chemotherapy induced damage to tumor niches promote the development of tumor therapy resistance in some instances [35,36]. Therefore, to evaluate the intrinsic cellular effect on treatment outcome, it would be more appropriate to have a model with a normal microenvironment. Instead of immunodeficient mice, we have established a mouse model with syngeneic transplantation of AML. By following an optimized Ara-C treatment protocol, we demonstrated that the portion of leukemic cells ($>1\times10^5$) with intrinsic drug resistance affected the survival of treated mice. The intrinsic sensitivity of AML cells affected the outcome of AML treatment with Ara-C. This may help explain the observations that AML cells from different patients showed differential sensitivity to chemotherapy in a xenograft model [5]. Furthermore, heavy tumor load may also give rise to an increased probability of having resistant cell clones or of deriving them during chemotherapy, and influencing leukemia treatment response. Interestingly, our molecular study found extensive changes between sensitive and resistant cells in the expression levels of many genes that are involved in the regulation of several important cellular properties, such as proliferation, survival, metabolism, etc. These results reinforce the idea of intrinsic cellular mechanisms contributing to the treatment outcome of AML. Whether the differentially expressed genes are directly involved in the regulation of leukemic drug response awaits further exploration.

When they become resistant to chemotherapeutics, leukemic cells may retain or even upregulate their intrinsic anti-apoptotic mechanisms. We found that the growth of both Ara-C sensitive and resistant leukemic cells could be inhibited by a Bcl-2-specific BH3 mimetic, called ABT-737. Interestingly, resistant B117HS cells were even more effectively treated by ABT-737 than B117P cells in vitro and in vivo, which may be at least in part explained by the so-called onco-addiction hypothesis. This was a surprise to us, initially, even it was within our conceptual assumptions beforehand, because, although the onco-addiction is an interesting concept which can be translated into efficacious therapy for tumors in some cases, this concept may not equally well suit into every cases. Therefore, based on these analyses, and given the fact that the Ara-C sensitive and resistant B117 cells have similar expression levels of BCL-XL but are different for BCL-2, it seems that the Ara-C resistant B117HS cells are now reliant on BCL-2 function, and that Ara-C resistant leukemic cells with increased BCL-2 expression can become more sensitive to BCL-2 inhibition. ABT-737 has previously been demonstrated to be effective against AML and other forms of hematologic malignancies [18,19,21,37–39]. The inhibition of resistant cells by ABT-737 suggests that AML cells with intrinsic resistance to Ara-C remain sensitive to the suppression of anti-apoptotic pathway. There may be potential benefit from using this novel therapy in combination with standard induction Ara-C. In consistence, Jordan and collaborators found that BCL-2 was upregulated in leukemia stem cells enriched primary AML populations, and that BCL-2 inhibitors (ABT-263 or ABT-737) induced cell death by targeting leukemia stem cell mitochondrial energy generation and showed in vivo therapeutic effects against engrafted primary human AML cells [40]. Recently, Abbott Laboratories developed a new Bcl-2-specific BH3 mimetic, ABT-199, which was shown to be efficacious against aggressive Myc-driven murine lymphomas with significantly reduced adverse side effects [41]. Although it seems to be an improved version, whether the new Bcl-2 inhibitory compound can also have in vivo activities against AML cells, especially those with intrinsic chemoresistance, merits further investigations using animal models such as the one that we developed and described in this study.

We have described a syngeneic engraftment mouse model for AML, and showed that this immunocompetent mouse system is valuable for investigating the therapeutic response. The leukemic cell load above certain range and cellular intrinsic chemosensitivity are important factors contributing to the outcome of therapy for AML.

Acknowledgments

We would like to thank Dr. David A. Largaespada for his critical review.

Author Contributions

Conceived and designed the experiments: BY ZJM. Performed the experiments: WZ LW DT. Analyzed the data: BY ZJM GS. Contributed reagents/materials/analysis tools: BY TPS. Assisted with the experiments: YZ CH.

References

1. Ipek Y, Hulya D, Melih A (2012) Disseminated exfoliative dermatitis associated with all-transretinoic Acid in the treatment of acute promyelocytic leukemia. Case Rep Med 2012: 236174.
2. Liu P, Han ZC (2003) Treatment of acute promyelocytic leukemia and other hematologic malignancies with arsenic trioxide: review of clinical and basic studies. Int J Hematol 78: 32–39.
3. Pulte D, Gondos A, Brenner H (2010) Expected long-term survival of patients diagnosed with acute myeloblastic leukemia during 2006–2010. Ann Oncol 21: 335–341.
4. Bin Yin, Largaespada DA (2006) Models of acute myeloid leukemia: Prospects for drug development and testing. Drug Discovery Today 3: 137–142.
5. Wunderlich M, Mizukawa B, Chou FS, Sexton C, Shrestha M, et al. (2013) AML cells are differentially sensitive to chemotherapy treatment in a human xenograft model. Blood 121: e90–97.
6. Coussens LM, Zitvogel L, Palucka AK (2013) Neutralizing tumor-promoting chronic inflammation: a magic bullet? Science 339: 286–291.
7. Connelly P, Quinn BP (2011) Manufacturing decline yields drug shortages. Science 333: 156–157.
8. Kaiser J (2011) Shortages of cancer drugs put patients, trials at risk. Science 332: 523–523.
9. Coenen EA, Raimondi SC, Harbott J, Zimmermann M, Alonzo TA, et al. (2011) Prognostic significance of additional cytogenetic aberrations in 733 de novo pediatric 11q23/MLL-rearranged AML patients: results of an international study. Blood 117: 7102–7111.
10. Marcucci G, Mrozek K, Ruppert AS, Maharry K, Kolitz JE, et al. (2005) Prognostic factors and outcome of core binding factor acute myeloid leukemia patients with t(8;21) differ from those of patients with inv(16): a Cancer and Leukemia Group B study. J Clin Oncol 23: 5705–5717.
11. Yin B, Morgan K, Hasz DE, Mao Z, Largaespada DA (2006) Nfl gene inactivation in acute myeloid leukemia cells confers cytarabine resistance through MAPK and mTOR pathways. Leukemia 20: 151–154.
12. Yin B, Kogan SC, Dickins RA, Lowe SW, Largaespada DA (2006) Trp53 loss during in vitro selection contributes to acquired Ara-C resistance in acute myeloid leukemia. Experimental hematology 34: 631–641.
13. Yu JL, Rak JW, Coomber BL, Hicklin DJ, Kerbel RS (2002) Effect of p53 status on tumor response to antiangiogenic therapy. Science 295: 1526–1528.
14. Jenkins NA, Copeland NG, Taylor BA, Bedigian HG, Lee BK (1982) Ecotropic murine leukemia virus DNA content of normal and lymphomatous tissues of BXH-2 recombinant inbred mice. Journal of virology 42: 379–388.
15. Largaespada DA, Shaughnessy JD Jr, Jenkins NA, Copeland NG (1995) Retroviral integration at the Evi-2 locus in BXH-2 myeloid leukemia cell lines disrupts Nf1 expression without changes in steady-state Ras-GTP levels. Journal of virology 69: 5095–5102.
16. Konoplev S, Huang X, Drabkin HA, Koeppen H, Jones D, et al. (2009) Cytoplasmic localization of nucleophosmin in bone marrow blasts of acute myeloid leukemia patients is not completely concordant with NPM1 mutation and is not predictive of prognosis. Cancer 115: 4737–4744.
17. Xu Z, Li Y, Mao ZJ, Yin B (2013) The development of APE-PCR for the cloning of genomic insertion sites of DNA elements. Biologia 68: 766–772.
18. Del Gaizo Moore V, Schlis KD, Sallan SE, Armstrong SA, Letai A (2008) BCL-2 dependence and ABT-737 sensitivity in acute lymphoblastic leukemia. Blood 111: 2300–2309.
19. Deng J, Carlson N, Takeyama K, Dal Cin P, Shipp M, et al. (2007) BH3 profiling identifies three distinct classes of apoptotic blocks to predict response to ABT-737 and conventional chemotherapeutic agents. Cancer cell 12: 171–185.
20. Kang MH, Kang YH, Szymanska B, Wilczynska-Kalak U, Sheard MA, et al. (2007) Activity of vincristine, L-ASP, and dexamethasone against acute lymphoblastic leukemia is enhanced by the BH3-mimetic ABT-737 in vitro and in vivo. Blood 110: 2057–2066.
21. High LM, Szymanska B, Wilczynska-Kalak U, Barber N, O'Brien R, et al. (2010) The Bcl-2 homology domain 3 mimetic ABT-737 targets the apoptotic machinery in acute lymphoblastic leukemia resulting in synergistic in vitro and in vivo interactions with established drugs. Molecular pharmacology 77: 483–494.
22. Gillies RJ, Verduzco D, Gatenby RA (2012) Evolutionary dynamics of carcinogenesis and why targeted therapy does not work. Nature reviews 12: 487–493.
23. Barabe F, Kennedy JA, Hope KJ, Dick JE (2007) Modeling the initiation and progression of human acute leukemia in mice. Science 316: 600–604.

24. Kumar AR, Sarver AL, Wu B, Kersey JH (2010) Meis1 maintains stemness signature in MLL-AF9 leukemia. Blood 115: 3642–3643.
25. Nardi V, Naveiras O, Azam M, Daley GQ (2009) ICSBP-mediated immune protection against BCR-ABL-induced leukemia requires the CCL6 and CCL9 chemokines. Blood 113: 3813–3820.
26. Omidvar N, Maunakea ML, Jones L, Sevcikova S, Yin B, et al. (2013) PML-RARalpha co-operates with Sox4 in acute myeloid leukemia development in mice. Haematologica 98: 424–427.
27. Malaise M, Neumeier M, Botteron C, Dohner K, Reinhardt D, et al. (2011) Stable and reproducible engraftment of primary adult and pediatric acute myeloid leukemia in NSG mice. Leukemia 25: 1635–1639.
28. Zhu H-H, Zhang X-H, Qin Y-Z, Liu D-H, Jiang H, et al. (2013) MRD-directed risk stratification treatment may improve outcomes of t (8; 21) AML in the first complete remission: results from the AML05 multicenter trial. Blood 121: 4056–4062.
29. Beran M (2000) Intensive chemotherapy for patients with high-risk myelodysplastic syndrome. Int J Hematol 72: 139–150.
30. Perez-Simon JA, Caballero D, Diez-Campelo M, Lopez-Perez R, Mateos G, et al. (2002) Chimerism and minimal residual disease monitoring after reduced intensity conditioning (RIC) allogeneic transplantation. Leukemia 16: 1423–1431.
31. Pratcorona M, Brunet S, Nomdedeu J, Ribera JM, Tormo M, et al. (2013) Favorable outcome of patients with acute myeloid leukemia harboring a low-allelic burden FLT3-ITD mutation and concomitant NPM1 mutation: relevance to post-remission therapy. Blood 121: 2734–2738.
32. Zhang B, Li M, McDonald T, Holyoake TL, Moon RT, et al. (2013) Microenvironmental protection of CML stem and progenitor cells from tyrosine kinase inhibitors through N-cadherin and Wnt-beta-catenin signaling. Blood 121: 1824–1838.
33. Straussman R, Morikawa T, Shee K, Barzily-Rokni M, Qian ZR, et al. (2012) Tumour micro-environment elicits innate resistance to RAF inhibitors through HGF secretion. Nature 487: 500–504.
34. Uy GL, Rettig MP, Motabi IH, McFarland K, Trinkaus KM, et al. (2012) A phase 1/2 study of chemosensitization with the CXCR4 antagonist plerixafor in relapsed or refractory acute myeloid leukemia. Blood 119: 3917–3924.
35. Sun Y, Campisi J, Higano C, Beer TM, Porter P, et al. (2012) Treatment-induced damage to the tumor microenvironment promotes prostate cancer therapy resistance through WNT16B. Nature medicine 18: 1359–1368.
36. Kessenbrock K, Plaks V, Werb Z (2010) Matrix metalloproteinases: regulators of the tumor microenvironment. Cell 141: 52–67.
37. Oltersdorf T, Elmore SW, Shoemaker AR, Armstrong RC, Augeri DJ, et al. (2005) An inhibitor of Bcl-2 family proteins induces regression of solid tumours. Nature 435: 677–681.
38. Szymanska B, Wilczynska-Kalak U, Kang MH, Liem NL, Carol H, et al. (2012) Pharmacokinetic modeling of an induction regimen for in vivo combined testing of novel drugs against pediatric acute lymphoblastic leukemia xenografts. PloS one 7: e33894.
39. Beurlet S, Omidvar N, Gorombei P, Krief P, Le Pogam C, et al. (2013) BCL-2 inhibition with ABT-737 prolongs survival in an NRAS/BCL-2 mouse model of AML by targeting primitive LSK and progenitor cells. Blood 122: 2864–2876.
40. Lagadinou ED, Sach A, Callahan K, Rossi RM, Neering SJ, et al. (2013) BCL-2 inhibition targets oxidative phosphorylation and selectively eradicates quiescent human leukemia stem cells. Cell stem cell 12: 329–341.
41. Vandenberg CJ, Cory S (2013) ABT-199, a new Bcl-2-specific BH3 mimetic, has in vivo efficacy against aggressive Myc-driven mouse lymphomas without provoking thrombocytopenia. Blood 121: 2285–2288.

5

Long Term Effectiveness on Prescribing of Two Multifaceted Educational Interventions: Results of Two Large Scale Randomized Cluster Trials

Nicola Magrini[1]*, Giulio Formoso[1], Oreste Capelli[2], Emilio Maestri[1], Francesco Nonino[1], Barbara Paltrinieri[1], Cinzia Del Giovane[3], Claudio Voci[1], Lucia Magnano[1], Lisa Daya[2], Anna Maria Marata[1], on behalf of the INDRA-NET study group¶

1 Drug Evaluation Area, Emilia-Romagna Regional Agency for Health and Social Care, Bologna, Italy, **2** Local Health Authority, Modena, Italy, **3** Department of Clinical and Diagnostic Medicine and Public Health, University of Modena and Reggio Emilia, Modena, Italy

Abstract

Introduction: Information on benefits and risks of drugs is a key element affecting doctors' prescribing decisions. Outreach visits promoting independent information have proved moderately effective in changing prescribing behaviours.

Objectives: Testing the short and long-term effectiveness on general practitioners' prescribing of small groups meetings led by pharmacists.

Methods: Two cluster open randomised controlled trials (RCTs) were carried out in a large scale NHS setting. Ad hoc prepared evidence based material were used considering a therapeutic area approach - TEA, with information materials on osteoporosis or prostatic hyperplasia - and a single drug oriented approach - SIDRO, with information materials on me-too drugs of 2 different classes: barnidipine or prulifloxacin. In each study, all 115 Primary Care Groups in a Northern Italy area (2.2 million inhabitants, 1737 general practitioners) were randomised to educational small groups meetings, in which available evidence was provided together with drug utilization data and clinical scenarios. Main outcomes were changes in the six-months prescription of targeted drugs. Longer term results (24 and 48 months) were also evaluated.

Results: In the TEA trial, one of the four primary outcomes showed a reduction (prescription of alfuzosin compared to tamsulosin and terazosin in benign prostatic hyperplasia: prescribing ratio −8.5%, p = 0.03). Another primary outcome (prescription of risedronate) showed a reduction at 24 and 48 months (−7.6%, p = 0.02; and −9,8%, p = 0.03), but not at six months (−5.1%, p = 0.36). In the SIDRO trial both primary outcomes showed a statistically significant reduction (prescription of barnidipine −9.8%, p = 0.02; prescription of prulifloxacin −11.1%, p = 0.04), which persisted or increased over time.

Interpretation: These two cluster RCTs showed the large scale feasibility of a complex educational program in a NHS setting, and its potentially relevant long-term impact on prescribing habits, in particular when focusing on a single drug. National Health systems should invest in independent drug information programs.

Trial Registration: Controlled-Trials.com ISRCTN05866587

Editor: Barbara Mintzes, University of British Columbia, Canada

Funding: Funding was provided by Agenzia Italiana del Farmaco, 2005 NHS fund for independent research on drugs. The funder had no role in study design, data collection and analysis, decision to publish, or preparation of the manuscript.

Competing Interests: The authors have read the journal's policy and have the following conflicts: Since 2001, the Authors have been involved in the implementation of a pharmacist outreach visit programs in a few Health Districts of Emilia-Romagna, receiving organizational support and NHS funding from the corresponding Local Health Authorities.

* Email: nmagrini@regione.emilia-romagna.it

¶ Membership of the INDRA-NET study group is provided in the Acknowledgments

Introduction

Information on benefits and risks of drug treatments is an important element affecting doctors' prescribing decisions though other factors such as clinical experience and therapeutic traditions, opinion leaders and local context influence, and also information coming from drug industry, play a role. Drug companies invest large sums in informing doctors through a wide range of activities: [1] promotion through drug representatives, sponsored events and symposia, and selective presentation of research findings,[2–5] which seem useful to the purpose of increasing sales, as companies spend on average a quarter of their revenues on marketing activities, almost twice as much as what they invest on research and development.[6–7].

As an international independent expert in drug policy expressed a few years ago "*a major challenge that remains is to reduce the imbalance between promotional and research expenditure, perhaps moving progressively towards a system in which health systems themselves provide the bulk of new drug information rather than indirectly funding, as they presently do, an army of company salesmen*". [8] Access to the best available information (critically appraised, made easy and brought into small groups) is an important step towards a more balanced view of the actual benefits and risks of drugs allowing a more realistic estimation of the magnitude of the clinically relevant outcomes. Educational outreach visits have been proposed since 1983 as an effective method to promote change in prescribing practices, [9] using either one-to-one meetings with prescribers [10] or group meetings. [11] These methods have been subsequently implemented in various countries, [12] either to provide information from research papers and systematic reviews, free of recommendations, or to favour the use of clinical practice guidelines. Though information is mostly presented in relative terms (RR, OR, HR) there is an increasing tendency of the evidence-based movement towards favouring a presentation of trials results using actual benefits and absolute differences, possibly taking patients baseline risk into account.[13–14] The GRADE approach represents a good example in this regard. [15].

Available evidence on the effectiveness of outreach visits shows variable results, indicating modest to moderate effects (with relatively short-term assessments at 6–12 months), mostly assessing the implementation of clinical practice guidelines. [16–17] There is paucity of evidence formally evaluating the feasibility on a large scale basis of implementing independent information programs, and their long-term prescribing impact – up to several years. Moreover, although specific methods to put these principles into practice have been well conceptualized since about thirty years ago, [10] they have been often applied to academic detailing settings or to single-doctor meetings.

We applied these general principles and methods to a NHS drug information program consisting of twice-a-year small group sessions led by a pharmacist, established in several provinces of the Emilia-Romagna region since 2001. We avoided clinical practice guidelines as supporting material to drive behaviour-change since they were frequently perceived as cost-containment tools. [18].

Two pragmatic cluster randomised trials designed within the same protocol were designed and funded within a public research program.[19–20] Specific aims were to evaluate, in the short and long term, whether an intervention carried out in a natural' NHS setting, consisting of small group meetings of all general practitioners (the clusters), using clear and appealing educational materials, may change doctors' prescribing behaviour. The two trials tested two different approaches: either relatively articulated and rich materials targeting a whole therapeutic area, or more focused materials targeting a newly approved single drug with rapidly increasing prescribing patterns.

Methods

Two consecutive cluster trials, stemming from the same study protocol, were carried out in spring 2007 and autumn-winter 2007–08, respectively, in five Provinces of the Emilia Romagna region (Bologna, Forlì, Modena, Parma and Reggio Emilia, totalling about 2,200,000 inhabitants) involving all practising NHS General Practitioners. [21].

It was initially planned to have also the participation of 40 primary care groups from another region in Northern Italy, Friuli Venezia Giulia (about 400 GPs corresponding to an assisted population of about 440,000 inhabitants), but no agreement was reached between the Regional Health Authority and general practitioners' organisations. For similar reasons, a parallel trial which had been planned in Sardinia was not implemented; such trial aimed to evaluate the effectiveness of different information formats delivered to single general practitioners and discussed by a pharmacist.

In order to evaluate and quantify the impact of such a program, we designed these randomised trials according to the following features:

- improving access to evidence-based clinically relevant information in a NHS setting using available resources;
- helping to assess the relevance and the limits of the available evidence, highlighting the role of systematic reviews and pitfalls due to publication bias, and also critically appraising the most relevant single studies;
- presenting benefit and risks clearly and effectively, [14] to provide better insight on their impact on clinical practice compared to market-driven interpretations from the drug industry; [22]
- integrating information from published studies with assessments from drug regulatory agencies [23] and other relevant contextual information;
- keeping in mind all the organisational factors and settings of what works in changing doctors' behaviour: audit and feedback using prescribing data; [24] strengthening the role of pharmacists as facilitators; [16] favouring active learning in small groups. [12]

We identified doctors' knowledge and attitudes as the main determinants of their prescription; therefore, we used the available resources to address these determinants through a dedicated information program. Specifically, the main principle embraced for our information campaign was the motto "doctor, we give you all the information, you decide".

Primary Care Groups (PCGs) are associations of about 10–15 general practitioners (GPs) constituted to improve the continuity and local provision of primary health care: PCGs were the unit of randomisation in the two cluster trials. All PCGs of the five provinces were asked to participate in two rounds of small group interactive information meetings (one in spring and one in autumn 2007). Within each round of visits, PCGs were randomised in two groups: those receiving information about a topic (A) and those receiving information about a different topic (B), unrelated to (A) (Fig. 1). Groups were compared using for each topic a set of specific prescribing outcomes: group receiving A compared to group "not receiving A" (actually receiving B) and vice versa, so two sets of comparisons were performed in each trial. Each group also received the presentation and discussion of 2 clinical scenarios for each topic and prescribing data concerning the group prescription vs the average prescription in the Local Health Authority (LHA). Feedback on individual prescriptions was avoided to favour a group evaluation rather than flattening the discussion on "who has prescribed what".

The two RCTs had the following distinctive features:

- the 1st RCT (ThErapeutic Area approach or TEA trial), randomised the PCGs in two groups receiving an educational session on a therapeutic topic (treatment of benign prostatic hyperplasia (BPH) or drugs used in the treatment of osteoporosis) using a fairly long information package of 12

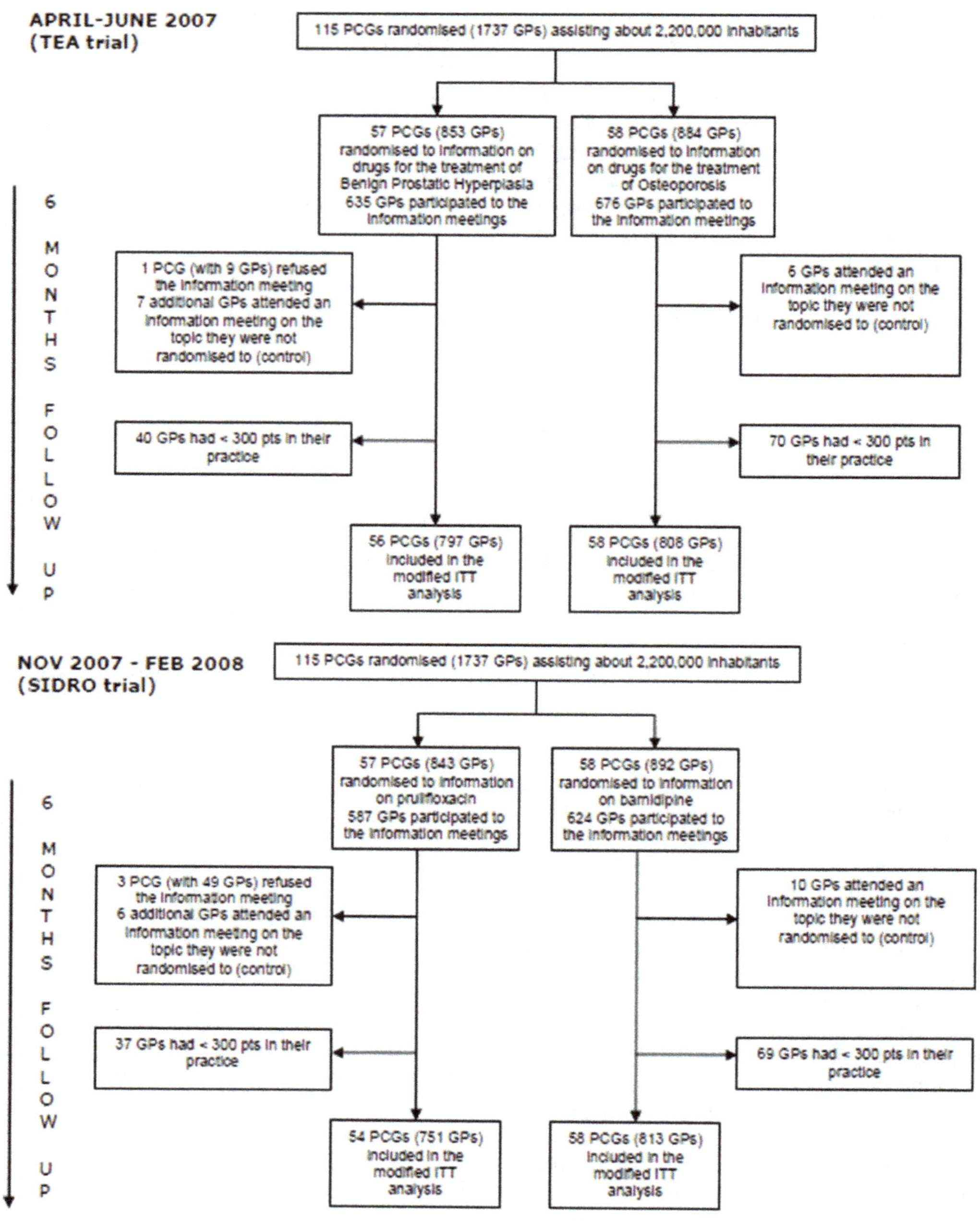

Figure 1. Flow-charts of the two cluster RCTs.

Table 1. The main components of the multifaceted educational intervention.

SETTING	bi-annual small group meetings (each lasting 3-4 hours) with a Primary Care Group (PCG)
TOOLS	ad hoc prepared information packages (pharmacists/referent GPs receive one three-day/half a day courses on the contents of that material); presentation and discussion of real life clinical scenarios; prescribing reports for each PCG comparing with local averages
METHODS	educational outreach visits (small group meetings); audit & feedback; problem-based learning: "we present to you the available evidence and some context, you decide"
ACTORS	a pharmacist acts as facilitator, presenting the evidence-based information packages and commenting on drug utilization data of PCG; a general practitioner acts as referent peer presenting real life clinical scenarios to be discussed in the light of available evidence

Table 2. TEA trial: GPs' mean baseline prescription (in the 3 months preceding the outreach visit) of drugs considered in the primary outcomes, expressed as DDD per 1000 patients.

Drugs considered	Group 1: information on drugs for the treatment of benign prostatic hyperplasia	Group 2: information on drugs for the treatment of osteoporosis
finasteride	5.35	5.46
dutasteride	4.09	4.30
alfuzosin	9.98	9.66
terazosin	4.64	4.73
tamsulosin	11.05	11.11
alendronate	7.35	7.29
risedronate	3.01	2.98

pages on benefits and risks of drugs, highlighting lack of superiority data of newer vs older (originator) drugs, availability of different drug classes and of generic drugs;

- the 2nd RCT (SIngle DRug Oriented – SIDRO trial, meaning cider in Italian), compared the same two groups of PCG, in a meeting occurring 3–4 months later, using more focused information material (4 pages information package) on a single

Table 3. TEA trial: differences in DDD per 1000 patients of prescribed drugs (intervention vs control: 1605 included GPs).

	Absolute mean prescription during follow-up in the 'intervention group' (DDD per 1000 assisted population/day)	Absolute difference at follow-up vs control group (change from baseline expressed as DDD per 1000 assisted population/day)	Relative % variation vs control: m-ITT (95% CI)
Primary outcomes (arm 1: BPH)			
finasteride+dutasteride	6.61	0.24	3.6% (−2.9 to 10.2%)
alfuzosin vs tamsulosin +terazosin †	0.71 (ratio)	−0.06	−8.5% (−16.9 to −0.7%)
Secondary outcomes (arm 1: BPH)			
finasteride	3.60	0.05	1.4% (−6.5 to 9.5%)
dutasteride	3.00	0.18	5.8% (−2.6 to 14.3%)
alfuzosin	6.82	−0.11	−1.7% (−8.9 to 5.6%)
tamsulosin	7.92	0.28	3.7% (−3.1 to 10.4%)
terazosin	3.21	0.17	5.4% (−4.1 to 14.6%)
Primary outcomes (arm 2: osteoporosis)			
alendronate	4.99	<0.01	0.1% (−7.3 to 7.5%)
risedronate	2.03	−0.11	−5.1% (−15.3 to 5.6%)
Secondary outcomes (arm 2: osteoporosis)			
ibandronate	0.48	−0.11	−19.6% (−33.9 to −5.4%)
alendronate vs risedronate + ibandronate §	2.89 (ratio)	0.27	10.4% (−3.5 to 24.6%)
strontium ranelate	0.59	0.03	4.8% (−12.9 to 21.0%)
raloxifene	0.13	<0.01	0.4% (−26.9 to 27.5%)
calcium	1.83	−0.11	−5.4% (−15.6 to 5.4%)
vitamin D	1.72	−0.06	−3.5% (−12.4 to 5.3%)

†56 physicians who had not prescribed tamsulosin or terazosin could not be included in the calculation since this is a ratio.
§300 physicians who had not prescribed risedronate or ibandronate could not be included in the calculation since this is a ratio.

"me too" drug recently approved and with rapidly increasing prescriptions: a calcium antagonist (barnidipine) or a fluoroquinolone (prulifloxacin) were the drugs chosen.

In fact these two RCTs offer two different models of approaching doctors' education: the first approach is disease oriented and closer to thematic courses, requires two ad-hoc trained professionals such as a pharmacist and a physician and tends to provide multiple key messages, often not straightforward for some of the various outcomes considered. The second one is closer to an anti-marketing strategy targeting a single drug, with a pharmacist as the main actor or facilitator of an easy-to-use evidence synthesis, and has more clear-cut outcomes based on prescribing difference of a single drug.

Though the main objective was to estimate the impact of such intervention on the prescribing profile of the various drugs, these two consecutive trials were also designed to allow us to consider differences (in terms of feasibility, acceptability and magnitude of effect) between the two approaches: either a more articulated and "therapeutic area" oriented approach, or a more focused "single drug" approach. They are jointly described in this paper to discuss and contrast these two different approaches, implemented using the same methodology.

The four information packages (the 2007 issues available at http://assr.regione.emilia-romagna.it/it/servizi/pubblicazioni/collane-cessate/archivio-pacchetti/intro) were developed in a clear, simple and appealing format, first reviewing the available evidence, then critically appraising the most relevant or largest among available studies, providing information on absolute benefits and harms of the chosen drugs and some contextual information (e.g. prescribing data and regulatory issues). [22] The idea was to "just present information", without recommending which of the addressed drugs should be prescribed. In particular, during the outreach visits, available evidence on targeted drugs was presented, highlighting the difference between a statistically significant effect on outcomes of questionable clinical relevance, and their meaning expressed in absolute terms (NNT/NNH, absolute reduction in risks, etc).

The small group meetings were organised by the Departments of Primary Care within each LHA and were part of a continuing medical education program (providing CME credits). They were led by a trained pharmacist, supported by a "referent" GP delegate by his/her PCG who had the main role to stimulate the "inter pares" discussion using *ad-hoc* clinical scenarios and a problem-based approach. Table 1 synthesizes the main components of the multifaceted intervention.

Approximately one pharmacist per 5–10 PCGs (80–150 GPs) was trained through one four-day intensive course (36 hours) on EBM methodology, a three-day course (about 20–22 hours) for each topic in TEA trial (osteoporosis and BPH) and 1 day course for each single drug in SIDRO trial. One GP for each PCG (referent) received a half-day training module on each topic their practice group had been randomised to. Pharmacists were assigned to each PCGs before randomization.

Stratified randomisation was carried out within each Local Health Authority (LHA), using the number of assisted population per PCG (under or over the mean for that LHA) as stratifying factor. Computer generated random numbers were used to assign PCGs to either group, in order to get the minimum possible difference between groups in terms of number of assisted population per PCG.

Outcomes

Main outcomes were referred to differences in NHS prescription of drugs under scrutiny (expressed as DDD per thousand patients) during the six months after the educational intervention, with a parallel comparison of individual doctors who had received the specific information topic versus those who received the other one, adjusted for the cluster effect. Baseline imbalances were taken into account calculating the change from baseline in the prescribing rate. Secondary analyses with 12, 24 and 48 months of follow-up were also performed, to assess the persistence of effects in absence of reminders.

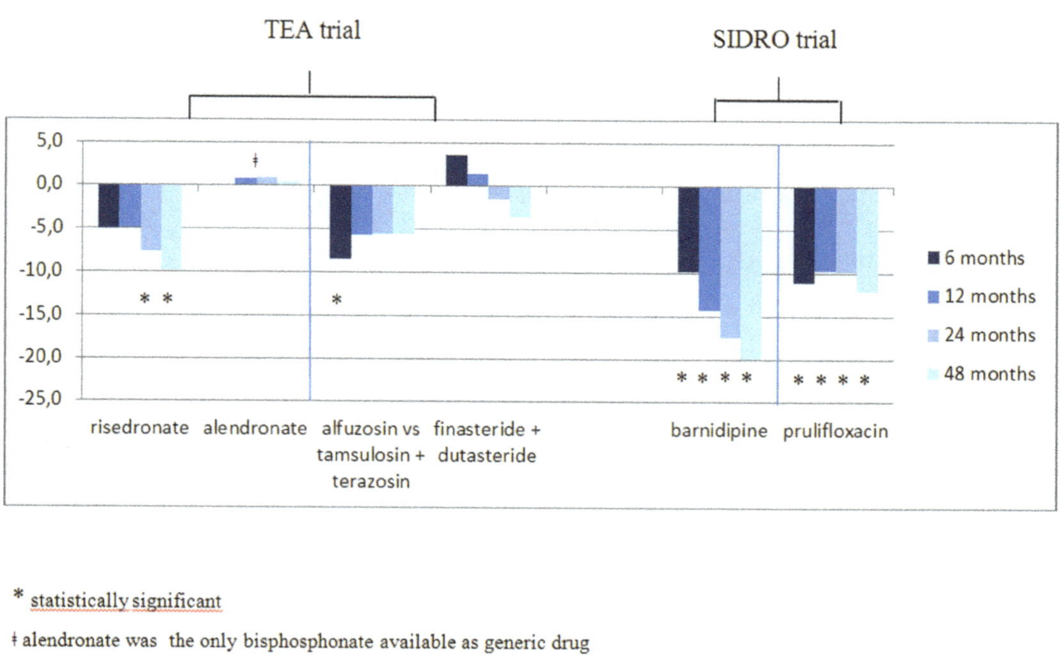

Figure 2. % differences in primary outcomes at 6 months (main analysis), 12, 24 and 48 months.

Table 4. SIDRO trial: GPs' mean baseline prescription (in the 3 months preceding the outreach visit) of considered drugs, expressed as DDD per 1000 patients.

Drugs considered:	Group 1: information on prulifloxacin	Group 2: information on barnidipine
prulifloxacin	0.19	0.18
barnidipine	1.07	1.06

Specifically, the TEA trial had four primary outcomes and 11 secondary outcomes (see results section). Some outcomes were designed to evaluate a shift toward off-patent drugs (such as tamsulosin and terazosin for BPH or alendronate for osteoporosis) which were also those with more robust evidence. In general, a prescribing reduction was expected since evidence-based data show that prescription of drugs in those therapeutic areas may be excessive.

In the SIDRO trial a reduction was expected for both the 2 two main outcomes (one for each arm), representing the prescription of me-too drugs.

All data were collected through a regional routine data collection system, containing information (including date of prescription) about all prescriptions written by each doctor to residents of Emilia-Romagna.

In addition to prescribing outcomes, a questionnaire exploring doctors' knowledge on the addressed topics and attitudes on the information materials was distributed before and after the information meetings. Questionnaires assessing knowledge were specifically designed for each topic and were nominal' (for receiving CME credits), whereas those assessing attitudes were anonymous for a more unbiased evaluation of opinions on completeness, balance and usefulness of the information.

Statistical considerations

From a sample of 40 clusters (about 600 general practitioners) and using a dedicated software (Cluster Randomisation Sample Size Calculator version 1.0.2, Health Services Research Unit, Aberdeen University) we estimated the intracluster correlation coefficients (ICC) and the sample size that would have been required to see a difference of 10–15% in the prescription of the specific drugs, assuming an average cluster (PCG) size of 15. [25].

With the recruitment of 115 PCGs, and using correction for multiplicity considering primary outcomes of both trials, we had 80% power to detect a 9–15% difference for the various drugs considered.

Doctors' prescriptions were analysed according to the randomisation scheme, independently of their participation in the outreach visits. A few exceptions leading to a modified intention-to-treat analysis (m-ITT) are described below. In particular, the following were excluded from the main analyses:

- general practitioners with fewer than 300 patients; these could have abnormal rates in the prescription of specific drugs if people using these drugs were over-represented among their patients, distorting the trial results; moreover, their practice populations may rapidly grow over time, since they are usually young doctors beginning their activity (in fact no prescribing reports are produced for these GPs since they would not be reliable);
- general practitioners who participated in a different information meeting (different topic) from the assigned one because they had moved to a different PCG after randomization. Since these cases occurred mostly for administrative reasons (rearranging of PCGs at LHA level) rather than through doctors' choice, we judged that this specific modification to the ITT would not limit generalizability, whereas keeping those doctors in the original randomization scheme even if receiving a different topic could have led to biased results;
- one PCG refused its consent to participate.

Generalised linear models (random effects models) were used to correct primary outcomes for baseline imbalances in the prescription of targeted drugs.

STATA version 11 was used for data analysis.

Ethics approval

The two RCTs have been approved by each of the Ethics Committees of the Local Health Authorities (Parma, Reggio Emilia, Modena, Bologna, Forlì) involved in the research. Randomized doctors were not asked to sign an informed consent form: their participation to the information meetings was part of a compulsory program set by the Local Health Authorities. Prescribing data are routinely collected and informed consent is not needed for their collection and analysis. Ethics Committees were of course aware of the recruitment procedure: one of the Committees (Modena) declared that a formal approval was not even necessary for the reasons described above.

Protocol publication and registration

The protocol has been published in a peer-reviewed journal and is openly accessible at http://www.biomedcentral.com/content/pdf/1472-6963-7-158.pdf.

Table 5. SIDRO trial: differences in DDD per 1000 patients of prescribed drugs (intervention vs control).

prescribing outcomes (primary)	Absolute mean prescription during follow-up in the 'intervention group' (DDD per 1000 patients)	Absolute difference at follow-up vs control group (change from baseline expressed as DDD per 1000 patients)	m-ITT (95% CI) (1564 included GPs)
prulifloxacin	0.17	−0.02	−11.1% (−0.5 to −22,2%)
barnidipine *	1.94	−0.21*	−9.8% (−1.9 to −18.2%)

*a lower increase was observed in the intervention group.

Table 6. Participants' opinions about usefulness of information received (question: Do you think the information you have received will be useful?).

Information package	Very much	Quite	Little	Not at all	No answer
Osteoporosis	42.5%	53.5%	1.8%	0.1%	2.1%
BPH	29.7%	62.3%	4.5%	0.9%	2.6%
Prulifloxacin	31.0%	43.6%	19.1%	3.1%	3.2%
Barnidipine	37.3%	35.8%	18.2%	6.3%	2.3%

Even if not strictly necessary (having randomized general practitioners and not patients) we registered the trials on the ISRCTN register (trial registration n.: ISRCTN05866587).

Results

First RCT: ThErapeutic Area approach (TEA) trial: Information on drugs for the treatment of benign prostatic hyperplasia (arm 1) and drugs for the treatment of osteoporosis (arm 2)

The flow charts of cluster participants is shown in Figure 1. All 115 PCGs, corresponding to 1737 GPs assisting about two millions inhabitants, were randomised. A total of 1605 GPs (92.4%) were included in the m-ITT analysis, excluding 110 GPs (6.3%) who had less than 300 subjects in their assisted population, one PCG (with 9 GPs –0,5%) refusing to participate to the study, and 13 single GPs (0,7%) who had moved to a different PCG after randomisation. A total of 1311 of the included GPs (81.7%) participated in the information meetings (per protocol population).

Table 2 shows GPs' mean baseline prescription of drugs considered in the primary outcomes. Limited imbalances between the two groups (less than 5%) had to be considered. Table S1 shows number and characteristics of PCGs and GPs in the ITT analysis.

Table 3 synthesizes differences in change from baseline between intervention and control groups in prescribing outcomes. In the ITT analysis, one BPH-related primary outcome showed a statistically significant reduction: specifically, the ratio between alpha blocker drugs alfuzosin (still under patent) and tamsulosin+ terazosin (off patent) decreased by 8.5% ($p = 0.03$; intracluster correlation coefficient or ICC of almost 0), suggesting a shift towards off patent drugs, as expected. The other BPH-related primary outcome, prescription of finasteride+dutasteride did not reach statistically significant differences (ICC = 0.06).

As for osteoporosis related outcomes, no primary outcome showed a statistically significant reduction in the ITT analysis (ICC for alendronic acid and risedronic acid were 0.04 and 0.31, respectively);

One secondary outcome, prescription of ibandronic acid, showed a statistically significant reduction (−19.6%; $p = 0.01$; ICC = 0.002), although its prescription was very limited in absolute terms. This drug was shown to lack evidence on primary prevention of osteoporotic fractures.

Fig. 2 provides a clear representation of results also related to longer term follow-ups (after 12, 24 and 48 months), allowing for an evaluation of persistence of effects: similar direction to 6-month results are showed, except for combined prescription of finasteride and dutasteride in BPH. Ratio between alpha blocker drugs alfuzosin and tamsulosin+terazosin lost statistical significance after 12 months. Surprisingly, prescription of risedronate in osteoporosis was further reduced and was statistically significant after 24 and 48 months (−7.6%, $p = 0.02$; and −9,8%, $p = 0.03$).

Second RCT: SIngle DRug Oriented (SIDRO) trial: A new antibiotic and a new antihypertensive (a calcium-channel blocker): prulifloxacin (arm 1) and barnidipine (arm 2)

In this subsequent trial, all 115 PCGs, corresponding to 1735 GPs, were randomised (two general practitioners retired in the period between the first and the second trial – Fig. 1).

A total of 1564 GPs (90.1%) were included in the ITT analysis, excluding 106 GPs (6.1%) who had fewer than 300 subjects in their assisted population, three PCGs (with 49 GPs –2,8%) refusing the small group meeting, and 16 single GPs (0,9%) who had moved to a different PCG after randomization receiving the "control" information (Fig. 1); 1211 of the included GPs (77,4%) participated in the information meetings (per protocol population).

Table 4 shows GPs' mean baseline prescription for the drugs of interest. Limited imbalances between the two groups (about 6%) had to be considered. Table S2 shows number and characteristics of PCGs and GPs in the ITT analysis.

Table 5 synthesizes differences in change from baseline between intervention and control groups in prescribing outcomes related to the prulifloxacin and barnidipine information meeting. In the modified ITT analysis, both the primary outcomes showed a statistically significant reduction of about 10%: prulifloxacin −11.1% ($p = 0.04$; ICC = 0.05); barnidipine −9.8% ($p = 0.02$; ICC = 0.08). This suggests that information focused on a single drug rather than on more complex therapeutic strategies can be successful in changing doctors' behaviours and this result is stable or even increasing over time (up to 4 years); however, caution is needed in interpreting these data, considering the limited prescription of these drugs in absolute terms (in particular of prulifloxacin).

Results after 12, 24 and 48 months showed, surprisingly, a progressively larger reduction in the prescription of barnidipine, doubled after 48 months, and similar reductions in the prescription of prulifloxacin, suggesting that the effect of the intervention might have persisted over time (Fig. 2).

Assessment of doctors' knowledge and attitudes

The majority of doctors could identify the correct answers to several questions and to improve their baseline knowledge after the intervention, although answers were given collectively in most of the information meetings, limiting the usefulness of such analysis. For this reason, those results are not shown.

As for doctors' opinions on completeness and usefulness of the information received, the vast majority of general practitioners evaluated it as "very much" or "quite", as shown in Table 6. Even if the more articulated information presented in the first RCT was associated with less evident changes in the prescribing outcomes, compared with the more focused information of the second RCT (as described above), such information was more appreciated by doctors: more than 90% considered information packages in the first RCT either "very" or "quite" useful compared to 72–75% in the second RCT.

Discussion

These two cluster RCTs confirm that pharmacists' outreach visits can be an effective way of promoting evidence-based prescribing in a large NHS setting and show that effects can persist in the long-term (up to 4 years). They are also the largest studies done in terms of number of doctors involved. A cluster design was used since group meetings are held regularly (at least twice a year) with Primary Care Groups in the intervention areas and because they represent a natural setting where to deliver information, stimulate analysis and discussion through a problem-based approach. [26–27].

In the first RCT (TEA trial) in which information materials addressed a therapeutic area and had broader clinical scope and extent (drugs in the treatment of benign prostatic hyperplasia/ osteoporosis), only one of the four predefined primary outcome showed a statistically significant reduction (prescription of alfuzosin compared to tamsulosin and terazosin in benign prostatic hyperplasia). The fairly ambitious quantitative hypothesis to be tested (10−15% difference in doctors' prescriptions) was thus substantially not demonstrated, in spite of the involvement of about 1800 general practitioners. Among the other three primary outcomes in the first RCT, one (prescription of risedronate) has become statistically significant after two years of follow-up, further reducing its prescription in the intervention group, and this finding is not easy to interpret; another primary outcome (prescription of alendronate) was affected by its availability as generic drug just before the start of the trial, as well as by its better assessed benefit-risk profile compared to the other bisphosphonates; this may have reduced the potential to show a difference between the two groups. As for bisphosphonates, the prescription of ibandronate (a secondary outcome) showed a reduction in the intervention group, but this drug was little prescribed.

Conversely, in the second RCT (SIDRO trial) which concerned information on a single drug, both primary outcomes showed clear and statistically significant prescribing reductions (10% or more) lasting a long time. Although doctors generally appreciated the therapeutic area approach used in the first RCT - addressing both diagnostic and therapeutic questions in a broad range of clinical scenarios - more than the more focused single drug approach, the latter seems to have affected doctors' prescribing behaviour more clearly.

These studies confirm findings from previous RCTs conducted mostly in Northern Europe and North America, showing that pharmacists delivering evidence-based information and prescribing data through outreach visits may influence doctors' prescribing behaviour in the short term. Our findings add that positive results are mostly obtained with an intervention focused on a single drug, suggesting that the more complex the information, the more complex and the less likely the related behaviour/prescribing change. Contrary to the findings of previous educational intervention trials, we found high persistence of the effects (measured initially as stated in the study protocol at 6 and 12 months, and in subsequent periods up to 48 months) even in absence of reminders. This result was particularly sharp for barnidipine, a calcium antagonist possibly suffering from the competition of many drugs in the same class.

The evaluation of educational interventions is fairly complex given the many different variables in play. [28] Among these, we did not consider patient demand as a main driver of drug prescription, giving priority to feasibility and replicability of the intervention. However, the pragmatic nature of these RCTs and their large-scale implementation in a natural setting strengthen the external validity of the results.

The context may determine the success of these educational programs, by hindering or facilitating the implementation of small group meetings. In this regard, general practitioners from Friuli Venezia-Giulia (another region in Northern Italy), initially supposed to take part in the RCTs, did not in the end do so because their representatives and the Regional Health Authority disagreed. Moreover, one more RCT was originally planned in Sardinia (a large island in Southern Italy), to compare three different strategies of information delivery to solo general practitioners: [21] this trial did not take place for similar reasons as in Friuli Venezia-Giulia. Involvement of doctors' organizations and strong endorsement of Health Authorities are crucial in implementing such an anti-promotional intervention; doctors may see these interventions as top-down, cost-saving approaches.

In conclusion, the confirmation of a positive impact of independent information programs in a large-scale natural setting, in particular when information on single drugs is provided, can be considered as a fairly relevant finding and the persistence of the observed differences for up to 4 years is quite a new one. If the organizational environment is "good enough" and a strong endorsement from Health Authorities (with the sole aim to promote public health optimizing treatments) is assured, information programs led by National Health Systems Agencies may provide a critical alternative to industry-led information to physicians. Future studies should focus on assessing whether positive findings are driven by how information is delivered (small groups versus one-to-one meetings) and presented, evaluating different formats and ways of presenting the actual magnitude of benefits and risks of drugs and other health interventions.

Supporting Information

Table S1 TEA trial: number and characteristics of PCGs and GPs in the ITT analysis.

Table S2 SIDRO trial: number and characteristics of PCGs and GPs in the ITT analysis.

Table S3 Primary data for the TEA trial.

Table S4 Primary data for the SIDRO trial.

Acknowledgments

We want to thank Prof. David Sackett (McMaster University, Canada) for useful suggestions and great encouragement in developing the research project.

Contributors

Members of the INDRA-NET (INformation on DRugs And NEw Therapies) study group are:

- Local Health Authority of Bologna: C. Castelvetri, P. Falcone, M. Magnani, M. Manzoli, P. Pagano, E. Pasi, G. Santilli, S. Scaramagli, P. Tomasi, L. Toni, P. Zuccheri.
- Local Health Authority of Forlì: F. Carnaccini, R. Consiglio.
- Local Health Authority of Modena: M. Ghelfi, C. Orsi, M. Pagani.
- Local Health Authority of Parma: M. Boffetti, G. Negri, F. Pinelli.
- Local Health Authority of Reggio Emilia: R. Ballestri, R. Montanari.

Steering Committee: M. Bobbio (Chairman); P. Malavasi, G. Negri, M. Salera, E. Sapigni (Emilia-Romagna); P. Carossino, G. Carta, M. Cicalò, D. Garau, G. Sanna (Sardinia); L. Crapesi, L. Marcuzzo, R. Paduano, G. Tosolini (Friuli Venezia Giulia); G. Formoso, N. Magrini, A. M. Marata (coordinating group).

Author Contributions

Conceived and designed the experiments: NM GF AMM. Analyzed the data: CDG CV. Wrote the paper: GF NM. Development of information tools: OC EM AMM GF BP LM LD FN. Coordination of educational meetings: AMM OC EM GF FN LM LD.

References

1. Collier J, Iheanacho I (2002) The pharmaceutical industry as an informant. Lancet 360: 1405–1409.
2. Melander H, Ahlqvist-Rastad J, Meijer G, Beermann B (2003) Evidence b(i)ased medicine – selective reporting from studies sponsored by pharmaceutical industry: review of studies in new drug applications. BMJ 326: 1171–1173.
3. Ridker PM, Torres J (2006) Reported outcomes in major cardiovascular clinical trials funded by for-profit and not-for-profit organizations: 2000–2005. JAMA 295: 2270–2276.
4. Dickersin K (2005) Publication bias: Recognizing the problem, understanding its origins and scope, and preventing harm. In: Rothstein H, Sutton A, Borenstein M (eds). Publication bias in meta-analysis: prevention, assessment, and adjustments. London: Wiley, p 11–33.
5. Chan AW (2008) Bias, spin, and misreporting: time for full access to trial protocols and results. PLoS Medicine 5(11): e230. DOI:10.1371/journal.pmed.0050230.
6. Light DW, Lexchin JR (2012) Pharmaceutical research and development: what do we get for all that money? BMJ 345: e4348.
7. The Congress of the United States – Congressional Budget Office (2006) Research and Development in the Pharmaceutical Industry.
8. Graham Dukes MN (2002) Accountability of the pharmaceutical industry. Lancet 360: 1682–1684.
9. Avorn J, Soumerai SB (1983) Improving drug-therapy decisions through educational outreach - a randomized controlled trial of academically based detailing. New Engl J Med 308: 1457–1463.
10. Soumerai SB, Avorn J (1990) Principles of educational outreach (academic detailing) to improve clinical decision making. JAMA 263: 549–556.
11. Simon SR, Majumdar SR, Prosser LA, Salem-Schatz S, Warner C, et al. (2005) Group versus individual academic detailing to improve the use of antihypertensive medications in primary care: a cluster-randomized controlled trial. Am J Med 118: 521–528.
12. O'Brien MA, Rogers S, Jamtvedt G, Oxman AD, Odgaard-Jensen J, et al. (2007) Educational outreach visits: effects on professional practice and health care outcomes. *Cochrane Database of Systematic Reviews*, Issue 4. Art. No.: CD000409. DOI: 10.1002/14651858.CD000409.pub2.
13. Woloshin S, Schwartz LM (2011) Communicating data about the benefits and harms of treatment: a randomized trial. Ann Intern Med 155: 87–96.
14. Woloshin S, Schwartz LM, Welch HG (2008) Know Your Chances. Understanding Health Statistics. Berkeley (CA): University of California Press 2008.
15. Guyatt GH, Oxman AD, Vist GE, Kunz R, Falck-Ytter Y, et al. (2008) GRADE: an emerging consensus on rating quality of evidence and strength of recommendations. BMJ 336: 924–926.
16. Nkansah N, Mostovetsky O, Yu C, Chheng T, Beney J, et al. (2010) Effect of outpatient pharmacists' non-dispensing roles on patient outcomes and prescribing patterns. Cochrane Database of Systematic Reviews Issue 7. Art. No.: CD000336. DOI: 10.1002/14651858.CD000336.pub2.
17. Grimshaw JM, Thomas RE, MacLennan G, Fraser C, Ramsay CR, et al. (2004) Effectiveness and efficiency of guideline dissemination and implementation strategies. Health Technol Assess 8: 1–352.
18. Formoso G, Liberati A, Magrini N (2001) Practice Guidelines: Useful and "Participative" Method? Survey of Italian Physicians by Professional Setting. Arch Intern Med 161: 2037–2042.
19. Italian Medicines Agency (AIFA) Research & Development Working Group (2010) Feasibility and challenges of independent research on drugs: the Italian Medicines Agency (AIFA) experience. Eur J Clin Invest 40: 69–86.
20. Garattini S, Chalmers I (2009) Patients and the public deserve big changes in evaluation of drugs. BMJ 338: b1025.
21. Magrini N, Formoso G, Marata AM, Capelli O, Maestri E, et al. (2007) Randomised controlled trials for evaluating the prescribing impact of information meetings led by pharmacists and of new information formats, in General Practice in Italy. BMC Health Services Research 7: 158.
22. Formoso G, Marata AM, Magrini N (2007) Social marketing: should it be used to promote evidence-based information? Soc Sci Med 64: 949–953.
23. Schwartz LM (2009) Lost in Transmission – FDA Drug Information That Never Reaches Clinicians. New Engl J Med 361: 1717–1720.
24. Ivers N, Jamtvedt G, Flottorp S, Young JM, Odgaard-Jensen J, et al. (2012) Audit and feedback: effects on professional practice and healthcare outcomes. Cochrane Database of Systematic Reviews Issue 6. Art. No.: CD000259. DOI: 10.1002/14651858.CD000259.pub3.
25. Donner A, Klar N (1996) Statistical considerations in the design and analysis of community intervention trials. J Clin Epidemiol 49: 435–439.
26. Norman G (2002) Research in medical education: three decades of progress. BMJ 324: 1560–1562.
27. Godwin M, Ruhland L, Casson I, MacDonald S, Delva D, et al. (2003) Pragmatic controlled clinical trials in primary care: the struggle between external and internal validity. BMC Medical Research Methodology 3: 28.
28. Craig P, Dieppe P, Macintyre S, Michie S, Nazareth I, et al. (2008) Developing and evaluating complex interventions: the new Medical Research Council guidance. BMJ 337: a1655 doi:10.1136/bmj.a1655.

6

Lack of Renoprotective Effect of Chronic Intravenous Angiotensin-(1-7) or Angiotensin-(2-10) in a Rat Model of Focal Segmental Glomerulosclerosis

Juan Carlos Q. Velez[1,2]*, Michael G. Janech[1], Megan P. Hicks[1], Thomas A. Morinelli[1], Jessalyn Rodgers[1], Sally E. Self[3], John M. Arthur[1,2], Wayne R. Fitzgibbon[1]

1 Division of Nephrology, Department of Medicine, Medical University of South Carolina, Charleston, South Carolina, United States of America, **2** Medical Service, Ralph H. Johnson Veterans Affairs Medical Center, Charleston, South Carolina, United States of America, **3** Department of Pathology, Medical University of South Carolina, Charleston, South Carolina, United States of America

Abstract

Unopposed angiotensin (Ang) II-mediated cellular effects may lead to progressive glomerulosclerosis. While Ang-II can be locally generated in the kidneys, we previously showed that glomerular podocytes primarily convert Ang-I, the precursor of Ang-II, to Ang-(1-7) and Ang-(2-10), peptides that have been independently implicated in biological actions opposing those of Ang-II. Therefore, we hypothesized that Ang-(1-7) and Ang-(2-10) could be renoprotective in the fawn-hooded hypertensive rat, a model of focal segmental glomerulosclerosis. We evaluated the ability of 8–12 week-long intravenous administration of either Ang-(1-7) or Ang-(2-10) (100–400 ng/kg/min) to reduce glomerular injury in uni-nephrectomized fawn-hooded hypertensive rats, early or late in the disease. Vehicle-treated rats developed hypertension and lesions of focal segmental glomerulosclerosis. No reduction in glomerular damage was observed, as measured by either 24-hour urinary protein excretion or histological examination of glomerulosclerosis, upon Ang-(1-7) or Ang-(2-10) administration, regardless of peptide dose or disease stage. On the contrary, when given at 400 ng/kg/min, both peptides induced a further increase in systolic blood pressure. Content of Ang peptides was measured by parallel reaction monitoring in kidneys harvested at sacrifice. Exogenous administration of Ang-(1-7) and Ang-(2-10) did not lead to a significant increase in their corresponding intrarenal levels. However, the relative abundance of Ang-(1-7) with respect to Ang-II was increased in kidney homogenates of Ang-(1-7)-treated rats. We conclude that chronic intravenous administration of Ang-(1-7) or Ang-(2-10) does not ameliorate glomerular damage in a rat model of focal segmental glomerulosclerosis and may induce a further rise in blood pressure, potentially aggravating glomerular injury.

Editor: Ariela Benigni, IRCSS - Istituto di Ricerche Farmacologiche Mario Negri, Italy

Funding: This work was partially funded by a grant from the National Institute of Diabetes and Digestive and Kidney Diseases of the National Institute of Health (DK080944) (JCV), American Recovery and Reinvestment Act supplement to DK080944 (MPH and WRF), and The Nephcure Foundation (MGJ), and Dialysis Clinics Incorporated (JCV and TAM). The funders had no role in study design, data collection and analysis, decision to publish, or preparation of the manuscript.

Competing Interests: The authors have declared that no competing interests exist.

* Email: velezj@musc.edu

Introduction

Angiotensin (Ang) II has been implicated in the pathogenesis of various glomerular diseases, such as diabetic glomerulopathy, focal segmental glomerulosclerosis (FSGS), IgA nephropathy, and others [1–3]. Ang-II is primarily formed after the cleavage of Ang-I by Ang-converting enzyme (ACE). In the kidney glomerulus and other organs, Ang-I can also be converted to other Ang fragments by the action of various peptidases. Neprilysin converts Ang-I into the heptapeptide Ang-(1-7), whereas aminopeptidase A converts it into the nonapeptide Ang-(2-10) [4,5]. Furthermore, Ang-(1-7) can also be generated by cleavage of Ang-II by ACE2, prolylcarboxypeptidase or prolylendopeptidase by other cell types that reside in the kidney [6,7].

It has been recognized that Ang-(1-7) may exert cellular actions by stimulation of a specific receptor, the *mas* receptor [8], that are antagonistic to those of Ang-II, including a vasodilatory [9], natriuretic [10], antiproliferative [11] and antifibrotic effect [12]. Those observations led others to postulate that Ang-(1-7) could be a protective peptide in glomerular diseases. Indeed, chronic subcutaneous administration of Ang-(1-7) was shown to be protective in rodent models of diabetic glomerulopathy [13] and anti-Thy1.1 nephritis [14]. In contrast, others have found that Ang-(1-7) is not protective in models of progressive glomerulosclerosis [15] and FSGS [16], and is detrimental in models of diabetic glomerulopathy [17]. Of note, most laboratories studied early stages of the disease and administered the heptapeptide for only 1–6 weeks [18]. Therefore, we opted to expand the investigation of the effect of Ang-(1-7) to advanced stages of glomerular disease and during longer duration of treatment.

Previous work demonstrated that rat glomeruli primarily convert Ang-I to Ang-(1-7) and Ang-(2-10) [4]. Studies from a single laboratory suggested that Ang-(2-10) may modulate the pressor actions of Ang-II [19]. However, the effects of chronic systemic administration of Ang-(2-10) have not been studied to date. In addition, Ang-(2-10) could be converted to Ang-III by ACE, and Ang-III has been proposed to promote natriuresis by virtue of being the predominant agonist of tubular Ang-II type 2 (AT_2) receptors [20]. Therefore, we also evaluated the effect of chronically infused Ang-(2-10) on kidney damage in a model of glomerular disease.

Thus, we hypothesized that Ang-(1-7) and/or Ang-(2-10) may ameliorate glomerular damage in a rat model of FSGS by diminishing the degree of Ang-II-mediated injury. To test our hypothesis, we selected the fawn-hooded hypertensive (FHH) rat, a well characterized model of spontaneous hypertension and proteinuria associated with a histological lesion of FSGS [21–23]. In addition, because stimulation of the Ang-II type 2 (AT_2) receptor has been reported to counteract some of the detrimental effects of Ang-II via the AT_1 receptor, we assessed the ability of Ang-(1-7) and Ang-(2-10) to bind to Ang receptors.

Materials and Methods

Ang peptide radioligand binding assay

HEK-293 cells stably expressing AT_{1a} receptor were maintained and characterized as previously described [24]. HEK-293 cells expressing AT_2 receptors were transfected with pcDNA3.1 plasmid containing human AT_2 receptor DNA using Lipofectamine 2000 at 1 µg DNA/well of a six-well plate according to manufacturer's protocol (Invitrogen, Carlsbad, CA). Transfected cells were maintained in Minimal Essential Medium (MEM) containing 10% fetal bovine serum and 1% antibiotic/fungizone/antimycotic with addition of geneticin (400 µg/ml) for stable transfectants. Confluent monolayers cells were deprived of serum (0.1% bovine serum albumin) for 2–24 hours before assay. Cells were placed on ice for 15 minutes followed by addition of assay buffer (50 mM Tris pH 7.4, 100 mM NaCl, 12 mM MgCl, 2 mM KCl, 1% BSA and freshly added bacitracin) or various concentrations of competing ligand and [^{125}I]-Ang-II (~200,000 cpm/well) in a total volume of 1 ml/well. After 90 min of incubation on ice, cells were gently washed 3 times with ice cold 0.9% sodium chloride followed by solubilization of the cell monolayer with 0.1 N NaOH/0.1% SDS. The solubilized sample was placed into a gamma counter for determination of cell-associated radioactivity. Log-logit analysis of the obtained competition curves was performed for determination of IC50 values.

Animal Procedures

Ethics statement. All animal procedures were conducted with approval from the Medical University of South Carolina Institutional Animal Care and Use Committee and in accordance with the procedures and practices of the *NIH Guide for the Care and Use of Laboratory Animals*.

Male FHH rats (In-house colony established from animals obtained from Charles River Laboratories, Wilmington, MA) were housed at a certified animal facility at 22°C and a 12:12 h light/dark cycle. The rats were allowed free access to tap water, fed a standard diet (Teklad #2918, Harlan Laboratories, Madison, FWI) and provided with environmental enrichment. All surgeries were performed under isoflurane anesthesia (5% induction, 2% maintenance), at 37°C, and perioperative buprenorphine.

Model of FSGS

A schematic of the animal protocols is shown in Figure 1. In order to accelerate the development of glomerulosclerosis [25], rats (95–205 g) underwent left nephrectomy at 6 weeks of age. Following anesthesia, an incision was made in the left flank; the kidney was exposed and excised after ligation of the pedicle. One (early disease) or 12 (late disease) weeks following single nephrectomy, the rats underwent implantation of osmotic mini-pumps (Alzet models 2004 or 2006 Alza Corp., Palo Alto, CA) for intravenous delivery of either isotonic saline (vehicle) or Ang peptides. Under anesthesia, a mini-pump was placed in a subcutaneous pocket. A catheter (PE 50) attached to the pump was then tunneled subcutaneously around the neck and cannulated into the right jugular vein. Pumps were replaced once during the treatment period. For the early disease model, five groups of rats were examined. Either saline (n = 4) or 100 ng/kg/min (low-dose, LD) of Ang II (n = 4), Ang-(1-7) (n = 4) or Ang-(2-10) (n = 4) was infused for a total of 8 weeks. An additional group (n = 5) received captopril (100 mg/kg/d) in the drinking water throughout the treatment period. For the late disease model, eight groups of rats were examined. Saline (n = 7) or 100 ng/kg/min (low-dose, LD) or 400 ng/kg/min (high-dose, HD) of either Ang-(1-7) or Ang-(2-10), or Ang II (LD), was infused for a total of 12 weeks (n = 9 per Ang peptide treatment). The dosages of the Ang peptides were selected based on previous studies where Ang-(1-7) was similarly administered using implanted osmotic mini-pumps [13,16,17,26]. Two further groups received captopril (100 mg/kg/d, n = 10) or losartan (20 mg/kg/d, n = 9) orally throughout the treatment period. Systemic blood pressure was measured by tail-cuff sphygmomanometer (Natume, Japan). Animals were placed on metabolic cages for urine collection at pre-specified time points. Urinary protein excretion was measured by the method of Lowry [27]. Urinary sodium concentration was measured by ion-selective electrodes. At sacrifice, kidneys were harvested for histological analysis and measurement of Ang peptide concentration.

Histological Analysis

Upon harvesting, kidneys were cleared of blood by transcardiac perfusion of iced-cold phosphate buffered saline, excised and fixed in 4% paraformaldehyde, embedded in paraffin and processed for microscopic examination. Kidney sections (2-µm) were stained with hematoxylin-eosin (H&E), Jones silver and Periodic Acid Schiff (PAS). Slides were reviewed by an experienced renal pathologist (S.S) in a blinded fashion. Index of glomerulosclerosis was evaluated by a semiquantitative score based on the percentage of the glomerular tuft occupied by sclerotic lesions (0: no lesions, 1: lesions affecting less than 25% of the glomerulus, 2-3-4: lesions affecting 25–50%, 50–75% and 75–100% of the glomerulus, respectively). Tubular injury was rated based on presence of tubular atrophy, microcystic tubular dilation and interstitial fibrosis, from 0 to 3 (0: none; 1: mild; 2: moderate; 3: severe).

Ang Peptide Content Determination

Stable isotope labeled peptide standards (SIS, ^{13}C ^{15}N, New England Peptide, Gardner, MA) were resuspended in water to 1 nM and stored at −80C in Lo-Bind microcentrifuge tubes (Eppendorf) with the exception of Ang-I, which was resuspended in 30% acetonitrile and stored at 0.4 nM final concentration. Ang-(1-7), Ang-II, and Ang-(2-10) contained isotopically labeled valine. Ang-I contained isotopically labeled valine and proline. Peptide concentration was determined by amino acid analysis.

Tissues were stored frozen at −80°C in 15 ml Falcon tubes. Whole kidney tissues were submerged in liquid nitrogen for 5 minutes and kidney tissue was processed in a biopulverizer (MidSci, St. Louis, MO) to a fine powder. Pulverized tissue was transferred to a 5-ml glass dounce with a chilled spatula. Approximately 200 mg of tissue was used for peptide extraction.

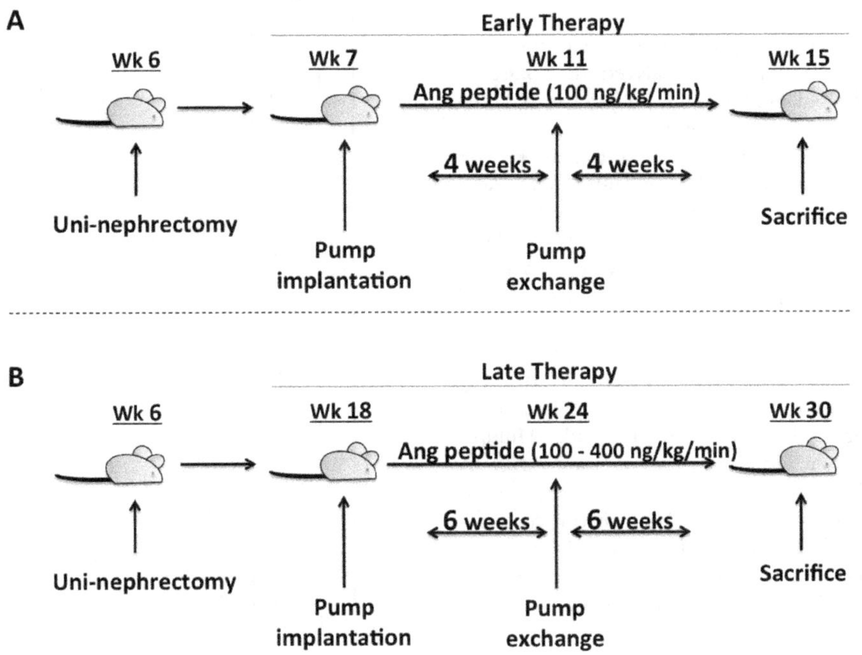

Figure 1. Experimental protocols. Schematic of treatment protocols employed to test the effect of early (Panel *A*) or late (Panel *B*) chronic intravenous administration of Ang-(1-7) and Ang-(2-10) on the progression of glomerulosclerosis in uni-nephrectomized FHH rats.

Four volumes of ice cold methanol (Burdick and Jackson, LC-MS Grade) were added to the tissue followed by a volume of water (Burdick and Jackson, LC-MS Grade) containing O-phenanthroline (Sigma Aldrich) and SIS peptides resulting in a final concentration of 1 mM and 1.8 nM, respectively. Tissue was homogenized in the dounce on ice for 1 minute. An aliquot of tissue homogenate was transferred to a 2-ml lo-bind microcentrifuge tube and stored at −20°C for at least 1 hour. Samples were further centrifuged for 10 minutes at 10,000×g at 4°C. An aliquot equal to approximately 60% of the total sample volume was transferred to a lo-bind tube equivalent to 100 mg of tissue (wet weight). From this aliquot, a volume equal to the wet weight of the starting tissue was transferred to a new lo-bind tube and diluted with ice cold water so that the final concentration of methanol was 40%. The total volume of this microcentrifuge tube was then transferred to a Microcon Ultracel YM-10 centrifugal filter (Milipore Ireland Ltd, Cork, IRL) following methods described by Lortie *et al.* [28]. Filters were preconditioned for 30 minutes with 40% methanol prior to use. Samples were filtered at 14,000×g for 1 hour at 4°C. The filtrate was transferred to a new lo-bind microcentrifuge tube. The filtrate volume was estimated by variable volume pipet and recorded to determine the fraction of starting volume collected. Two volumes of 0.1% formic acid were added to each sample. A solid phase extraction cartridge (Phenomenex Strata-x reversed phase, 60 mg, Torrance, CA) was conditioned with 1 ml acetonitrile and washed with 1 ml 0.1% formic acid. Peptides were bound to the column and washed with 1 ml 0.1% formic acid. Peptides were eluted sequentially in 12% Mobile Phase B [MPB, 95% acetonitrile (v/v), 0.2% formic acid (v/v)]/88% Mobile Phase A [MPA, 0.2% formic acid] and then 30% MPB/70% MPA to separate Ang-(1-7) from Ang-II [Ang-(1-8)], Ang-(2-10), and Ang-I [Ang-(1-10)]. Eluted peptides were flash frozen in liquid nitrogen, placed in a speedvac concentrator and dried. Peptides from the 12% MPB fraction were resuspended in MPA to a volume equivalent to 0.18 mg of starting kidney weight per microliter (approximately 100–150 microliters). Peptides from the 30% MPB fraction were resuspended in 10% MPB to the same volume equivalent. For each fraction, 10 µl of resuspended peptides were injected onto a 100 µm×2 cm C18 (100 Å with 5-µm particles) trap column (Acclaim PepMap 100; Thermo Fisher Scientific), and separated on a 75 µm×15 cm C18 (300 Å with 3 µm particles) analytical column (Acclaim PepMap 100; Thermo Fisher Scientific). Reverse phase separation was performed with a gradient of 0% to 40% MPB over 42 minutes on a 2D+ NanoLC system (Eksigent, Dublin, CA). The nanoLC was coupled to a TripleTOF 5600 mass spectrometer (AB Sciex, Foster City, CA) through a nanospray source. Declustering potential was set at 80 V. For parallel reaction monitoring (PRM) quantification, the dominant charge state of each peptide was determined and collision energies were optimized manually for SIS peptides (Table 1). Peptide data was collected in positive ion mode using product ion scans (set at 1 unit resolution). External calibration curves were constructed for each SIS peptide. Seven concentrations were injected from 0.3 fmols to 25 fmols in duplicate, with the exception of Ang-II where 20 fmols was injected as the highest concentration. Measurements were calculated by using area under the curve for ion pairs using the MQ4 algorithm built in to MultiQuant (v 2.0.2, AB Sciex). Fragment ions were extracted from each product scanusing a monoisotopic mass ±0.1 m/z. Regression was performed using peak areas with linear fit and 1/x weighting. Limit of detection and lower limit of quantification (LLOQ) were calculated for SIS peptides as 3 and 10 standard deviations of the mean from triplicate kidney lysate preps without SIS peptides. Percent coefficient of variation was calculated for a single sample injected in triplicate.

Statistical analyses

Blood pressure data were analyzed by repeated measures ANOVA. Differences within groups were analyzed using paired t-tests adjusted with Bonferroni modification. Differences between group means at each time point were tested using one-way ANOVA followed by Tukey-Kramer *post-hoc* test. Urinary protein excretions were log10 transformed and tested using a two-way ANOVA for repeated measures followed by Scheffe *post hoc* test for differences between the groups. Untransformed 24-hour urinary protein excretions at each time point were then tested using Kruskal-Wallis test. If a significant main effect was detected then differences between groups were tested using the Mann-Whitney U test with the probability adjusted using the Bonferroni modification. Urine sodium was also assessed by two-way ANOVA for repeated measures and pairwise multiple comparisons were made using the Holm-Sidak method. Multiple comparisons of Ang peptide levels were made using ANOVA when data were normally distributed and with log10 transformation when non-normally distributed. *Post-hoc* pairwise comparisons were made using the Holm-Sidak method. Correlations were assessed using Spearman Rank Order correlation. For Ang peptide measurements by LC/MS/MS, only values above the LLOQ were utilized for statistical comparisons.

Results

Ang Peptide Binding

As illustrated in Figure 2, all three ligands demonstrated concentration-dependent displacement of radiolabeled Ang-II from both AT_1 and AT_2 receptors indicating specific interaction with the receptors in HEK-293 cells. However, the rank order potency for the ligands differed between the two expressed receptors. For the AT_1 receptor, the rank order for affinity was: Ang-II>Ang-(2-10)>>Ang-(1-7). On the other hand, for the AT_2 receptor, Ang-II and Ang-(2-10) demonstrated similar affinity for the receptor, which was approximately 6–10 greater than that of Ang-(1-7). In addition, Ang-(1-7) appeared to demonstrate a greater affinity for the AT_2 receptor than for the AT_1 receptor, as reflected by an IC50 value approximately 60-fold higher for the AT_1 receptor.

Effect of Ang-(1-7) and Ang-(2-10) on a rat model of FSGS

In accordance to previous studies utilizing the uni-nephrectomized FHH rat model [25,29], all animals exhibited a progressive increase over time in systemic blood pressure, urinary protein excretion and parenchymal injury characterized by focal segmental glomerulosclerosis and microcystic tubular dilatation. In the late disease model, approximately 80% of the glomeruli were affected with some degree of glomerulosclerosis, either segmental or global, demonstrating the robustness of the animal model. The changes observed in systolic blood pressure during the early and late disease models are shown in Figure 3. Data on changes in body weight, kidney weight and urine volume are presented in Table 2.

In the early disease model, rats in all groups exhibited a small but consistent elevation in systolic blood pressure one week after single nephrectomy. Four weeks after initiation of therapy, systolic blood pressure in vehicle-treated rats increased (from 144±5, 161±4 mmHg, p = 0.01) and it remained elevated at 8 weeks (162±4 mmHg). A similar rise in arterial blood pressure was observed among animals treated with either low-dose Ang-(1-7) or low-dose Ang-(2-10). Ang-II induced a broader rise in mean systolic blood pressure compared to that in vehicle-treated rats after both 4 and 8 weeks of treatment. As expected, captopril

Table 1. LC/MS/MS peptide transition ions, optimized collision energy and standard curve correlation coefficients.

Peptide	Peptide Sequence	Charge state	Product scan (m/z)	Extracted Ion Monitored	Collision Energy (V)	*R*	LOD (fmol)	LLOQ (fmol)	CV%
Ang-I	DRVYIHPFHL	(M+3H)+3	432.9	b5, 647.35	25				14.4
Ang-I^	DRV^YIHP^FHL	(M+3H)+3	438.2	b5, 657.35	25	0.995	0.012	0.030	
Ang-(2-10)	RVYIHPFHL	(M+3H)+3	394.6	b4, 532.32	23				2.1
Ang-(2-10)^	RV^YIHPFHL	(M+3H)+3	396.6	b4, 538.32	23	0.991	1.367	3.809	
Ang-II	DRVYIHPF	(M+3H)+3	349.5	b3, 371.20	14				5.9
Ang-II^	DRV^YIHPF	(M+3H)+3	351.5	b3, 377.20	14	0.993	0.005	0.015	
Ang-(1-7)	DRVYIHP	(M+3H)+3	300.5	b3, 371.20	14				18.4
Ang-(1-7)^	DRVYIHP	(M+3H)+3	302.5	b3, 377.20	14	0.986	0.017	0.046	

On column limit of detection (LOD), On column lower limit of quantification (LLOQ) and concentration range measured for peptides in this study. ^ indicates $^{13}C/^{15}N$ SIS peptide. CV = coefficient of variation.

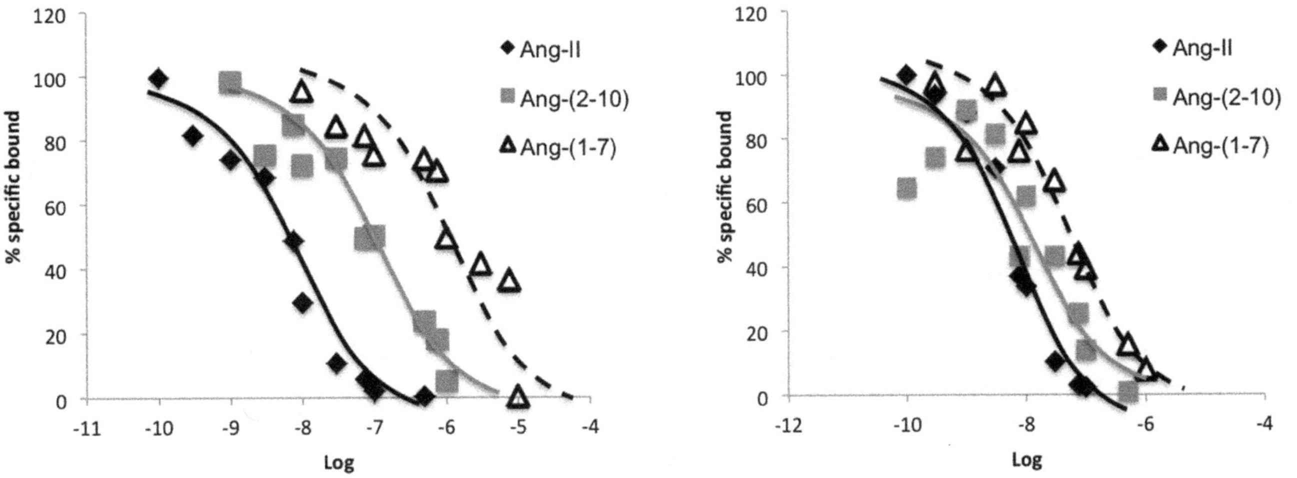

AT1R/HEK IC50 (nM)

	Average	SEM	n
Ang-II	3.1	1.6	4
Ang-(2-10)	47.8	28	5
Ang-(1-7)	3789	900	4

AT2R/HEK IC50 (nM)

	Average	SEM	n
Ang-II	10.2	2.8	8
Ang-(2-10)	6.6	4.5	3
Ang-(1-7)	60.9	16.6	4

Figure 2. Displacement curves of competition radioligand binding studies. Representative curves are shown for each peptide from studies performed on cells expressing the indicated Ang receptor. Average IC50 values ± SEM from the indicated number of studies (n) are shown.

decreased systolic blood pressure after 4 and 8 weeks of therapy (117±5 and 134±3, respectively); ($p<0.0001$ vs. vehicle) (Fig. 3A). Urine sodium excretion did not change over time in any of the groups, nor was a difference found between groups (Table S1). Urinary protein excretion increased between 4 and 8 weeks after the commencement of treatment ($p<0.001$). Median proteinuria in vehicle-treated rats was 89 (31–188) and 243 (91–402), mg/day, after 4 and 8 weeks, respectively (Fig. 4). Captopril significantly mitigated the development of proteinuria [14 (13–17) and 30 (25–33) mg/day, after 4 and 8 weeks of therapy, respectively; $p=0.014$ vs. vehicle]. In contrast, proteinuria was not modified by either Ang-(1-7) or Ang-(2-10) at the doses tested and it was increased by Ang-II. Ang-II significantly worsened the degree of glomerulosclerosis (1.4±0.4 vs. 0.4±0.1; $p<0.01$) and tubular injury (1.6±0.2 vs. 0.8±0.2; $p<0.05$) compared to vehicle, whereas neither Ang-(1-7) nor Ang-(2-10) infusion changed the degree of structural damage. Captopril caused a significant reduction in glomerulosclerosis (0.1±0.1 vs. 0.4±0.1; $p<0.05$) but a non-significant reduction in tubular injury (Fig. 5).

In the late disease model, all animals exhibited a substantial increase in systolic blood pressure 12 weeks after single nephrectomy (Fig. 3B). Thereafter, vehicle-treated rats continued to increase their blood pressure, raising it from 167±8 (at pump implantation) to 179±2 mmHg (after 6 weeks) ($p<0.005$) and maintaining it elevated at 185±3 mmHg after 12 weeks. Captopril and losartan decreased systolic blood pressure (156±7 and 155±5 mmHg at 6 weeks, and 145±5 and 146±5 mmHg after 12 weeks; for captopril and losartan, respectively; $p<0.0001$ vs. vehicle), suggesting that hypertension in FHH rats is partially Ang-II mediated. In contrast, low-dose Ang-(1-7) had no effect on blood pressure, low-dose Ang-(2-10) raised blood pressure after 12 weeks (194±3 mmHg; $p<0.01$ vs. vehicle), and both high-dose Ang-(1-7) and high-dose Ang-(2-10) raised blood pressure throughout the study (188±3 and 187±3 mmHg after 6 weeks, and 197±3 and 196±4 mmHg; for high-dose Ang-(1-7) and high-dose Ang-(2-10), respectively; $p<0.001$ vs. vehicle). However, only 2 high-dose Ang-(2-10)-treated rats survived until the end of the study. Ang-II-treated rats also exhibited increased blood pressure after 6 weeks, but no rats in this group survived beyond that time mark. Although the urine sodium excretion decreased in all groups after the 12-week therapy, no differences were found between groups (Table S1). Median proteinuria in vehicle-treated rats was 2 (1–5), 537 (184–862), 978 (433–2839) and 738 (622–2032) mg/day, at baseline (week 6), at the time of pump implantation (week 18), at week 24 and at week 30, respectively (Fig. 6). There was no change in 24-hour urinary protein excretion over the 12 weeks of treatment for any of the groups. However, the progression of the degree of proteinuria between weeks 18 and 24 was significantly attenuated by captopril (+342±289 vs. −225±453 mg/day, vehicle vs. captopril, respectively; $p=0.012$). Proteinuria was not modified by either Ang-(1-7) or Ang-(2-10), regardless of dosing. Captopril significantly reduced the degree of glomerulosclerosis (0.88±0.2 vs. 2.29±0.9, $p<0.0001$) and tubular injury score (2.6±0.4 vs. 1.3±0.4, $p<0.05$) compared to vehicle, whereas losartan only reduced glomerulosclerosis (1.28±0.7 vs. 2.29±0.9, $p<0.0005$). None of the Ang-(1-7) and Ang-(2-10) treatments had an effect on structural damage (Fig. 7).

Ang Peptide Content

The concentration of Ang peptides in kidney tissue was measured in kidneys harvested upon completion of the late disease model protocol, i.e., at 30 weeks of age, after 12 weeks of therapy. LC/MS/MS assay performance measures and peptide concentrations are summarized in Table 1 and Figure 8. Kidney Ang-I and Ang-(1-7) concentrations were different between groups, but evaluation by *post-hoc* comparison did not reveal any significant differences. Kidney levels of Ang-II and Ang-(2-10) were not different between groups. The statistical power of the test

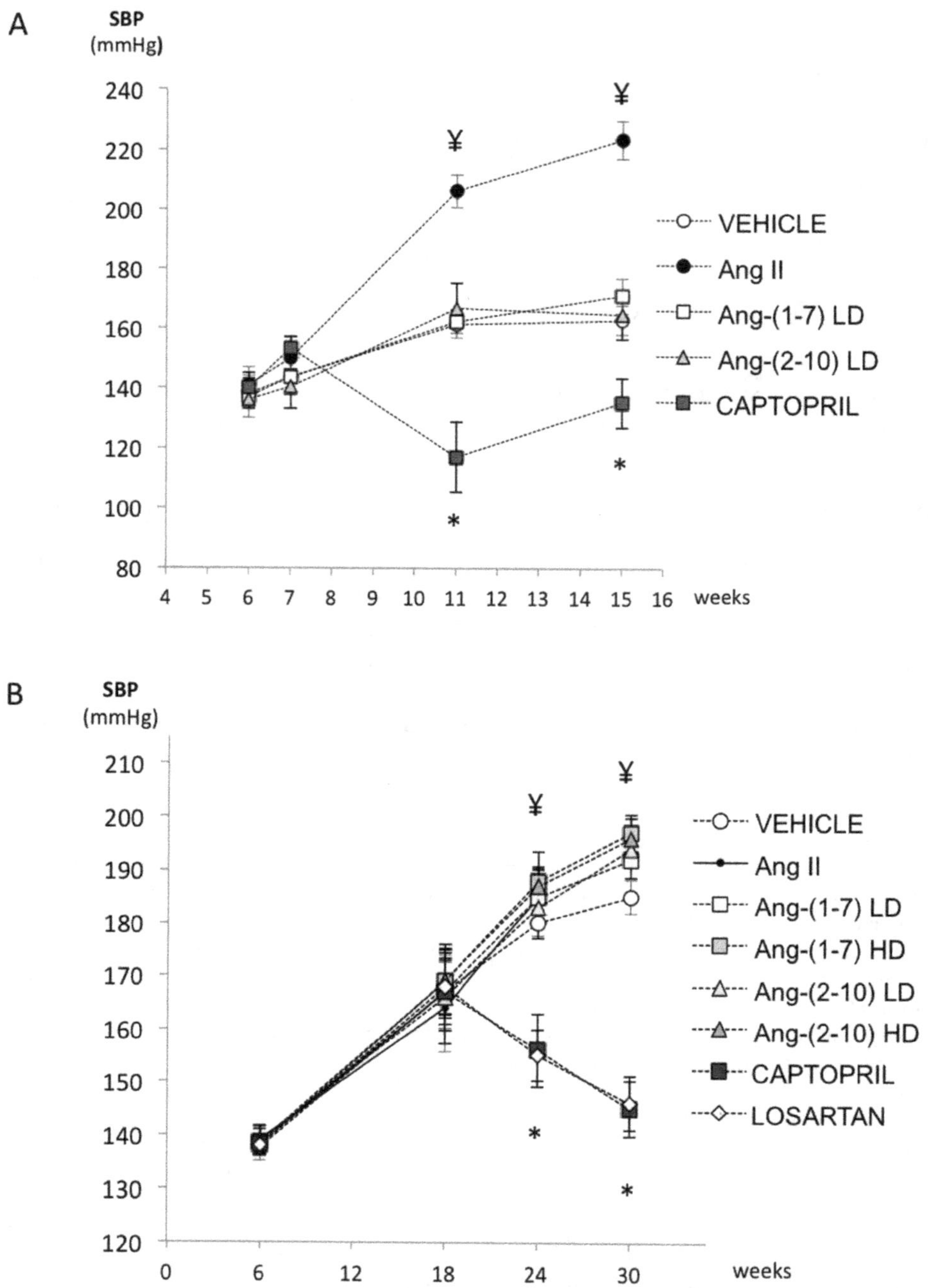

Figure 3. Effect of Ang peptides on blood pressure. Tail-cuff systolic blood pressure readings in uni-nephrectomized FHH rats obtained in *A: early disease protocol [n = 4/group, except captopril group (n = 5)]:* at the time of uni-nephrectomy (week 6), initial mini-pump implantation (week 7), mini-pump exchange (week 11), and sacrifice (week 15); or *B: late disease protocol [n = 9/group, except vehicle group (n = 7)]:* at the time of uni-nephrectomy (week 6), initial mini-pump implantation (week 18), mini-pump exchange (week 24), and sacrifice (week 30). * = significantly lower than vehicle (p = 0.014); ¥ = significantly higher than vehicle (p<0.001). Only 2 rats from the Ang-(2-10) HD group and none of the Ang-II group were alive at week 30. Data are in means ± SEM. SBP = systolic blood pressure, LD = low-dose, HD = high-dose.

for both Ang-II and Ang-(2-10) were 0.27 and 0.05, respectively. When Ang-II levels were compared separately between vehicle and captopril groups using a Mann-Whitney U test, they were found to be lower in captopril-treated rats (p = 0.002) suggesting that the multi-group comparisons were underpowered. Because the majority of rats treated with high-dose Ang-(2-10) did not survive, we were unable to determine the effect of high-dose Ang-(2-10) treatment on Ang-(2-10) kidney content. Table S2 shows the range of previously reported intrarenal Ang peptide concentration in comparison to this study [17,30–34].

Although individual Ang-(1-7) peptide levels were not elevated in the Ang-(1-7) infused groups, the ratio of Ang-(1-7)/Ang-II content was higher in both the low dose and high dose groups compared to vehicle (Figure 9), suggesting an effect of Ang-(1-7) infusion on Ang peptide balance in the kidney, but were not different from captopril treatment, a finding that is in line with a known effect of ACE inhibition on Ang-(1-7) degradation and

Table 2. Body weight, kidney weight and urine volumes at initiation of therapy and study end.

	Body Wt (g)		Kidney Wt (g)	Kid. Wt/B. Wt (g/100 g b.wt)	Urine Volume (ml/day)	
Early Disease Model [n = 4/group, except captopril group (n = 5)]						
	Baseline (week 7)	Final (week 15)	Final (week 15)		Baseline (week 7)	Final (week 15)
Vehicle (0.9% NaCl)	175 (13)	320 (18)	1.9 (0.3)	0.6 (0.0)	31.4 (6.2)	28.4 (2.7)
Ang-II	185 (43)	323 (18)	2.0 (0.2)	0.7 (0.1)	39.7 (15.1)	37.6 (14.1)
Ang-(1-7) LD	176 (23)	317 (22)	2.0 (0.2)	0.6 (0.1)	34.8 (10.4)	28.5 (2.3)
Ang-(2-10) LD	160 (17)	299 (23)	1.9 (0.2)	0.7 (0.1)	30.9 (6.3)	30.9 (5.3)
Captopril	158 (3)	284 (10)	1.6 (0.1)	0.5 (0.0)	30.9 (2.3)	31.5 (1.0)
Late Disease Model [n = 9/group, except vehicle (n = 7) and final Ang-(2-10) HD group (n = 2)]						
	Baseline (week 18)	Final (week 30)	Final (week 30)		Baseline (week 18)	
Vehicle (0.9% NaCl)	340 (16)	340 (43)	2.0 (0.4)	0.6 (0.1)	27.9 (5.4)	37.6 (6.4)
Ang-(1-7) LD	342 (13)	344 (21)	2.1 (0.2)	0.6 (0.1)	32.6 (7.6)	36.7 (11.4)
Ang-(1-7) HD	341 (23)	340 (22)	2.0 (0.3)	0.6 (0.0)	31.5 (5.6)	40.4 (9.7)
Ang-(2-10) LD	340 (33)	336 (41)	2.1 (0.2)	0.6 (0.1)	32.1 (6.7)	43.5 (5.5)
Ang-(2-10) HD	350 (22)	339 (8)	1.6 (0.6)	0.5 (0.4)	30.7 (6.6)	40.2 (7.8)
Captopril	338 (15)	354 (16)	1.9 (0.1)	0.5 (0.1)	28.5 (5.3)	31.6 (11)
Losartan	339 (14)	351 (22)	2.1 (0.1)	0.6 (0.1)	29.0 (4.8)	35.1 (8)

Data are in means (SD). Wt: weight, B: body, Kid: kidney, LD: low-dose, HD: high-dose.

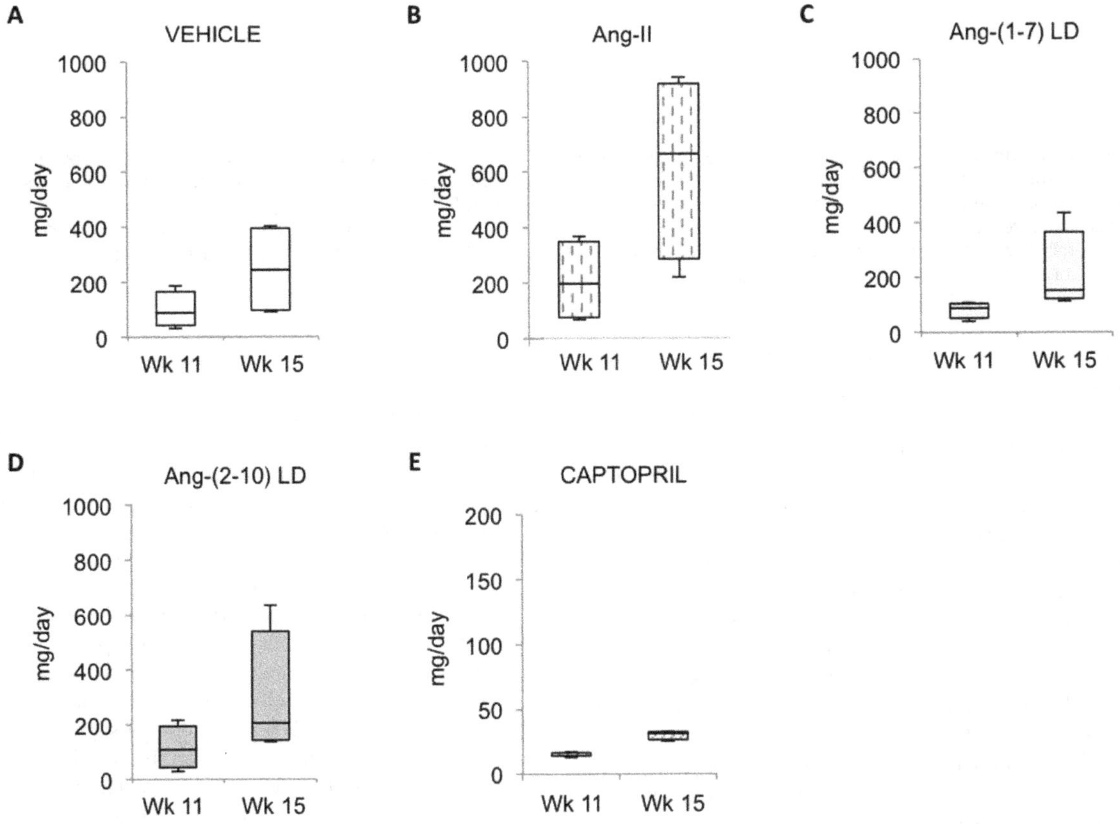

Figure 4. Effect of Ang peptides on proteinuria during the early disease protocol. Urinary protein excretion measured in uninephrectomized FHH rats treated with: *A*: vehicle; *B*: Ang-II; *C*: low-dose Ang-(1-7); *D*: low-dose Ang-(2-10); and *E*: captopril; for 8 weeks, i.e., between weeks 7 and 15 after birth; n = 4/group, except captopril group (n = 5). LD = low-dose, HD = high-dose.

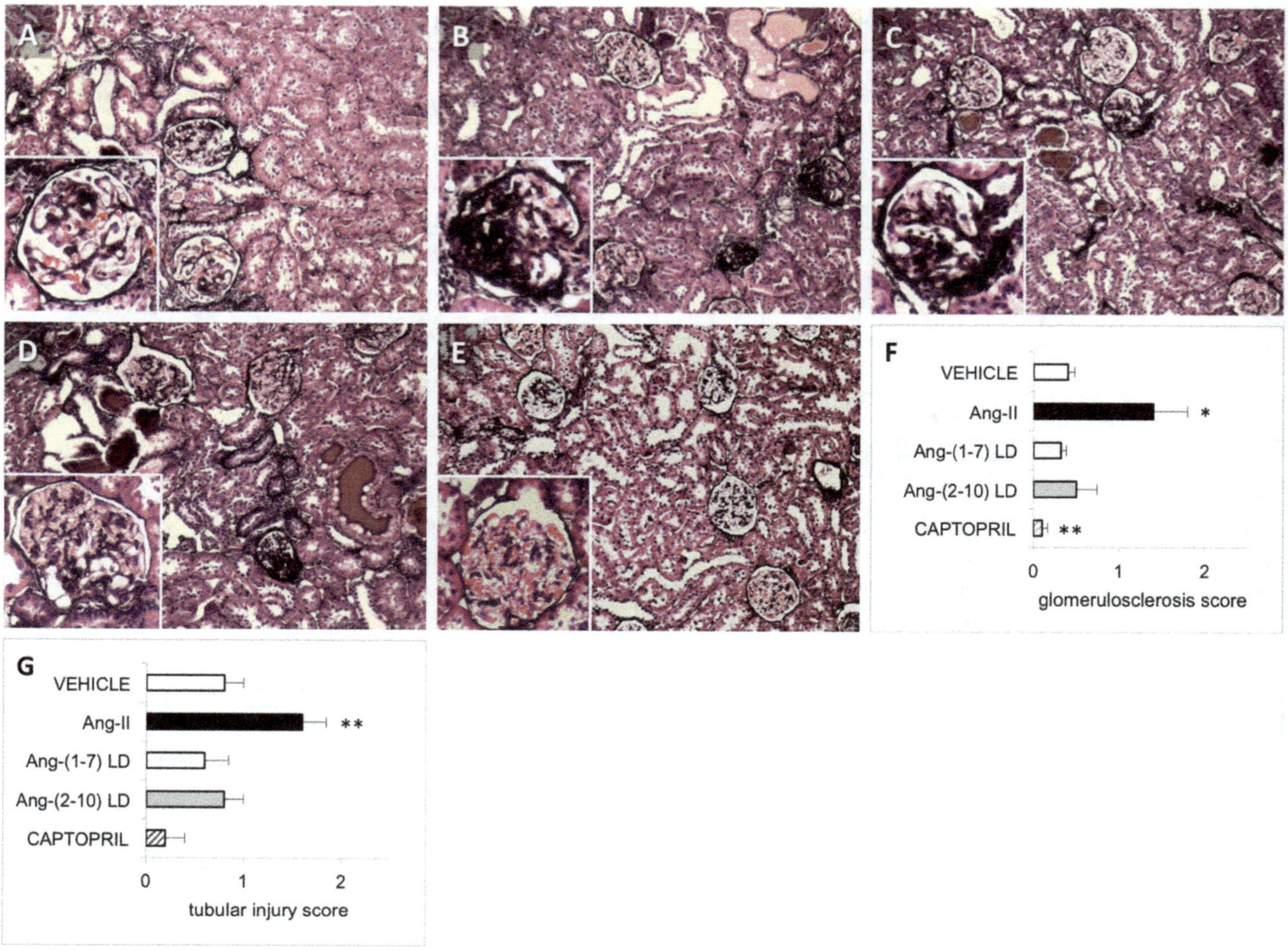

Figure 5. Effect of Ang peptides on renal histology during the early disease protocol. Representative light microscopy (10×) images of kidney cortex specimens of uni-nephrectomized FHH rats double-stained with hematoxylin-eosin (H&E) and Jones silver stain. Tissue was harvested at the end of the early disease protocol, i.e., after 8 weeks of treatment with: *A*: vehicle; *B*: Ang II; *C*: Ang-(1-7) LD; *D*: Ang-(2-10) LD; and *E*: captopril. *F*: Glomerulosclerosis scores. *G*: Tubular injury scores. Insets show a representative glomerulus. Segmental glomerulosclerosis and microcystic tubular dilatation is appreciated in all treatment groups. * = $p<0.01$ compared to vehicle; ** = $p<0.05$ compared to vehicle n = 4/group, except captopril group (n = 5). Data are in means ± SEM. LD = low-dose.

Ang-II generation [32]. Low-dose Ang-(1-7) infusion also resulted in an elevation in the Ang-I/Ang-II and Ang-(2-10)/Ang-II ratios compared to vehicle-infused controls ($p = 0.01$) but was not different from captopril-treated animals. The effects of Ang-(1-7) and captopril on Ang-(1-7)/Ang-I and Ang-(2-10)/Ang-I ratios could not be discerned by *post hoc* comparison, despite the fact that significant differences between groups were detected (ANOVA, $p<0.05$). Infusion of low-dose Ang-(2-10) did not significantly change any ratio compared to vehicle.

In agreement with the pathogenesis of FSGS, we found a significant correlation between proteinuria and increase in kidney size, likely from glomerulomegaly (Table S3). We also found a significant correlation between systolic blood pressure and urinary volume, possibly reflecting pressure natriuresis. In terms of Ang peptide content, higher Ang-II abundance was associated with increased kidney size and urinary volume, whereas Ang-(1-7) exhibited an even stronger correlation with urinary volume, possibly due to its reported aquaretic property [35]. No Ang peptide level correlated with the degree of proteinuria.

Discussion

Our study demonstrates that chronic intravenous administration of Ang-(1-7) or Ang-(2-10) does not ameliorate glomerulosclerosis in a spontaneous rat model of FSGS. The lack of benefit of these alternative Ang peptides was observed regardless of the delivered dose or the stage of the disease studied. We opted to infuse the peptides longer that previously done by others in order to allow more time for the peptide to elicit a measurable effect. However, no reduction in glomerular injury was observed after 8 weeks of infusion during the early disease protocol or after 12 weeks of infusion during the late disease protocol, for either Ang-(1-7) or Ang-(2-10). Our study is the first to evaluate the long-term effect of 2 doses of Ang-(1-7) in a model of spontaneous FSGS.

Significant enthusiasm was raised by a body of evidence suggesting potentially beneficial cardiovascular effects of Ang-(1-7) in various *in vitro* and *in vivo* models of heart and kidney disease [36,37]. Those studies demonstrated that Ang-(1-7) can elicit biological actions that are antagonistic to those of Ang-II. Stimulated by those observations, many laboratories have searched for a renoprotective effect of Ang-(1-7) in various rodent

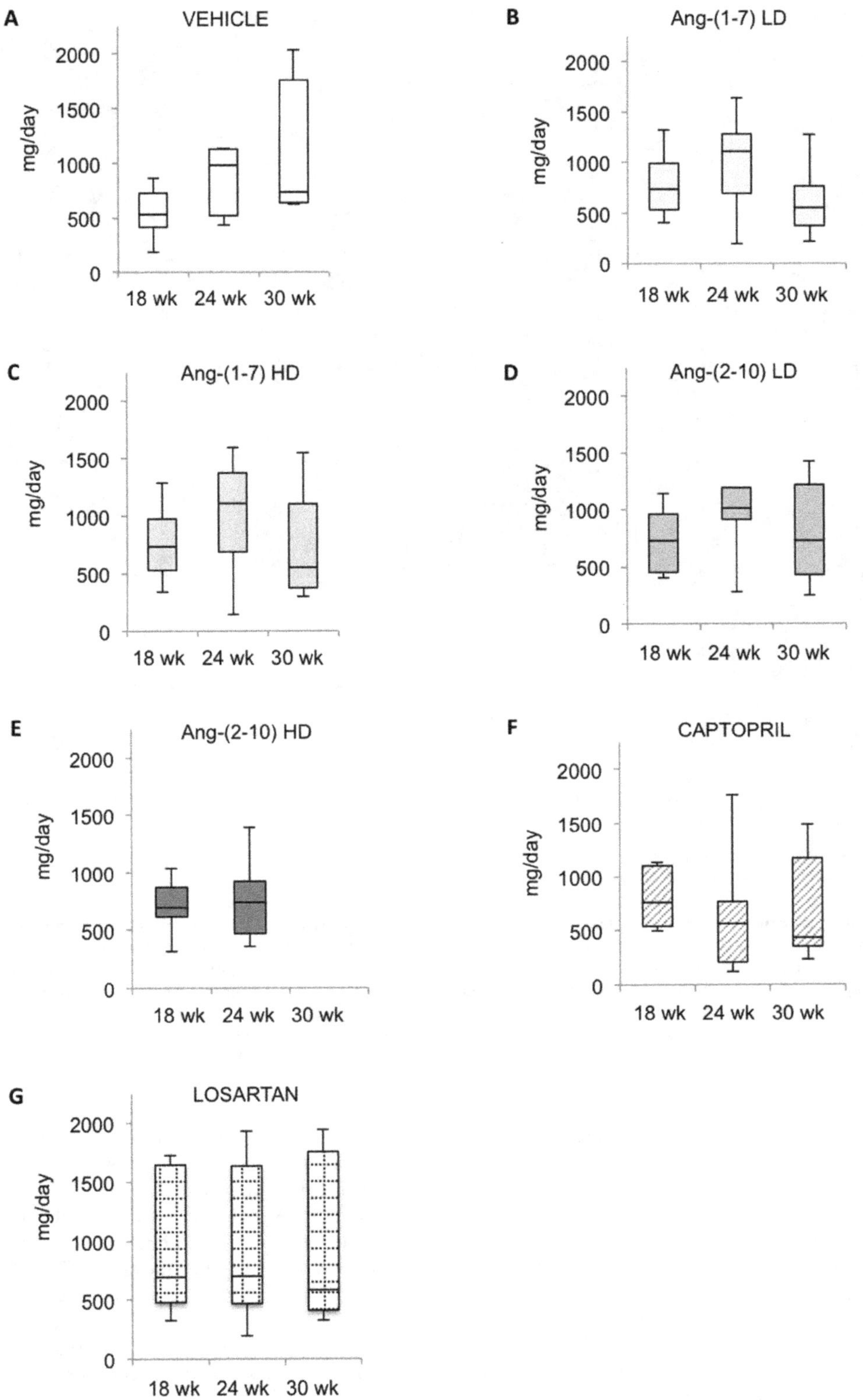

Figure 6. Effect of Ang peptides on proteinuria during the late disease protocol. Urinary protein excretion measured in uni-nephrectomized Fawn-Hooded Hypertensive rats treated with: *A:* vehicle; *B:* low-dose Ang-(1-7); *C:* high-dose Ang-(1-7); *D:* low-dose Ang-(2-10); *E:* high-dose Ang-(2-10); *F:* captopril and *G:* losartan for 12 weeks, i.e., between weeks 18 and 30 after birth; n = 9/group, except vehicle group (n = 7). LD = low-dose, HD = high-dose.

models of human glomerular disease [18]. The majority of those studies administered Ang-(1-7) via osmotic mini-pump at a dose of 400 ng/kg/min, whereas others used 100 ng/kg/min, doses that we categorized as high and low, respectively. Overall, the results obtained across all studies have not been uniform. In a study where Ang-(1-7) was delivered via a route similar to that employed

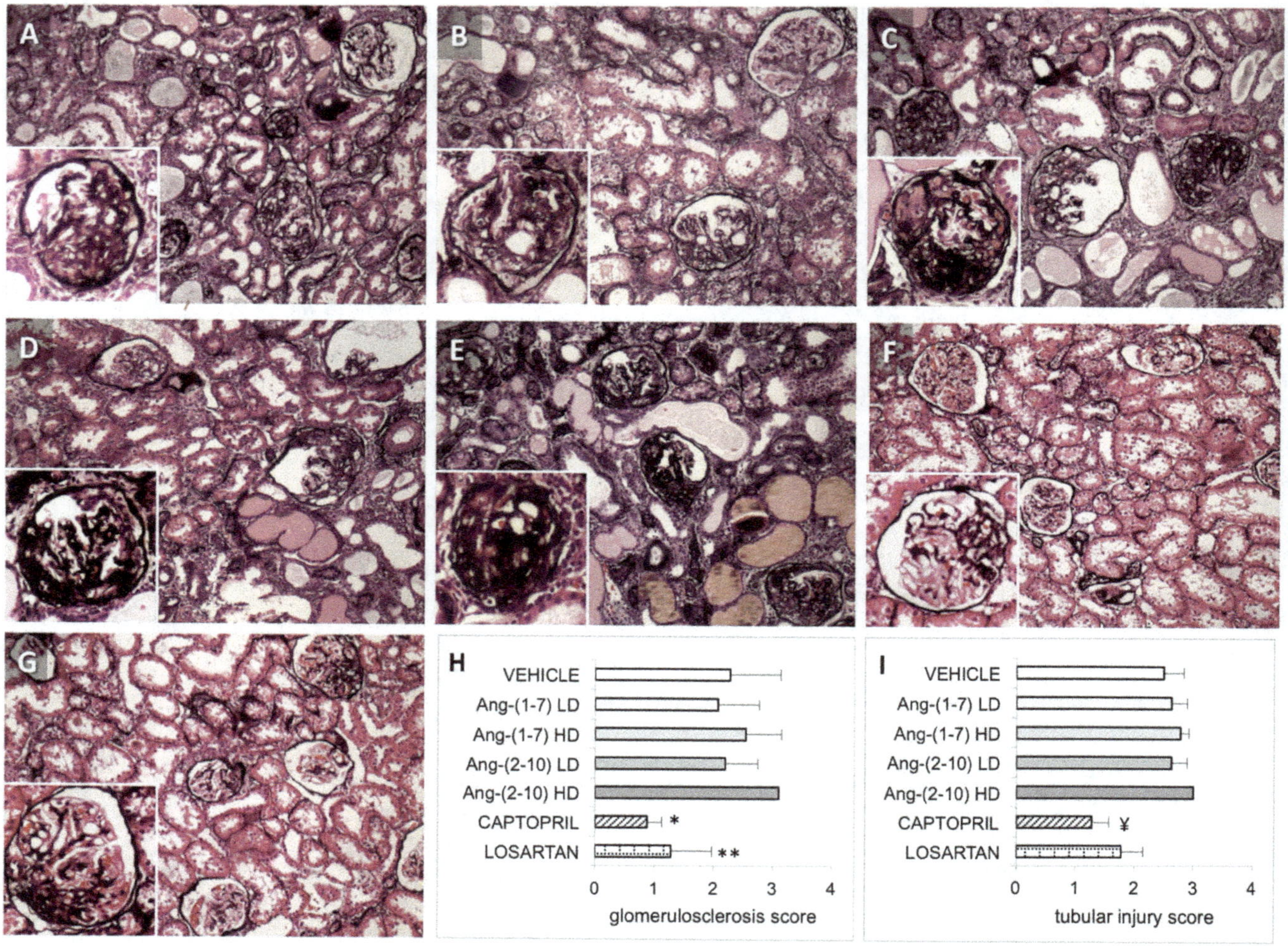

Figure 7. Effect of Ang peptides on renal histology during the late disease protocol. Representative light microscopy (10×) images of kidney cortex sections of uni-nephrectomized Fawn-Hooded Hypertensive rats double-stained with hematoxylin-eosin (H&E) and Jones silver stain. Tissue was harvested at week 30, i.e., after 12 weeks of treatment with: *A:* vehicle; *B:* Ang-(1-7) LD; *C:* Ang-(1-7) HD; *D:* Ang-(2-10) LD; *E:* Ang-(2-10) HD; *F:* captopril; *G:* losartan; *H:* glomerulosclerosis scores; *I:* tubular injury scores. Insets show a representative glomerulus. Significant segmental and global glomerulosclerosis, glomerular collapse and microcystic tubular dilatation is appreciated in all treatment groups, except in captopril-treated and losartan-treated rats. * = $p<0.0001$ compared to vehicle; ** = $p<0.005$ compared to vehicle; ¥ = $p<0.05$ compared to vehicle; n = 9/group except for vehicle group (n = 7) and Ang-(2-10) HD (n = 2). Data are in means ± SEM. LD = low-dose, HD = high-dose.

in this study, i.e., intravenously, for 2 weeks, Ang-(1-7) had no effect on either blood pressure or proteinuria in a rat model of adriamycin-induced nephrosis [16]. In a mouse remnant kidney model of progressive glomerulopathy, mesangial expansion was worsened after 4 weeks of subcutaneous administration of Ang-(1-7), while blood pressure remained unaffected [4]. In a rat remnant kidney model, blood pressure was increased by Ang-(1-7) delivered subcutaneously [38]. Proteinuria was not altered in either of the remnant kidney studies. In contrast, in a model of mesangioproliferative glomerulonephritis, anti-Thy1.1 nephritis, Ang-(1-7) ameliorated the degree of glomerular scarring and decreased proteinuria [14]. Furthermore, the reported effects of Ang-(1-7) infusion on models of diabetic kidney disease have been conflicting. Benter *et al.* reported a decrease in blood pressure and proteinuria after 4 weeks of intraperitoneal Ang-(1-7) in spontaneously hypertensive rats injected with streptozotocin [39], whereas Shao *et al.* observed worsening proteinuria and transforming growth factor beta accumulation after 6 weeks of intravenous Ang-(1-7) in streptozotocin-induced diabetic rats [17]. Differences in methodology may account for some of the discrepancy among studies, including dose of the peptide, route of administration, duration of therapy and disease model. However, it remains difficult to reconcile the findings across laboratories. Furthermore, Ang-(1-7) has been reported to both attenuate [40] and promote [41] profibrotic pathways though *mas* receptor stimulation in cultured mesangial cells. Therefore, glomerular cells may exhibit variable responses to Ang-(1-7) depending on the experimental conditions.

Despite the vasodilatory effect of Ang-(1-7) reported by others [42,43], we did not observe a reduction in systolic blood pressure in Ang-(1-7)-infused animals. On the contrary, animals treated with high-dose Ang-(1-7) experienced an increase in blood pressure. Previous studies also found pressor effect of Ang-(1-7) in rat models of kidney disease [38,44]. Our radioligand binding curves indicate that Ang-(1-7) has low affinity for the AT_1 receptor. However, it is conceivable that at the administered pharmacological doses, Ang-(1-7) may have elicited some degree of AT_1 receptor stimulation, thereby explaining the observed rise in systolic blood pressure. However, such mechanism remains speculative. Alternatively, binding affinity might change in disease

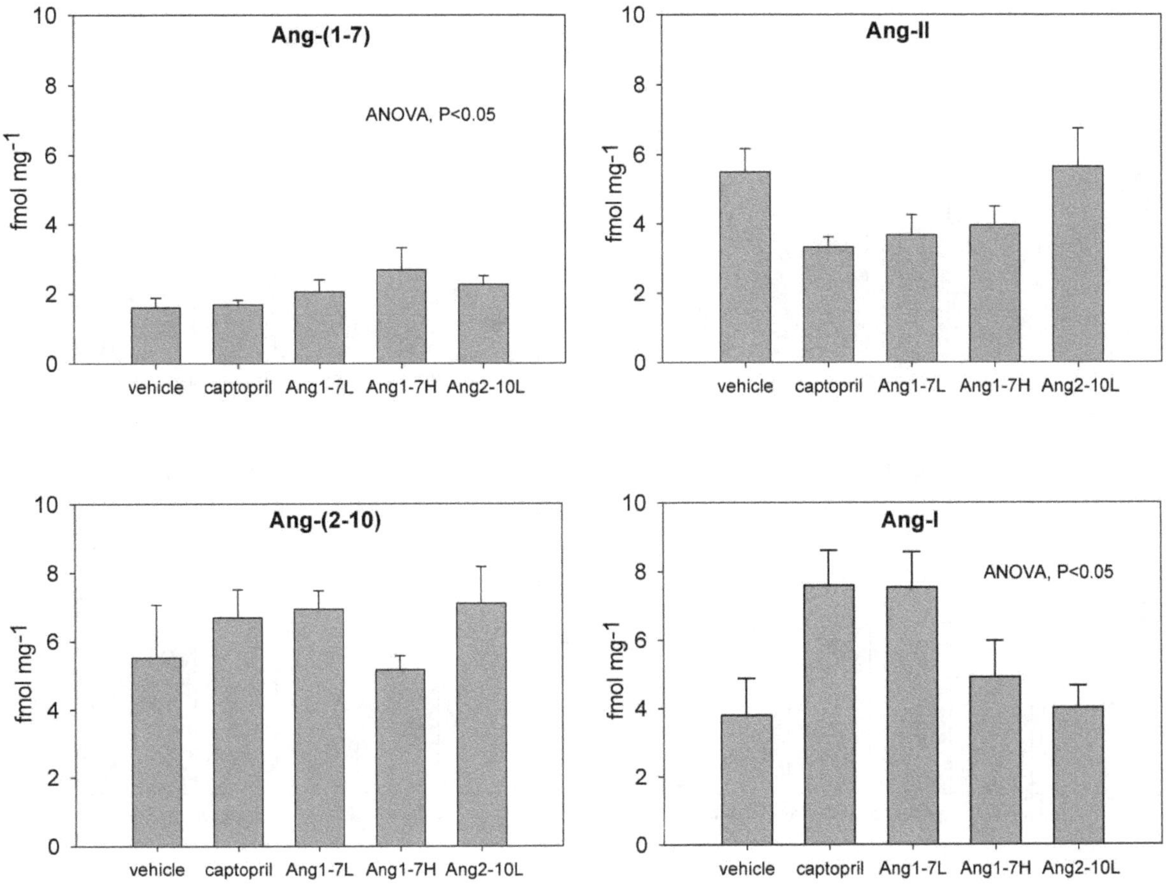

Figure 8. Intrarenal Ang peptide content as measured by Parallel Reaction Monitoring. Kidneys were harvested at the end of the late disease protocol (after 12 weeks of therapy). Treatment arms are listed in the *x*-axes. ANOVA ($p<0.05$) indicates differences between groups that were detected, but no pairwise differences were significant; n = 5/group Data are in means ± SEM. L = low-dose, H = high-dose.

states. Others have reported that Ang-(1-7) is capable of binding the AT_1 receptor [45]. We did not treat animals simultaneously with Ang-(1-7) and losartan to determine if the pressor effect of Ang-(1-7) could be reduced by AT_1 receptor blockade. However, even under those circumstances, it would be difficult to ascertain whether the observed pressor effect of Ang-(1-7) is indeed AT_1 receptor-mediated because losartan alone reduced blood pressure in our animals. Because a *mas* receptor antagonist was not utilized, it cannot be determined whether the observed pressor effect of Ang-(1-7) was *mas* receptor-mediated.

Stimulation of the AT_2 receptor may mitigate parenchymal injury in models of renal disease by antagonizing the pro-inflammatory effects of Ang-II [46]. Thus, the observed higher affinity of Ang-(2-10) for the AT_2 receptor compared to the AT_1 receptor led us to postulate that preponderance of AT_2 stimulation may result in a renoprotective effect in our rat model of FSGS. However, there was no significant effect of Ang-(2-10) infusion at a dose of 100 ng/kg/min, neither early nor late in the disease, on blood pressure, proteinuria or histology. Furthermore, when given at a higher dose of 400 ng/kg/min, Ang-(2-10) raised systolic blood pressure and led to the demise of 7 out of the 9 treated animals. Therefore, we speculate that at the higher administered pharmacological doses, Ang-(2-10) could potentially stimulate AT_1 receptors. However, further studies will be necessary to verify this hypothesis.

Because this investigation aimed to induce a local effect in the kidneys by infusion of Ang-(1-7) or Ang-(2-10), we quantified the kidney content of a panel of Ang peptides to determine whether the intravenous delivery of the Ang peptides led to a corresponding increase in their concentration in the kidney. We utilized PRM (nano-flow LC-MS/MS) as an analytical technique for peptide quantification because of its superior specificity compared to antibody-based methods. Although there appear to be a dose-dependent increase in Ang-(1-7) kidney content in Ang-(1-7)-treated rats, no significant difference was found when the content of the heptapeptide was compared to that of vehicle-treated rats. Therefore, the intravenous route may be an inadequate strategy to elevate Ang peptide content in the kidney. However, because whole kidney homogenates were analyzed, our measurements may have underestimated actual changes in cortical Ang peptide concentrations. In addition, plasma Ang peptide concentration was not measured to verify whether pharmacological concentrations of the delivered peptides were reached. Furthermore, it is not known whether the local concentration of Ang peptides is altered in FHH rat kidneys as the kidney disease evolves. Therefore, intrinsic abundance of endogenous Ang peptides in injured FHH rat kidneys may comprise a large fraction of Ang peptide concentration relative to the delivered amount of Ang-(1-7) or Ang-(2-10).

In summary, chronic intravenous administration of Ang-(1-7) or Ang-(2-10) failed to ameliorate glomerular damage in a rat model

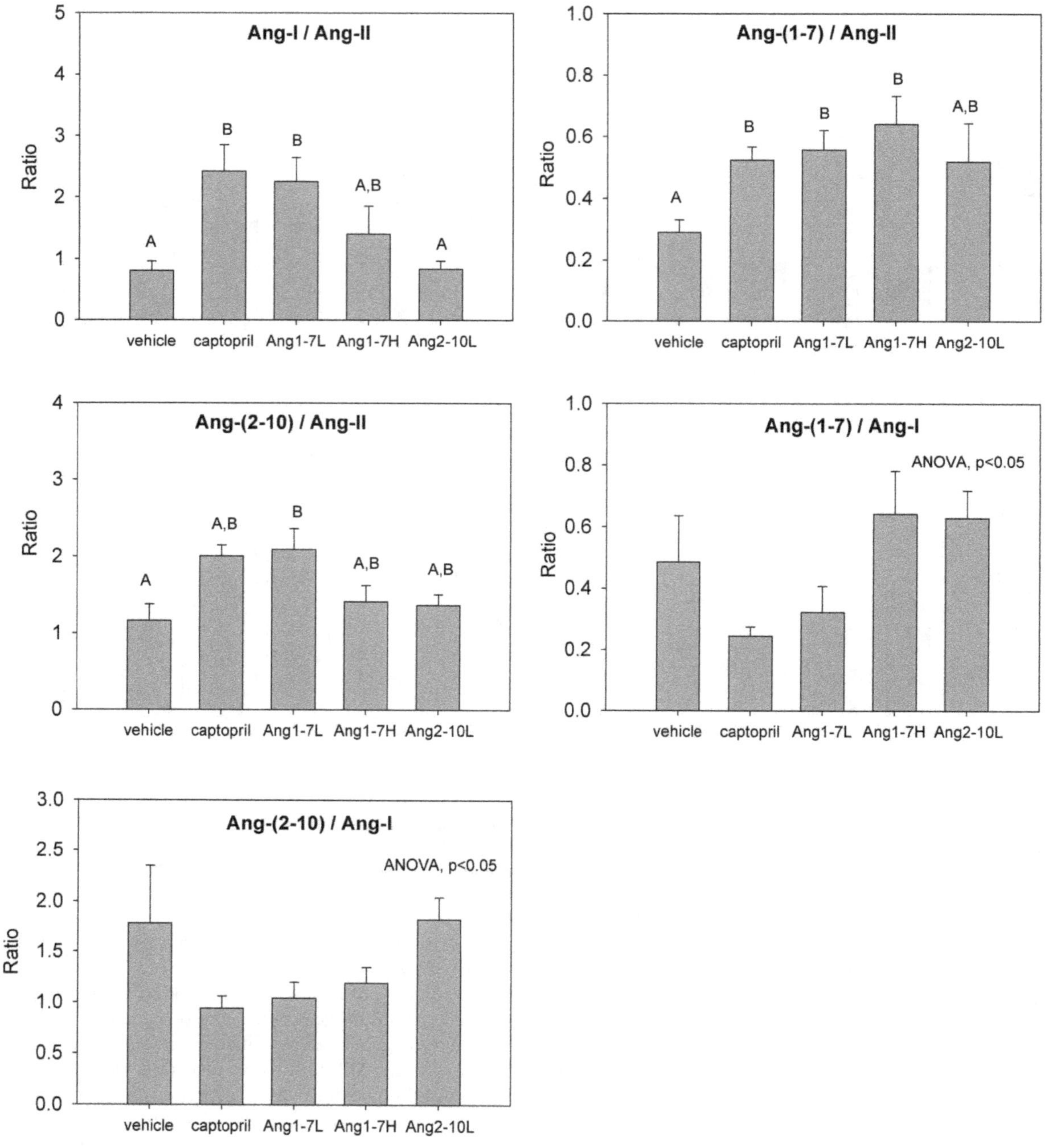

Figure 9. Ratios of intrarenal Ang peptide abundance. Kidneys were harvested at the end of the late disease protocol (after 12 weeks of therapy). Treatment arms are listed in the *x*-axes. Group specific *post-hoc* pairwise differences ($P<0.05$) are indicated by letters. Equivalent letters indicate groups that are not significantly different from each other and different letters indicate a significant difference was detected between groups. ANOVA ($p<0.05$) indicates if differences between groups were detected, but no pairwise differences were significant; n = 5/group Data are in means ± SEM. L = low-dose, H = high-dose.

of FSGS. The lack of benefit might be related to an undesired hypertensive effect of the peptides and/or suboptimal peptide delivery to the kidney attained with intravenous delivery.

Supporting Information

Table S1 Urine sodium excretion rates.

Table S2 Intrarenal Ang peptide concentrations gathered from previous publications for comparison with this study. Data from Nishiyama et al. were extracted from supplementary table and from the text of the results section and included all pharmacological manipulations. Range of means ± SE were extracted when possible. RIA, Radioimmunoassay; LC/MS/MS, liquid chromatography tandem mass spectrometry; HPLC, High Performance Liquid Chromatography. * Seikaly et al. reported immunoreactive angiotensin peptides of which 23% was considered to be Ang-II.

Table S3 Spearman Rank correlations between Ang peptide content and phenotypical parameters. Significant correlations are listed for $p<0.05$.

Acknowledgments

We wish to thank Alison Bland for her assistance preparing lysates for MS/MS. We also wish to thank Dr. Mark Lortie for his helpful advice during the design of the MS/MS protocol.

Portions of this work were presented in abstract form at the annual meeting of the American Society of Nephrology (Renal Week) in San Diego, CA, in November, 2012.

Author Contributions

Conceived and designed the experiments: JCV MGJ JMA WRF. Performed the experiments: MGJ MPH JR. Analyzed the data: JCV MGJ TAM SES WRF. Contributed reagents/materials/analysis tools: JCV TAM JMA SES. Wrote the paper: JCV MGJ WRF. Reviewed and approved the manuscript: JCV MGJ MPH TAM JR SES JMA WRF.

References

1. Ibrahim HN, Rosenberg ME, Hostetter TH (1997) Role of the renin-angiotensin-aldosterone system in the progression of renal disease: a critical review. Seminars in nephrology 17: 431–440.
2. Colucci JA, Yuri Arita D, Sousa Cunha T, Seno Di Marco G, Vio CP, et al. (2011) Renin-angiotensin system may trigger kidney damage in NOD mice. Journal of the renin-angiotensin-aldosterone system: JRAAS 12: 15–22.
3. Fukuda A, Wickman LT, Venkatareddy MP, Sato Y, Chowdhury MA, et al. (2012) Angiotensin II-dependent persistent podocyte loss from destabilized glomeruli causes progression of end stage kidney disease. Kidney international 81: 40–55.
4. Velez JC, Ryan KJ, Harbeson CE, Bland AM, Budisavljevic MN, et al. (2009) Angiotensin I is largely converted to angiotensin (1-7) and angiotensin (2-10) by isolated rat glomeruli. Hypertension 53: 790–797.
5. Velez JC, Bland AM, Arthur JM, Raymond JR, Janech MG (2007) Characterization of renin-angiotensin system enzyme activities in cultured mouse podocytes. American journal of physiology Renal physiology 293: F398–407.
6. Velez JC, Ierardi JL, Bland AM, Morinelli TA, Arthur JM, et al. (2012) Enzymatic processing of angiotensin peptides by human glomerular endothelial cells. American journal of physiology Renal physiology 302: F1583–1594.
7. Grobe N, Weir NM, Leiva O, Ong FS, Bernstein KE, et al. (2013) Identification of prolyl carboxypeptidase as an alternative enzyme for processing of renal angiotensin II using mass spectrometry. American journal of physiology Cell physiology 304: C945–953.
8. Santos RA, Simoes e Silva AC, Maric C, Silva DM, Machado RP, et al. (2003) Angiotensin-(1-7) is an endogenous ligand for the G protein-coupled receptor Mas. Proceedings of the National Academy of Sciences of the United States of America 100: 8258–8263.
9. Haulica I, Bild W, Mihaila CN, Ionita T, Boisteanu CP, et al. (2003) Biphasic effects of angiotensin (1-7) and its interactions with angiotensin II in rat aorta. Journal of the renin-angiotensin-aldosterone system: JRAAS 4: 124–128.
10. Simoes e Silva AC, Bello AP, Baracho NC, Khosla MC, Santos RA (1998) Diuresis and natriuresis produced by long term administration of a selective Angiotensin-(1-7) antagonist in normotensive and hypertensive rats. Regulatory peptides 74: 177–184.
11. Tallant EA, Ferrario CM, Gallagher PE (2005) Angiotensin-(1-7) inhibits growth of cardiac myocytes through activation of the mas receptor. American journal of physiology Heart and circulatory physiology 289: H1560–1566.
12. Yoshida M, Naito Y, Urano T, Takada A, Takada Y (2002) L-158,809 and (D-Ala(7))-angiotensin I/II (1-7) decrease PAI-1 release from human umbilical vein endothelial cells. Thrombosis research 105: 531–536.
13. Giani JF, Burghi V, Veiras LC, Tomat A, Munoz MC, et al. (2012) Angiotensin-(1-7) attenuates diabetic nephropathy in Zucker diabetic fatty rats. American journal of physiology Renal physiology 302: F1606–1615.
14. Zhang J, Noble NA, Border WA, Huang Y (2010) Infusion of angiotensin-(1-7) reduces glomerulosclerosis through counteracting angiotensin II in experimental glomerulonephritis. American journal of physiology Renal physiology 298: F579–588.
15. Dilauro M, Zimpelmann J, Robertson SJ, Genest D, Burns KD (2010) Effect of ACE2 and angiotensin-(1-7) in a mouse model of early chronic kidney disease. American journal of physiology Renal physiology 298: F1523–1532.
16. van der Wouden EA, Henning RH, Deelman LE, Roks AJ, Boomsma F, et al. (2005) Does angiotensin (1-7) contribute to the anti-proteinuric effect of ACE-inhibitors. Journal of the renin-angiotensin-aldosterone system: JRAAS 6: 96–101.
17. Shao Y, He M, Zhou L, Yao T, Huang Y, et al. (2008) Chronic angiotensin (1-7) injection accelerates STZ-induced diabetic renal injury. Acta pharmacologica Sinica 29: 829–837.
18. Zimmerman D, Burns KD (2012) Angiotensin-(1-7) in kidney disease: a review of the controversies. Clinical science 123: 333–346.
19. Min L, Sim MK, Xu XG (2000) Effects of des-aspartate-angiotensin I on angiotensin II-induced incorporation of phenylalanine and thymidine in cultured rat cardiomyocytes and aortic smooth muscle cells. Regulatory peptides 95: 93–97.
20. Kemp BA, Bell JF, Rottkamp DM, Howell NL, Shao W, et al. (2012) Intrarenal angiotensin III is the predominant agonist for proximal tubule angiotensin type 2 receptors. Hypertension 60: 387–395.
21. Kuijpers MH, Gruys E (1984) Spontaneous hypertension and hypertensive renal disease in the fawn-hooded rat. British journal of experimental pathology 65: 181–190.
22. de Keijzer MH, Provoost AP, Molenaar JC (1989) Proteinuria is an early marker in the development of progressive renal failure in hypertensive fawn-hooded rats. Journal of hypertension 7: 525–528.
23. Kreisberg JI, Karnovsky MJ (1978) Focal glomerular sclerosis in the fawn-hooded rat. The American journal of pathology 92: 637–652.
24. Morinelli TA, Raymond JR, Baldys A, Yang Q, Lee MH, et al. (2007) Identification of a putative nuclear localization sequence within ANG II AT(1A) receptor associated with nuclear activation. American journal of physiology Cell physiology 292: C1398–1408.
25. Simons JL, Provoost AP, De Keijzer MH, Anderson S, Rennke HG, et al. (1993) Pathogenesis of glomerular injury in the fawn-hooded rat: effect of unilateral nephrectomy. Journal of the American Society of Nephrology: JASN 4: 1362–1370.
26. Grobe JL, Mecca AP, Lingis M, Shenoy V, Bolton TA, et al. (2007) Prevention of angiotensin II-induced cardiac remodeling by angiotensin-(1-7). American journal of physiology Heart and circulatory physiology 292: H736–742.
27. Lowry OH, Rosebrough NJ, Farr AL, Randall RJ (1951) Protein measurement with the Folin phenol reagent. The Journal of biological chemistry 193: 265–275.
28. Lortie M, Bark S, Blantz R, Hook V (2009) Detecting low-abundance vasoactive peptides in plasma: progress toward absolute quantitation using nano liquid chromatography-mass spectrometry. Analytical biochemistry 394: 164–170.
29. Oliver JD 3rd, Simons JL, Troy JL, Provoost AP, Brenner BM, et al. (1994) Proteinuria and impaired glomerular permselectivity in uninephrectomized fawn-hooded rats. The American journal of physiology 267: F917–925.
30. Nishiyama A, Seth DM, Navar LG (2002) Renal interstitial fluid concentrations of angiotensins I and II in anesthetized rats. Hypertension 39: 129–134.
31. Seikaly MG, Arant BS Jr, Seney FD Jr (1990) Endogenous angiotensin concentrations in specific intrarenal fluid compartments of the rat. The Journal of clinical investigation 86: 1352–1357.
32. Campbell DJ, Lawrence AC, Towrie A, Kladis A, Valentijn AJ (1991) Differential regulation of angiotensin peptide levels in plasma and kidney of the rat. Hypertension 18: 763–773.
33. Navar LG, Lewis L, Hymel A, Braam B, Mitchell KD (1994) Tubular fluid concentrations and kidney contents of angiotensins I and II in anesthetized rats. Journal of the American Society of Nephrology: JASN 5: 1153–1158.
34. Prieto MC, Gonzalez-Villalobos RA, Botros FT, Martin VL, Pagan J, et al. (2011) Reciprocal changes in renal ACE/ANG II and ACE2/ANG 1-7 are associated with enhanced collecting duct renin in Goldblatt hypertensive rats. American journal of physiology Renal physiology 300: F749–755.
35. Joyner J, Neves LA, Stovall K, Ferrario CM, Brosnihan KB (2008) Angiotensin-(1-7) serves as an aquaretic by increasing water intake and diuresis in association with downregulation of aquaporin-1 during pregnancy in rats. American journal of physiology Regulatory, integrative and comparative physiology 294: R1073–1080.
36. Handa RK, Ferrario CM, Strandhoy JW (1996) Renal actions of angiotensin-(1-7): in vivo and in vitro studies. The American journal of physiology 270: F141–147.
37. Ferrario CM, Varagic J (2010) The ANG-(1-7)/ACE2/mas axis in the regulation of nephron function. American journal of physiology Renal physiology 298: F1297–1305.
38. Velkoska E, Dean RG, Griggs K, Burchill L, Burrell LM (2011) Angiotensin-(1-7) infusion is associated with increased blood pressure and adverse cardiac remodelling in rats with subtotal nephrectomy. Clinical science 120: 335–345.
39. Benter IF, Yousif MH, Dhaunsi GS, Kaur J, Chappell MC, et al. (2008) Angiotensin-(1-7) prevents activation of NADPH oxidase and renal vascular dysfunction in diabetic hypertensive rats. American journal of nephrology 28: 25–33.
40. Moon JY, Tanimoto M, Gohda T, Hagiwara S, Yamazaki T, et al. (2011) Attenuating effect of angiotensin-(1-7) on angiotensin II-mediated NAD(P)H oxidase activation in type 2 diabetic nephropathy of KK-A(y)/Ta mice. American journal of physiology Renal physiology 300: F1271–1282.
41. Zimpelmann J, Burns KD (2009) Angiotensin-(1-7) activates growth-stimulatory pathways in human mesangial cells. American journal of physiology Renal physiology 296: F337–346.

42. Benter IF, Diz DI, Ferrario CM (1993) Cardiovascular actions of angiotensin(1-7). Peptides 14: 679–684.
43. Benter IF, Ferrario CM, Morris M, Diz DI (1995) Antihypertensive actions of angiotensin-(1-7) in spontaneously hypertensive rats. The American journal of physiology 269: H313–319.
44. Ji H, Menini S, Zheng W, Pesce C, Wu X, et al. (2008) Role of angiotensin-converting enzyme 2 and angiotensin(1-7) in 17beta-oestradiol regulation of renal pathology in renal wrap hypertension in rats. Experimental physiology 93: 648–657.
45. Bosnyak S, Jones ES, Christopoulos A, Aguilar MI, Thomas WG, et al. (2011) Relative affinity of angiotensin peptides and novel ligands at AT1 and AT2 receptors. Clinical science 121: 297–303.
46. Dhande I, Ali Q, Hussain T (2013) Proximal tubule angiotensin AT2 receptors mediate an anti-inflammatory response via interleukin-10: role in renoprotection in obese rats. Hypertension 61: 1218–1226.

7

miR-375 Mediated Acquired Chemo-Resistance in Cervical Cancer by Facilitating EMT

Yuanming Shen, Jiansong Zhou, Yang Li, Feng Ye, Xiaoyun Wan, Weiguo Lu, Xing Xie, Xiaodong Cheng*

Department of Gynecologic Oncology, Women's Hospital, School of Medicine, Zhejiang University, Hangzhou, China

Abstract

Acquired chemo-resistance is one of the key causal factors in cancer death. Emerging evidences suggest that miRNA and epithelial–mesenchymal transition play critical roles in the chemo-resistance in cancers. Here, we showed the association of paclitaxel-resistance with miR-375 over-expression and epithelial–mesenchymal transition inducement in cervical cancer. Using different cervical cancer cell models, we found that paclitaxel transiently induced up-regulation of miR-375 expression, proliferation inhibition, transition from epithelial to mesenchymal phenotype, and consequently impaired paclitaxel sensitivity. Forced over-expression of miR-375 may suppress Ecadherin expression by a directly targeting pathway, which led to paclitaxel resistance. Contrarily, re-expression of Ecadherin partly reversed epithelial–mesenchymal transition phenotype and miR-375 induced paclitaxel-resistance. Our findings suggest that paclitaxel-induced miR-375 over-expression facilitates epithelial–mesenchymal transition process via directly targeting Ecadherin, proliferation inhibition, and consequently results in chemo-resistance in cervical cancer cells. A reversion of miR-375 or Ecadherin expression may be a novel therapeutic approach for overcoming chemo-resistance in cervical cancer.

Editor: Zhi-Ming Zheng, National Institute of Health - National Cancer Institute, United States of America

Funding: The authors would like to acknowledge the continuous financial support from the National Natural Science Foundation of China (grant No. 81172475 and 81172474), the Natural Science Foundation of Zhejiang Province of China (grant No. Z2110056, LQ13H160005 and Y2110206). The funders had no role in study design, data collection and analysis, decision to publish, or preparation of the manuscript.

Competing Interests: The authors have declared that no competing interests exist.

* Email: chengxd@zju.edu.cn

Introduction

Emerging evidences have revealed that chemo-resistance is associated with epithelial mesenchymal transition (EMT) in cancer cells, and the acquisition of chemo-resistance in cancer cells is accompanied by a transition from an epithelial to a mesenchymal phenotype [1–3]. For instance, various drug-resistant cancers, including oxaliplatin-resistant colorectal cancer cells [4], paclitaxel-resistant ovarian cancer cells [5], and gefitinib-resistant lung cancer cells [6], present the transition from epithelial to mesenchymal phenotype along with a loss of epithelial adhesion molecule Ecadherin and a gain of mesenchymal markers such as vimentin, Ncadherin, and fibronectin. More recent studies also have shown that chemotherapy agents can facilitate the epithelial to a mesenchymal phenotypic transformation in residual surviving cancer cells which may be one of the critical steps in acquired drug resistance in cancers [7,8]. Thus, acquirement of EMT becomes a key process contributing to the malignant phenotypes of cancer cells in resistance to chemotherapy. Therefore, the intervention of EMT process has been proposed as a therapeutic approach against acquired chemo-resistance.

MicroRNAs (miRNAs) act as important gene regulators in human genomes and their aberrant expression may promote not only tumori-genesis and tumor aggressiveness but also resistance to chemotherapy [9]. More recently, the studies have revealed that miRNAs play an integral role in modulating EMT, such as miR-200s that regulates EMT through inhibiting ZEB1/2, a transcription repressor of Ecadherin [1,10,11]. We recently reported that the expression of miR-375 was reduced in cervical cancer cells [12] and enforced over-expression of miR-375 significantly inhibited proliferation and blocked G1-S cell cycle transition [13]. In another study, we further observed that miR-375 was up-regulated in paclitaxel-treated cervical cells and tissues, and forced over-expression of miR-375 decreased paclitaxel sensitivity in cervical cancer [14]. However, the precise molecular mechanism underling miR-375 regulated drug resistance remains to be explored. By the miRNA targets gene prediction, we found a binding site between miR-375 and Ecadherin 3′-UTR, which indicated that Ecadherin was a potential direct target of miR-375. Therefore, we assume that miR-375 may participate in EMT regulation and acquired paclitaxel-resistance in cervical cancer cells.

In the present study, we found for the first time that paclitaxel inhibits proliferation, induces EMT, and up-regulates miR-375 expression simultaneously in cervical cancer cells. And miR-375 over-expression directly inhibited Ecadherin expression and facilitated paclitaxel-resistance. Thus, there is a distinct positive feedback mechanism among paclitaxel, miR-375, and EMT that leads to acquired chemo-resistance phenotypes in cervical cancer cells. Such a regulatory feedback loop results in miR-375 over-expression, the epithelial to a mesenchymal phenotypic transformation, and consequently acquirement of paclitaxel-resistance. Anyway, it could be believed that a break of such a feedback loop would, at least partly, overcome chemo -resistance in cervical cancer.

Materials and Methods

Patients and samples

The samples of cancer tissue were collected from 23 cervical squamous cell carcinoma patients with FIGO (2009) stage IB_2 or IIA_2 who underwent neo-adjuvant chemotherapy followed by type III radical hysterectomy between November 1, 2008 and May 30, 2010 in Women's Hospital, School of Medicine, Zhejiang University. The collection of all samples was approved by the Ethical Committee for Clinical Research from the Women's Hospital, School of Medicine, Zhejiang University and written informed consents were obtained.

All patients underwent 2 cycles of intravenous neo-adjuvant chemotherapy (paclitaxel 135 mg/m^2 and cisplatin 75 mg/m^2, 3-week interval) before surgery. The effect of chemotherapy was evaluated according to the Response Evaluation Criteria in Solid Tumors (RECIST) [15] as previously described[14]. Of all 23 patients, mean age was 36.5 years (range 20 to 65 years), had pre- and post-chemotherapy cervical tumor samples. The specified composition of each samples were determined by an experienced pathologist.

Cell culture and EMT inducement

Two human cervical cancer cell lines, SiHa and CaSki were cultured as previously described[14]. Human recombinant TGF-β1 and EGF-β were obtained from ProSpec-Tany Techno Gene Ltd (Israel), respectively used at a final concentration of 5 ng/ml and 2 ng/ml. The cancer cell lines were seeded 1×10^5/well in 6-well plates and incubated in serum-free medium overnight, and then treated with TGF-β1 or EGF-β for 72 h respectively, to induce the EMT.

RNA Extraction and Real-Time RT-PCR

Total RNAs containing miRNAs were extracted from liquid nitrogen preserved tissues or the harvested cells using 1 ml TRIZOL reagent (Invitrogen, Carlsbad, CA, USA) following the manufacturer's instructions. cDNA was synthesized with the PrimeScript RT reagent Kit (TaKaRa Otsu, Shiga, Japan). Quantitative RT-PCR (qRT-PCR) for miRNA and mRNA was performed as described previously[14]. The sequences of all primers are given in Table 1.

Cell Proliferation Assay and MTS Assay

To determine the effect of miR-375 and paclitaxel on proliferation of cervical cell lines, the cell proliferation was determined with MTT assay and CellTrace CFSE cell proliferation assay at 24, 48, 72, 96 hours and 5 days respectively. For viability experiments, cervical cancer cells with or without 10 nM paclitaxel treatment 72 hours were plated (SiHa, 3×10^3/well in 96-well plate and 2×10^5/well in 6-well plate; CaSki, 2×10^3/well in 96-well plate and 1×10^5/well in 6-well plate) and cultured overnight. In MTT assay the absorbance of samples was measured with a spectrophotometer reader at 490 nm. CellTrace CFSE cell proliferation assay was performed by staining activated cervical cancer with CellTrace CFSE cell proliferation dye (2.5 μM) (Invitrogen) and analyze using by flow cytometry with 488 nm excitation and emission filters. An in vitro paclitaxel chemosensitivity of cervical cancer cells was evaluated using MTS assay (Promega, Madison, WI) as previously described [12]. Four replicate wells were used for each analysis, and at least three independent experiments were performed.

Western Blot Analysis

A total of 50 mg protein was separated by denaturing 8–15% SDS–polyacrylamide gel electrophoresis. Western analysis was conducted as previously described [12]. The films were analyzed by densitometry with a VersaDoc Imaging System; Model 3000 (BioRad) using Quantity One software. Analysis of variance with Bonferroni correction for multiple tests was used to determine significance. The primary antibodies used were anti-Ncadherin (1:5000), anti-Ecadherin (1:2000), anti-fibronectin (1:1000), anti-vimentin (1:1000) and anti-actin (1:2000) as an endogenous control, all from Epitomics Biotechnology (Epitomics).

Immunohistochemistry

Sections (6 μm thick) of tumor tissue were cut from paraffinised 23 couples of self-paired pre-and post-chemotherapy cervical cancer samples, and immunohistochemistry analysis and scoring were described previously[12]. The primary antibodies used for immunohistochemistry analysis were anti-Ecadherin antibody (1:1000) and anti-actin antibody as an endogenous control (1:2000), both from Epitomics Biotechnology (Epitomics).

Lentivirus construction and transfection

To generate miR-375 and Ecadherin over-expression stable transfectants, cervical cancer cells were transfected with lentiviral expressing vectors. The plasmid construction and lentivirus package were complete in GENECHEM Company. The pre-miR-375 sequences were amplified and cloned into the pGCsil-GFP vector using the following primers: (Forward) hsa-pre-miR-375-XhoI-F, ACCGCTC GAGCCCCGCGAC-GAGCCCCTCGC; (Reverse) hsa-pre-mi-R-375-MfeI-R, AC-CGCAATTGAAAAAGCCTCACGCGAGCCGAACG. The hsa-CDH1 (CDS) gene was amplified and cloned into a pGC-FU-GFP vector using the following primers: (Forward) 5′-GAGGATCCCCGGGTACCGGTCGCCAC-

Table 1. Sequences of primers for miRNAs, RNU6, and EEF1A1.

miR-375 RT	5′-GTCGTATCCAGTGCAGGGTCCGAGGTATTCGCACTGGATACGACTCACGC-3′
miR-375 forward	5′-AGCCGTTTGTTCGTTCGGCT-3′
miR-375 reverse	5′-GTGCAGGGTCCGAGGT-3′
U6 snRNA RT	5′-AACGCTTCACGAATTTGCGT-3′
U6 snRNA forward	5′-CTCGCTTCGGCAGCACA-3′
U6 snRNA reverse	5′-AACGCTTCACGAATTTGCGT-3′
EEF1A1 forward	5′-TGCGGTGGGTGTCATCAAA-3′
EEF1A1 reverse	5′-AAGAGTGGGGTGGCAGGTATTG-3′

CATGGGCCCTTGGAGCCGCAG-3′, (Reverse) 5′-TCATCCTTGTAGTCGC-TAGCGTCGTCCTCGCCGCCTCCGTACATG-3′. Viruses packaging were performed in HEK 293 T cells after the cotransfection of 20 mg pGCsil-GFP-pre-miR-375 vector or pGC-GFP-CDH1 vector with 15 mg of the packaging plasmid pHelper 1.0 Vector and 10 mg of the envelope plasmid pHelper 2.0 vector using Lipofectamine 2000. Viruses were harvested 48 h after transfection, and viral titers were determined. The titers of the viral used in this study were in the range of $5\times10^{8}\sim2\times10^{9}$ TU/mL.

To generate miR-375 and Ecadherin over-expression stable transfectants, cervical cancer cells were transfected with lentiviral expressing vectors as previously described [12]. An MOI = 5 was used for SiHa and MOI = 10 was used for CaSki. After 4~7 d of transfection, stable clones were selected with GFP by flow cytometry and harvested for further experimentation. An empty pGC FU-GFP-NC-LV vector was used as a negative control.

Luciferase Activity Assay

To investigate whether CDH1 expression was regulated by miR-375, a psicheck-2 dual-luciferase miRNA target expression vector (psicheck-2 -UTR vector) was used to perform the luciferase activity assay. The wild and mutant type 3′-UTR of CDH1 containing predicted miR-375 binding site was synthesized and inserted into the 3′-UTR region downstream of the firefly luciferase gene of psicheck-2 vector (psicheck-2 -UTR) using the Xho I and NotI I restriction sites. All constructs were verified by sequencing. After cotransfected with miR-375 mimics (20 uM) and reporter vectors (0.2 μg/mL), luciferase activities were measured at 24 hours using a Dual-Glo luciferase assay system (Promega). Relative luciferase activity in all figures refers to firefly luciferase activities normalized to Renilla luciferase. Values cells with empty psicheck-2 vector were set equally to 1.

Statistical Analysis

The experiments were repeated at least three times. Results are expressed as mean ± s.e.m. An independent Student's t-test or an ANOVA was used to compare continuous variables. Pearson's correlation coefficient test was used to assess the correlation between two continuous variables. $P<0.05$ was considered statistically significant.

Results

Paclitaxel induced EMT and inhibited proliferation simultaneously in cervical cancer cells

When the morphology of routinely cultured cervical cancer cells treated with or without paclitaxel were examined by microscopy, we observed that SiHa cell grew as tightly-packed "cobblestone"-like epithelial cells, whereas cells treated with paclitaxel seemed a spindle-like shape flattened and lost the majority of their cell-cell contacts. (Figure 1a) Meanwhile, the expression of Ecadherin protein was decreased (10.5%~66.6% and 43.75%~67.6% under 5 nM to 20 nM paclitaxel treatment respectively) and the expressions of Ncadherin and fibronectin protein were increased in a dose-responsive manner. (Figure 1b) Similar effects were also observed in CaSki cells. (Figure 1b, Figure S1).

Further, a transient cell proliferation inhibition induced by paclitaxel was observed by flow cytometry and MTT. SiHa and CaSki cells were routinely cultured with 10 nM paclitaxel, after 72 hours, the paclitaxel were removed and the cells were cultured with complete medium continuously, subsequently the proliferation changes in SiHa and CaSki cells before and after paclitaxel administration revealed at 24 h, 72 h, 96 h, day 5, day 7, day 14, and day 21, respectively. As showed in Figure 1c, 1d, the proliferation rate of paclitaxel treated SiHa and CaSki cells at day 7 was significantly reduced (SiHa, $p=0.002$ and $p=2.3\times10^{-5}$; CaSki, $p=3.1\times10^{-4}$ and $p=1.2\times10^{-5}$ respectively), compared with that of blank control, and restored to the levels before drug treatment at day 21. At the same time, the "cobblestone"-like morphological changes induced by paclitaxel in survived cells were also restored to normal morphology at day 21. These facts indicate that paclitaxel transiently inhibits proliferation and induces EMT simultaneously in cervical cancer cells, but all these paclitaxel-induced changes reversed after drug withdrawal.

Paclitaxel up-regulates miR-375 during inducing EMT and proliferation inhibition

We had explored miR-375 expression changing involved in paclitaxel induced EMT and proliferation inhibition in cervical cancer cells, and the clear dose dependent effect of paclitaxel on miR-375 over-expression was observed[14]. Moreover, the progressive up-regulated expression of miR-375 reached a peak at day 7 after paclitaxel administration, gradually declined after paclitaxel removed and restored to the level before drug treatment at about day 21[14]. In addition, there was a strong negative correlation between the expression of miR-375 and the relative proliferation proportion of cervical cancer cells (SiHa, $r=-0.472$, $P=1.52\times10^{-3}$; CaSki, $r=-0.835$, $P=3.03\times10^{-4}$). (Figure S2) Our data revealed that paclitaxel up-regulated miR-375 expression and inhibited proliferation simultaneously in cervical cancer cells but both paclitexel-induced changes reversed after drug withdrawal, suggesting that some of cervical cancer cells survive in paclitaxel, probably though up-regulating miR-375 expression and acquiring malignant mesenchymal phenotypes, then developing a potential to decrease proliferation and resist drug toxicity. These correlation suggest that miR-375 over-expression might have a causal role in chemotherapy induced EMT.

MiR-375 mediates EMT by directly targeting Ecadherin

By miRDB and TargetScan search programs analysis, we found a predicted binding of miR-375 with CDH1 (Ecadherin) 3′-UTR, which indicated that Ecadherin was a potential direct target of miR-375 (Figure 2c). To further ascertain that Ecadherin is a target gene of miR-375, we firstly analyze the relationship between Ecadherin and miR-375 expression in cervical cancer cells under different amounts of paclitaxel treatment. As showed in Figure 1b and Figure S2, miR-375 expression in cells was markedly unregulated in a dose dependent manner during paclitaxel-induced EMT process, as well as Ecadherin protein and miR-375 expression were reversely correlated ($r=-0.752$, $P=2.32\times10^{-4}$). Then we further used the Luciferase Activity Assay to confirm the binding of miR-375 to the 3′-UTR of Ecadherin. (Figure 2c).

To test whether the up-regulation of miR-375 contributed to paclitaxel -induced EMT, the effects of miR-375 over-expression on these events were evaluated. The expression of miR-375 was analyzed by Real-time PCR at the second week, third week and first month after pre-miRNA lentiviral stable transfection. As shown in Figure 2a and 2b, the forced over-expression of miR-375 induced EMT process in cervical cancer cells, characterized by acquisition of fibroblast-like cell morphology, suppression of Ecadherin expression (65%~69.2%), and enhancement of vimentin, Ncadherin, and fibronectin expression, similar to the effects observed in the paclitaxel treated cells.

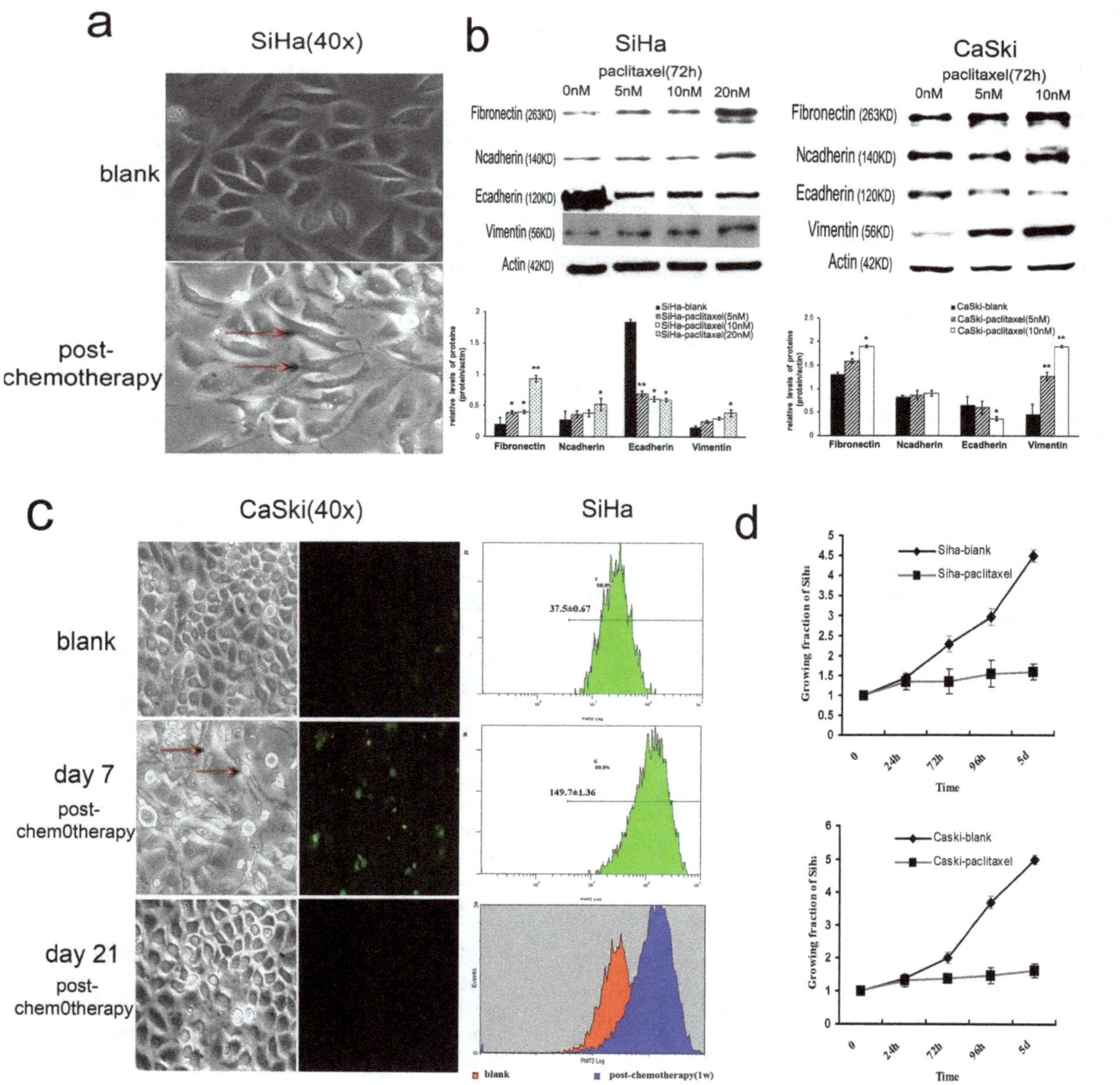

Figure 1. Paclitaxel inhibits proliferation, induces EMT, and up-regulates miR-375 expression simultaneously in cervical cancer cells. (**a**) Visible morphological changes from "cobblestone"-like to "fibroblast"-like cells was observed in SiHa after 72 h paclitaxel treatment. The representative cells with morphological changes were labeled (**b**) Immunoblotting measured the expression of Ecadherin and other EMT related proteins (vimentin, Ncadherin, and fibronectin) in cervical cancer cells (SiHa and CaSki) under different amounts (0, 5, 10, 20 nM) of paclitaxel treatment. The expression of Ecadherin protein was decreased and the expressions of vimentin, Ncadherin, and fibronectin protein were increased in cells treated with paclitaxel for 72 hours in a dose-responsive manner. All the expressions of the proteins were normalized to ß-actin and the data in bar graphs are presented as mean of triple samples from three independent experiments. All error bars indicated s.e.m. (**$p \le 0.01$, *$p \le 0.05$). (**c, d**) The transient cell proliferation inhibition and morphological changes induced by paclitaxel were observed. The proliferation changes in SiHa and CaSki cells after paclitaxel administration were analyzed by CellTrace CFSE cell proliferation (**c**) and MTT assay (**d**) at 24 h, 72 h, 96 h, day 5, day 7, day 14, and day 21, respectively. The proliferation rate of paclitaxel treated SiHa and CaSki cells was significantly reduced at day 7 and restored at day 21 after paclitaxel administration. The survived CaSki cells were restored into normal morphology at day 21 after paclitaxel administration.

Thus, our findings indicate that miR-375 over-expression promotes paclitaxel-induced EMT partly by directly targeting Ecadherin in cervical cancer cells.

EMT regulates the paclitaxel sensitivity but not miR-375 expression

To determine whether EMT may regulate miR-375 expression inversely, the next set of experiments was carried out. We induced EMT by TGF-β1 or EGF-β in cervical cancer cells (SiHa and CaSki) and observed the influence of EMT on paclitaxel sensitivity and miR-375 expression. Stimulated by TGF-β1 or EGF-β, cervical cancer cells underwent EMT accompanying visible morphological changes (Figure 3a), such as appearance of a spindle-like shape in cells, and EMT marker alteration, including decreased Ecadherin protein expression (28.5%~65.8% for TGF-β1 and 47.5%~67.6% for EGF-β), as well as increased

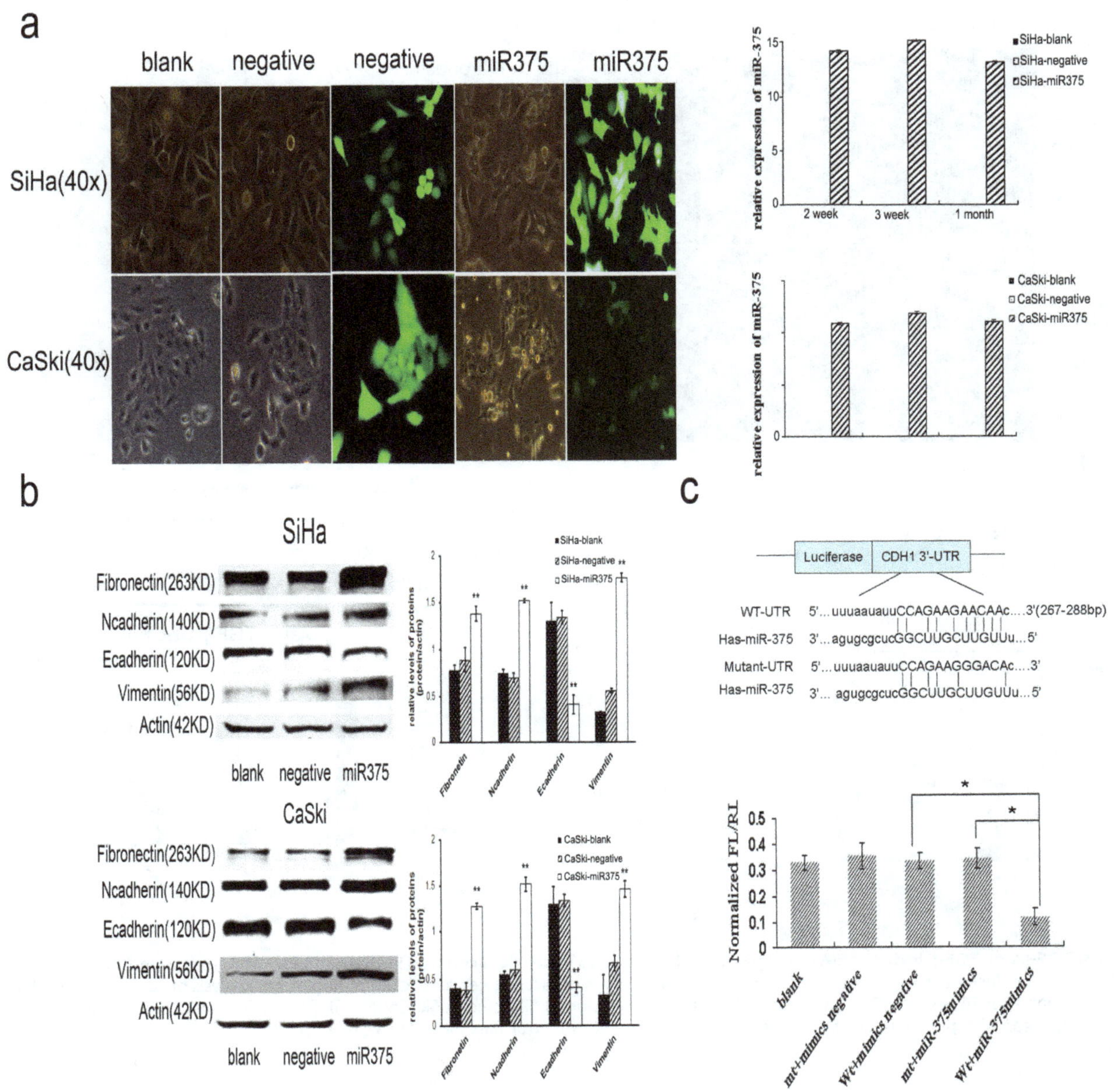

Figure 2. Conditionally over-expressed miR-375 induces EMT via targeting Ecadherin in cervical cancer cells. (a) Phase contrast images of cervical cancer cells infected with the pre-miR-375 or negative lentivirus vector and blank control. (b) Immunoblotting measurement of Ecadherin and EMT related proteins in cervical cancer tercells infected with the pre-miR-375 or negative lentivirus vector. (c) A predicted duplex formation between human CDH1 (Ecadherin) 3′-UTR and miR-375. A reduced luciferase activity was observed after cotransfection of Ecadherin 3′-UTR wild type vector with miR-375, but not mutated or empty vector (p = 0.014). Data in a–c were presented as the mean of triplets samples from independent experiments. All error bars indicated s.e.m. (**p≤0.01, *p≤0.05).

Ncadherin, vimentin, and fibronectin protein expression (Figure 3c). However, the expression of miR-375 was not changed during TGF-β1 or EGF-β induced EMT process in cervical cancer cells (SiHa, $p = 0.538$; CaSki $p = 0.542$) (Figure 3d).

Further, we delineated the drug sensitivity of cells undergoing EMT using MTS assay. The paclitaxel sensitivity was significantly decreased in SiHa and CaSki cells after TGF-β1 or EGF-β stimulation compared with serum-free culture controls (Figure 3b). The IC50 values were increased in SiHa and CaSki with 5 ng/ml TGF-β1 (95.81±2.53 nM and 66.66±2.32 nM respectively, SiHa, $p = 0.032$; CaSki, $p = 0.023$) or 2 ng/ml EGF-β stimulation (96.74±2.47 nM and 94.78±1.72 nM respectively, SiHa, $p = 0.038$; CaSki $p = 0.028$) compared with serum-free culture controls (24.54±1.37 nM, and 23.98±2.62 nM respectively).

Our findings indicate that TGF-β1 or EGF-β induces EMT but dose not alter miR-375 expression in cervical cancer cells, and mesenchymal cell-like cervical cancer cells induced by TGF-β1 or EGF-β are typically paclitaxel resistant. The significantly upregulated expression of miR-375 in paclitaxel treated cervical caner cells is induced by paclitaxel but not EMT.

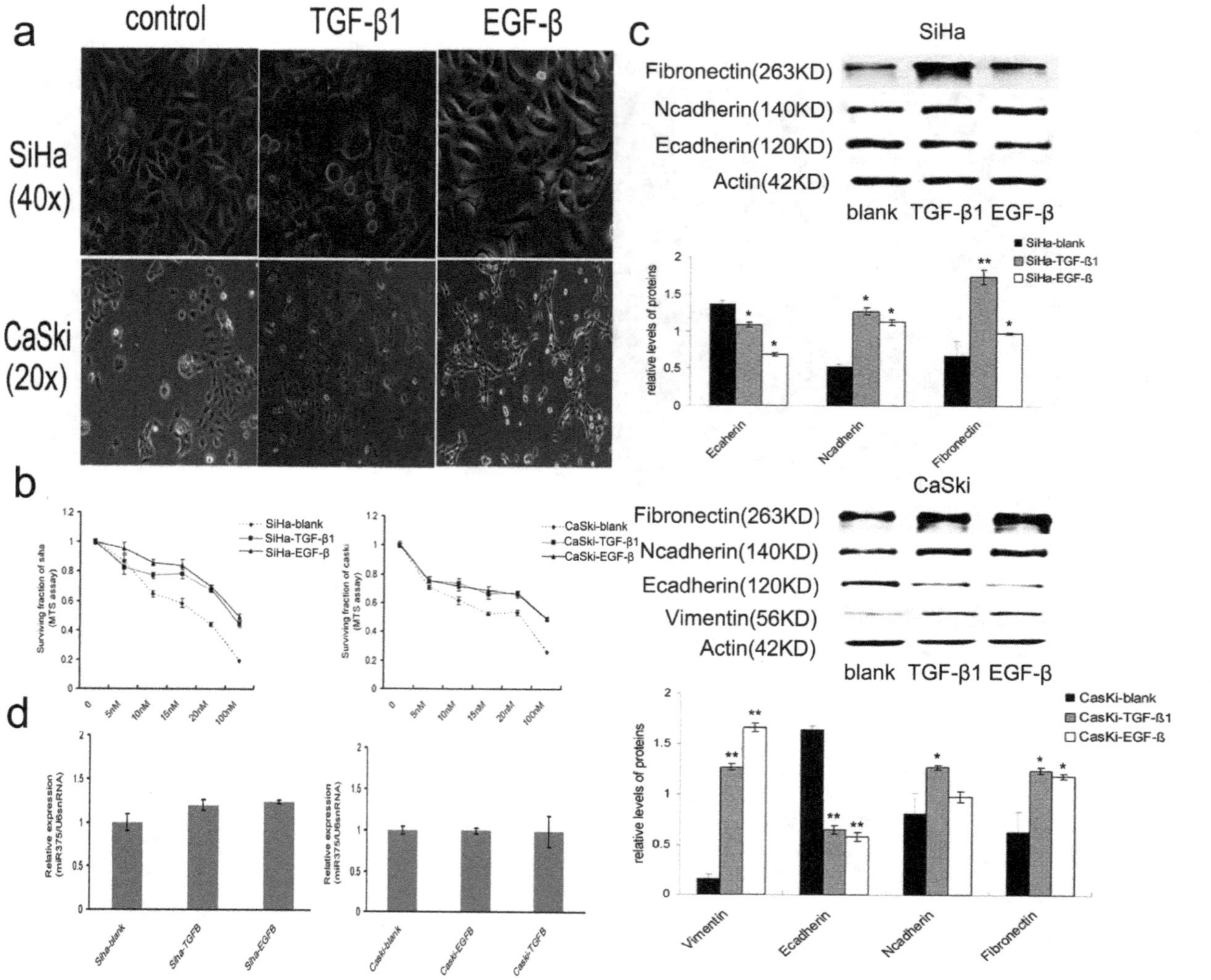

Figure 3. TGF-β1 or EGF-β induces EMT and paclitaxel resistance in cervical cells. (a) Visible morphological changes in SiHa and CaSki under TGF-β1 or EGF-β inducement. (b) MTS analysis of paclitaxel-sensitivity in cervical cancer cells. (c) Immunoblotting analysis of Ecadherin and other EMT related proteins after TGF-β1 or EGF-β induction. (d) miR-375 expression in SiHa and CaSki under TGF-β1 or EGF-β inducement. Data in b–d were presented as mean of triplets samples from independent experiments. All error bars indicated s.e.m. (**p≤0.01, *p≤0.05).

Ecadherin over-expression attenuates the ability miR-375 to mediate EMT and paclitaxel-resistance

Ecadherin is not only an important molecule in the initiation of EMT but also a hallmark for EMT and miR-375 mediates EMT by directly targeting Ecadherin.To investigate the role of Ecadherin in EMT and paclitaxel sensitivity and to test whether the up-regulation ofEcadherin can attenuates the effect of miR-375 on EMT and paclitaxel-resistance in cervical cancer cells; the Ecadherin over-expressed lentviral pGC-flag-CDH1 vector was used. We respectively transfected Ecadherin over-expressed lentviral vector and negative control into SiHa and CaSki cells with and without miR-375 over-expression, and observed that the effect of forced over-expression Ecadherin on EMT and paclitaxel-resistance. In Ecadherin over-expressing clones with and without miR-375 over-expression, there was a pronounced and significant increase in the expression of Ecadherin (Figure 4a). In cells without miR-375 over-expression, no remarkable differences of morphology and mesenchymal markers were observed in SiHa and CaSki cells after Ecadherin over-expression, which is probably because their parental cells already exhibited an epithelial phenotype. Contrarily, in cells with miR-375 over-expression, there was a transition from isolated fibroblastic cells to "cobblestone"-like epithelial cells. Meanwhile, the expressions of Ncadherin, vimentin, and fibronectin were significantly decreased after Ecadherin over-expression (Figure 4a, 4c).

The paclitaxel chemo-sensitivity was then evaluated by MTS assays. As expected, paclitaxel sensitivity was significantly increased in Ecadherin lentvirus-transfected cells with and without miR-375 overexpression compared with control cells. The IC50 values were decreased in SiHa and CaSki with Ecadherin overexpression (12.82±2.54 nM and 7.62±0.93 nM respectively, SiHa, $p = 0.043$; CaSki, $p = 0.038$) compared with negative controls (20.73±1.23 nM and 11.68±0.62 nM respectively, SiHa, $p = 0.028$; CaSki, $p = 0.021$). Moreover, the paclitaxel resistance was significantly attenuated after Ecadherin was effectively over-expressed in cervical cells with over-expressed miR-375 compared with negative control (Figure 4b). The IC50 values were decreased in SiHa and CaSki with Ecadherin and miR-375 cotransfection (22.82±3.54 nM and 13.68±0.64 nM respectively, SiHa, $p = 0.033$; CaSki, $p = 0.038$) compared with SiHa and CaSki with negative control and miR-375 cotransfection (82.83±2.23 nM and 20.31±3.01 nM respectively, SiHa, $p = 0.032$; CaSki,

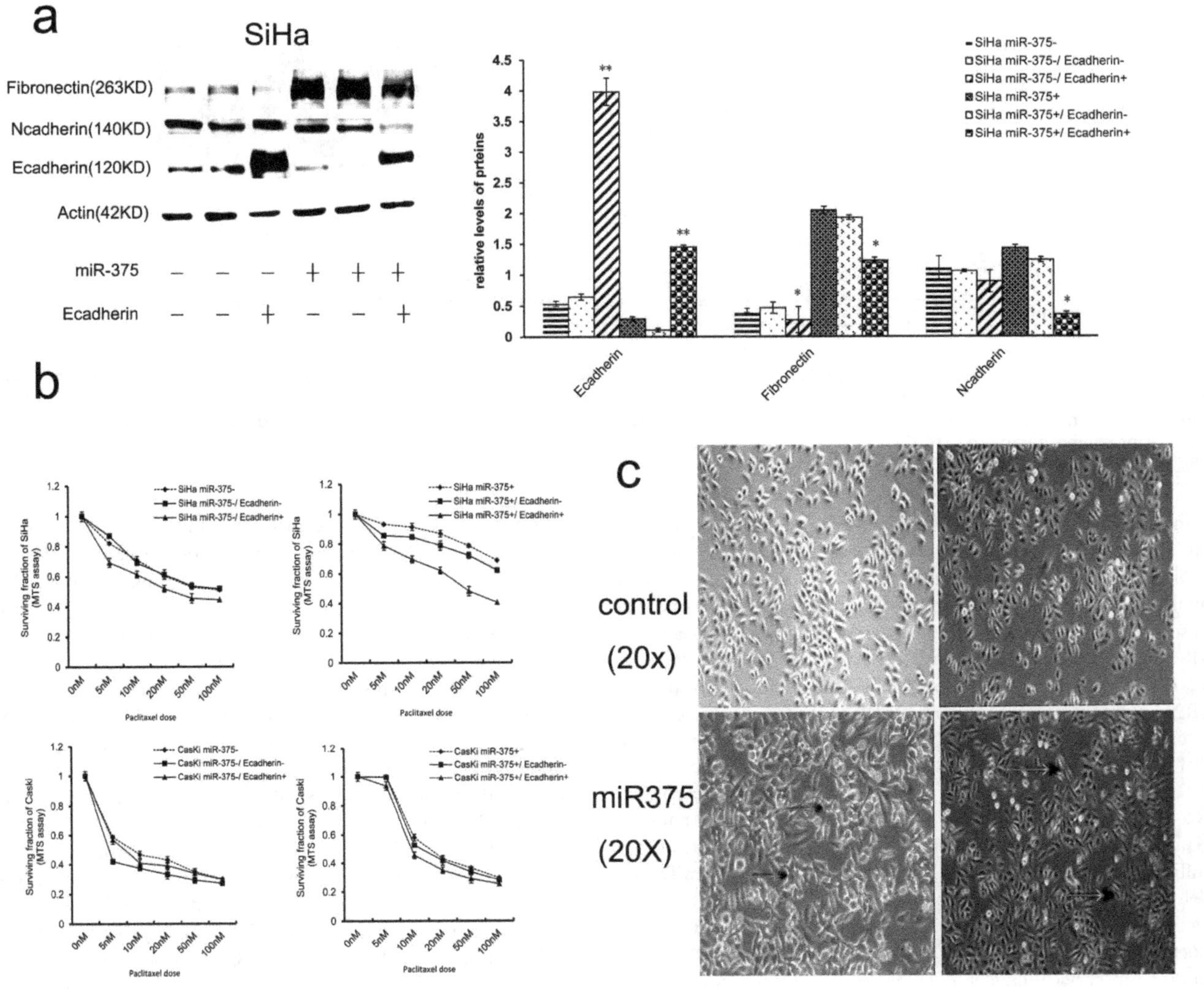

Figure 4. Forced expression of Ecadherin attenuates the ability miR-375 to mediate EMT and paclitaxel-resistance. Immunoblotting (a) and MTS (b) analysis of Ecadherin and other EMT related proteins in SiHa with and without miR-375 overexpression after the Ecadherin-expressing or negative lentivirus vector transfection. Data in (a) and (b) were presented as the mean of triplets samples from independent experiments. All error bars indicated s.e.m. (**p≤0.01, *p≤0:05). (c) Morphological changes in SiHa with and without miR-375 over-expression after the Ecadherin-expressing or negative lentivirus vector transfection. The representative cells with morphological changes had been labeled.

$p = 0.025$). Our results revealed that Ecadherin over-expression significantly enhanced paclitaxel sensitivity in cervical cancer cells with or without miR-375 over-expression, suggesting that Ecadherin over-expression dramatically enhances paclitaxel sensitivity, further, re-expression of Ecadherin reverses, at least partly, the EMT phenotype and paclitaxel-resistance mediated by miR-375 in cervical cancer cells.

miR-375 over-expression correlates with Ecadherin expression in post-chemotherapy human cervical carcinoma tissues

To establish the clinical relevance of miR-375 between Ecadherin expressions under chemotherapy effects, we assessed miR-375 and Ecadherin expression in 23 couples of self paired pre- and post-chemotherapy human cervical cancer tissues. The immunostaining for Ecadherin revealed more extensive and stronger expression in pre-chemotherapy than that in post-chemotherapy tumor tissues (Figure 5). At the same time, miR-375 was markedly upregulated (4.67 fold) in paclitaxel-treated cervical samples, Ecadherin and miR-375 expression were reversely correlated in all tissues including pre- and post-chemotherapy ($r = -0.905$, $P = 1.81 \times 10^{-3}$) (Table S1).

Of all 23 patients, 19 were chemo-sensitive and 4 chemo-resistance, the upregulated expression of miR-375 is more significantly in chemo-resistance patients when compared post-chemotherapy tissues with their self paired pre-chemotherapy tissues (6.7±2.3 fold in chemo-resistance and 4.35±0.63 fold in chemosensitive patients respectively, $p = 0.033$). But it should be noted that there is no enough power to conclude that miR-375 expression is higher in chemo-resistance patients, partially due to the small sample size for the chemo-resistance patients (N = 4).

Discussion

Chemo-resistance is one of the key causal factors in cancer relapses and progression. The majority of cancer cells responds well initially to chemotherapy, but eventually develops resistance following drug exposure. Emerging evidences have revealed that cancer cells undergo EMT promotes cell survival and resistance to

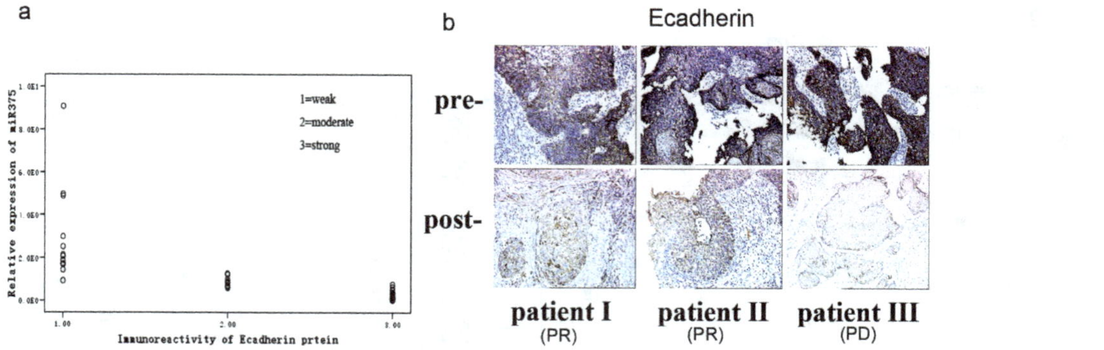

Figure 5. miR-375 over-expression correlates with Ecadherin expression in post-chemotherapy human cervical carcinoma tissues. (a) Ecadherin and miR-375 expression were reversely correlated in all tissues including pre- and post-chemotherapy ($r = -0.905$, $P = 1.81 \times 10^{-3}$). (b) Staining of human-specific Ecadherin expression in three representatives (1 PD and 2 PR) (×200). A decreased Ecadherin expression was shown in the tissues after chemotherapy ($p = 0.0023$).

chemotherapy [3]. Although it has been reported that miRNAs may play an integral role in modulating EMT [16]; however, detailed regulatory procedure remains unexplored. miR-375 was initially found to be expressed in pancreatic islet, where it regulates the secretion of insulin and metabolism of glucose [17]. Recently, miR-375 was identified as an important regulator in tumorgenesis and cancer progression; however, the precise functions of this miRNA remain largely obscure. miR-375 was identified as a tumor suppressor in most of cancers, such as gastric cancer [18,19], liver cancer [20], head and neck squamous cell carcinoma [21] and prostate cancers [22], but plays an oncogenic role in ERα-positive breast cancer [23], in lung adenocarcinoma patients [24], and in HBV positive HCC patients [25]. Thus, these conflicting reports regarding the association between miR-375 level and cancer suggested a more complex and possibly cancer specific relationship. In another study of ours, we observed the association between miR-375 over-expression and paclitaxel - resistance in cervical cancer[16]. Here, we directly link miR-375 to chemotherapy-induced EMT process in cervical cancer. We found for the first time that paclitaxel inhibits proliferation, induces EMT, and up-regulates miR-375 expression in a dose-dependent manner simultaneously in cervical cancer cells, but all these paclitaxel-induced changes reversed after drug withdrawal. Mechanistically, ectopic over-expression of miR-375 resulted in reduced Ecadherin expression and accompanied by acquired mesenchymal characteristics and chemo-resistance in cervical cancer cells. Thus, our findings suggested that paclitaxel does not eliminate all cervical cancer cells and some of residual cells can survive under drug exposure. During this procedure, those residual cervical cancer cells with up-regulated miR-375 expression probably possess a potential to acquire mesenchymal phenotypes, slow down proliferation, and resist to drug toxicity. Thus, miR-375 induced EMT might play a key role in paclitaxel resistance in cervical cancer cells. Both cell proliferation inhibition and mesenchymal phenotype have been regarded as features of dormant tumor cells that are resistant to chemotherapy [26,27]. It is possible that residual surviving cells go into the status of tumor dormancy. More importantly, those dormant-like cells escaping from killing by drug can *de novo* down-regulate miR-375 expression and reconvert proliferation after drug withdrawal. Clinically, it is those revival cells that present the progression or recurrence and consequently contribute to poor prognosis of cancer patients. There are only few reports associating miR-375 with chemo-resistance. However, recently a reduced expression of miR-375 was found in tamoxifen resistant cell lines and re-expression of miR-375 reverses both tamoxifen resistance and accompanying EMT-like properties in breast cancer [28]. This conflicting report indicated that the role of miR-375 in regulating drug-sensitivity is possibly cancer and anticancer agents' specific relationship such as in regulating tumorgenesis and cancer progression.

Previous studies showed that miRNAs regulated EMT process but EMT in turn regulated miRNA expression. For example, miR-200 family members regulate EMT, through targeting and suppressing ZEB, and they are in turn repressed in a timely correlated manner during Snail-induced EMT in MCF7 breast cancer cells [29]. To exclude the possibility that miR-375 was regulated by EMT, we examined miR-375 expression during EMT process induced by transforming growth factor-b (TGF-β) and epidermal growth factor-b (EGF-β) treatment in cervical cancer cells. Both factors are multifunctional cytokines that induce EMT in multiple cell types [30,31]. Our results showed that miR-375 was regulated only during paclitaxel induced EMT but not TGF-β and EGF induced EMT. Thus, our findings recognize that the upregulated expression of miR-375 in paclitaxel treated cervical caner cells is only induced by paclitaxel but not EMT.

Ecadherin is a calcium dependent cell adhesion molecule which plays an important role in the growth and development of cells via controlling tissue architecture and maintaining tissue integrity [32]. Recently some studies have demonstrated that reduction and/or loss of Ecadherin expression is a hallmark of the EMT process, which is required for enhancing drug resistance of cancer cells [33]. Here, we observed that Ecadherin is a direct target of miR-375 in cervical cancer cells; moreover, re-expression of Ecadherin partly reversed the EMT phenotype and paclitaxel - resistance induced by miR-375 in cervical cancer cells. These data suggest that Ecadherin is a major molecule in regulating chemo-sensitivity.

In summary, our findings for the first time, to our knowledge, suggest that paclitaxel up-regulates miR-375 expression and over-expressed miR-375 induces EMT process via directly targeting Ecadherin, proliferation inhibition, and consequently results in chemo-resistance in cervical cancer cells. A reversion of miR-375 or Ecadherin expression may be a novel therapeutic approach for overcoming chemo-resistance in cervical cancer.

Supporting Information

Figure S1 Visible morphological changes in CaSki after chemotherapy. Visible morphological changes from "cobblestone"-like to "fibroblast"-like cells were observed in CaSki after 72 h paclitaxel treatment.

Figure S2 The correlation between miR-375 and proliferation. (a) miR-375 inhibited proliferation in cervical cancer cells. (b) The progressive up-regulated expression of miR-375 reached a peak at day 7 after paclitaxel administration, gradually declined after paclitaxel removed and restored to the level before drug treatment at about day 21. (c) miR-375 expression in cells was markedly unregulated in a dose dependent manner during paclitaxel treatment.

Table S1 miR-375 over-expression correlates with Ecadherin expression in cervical cancer tissues. Staining of human-specific Ecadherin expression in paraffin embedded 23 couples of self-paired pre-and post-chemotherapy cervical cancer samples (19 chemo-sensitive, 4 chemo-resistance). Ecadherin and miR-375 expression were reversely correlated ($r = -0.905$, $P = 1.81 \times 10-3$).

Acknowledgments

All authors declare that the material is an original research, has not been previously published and has not been submitted for publication elsewhere while under consideration.

Author Contributions

Conceived and designed the experiments: YS XDC YL. Performed the experiments: YS JSZ. Analyzed the data: YS FY. Contributed reagents/materials/analysis tools: XYW WGL XX. Wrote the paper: YS XX XDC.

References

1. Adam L, Zhong M, Choi W, Qi W, Nicoloso M, et al. (2009) miR-200 expression regulates epithelial-to-mesenchymal transition in bladder cancer cells and reverses resistance to epidermal growth factor receptor therapy. Clin Cancer Res 15: 5060–5072.
2. Cannito S, Novo E, di Bonzo LV, Busletta C, Colombatto S, et al. (2010) Epithelial-mesenchymal transition: from molecular mechanisms, redox regulation to implications in human health and disease. Antioxid Redox Signal 12: 1383–1430.
3. Wang Z, Li Y, Ahmad A, Azmi AS, Kong D, et al. (2010) Targeting miRNAs involved in cancer stem cell and EMT regulation: An emerging concept in overcoming drug resistance. Drug Resist Updat 13: 109–118.
4. Yang AD, Fan F, Camp ER, van Buren G, Liu W, et al. (2006) Chronic oxaliplatin resistance induces epithelial-to-mesenchymal transition in colorectal cancer cell lines. Clin Cancer Res 12: 4147–4153.
5. Kajiyama H, Shibata K, Terauchi M, Yamashita M, Ino K, et al. (2007) Chemoresistance to paclitaxel induces epithelial-mesenchymal transition and enhances metastatic potential for epithelial ovarian carcinoma cells. Int J Oncol 31: 277–283.
6. Rho JK, Choi YJ, Lee JK, Ryoo BY, Na, II, et al. (2009) Epithelial to mesenchymal transition derived from repeated exposure to gefitinib determines the sensitivity to EGFR inhibitors in A549, a non-small cell lung cancer cell line. Lung Cancer 63: 219–226.
7. Dean M, Fojo T, Bates S (2005) Tumour stem cells and drug resistance. Nat Rev Cancer 5: 275–284.
8. Ranganathan AC, Zhang L, Adam AP, Aguirre-Ghiso JA (2006) Functional coupling of p38-induced up-regulation of BiP and activation of RNA-dependent protein kinase-like endoplasmic reticulum kinase to drug resistance of dormant carcinoma cells. Cancer Res 66: 1702–1711.
9. Li Y, Kong D, Wang Z, Sarkar FH (2010) Regulation of microRNAs by natural agents: an emerging field in chemoprevention and chemotherapy research. Pharm Res 27: 1027–1041.
10. Gregory PA, Bert AG, Paterson EL, Barry SC, Tsykin A, et al. (2008) The miR-200 family and miR-205 regulate epithelial to mesenchymal transition by targeting ZEB1 and SIP1. Nat Cell Biol 10: 593–601.
11. Mongroo PS, Rustgi AK (2010) The role of the miR-200 family in epithelial-mesenchymal transition. Cancer Biol Ther 10: 219–222.
12. Li Y, Wang F, Xu J, Ye F, Shen Y, et al. (2011) Progressive miRNA expression profiles in cervical carcinogenesis and identification of HPV-related target genes for miR-29. J Pathol 224: 484–495.
13. Wang F, Li Y, Zhou J, Xu J, Peng C, et al. (2011) miR-375 is down-regulated in squamous cervical cancer and inhibits cell migration and invasion via targeting transcription factor SP1. Am J Pathol 179: 2580–2588.
14. Shen Y, Wang P, Li Y, Ye F, Wang F, et al. (2013) miR-375 is upregulated in acquired paclitaxel resistance in cervical cancer. Br J Cancer.
15. Eisenhauer EA, Therasse P, Bogaerts J, Schwartz LH, Sargent D, et al. (2009) New response evaluation criteria in solid tumours: revised RECIST guideline (version 1.1). Eur J Cancer 45: 228–247.
16. Ma L, Young J, Prabhala H, Pan E, Mestdagh P, et al. (2010) miR-9, a MYC/MYCN-activated microRNA, regulates E-cadherin and cancer metastasis. Nat Cell Biol 12: 247–256.
17. Poy MN, Hausser J, Trajkovski M, Braun M, Collins S, et al. (2009) miR-375 maintains normal pancreatic alpha- and beta-cell mass. Proc Natl Acad Sci U S A 106: 5813–5818.
18. Ding L, Xu Y, Zhang W, Deng Y, Si M, et al. (2010) MiR-375 frequently downregulated in gastric cancer inhibits cell proliferation by targeting JAK2. Cell Res 20: 784–793.
19. Tsukamoto Y, Nakada C, Noguchi T, Tanigawa M, Nguyen LT, et al. (2010) MicroRNA-375 is downregulated in gastric carcinomas and regulates cell survival by targeting PDK1 and 14-3-3 zeta. Cancer Res 70: 2339–2349.
20. Liu AM, Poon RT, Luk JM (2010) MicroRNA-375 targets Hippo-signaling effector YAP in liver cancer and inhibits tumor properties. Biochem Biophys Res Commun 394: 623–627.
21. Hui AB, Lenarduzzi M, Krushel T, Waldron L, Pintilie M, et al. (2010) Comprehensive MicroRNA profiling for head and neck squamous cell carcinomas. Clin Cancer Res 16: 1129–1139.
22. Szczyrba J, Nolte E, Wach S, Kremmer E, Stohr R, et al. (2011) Downregulation of Sec23 A protein by miRNA-375 in prostate carcinoma. Mol Cancer Res 9: 791–800.
23. de Souza Rocha Simonini P, Breiling A, Gupta N, Malekpour M, Youns M, et al. (2010) Epigenetically deregulated microRNA-375 is involved in a positive feedback loop with estrogen receptor alpha in breast cancer cells. Cancer Res 70: 9175–9184.
24. Yu L, Todd NW, Xing L, Xie Y, Zhang H, et al. (2010) Early detection of lung adenocarcinoma in sputum by a panel of microRNA markers. Int J Cancer 127: 2870–2878.
25. Li LM, Hu ZB, Zhou ZX, Chen X, Liu FY, et al. (2010) Serum microRNA profiles serve as novel biomarkers for HBV infection and diagnosis of HBV-positive hepatocarcinoma. Cancer Res 70: 9798–9807.
26. Lu Z, Luo RZ, Lu Y, Zhang X, Yu Q, et al. (2008) The tumor suppressor gene ARHI regulates autophagy and tumor dormancy in human ovarian cancer cells. J Clin Invest 118: 3917–3929.
27. Yu Y, Zhu Z (2013) Cell dormancy and tumor refractory. Anticancer Agents Med Chem 13: 199–202.
28. Ward A, Balwierz A, Zhang JD, Kublbeck M, Pawitan Y, et al. (2013) Re-expression of microRNA-375 reverses both tamoxifen resistance and accompanying EMT-like properties in breast cancer. Oncogene 32: 1173–1182.
29. Moes M, Le Bechec A, Crespo I, Laurini C, Halavatyi A, et al. (2012) A novel network integrating a miRNA-203/SNAI1 feedback loop which regulates epithelial to mesenchymal transition. PLoS One 7: e35440.
30. Doerner AM, Zuraw BL (2009) TGF-beta1 induced epithelial to mesenchymal transition (EMT) in human bronchial epithelial cells is enhanced by IL-1beta but not abrogated by corticosteroids. Respir Res 10: 100.
31. Shinto O, Yashiro M, Kawajiri H, Shimizu K, Shimizu T, et al. (2010) Inhibitory effect of a TGFbeta receptor type-I inhibitor, Ki26894, on invasiveness of scirrhous gastric cancer cells. Br J Cancer 102: 844–851.
32. von Burstin J, Eser S, Paul MC, Seidler B, Brandl M, et al. (2009) E-cadherin regulates metastasis of pancreatic cancer in vivo and is suppressed by a SNAIL/HDAC1/HDAC2 repressor complex. Gastroenterology 137: 361–371, 371 e361–365.
33. Rosano L, Cianfrocca R, Spinella F, Di Castro V, Nicotra MR, et al. (2011) Acquisition of chemoresistance and EMT phenotype is linked with activation of the endothelin A receptor pathway in ovarian carcinoma cells. Clin Cancer Res 17: 2350–2360.

8

Treatment Effect and Drug-Resistant Mutations in Chinese AIDS Patients Switching to Second-Line Antiretroviral Therapy

Min Zhang[1,2]☯, Mingquan Shang[1,2], Weiwei Yang[1,2], Junli Chen[1,2], Zhe Wang[3], Hong Shang[1,2]*☯

1 Key Laboratory of AIDS Immunology of National Health and Family Planning Commission, Department of Laboratory Medicine, The First Affiliated Hospital, China Medical University, Shenyang, China, 2 Collaborative Innovation Center for Diagnosis and Treatment of Infectious Diseases, Hangzhou, China, 3 Disease Prevention and Control Center of Henan Province, Zhengzhou, China

Abstract

This study aimed to investigate treatment effect, drug resistance changes, and their influencing factors in Chinese AIDS patients after switching to second-line antiretroviral therapy, and thus provide important information for the scale-up of second-line antiretroviral treatment in China. In Weishi county of Henan province, where second-line antiretroviral therapy was introduced early in China, 195 AIDS patients were enrolled, of which 127 patients met the switching criterion and 68 patients volunteered to switch drugs without meeting the switching criterion. CD4 cell count, viral load and in-house PCR genotyping for drug resistance were measured for all 195 subjects before drug switch, as well as 6 and 12 months after drug switch. Extensive secondary mutations to the protease inhibitor were observed, which suggested that long-term drug resistance surveillance is necessary for patients switching to second-line antiretroviral therapy. Multidrug resistance and cross-resistance were extensive in Chinese patients that experienced first-line treatment failure. Patients need timely CD4 count, viral load, and drug resistance monitoring in order to switch to second-line therapy under conditions of relatively good immunity and low viral duplication levels.

Editor: Xia Jin, University of Rochester, United States of America

Funding: This study was supported by the Twelfth Five-Year Project on Tackling Key Problems of National Science and Technology (2012ZX10001002-002-013) and National Natural Science Foundation of China (81171619). The funders had no role in study design, data collection and analysis, decision to publish, or preparation of the manuscript.

Competing Interests: The authors have declared that no competing interests exist.

* Email: hongshang100@hotmail.com

☯ These authors contributed equally to this work.

Introduction

Highly active antiretroviral therapy (HAART) is currently the most effective therapy for the treatment of acquired immune deficiency syndrome (AIDS) [1]. However, the characteristic high mutation level of human immunodeficiency virus (HIV), along with selection pressure of antiretroviral drugs, usually cause rapid occurrence of drug resistance of HIV, which has been the main reason for clinical failure of antiretroviral treatment. In America and Europe, drug resistance of HIV existed in more than 60% of patients who were antiretroviral treatment failure [2].

China initiated a large-scale program for free antiretroviral treatment in 2003, with zidovudine (AZT)/stavudine (D4T) + didanosine (DDI) + nevirapine (NVP) as the main first-line therapy regimen. By October 2011, more than 130,000 patients with AIDS had received HAART. The increase in availability and access to free antiretroviral treatment had resulted in considerably prolonged survival time, improved quality of life and decreased mortality rate in AIDS patients [3]. But with the increase of HAART treatment duration, treatment failure and drug resistance occurred in more and more patients. In a cross-sectional survey conducted in 2007, Min Zhang et al. [4] studied HIV infected patients living in 7 provinces in China and reported that the rate of drug resistance was significantly higher in patients receiving first-line treatment for more than 6 months than that in patients receiving treatment for less than 6 months. In 2008, Min Zhang [5] conducted a cohort study on HIV infected patients living in Weishi county of Hunan province of China. The results showed that, among 88 patients who had received the first-line antiretroviral treatment, only 1% of patients had drug resistance before treatment. The rate increased to 15% after the patients received treatment for 12 months, and increased to 17% after 36 months. As the increasing rate of drug resistance resulted in diminishing efficacy of the free antiretroviral treatment, in 2009 China initiated the switch to second-line antiretroviral therapy for patients with failure of first-line treatment.

Some foreign researchers reported that extensive drug-resistant mutations were observed before switching therapy regimens. Regarding treatment results after switching to second-line antiretroviral regimens, there is variance among reports from different regions and countries [6–8]. In China, with the expanding of the free antiretroviral treatment and the extending of treatment duration, the rate of drug resistance increases over time. What would be the treatment results after patients switch to second-line antiretroviral therapy? Would accumulation of drug-resistant mutations during the first-line treatment have an impact on the second-line treatment results? Would new drug-resistant mutations appear soon after the administration of second-line regimens? In China, no study has examined efficacy and drug resistance after patients switch to second-line regimens. In Weishi county of Henan province, where antiretroviral treatment started early, more than 2,000 HIV infected individuals had received antiretroviral treatment, and rates of treatment failure and drug resistance were increasing annually [5]. From August 2009, some patients began to switch to second-line therapy. We conducted a prospective observational cohort follow-up study on these AIDS patients in Weishi county who switched to second-line therapy.

Materials and Methods

Ethics statement

This study was approved by the Institutional Review Board of the First Affiliated Hospital of China Medical University (Shen Yang, China). All participants ≥18 years of age, written informed consent was obtained from all subjects.

Study subjects

Our research is an observational study; we did not determine or influence the course of treatment. We just collected the therapy information and blood samples of patients in the second-line antiretroviral therapy pilots in Henan province.

One hundred and ninety-five AIDS patients living in Weishi county of Henan province were enrolled in August 2009 and February 2010, respectively. In accordance with Chinese National Free AIDS Antiretroviral Therapy Manual issued in 2009 [9] and WHO antiretroviral therapy for HIV infection in adults and adolescents [10], virological failure defines as plasma HIV-1 RNA level >400 copies/mL after 6 months of treatment or HIV-1 RNA level >1000 copies/mL after initial virological suppression. Virological failure of first-line therapy was the main reason to switch to second-line treatment. 127 patients were first-line virological failure, after first-line virological failure happened, the patients continued the old treatment for one month with rectified treatment compliance. After that, if the viral load of the patient was higher than 1000 copies/mL, the patient switched to second-line therapy. As a result, viral loads of all the 127 subjects were higher than 1000 copies/mL. The remaining 68 patients who were virological suppression after first-line therapy, but they requested to switch to the second-line drugs due to significant toxicity and side effects of their first-line drugs.

The second-line antiretroviral regimen used was Lamivudine (3TC) + tenofovir (TDF) and lopinavir + ritonavir (LPV/r), as recommended by WHO [9]. Patients were followed up and their CD4, viral loads and drug resistance were measured 6 and 12 months after starting second-line treatment. Peripheral venous blood was obtained from each patient using an EDTA-3 K tube containing anticoagulants. CD4+T lymphocytes were counted within 24 hours. Blood for measurement of viral loads and drug resistance was centrifuged for 15 minutes, and plasma separated from blood was stored at −80°C.

CD4+T lymphocyte count

Absolute CD4+, CD8+, and CD3+T lymphocytes were counted with the FACSCalibur flow cytometer (Becton Dickinson, USA).

Viral load measurement

Viral loads were measured using COBAS AmpliPrep/COBAS TaqMan HIV-1 Test (Roche, Switzerland).

Drug-resistant mutation analysis

HIV-1 viral RNA was extracted from 140 ul plasma with the QIAamp Viral RNA Mini Kit (Qiagen Inc, USA). Reverse transcription-polymerase chain reaction (RT-PCR) was carried out with the One-step RNA PCR Kit (AMV) within 4 hours, and 1300 bp of reverse transcriptase (RT) and protease (PR) genes of HIV-1 were amplified with nested PCR, including the whole PR and the first 300 amino acids of RT [5]. The PCR product was then analyzed with ABI 3130 Genetic Analyzers (ABI, USA) using the chain termination method.

Sequence analysis and statistical analysis

Sequencher 4.10.1, NTI advance 9 and ContigExpress were used for sequence editing, assembly and rectification. The resulting sequences were compared with the Stanford University HIV drug resistance database (http://hivdb.stanford.edu) version 6.1.1. for analysis of HIV drug-resistant mutations and drug resistance. Statistical Package for Social Sciences (SPSS) version 15.0 was used for statistical analysis; data are shown as means ± standard deviation. Differences between groups were compared with chi-square tests and Fisher exact probability tests. Logistic regression analysis was used to identify the influencing factors of viral inhibition failure (viral load <400 copies/mL) 12 months after switching to second-line treatment, and odds ratios (OR) and confidence intervals (CI) were used to express the relative strength of association. A P value <0.05 was considered statistically significant. Viral loads <400 copies/mL after treatment were considered to have virological inhibition. The average viral load was expressed with the logarithmic (log_{10}) form.

Results and Discussion

General information and drug resistance of patients before drug switches

Of 127 patients who met the second-line treatment criterion, 71 patients (61.5%) were male and 56 patients (38.5%) were female. The average age was 45 (32–60) years. Among these 127 patients, 88 patients (69.3%) were drug resistant, 108 patients (85%) had CD4 cell counts <350 cells /mm^3, and all patients had viral loads >1,000 copies/mL (Table 1). Before drug switches, the average first-line treatment duration of 127 patients was 54.8 (13–73) months. The first-line regimens used included AZT+DDI+NVP (70.0%), AZT+DDI+3TC (4.3%), AZT+3TC+NVP (8.6%), D4 T+DDI+NVP (8.6%) and others (8.5%).

Of 68 patients who did not meet the second-line treatment criterion, 42 patients (61.8%) were male and 26 patients (38.2%) were female. The average age was 44 (33–59) years. Among these 68 patients, 7 patients (10.3%) were drug resistant, 42 patients (61.8%) had CD4 cell counts <350 cells /mm^3, and all patients had viral loads <1,000 copies/mL (Table 1). Before drug switches, the average first-line treatment duration of 68 patients was 50.8 (24–70) months. The first-line regimens used included AZT+DDI+NVP (67.6%), AZT+DDI+3TC (6.0%), AZT+3TC+NVP (8.8%), D4 T+DDI+NVP (8.8%) and others (8.8%).

Treatment results after drug switches

All patients were 95% or more adherent to therapy after switching to second-line therapy according to the questionnaire results. One hundred and fifty-six patients were followed up 6

Table 1. General information of subjects before drug switch.

		Patients meeting drug switching criterion (127 patients)	Percent	Patients failing to meet Drug switching criterion (68 patients)	Percent
Gender	Male	71	61.50%	42	61.80%
	Female	56	38.50%	26	38.20%
CD4 cell count (cells /μl)	<200	72	56.70%	22	32.40%
	200–350	36	28.30%	20	29.40%
	≥350	19	15.00%	26	37.20%
viral loads (copies/mL)	>1,000	127	100%	0	0
Drug resistance	NRTI	69	54.30%	5	7.40%
	NNRTI	88	69.30%	7	10.30%
No. of sequence		122	96.10%	8	11.80%

months after switching to second-line therapy and one hundred and sixty-seven patients were followed up at 12 months.

Of 127 patients who met the second-line treatment criterion, 98 and 113 patients were followed up at 6 and 12 months. At 6 months, 29 subjects were loss-of-follow-ups during the study, 15 of these patients were migrant workers, when we went to collect the blood samples and therapy information they were away from Weishi county of Henan province, but according to the drug receiving records in CDC, they continued second-line therapy; The remaining 14 patients, we totally can not contact with them. At 12 months, we got the 15 migrant workers' blood samples and therapy information, but the 14 patients who we did not contact with at 6 months were still lost contact. After switching to second-line treatment, the CD4 average increased to 220.0±137.2 at 6 months with an increase of 16.6 cells/μl, and 280.0±160.0 ($P<0.01$) at 12 months with an increase of 76.6 cells/μl, showing a gradual increase trend. Percentage of patients with CD4 <350 cells/μl reduced to 70% (79/113) at 12 months. At 6 months, the percentage of patients with viral loads <400 copies/mL increased from 0% before drug switches to 60.8%, and the viral load average VL($\log_{10}$) decreased from 4.6±0.8 before drug switches to 2.3±1.7; at 12 months, the percentage of patients with viral loads <400 copies/mL increased to 67.3%, and the viral load average VL ($\log_{10}$) decreased to 2.0±1.7 (Table 2) ($P<0.01$).

Of 68 patients who volunteered for second-line treatment, 58 and 54 patients were followed up at 6 and 12 months. The 14 loss-of-follow-up patients were migrant workers, they were away from Weishi county of Henan province that we can not contact with them. After switching to second-line treatment, the CD4 average was 322.2±164.8 at 6 months with an increase of 61.2 cells/μl, and 329.4±134.0 ($P>0.05$) at 12 months with an increase of 68.4 cells/μl, showing insignificant difference compared to that before drug switches. The percentage of patients with viral loads <400 copies/mL decreased from 89.7% before drug switches to 83.1% at 6 months, and increased to 90.7% at 12 months ($P>0.05$); the viral load average VL ($\log_{10}$) increased from 1.2±0.6 before drug switches to 1.6±1.4 at 6 months, and then decreased to 1.3±1.1 at 12 months (Table 2) ($P>0.05$).

Drug resistance in patients after drug switches

Of 127 patients, the rate of drug resistance was 69.3% (88/127) before second-line treatment, 23.5% (23/98) and 8.8% (10/113) after 6 and 12 months after drug switches, showing a significant decrease ($P<0.001$) compared to that before drug switches.

Of 68 patients who volunteered to participate in second-line treatment, drug-resistant mutations existed in 7 patients before drug switches. At 6 months, 58 patients were followed-up and 4 patients were found to have drug resistance, of which 2 patients were new to carry drug resistance. At 12 months, 54 patients were followed-up and 1 new patient was found to have drug resistance. All drug resistance found were high drug resistance to nonnucleoside reverse transcriptase inhibitor (NNRTI). No significant

Table 2. CD4 count, viral load and viral inhibition rates before, 6 months after, and 12 months after drug switch.

	CD4 count		Viral load (lg)		Viral inhibition	
Treatment duration	Patients meeting switching criteria	Patients failing to meet switching criteria	Patients meeting switching criteria	Patients failing to meeting switching criteria	Patients meet switching criteria	Patients failing to meet switching criteria
Before drug switch	203.4±153.0	261.0±127.0	4.8±0.8	1.2±0.6	0	89.7%
At 6 months	220.0±137.2	322.2±164.8	2.3±1.7	1.6±1.4	60.8%	83.1%
At 12 months	280.0±160.0	329.4±134.0	2.0±1.7	1.3±1.1	67.3%	90.7%

difference was observed between drug resistance before and after second-line treatment (P>0.05).

Cross-resistance and multidrug resistance before and after drug switches

Before second-line treatment, rates of cross-resistance and multidrug resistance were high. The rates of drug resistance to NRTI and cross-resistance to AZT/D4 T/DDI were 54.3% (69/127) and 51.2% (65/127), respectively. Rates of drug resistance to NRTI significantly decreased to 17.3% (17/98) and 7.1% (8/113) at 6 and 12 months (P<0.001) after second-line drug switches; Rates of cross-resistance to AZT/D4 T/DDI significantly decreased to 16.3% (16/98) and 7.1% (8/113) at 6 and 12 months (P<0.001), respectively. Before drug switches, the rate of drug resistance to NNRTI was 69.3% (88/127), it decreased to 23.5% (23/98) and 11.5% (13/113) at 6 and 12 months after drug switches, respectively. The multidrug resistance rate to NRTI and NNRTI decreased from 54.3% (69/127) to 7.1% (8/113) after one year of second-line treatment (Table 3).

Drug resistance to 3TC and TDF before and after drug switches

3TC and TDF, which were included in second-line therapy regimens, are NRTI. Rates of drug resistance to 3TC and TDF before drug switches were 30.7% (39/127) and 45.7% (58/127), respectively. After 6 and 12 months of second-line treatment, rates of drug resistance to 3TC decreased to 11.2% (11/98) and 2.7% (3/113) respectively, and rates of drug resistance to TDF decreased to 15.3% (15/98) and 6.2% (7/113) respectively (Table 4). At 6 and 12 months, rates of cross-resistance to 3TC and TDF also decreased from 28.3% (36/128) before second-line treatment to 9.2% (9/98) and 1.8% (2/113), respectively (Table 4). In which, there were 3 cases of new cross-resistance at 6 months, and 1 new case at 12 months. At 12 months, 86.1% (31/36) of patients who showed cross-resistance to 3TC and TDF had a HIV RNA <400 copies/mL.

Analysis of associated factors of treatment results

All patients were 95% or more adherent to therapy 6 and 12 months after second-line treatment initiation. At 12 months, viral loads in 32.7% (37/113) of patients were not inhibited under 400 copies/mL. Results of univariate analysis showed that HIV-1 RNA >100,000 copies/mL before drug switches correlated with ineffective inhibition of viral loads after regimen change, the OR values was 3.95 (95% CI: 1.20, 13.0) (P<0.05). The OR of CD4< 100 cells/μl was 5.14 (95% CI: 0.99, 26.71), however, the P value were insignificance statistical (P>0.05) (Table 5). The OR values of virological inhibition failure in female patients and 45 years old patients were 1.19 (95% CI: 0.34, 4.18) (P>0.05) and 2.11 (95% CI: 0.64, 6.95) (P>0.05) respectively. The second-line regimen with only 1 NRTI drug changed compared to the first-line regimen, OR = 1.31 (95% CI: 0.13, 13.74) (P>0.05). The OR of more than 3 years of first-line antiretroviral treatment duration was 1.01 (95% CI: 0.46, 1.68) (P>0.05) (Table 5).

In this study, 127 patients with first-line antiretroviral treatment failure switched to the second-line regimen after an average of 54.8 months of first-line treatment. Before second-line treatment, viral loads in all patients were higher than 1000 copies/mL. The patients had low immunity, 85% of which had a CD4 count lower than 350 cells/μl, and 69.3% harbored drug resistance. After switching to second-line regimen (3TC+TDF+LPV/r) for 12 months, 67.3% of patients had effective viral inhibition; the average of CD4 cell count had an increase of 76.6 cells/μl; the rate of CD4<350 cells/μl decreased to 70%; and the rate of drug resistance decreased to 8.8%. The significant improvement indicated that switching to second-line antiretroviral drugs led to good treatment effect.

Chinese second-line antiretroviral therapy is the first treatment choice in Europe and America, which produced satisfactory results in antiretroviral-naïve patients with AIDS [8,11]. While in most developing countries, second-line antiretroviral therapy is a substitute when first-line treatment fails. Extensive drug-resistant mutations accumulate in bodies of patients who experienced first-line treatment failure. MC Hosseinipour et al. [7] reported that 85.2% of 88 patients had viral loads lower than 400 copied/mL after one year treatment with (AZT+3TC+TDF+LPV/r) second-line therapy regimen, despite the extensive drug resistance at baseline. In a large multicenter study of 632 patients receiving second-line therapy for 16.6 months in Africa and Asia, only 54% of patients had effective inhibition of virus loads [8]. Possible reasons for significantly different efficacy of second-line therapy are accumulation of drug resistance before drug change or poor adherence to therapy. In this study, 67.3% inhibition rate of viral load was achieved 12 months after drug change, despite the 69.3% in drug-resistant mutation before second-line therapy. As second-line antiretroviral drugs are relatively costly, in addition to the timely switch to second-line drugs after first-line treatment failure, it is essential to strengthen the education of treatment adherence for patients to fully utilize the limited drug sources and obtain good treatment effect.

In our study, before switching to second-line antiretroviral therapy, drug resistance existed in 69.3% of patients who met drug switching criteria. Cross-resistance and multidrug resistance also existed severely. The rates of cross-resistance and multidrug resistance to NRTI and NNRTI were 69.3% and 54.3%,

Table 3. Drug resistance analysis before and after second-line treatment.

	NRTI		NNRTI		NRTI and NNRTI	
	Drug resistance	High drug resistance*	Drug resistance	High drug resistance	Drug resistance	High drug resistance
Before drug switch(N = 127)	54.3% (69)	42.5% (54)	69.3% (88)	66.1% (84)	54.3% (69)	42.5% (54)
At 6 months (N = 98)	17.3% (17)	14.3% (14)	23.5% (23)	23.5% (23)	17.3% (17)	14.3% (14)
At 12 months (N = 113)	7.1% (8)	4.4% (5)	11.5% (13)	11.5% (13)	7.1% (8)	4.4% (5)

*A score >60 get from Stanford University drug resistance database was regarded as high drug resistance.

Table 4. Resistance to 3TC and TDF before and after drug switch.

	3TC	TDF	3TC & TDF
Before drug switches (N = 127)	30.7% (39)	45.7% (58)	28.3% (36)
At 6 months (N = 98)	11.2% (11)	15.3% (15)	9.2% (9)
At 12 months(N = 113)	2.7% (3)	6.2% (7)	1.8% (2)

respectively. However, after one year of second-line treatment, the overall drug resistance rate decreased to 8.8%, and rates of cross-resistance and multidrug resistance also decreased to 11.5% and 7.1%. Our results showed that, although severe cross-resistance and multidrug resistance existed after first-line treatment failure, second-line therapy effectively decreased the rate of drug resistance, as well as the epidemic risk of drug-resistant bacterial strains. Analysis of cross-resistance to NRTI (3TC and TDF), the main drug in the second-line antiretroviral regimen, showed that before drug change, 28.3% of patients had cross-resistance to 3TC and TDF, along with viral loads >1000 copies/mL. After 12 months of second-line treatment, viral loads in 86.1% of patients were effectively inhibited. In these patients, although there was only LPV/r playing a role, satisfying effect were observed and the cross-resistance rate to the 3TC and TDF decreased to 1.8%. It was noticeable that in our study, although drug resistance to the protease inhibitor (PI) was not found, extensive PI secondary drug-resistant mutations were detected. In case PIs primary drug-resistant mutations occur, it will lead to high PI drug resistance. Considering that there were new patients found to have drug-resistant mutations at 6 and 12 months, drug resistance surveillance should be continued to observe the cross-resistance, multidrug resistance and PI drug-resistant mutations after long-term second-line treatment.

Among patients meeting drug switching criteria, we performed a regression analysis of those patients whose virus loads were not inhibited under 400 copies/mL after drug change. The results showed that viral load higher than 100,000 copies/mL before drug change was a risk factor of virological inhibition failure. Similarly, a European study demonstrated that after switching to second-line antiretroviral regimen (including the protease inhibitor); levels of viral loads were more easily inhibited in patients with lower viral loads [8]. Similar findings have been reported that factor associated with HIV-1 RNA >400 copies/mL at 12 months on univariate analysis included having a presenting CD4 count <50 cells/µl and HIV-1 RNA >100,000 copies/mL [7]. However, in our research, lower CD4 count was not a significant factor associated with virological failure. This may be affected by the loss-of-follow-up subjects. In our study, 68 patients did not meet drug switching criteria and volunteered to change drugs. Before second-line treatment, the CD4 count average was 261.0 cells/µl, the rate of viral loads <400 copies/mL was 89.7%, and there were 7 cases of drug resistance; after 12 months of second-line treatment, the CD4 count average was 329.4 cells/µl, the rate of viral load inhibition was 90.7%, and there was 1 case of drug resistance. Although after second-line treatment, no significant differences were observed in virological immunological performance compared to that before drug change, ability of immunity and viral inhibition were still maintained in relatively high levels. These results suggested that in order to fully and effectively utilize the limited second-line drug sources and obtain good clinical effect, it is important to increase the measuring viral loads of treated patients.

Conclusions

Multidrug resistance and cross-resistance existed severely in Chinese patients that experienced first-line treatment failure.

Table 5. Associated factors of virological inhibition failure 12 months after second-line treatment initiation with logistic regression analysis.

Associated factors		OR (95% CI)
Female		1.19 (0.34, 4.18)
>45 years old		2.11 (0.64, 6.95)
CD4 cell count before second-line treatment	<100 cells/mL	5.14 (0.99, 26.71)
	100–200 cells/mL	1.72 (0.35, 8.48)
	≥200 cells/mL	1.0
Viral loads before second-line treatment	1000–10000 copies/mL	1.0
	10000–100000 copies/mL	0.87 (0.24, 3.08)
	≥100000 copies/mL	3.95 (1.20, 13.0)*
No. of NRTI drugs changed compared to the first-line regimen	1 NRTI drug	1.31 (0.13, 13.74)
	2 NRTI drugs	0.76 (0.07, 7.98)
Treatment duration of first-line therapy	<3 years	1.0
	≥3 years	1.01 (0.46, 1.68)

*P<0.05, which were considered statistical significance.

These patients need to be monitored timely on viral loads and drug resistance and switch to second-line therapy under conditions of relatively low viral duplication levels. Satisfactory results were observed in patients treated with Chinese second-line antiretroviral therapy regimen (3TC+TDF+LPV/r) for 12 months, with no drug resistance to PI found. However, extensive secondary mutations to PI were observed, which suggested that the long-term drug resistance surveillance is necessary for patients switching to second-line antiretroviral therapy.

Acknowledgments

We thank Serena Fuller, Wen Xiaoning of USCDC GAP and professor Ping Zhong of Shanghai CDC for their comments and suggestions which help to improve the presentation of the paper.

Author Contributions

Conceived and designed the experiments: MZ HS. Performed the experiments: MZ MS WY. Analyzed the data: MZ MS JC. Contributed reagents/materials/analysis tools: MZ HS ZW. Contributed to the writing of the manuscript: MZ JC.

References

1. Galárraga O, O'Brien ME, Gutiérrez JP, Renaud-Théry F, Nguimfack BD, et al. (2007) Forecast of demand for antiretroviral drugs in low and middle-income countries: 2007–2008. AIDS 21: S97–S103.
2. Boyd MA, Cooper DA (2007) Second-line combination antiretroviral therapy in resource-limited settings: facing the challenges through clinical research. AIDS 21: S55–S63.
3. Zhang F, Dou Z, Ma Y, Zhang Y, Zhao Y, et al. (2011) Effect of earlier initiation of antiretroviral treatment and increased treatment coverage on HIV-related mortality in China: a national observational cohort study. Lancet Infect Dis 11: 516–524.
4. Zhang M, Han XX, Cui WG, Jia MH, Meng XD, et al. (2008) The impacts of current antiretroviral therapy regimens on Chinese AIDS patients and their implications for HIV-1 drug resistance mutation. JPN J INFECT DIS 61: 361–365.
5. Zhang M, Han X, Hu Q, Cui W, Zhao B, et al. (2008) Cohort study of highly active antiretroviral therapy and drug resistant mutation in Henan Province, China. Chineses Journal of Laboratory Medicine 31: 1101–1104.
6. Pujades-Rodríguez M, O'Brien D, Humblet P, Calmy A (2008) Second-line antiretroviral therapy in resource-limited settings: the experience of Médecins Sans Frontières. AIDS 22: 1305–1312.
7. Hosseinipour MC, Kumwenda JJ, Weigel R, Brown LB, Mzinganjira D, et al. (2010) Second-line treatment in the Malawi antiretroviral programme: high early mortality, but good effect in survivors, despite extensive drug resistance at baseline. HIV Medicine 11: 510–518.
8. Pujades-Rodríguez M, Balkan S, Arnould L, Brinkhof MA, Calmy A, et al. (2010) Treatment failure and mortality factors in patients receiving second-line HIV therapy in resource-limited countries. JAMA 304: 303–312.
9. (2009) Chinese National Free AIDS Antiretroviral Therapy Manual.
10. WHO (2009) Rapid advice: antiretroviral therapy for HIV infection in adults and Adolescents.
11. Kempf DJ, King MS, Bernstein B, Cernohous P, Bauer E, et al. (2004) Incidence of resistance in a double-blind study comparing lopinavir/ritonavir plus stavudine and lamivudine to nelfinavir plus stavudine and lamivudine. J Infect Dis 189: 51–60.

9

The Long-HER Study: Clinical and Molecular Analysis of Patients with HER2+ Advanced Breast Cancer Who Become Long-Term Survivors with Trastuzumab-Based Therapy

Angelo Gámez-Pozo[1], Ramón M. Pérez Carrión[2], Luis Manso[3], Carmen Crespo[4], Cesar Mendiola[3], Rocío López-Vacas[1], Julia Berges-Soria[1], Isabel Álvarez López[5], Mireia Margeli[6], Juan L. Bayo Calero[7], Xavier González Farre[8], Ana Santaballa[9], Eva M. Ciruelos[3], Ruth Afonso[10], Juan Lao[11], Gustavo Catalán[12], José V. Álvarez Gallego[13], José Miramón López[14], Francisco J. Salvador Bofill[15], Manuel Ruiz Borrego[16], Enrique Espinosa[17], Juan A. Fresno Vara[1], Pilar Zamora[17]*

1 Instituto de Genética Médica y Molecular (INGEMM) – IdiPAZ, Hospital La Paz, Madrid, Spain, **2** Medical Oncology Department, Hospital Quirón, Pozuelo de Alarcón, Madrid, Spain, **3** Medical Oncology Department, Hospital 12 de Octubre, Madrid, Spain, **4** Medical Oncology Department, Hospital Ramón y Cajal, Madrid, Spain, **5** Medical Oncology Department, Hospital de Donostia, San Sebastián, Pais Vasco, Spain, **6** Medical Oncology Department, Hospital Germans Trias i Pujol, Badalona, Barcelona, Spain, **7** Medical Oncology Department, Hospital Juan Ramón Jiménez, Huelva, Spain, **8** Medical Oncology Department, Hospital Clinic de Barcelona, Barcelona, Spain, **9** Medical Oncology Department, Hospital La Fe, Valencia, Spain, **10** Medical Oncology Department, Hospital Nuestra Señora de la Candelaria, Santa Cruz de Tenerife, Spain, **11** Medical Oncology Department, Hospital Miguel Servet, Zaragoza, Spain, **12** Medical Oncology Department, Hospital Son Llàtzer, Palma de Mallorca, Spain, **13** Medical Oncology Department, Complejo Hospitalario de Zamora, Zamora, Spain, **14** Medical Oncology Department, Hospital Serranía de Ronda, Ronda, Málaga, Spain, **15** Medical Oncology Department, Hospital Virgen de Valme, Sevilla, Spain, **16** Medical Oncology Department, Hospital Virgen del Rocío, Sevilla, Spain, **17** Medical Oncology Department, Hospital La Paz, Madrid, Spain

Abstract

Background: Trastuzumab improves survival outcomes in patients with HER2+ metastatic breast cancer. The Long-Her study was designed to identify clinical and molecular markers that could differentiate long-term survivors from patients having early progression after trastuzumab treatment.

Methods: Data were collected from women with HER2-positive metastatic breast cancer treated with trastuzumab that experienced a response or stable disease during at least 3 years. Patients having a progression in the first year of therapy with trastuzumab were used as a control. Genes related with trastuzumab resistance were identified and investigated for network and gene functional interrelation. Models predicting poor response to trastuzumab were constructed and evaluated. Finally, a mutational status analysis of selected genes was performed in HER2 positive breast cancer samples.

Results: 103 patients were registered in the Long-HER study, of whom 71 had obtained a durable complete response. Median age was 58 years. Metastatic disease was diagnosed after a median of 24.7 months since primary diagnosis. Metastases were present in the liver (25%), lungs (25%), bones (23%) and soft tissues (23%), with 20% of patients having multiple locations of metastases. Median duration of response was 55 months. The molecular analysis included 35 patients from the group with complete response and 18 patients in a control poor-response group. Absence of trastuzumab as part of adjuvant therapy was the only clinical factor associated with long-term survival. Gene ontology analysis demonstrated that PI3K pathway was associated with poor response to trastuzumab-based therapy: tumours in the control group usually had four or five alterations in this pathway, whereas tumours in the Long-HER group had two alterations at most.

Conclusions: Trastuzumab may provide a substantial long-term survival benefit in a selected group of patients. Whole genome expression analysis comparing long-term survivors vs. a control group predicted early progression after trastuzumab-based therapy. Multiple alterations in genes related to the PI3K-mTOR pathway seem to be required to confer resistance to this therapy.

Editor: Joseph Najbauer, University of Pécs Medical School, Hungary

Funding: The Long-HER study was supported by an unrestricted grant from Roche. AGP (CA12/00258) and RLV (CA12/00264) are supported by Instituto de Salud Carlos III, Spain. The funders had no role in study design, data analysis, decision to publish, or preparation of the manuscript.

* Email: zamorapilar@gmail.com

Introduction

Metastatic breast cancer is an incurable disease, with a median overall survival of approximately 3 years. However, patients' outcome varies widely depending on a number of prognostic factors, such as visceral involvement, time from initial diagnosis, hormonal receptors and HER-2 status.

HER2 positive disease accounts for 15–20% of all cases and entails a poor prognosis [1]. Trastuzumab is a recombinant humanized monoclonal antibody that selectively targets the extracellular domain of the HER2 receptor. The prognosis of patients with HER2-positive metastatic breast cancer has dramatically changed since the advent of this drug [2,3,4,5,6]. Phase II and III studies have shown an advantage in response rate, disease-free survival and overall survival when the antibody is added to chemotherapy. Median overall survival was 25 months in the first reported trial of trastuzumab in advanced disease [2], and exceeded 37 months in a recent study [7]. In general, better results are seen in first-line as compared with subsequent lines of therapy [3].

Long-term survival can be achieved with trastuzumab and durable complete responses have occasionally been reported. Some of these women remain alive and disease-free after five to ten years from the diagnosis of metastases, which leads to hypothesize that cure could be possible in a small subset of patients. The Long-HER study was designed to analyse the clinical and molecular characteristics of HER2-positive advanced breast cancer in patients who obtained long-term responses with trastuzumab.

Microarray analysis is a widely used technology for studying gene expression on a global scale. Gene expression profiling is contributing important advances in clinical oncology, providing a basis for understanding the complex biology of tumours, improving the accuracy of disease diagnosis as well as disease prognosis, and providing tools to determine which targeted therapeutic agents are likely to be effective in the treatment of particular tumours. However, the requirement of frozen tissues for microarray experiments limits the clinical use of these gene signatures. Many laboratories are developing methods to assess gene expression profiling using formalin-fixed, paraffin-embedded (FFPE) samples [8,9,10].

In this work, we used genome-wide expression profiling of FFPE samples to study the molecular characteristics of breast cancers from patients with long-term complete response to trastuzumab. The aim of the study was to find clinical and molecular factors that would differentiate this population from patients developing treatment failure.

Materials and Methods

Ethics statement

Institutional approval from our ethical committee was obtained for the conduct of the study (Ethics Committee for Clinical Investigations, Hospital Universitario La Paz). The study was also approved by ethics committees from Área Sanitaria de Guipúzcoa and Hospital La Fe. Data were analyzed anonymously. Patients provided written consent so that their samples and clinical data could be used for investigational purposes.

Study design

This was a multi-institutional retrospective study. Investigators searched their local databases to find patients with HER2 positive metastatic breast cancer who were long-term survivors. Participants had to fulfil all the following criteria: a confirmed diagnosis of metastatic breast cancer; HER2 positive disease, as determined by 3+ immunohistochemistry or positive fluorescence in situ hybridization (FISH); treatment with chemotherapy plus trastuzumab; stable disease or a sustained partial or complete response lasting at least 3 years; and availability of clinical data and tumour FFPE block. Clinical and radiological responses were assessed by local investigators using the Response Evaluation Criteria In Solid Tumors (RECIST) 1.1 (Eisenhower, EJC 2009; 45:228). Treatment with anti-HER2 therapy other than trastuzumab was not allowed. Clinical characteristics were introduced in a database and the FFPE blocks were sent to a central laboratory. Molecular analysis would be performed in available samples from patients obtaining a complete response. A control group was also created with patients who had had a progression within the first 12 months of first-line trastuzumab-based therapy: molecular analysis was also performed in samples from this control group (poor-response group, hereafter). Patients from the control group came from a single institution (reference centre) and availability of tumour sample was required for these cases.

RNA isolation and gene expression analysis

Selected FFPE tumour specimens were cut into serial sections with a thickness of 10 µm. RNA was then extracted with the RecoverAll Total Nucleic Acid Isolation Kit (Life Technologies). Since a significant part of RNA isolated from FFPE samples is not suitable for enzymatic reactions [11], we decided to use Pico Profiling [12], a novel method optimized for whole transcriptome amplification. Briefly, 100 ng RNA was subject to library synthesis and amplification for 23 cycles using WTA2 (Sigma Aldrich). 10 µg cDNA was subsequently fragmented by DNAseI and biotinylated by terminal transferase obtained from GeneChip Mapping 10Kv2 Assay Kit (Affymetrix). Hybridization, washing, staining and scanning of Affymetrix Human Genome U219 arrays were performed following the manufacturer's recommendations. Scanned images (DAT files) were transformed into intensities (CEL files) by GCOS (Affymetrix). The raw intensity values were background corrected, log2 transformed, quartile normalized and summarized using the RMA algorithm in Genomics Suite 6.6 (Partek). Microarray data and clinical info are available at the Gene Expression Omnibus (GSE44272).

Statistical analyses

Univariate analysis was used to assess the value of clinical and pathological variables: grade of differentiation, expression of hormonal receptors, size of the primary tumour, stage at diagnosis, number of metastatic sites, location of metastases, use of adjuvant chemotherapy, use of adjuvant trastuzumab, and time from initial diagnosis to relapse. Multivariate logistic regression was to be used with variables significant at univariate analysis.

Genes that were significantly up- or down-regulated between patient groups were identified using Significance Analysis of Microarrays (SAM) [13]. SAM assigns a score to each gene on the basis of a change in gene expression relative to the standard deviation of repeated measurements. For genes with scores greater than an adjustable threshold, SAM uses permutations of the repeated measurements to estimate the percentage of genes identified by chance – the false discovery rate (FDR). Analysis parameters (delta) were set to result in a FDR≤5%. Differentially expressed genes were investigated for network and gene functional interrelation using different bioinformatics tools [13]. Predictive models were built using a discriminant analysis approach in SPSS 16. SAM, hierarchical clustering analyses and mutations graphs were carried out with TIGR MeV v.4.7.4 [14]. Boxplots and univariant analyses were performed in GraphPad Prism 5.1.

Table 1. Summary of patients' characteristics.

	All Long-HER, n = 103	Complete responders n = 71	Complete responders with molecular analysis, n = 35	Control poor-response group, n = 18
Median age (years)	58 (36–87)	58 (40–87)	59 (40–87)	57 (41–83)
Hormone receptors +	49%	47%	49%	56%
Location of mets.				
Liver	14 (13%)	18 (25%)	6 (11%)	2 (11%)
Lung	24 (23%)	18 (25%)	15 (43%)	6 (33%)
Bones	15 (14%)	16 (23%)	11 (31%)	3 (17%)
Soft tissues	6 (6%)	16 (23%)	10 (29%)	6 (33%)
Multiple sites	32 (31%)	14 (20%)	8 (23%)	6 (33%)
Adjuvant or neoadjuvant therapy	90 (91%)	66 (94%)	32 (93%)	14 (78%)
First-line therapy				
Anthracycline-based	9 (9%)	4 (6%)	2 (6%)	0
Taxane-based	41 (40%)	35 (49%)	22 (63%)	13 (72%)
Anthracycline+taxane	34 (33%)	19 (27%)	8 (23%)	1 (6%)
Other chemotherapy	11 (10%)	8 (11%)	3 (8%)	4 (22%)
Hormonal therapy	8 (8%)	5 (7%)	0	0
Trastuzumab duration	61 months (6–148)	62 months (12–138)	62 months (12–138)	10 months (3–15)

The whole population of long-term responders included 103 patients, of who 71 achieved a complete response. Molecular analysis was performed in 35 out of 71 patients with complete response.

Gene ontology analyses

Gene ontology analyses including pathways, biological processes and molecular functions of genes related with trastuzumab response were performed in PANTHER [15]. Signalling pathway enrichment analyses were performed in SPEED [16].

PI3K-mTOR pathway analysis

Genes related with PI3K pathway were selected from previous works [17,18,19]. For each gene all probes were selected and z-scored. Final expression values were the mean of all probes for each gene. Differences were assessed using the Mann Whitney test; significance was set at $p<0.01$.

Mutations in Her2 breast cancer samples

To assess the mutational background of HER2 breast cancer samples, we used online available information about the mutations identified in 30 HER2 positive samples previously analysed [20]. We selected all mutations and copy number variants in these samples, then we investigated which genes differentially expressed in our study had any mutation or copy number variant. Finally, we performed the same analysis with genes from the PI3K-mTOR pathways.

Results

Clinical data

A total of 103 long-term survivors were identified, of whom 71 had achieved a durable complete response. Median age was 58 years. Median duration of response for the group of 103 survivors was 55 months (35–127) and median overall survival was 59 months (36–130). Two thirds of the tumours were poorly differentiated and 51% did not express oestrogen or progesterone receptors. HER2 status had been determined by immunohistochemistry in 98% of cases and by FISH in 21%. At the time of initial diagnosis, 21% of patients had received neoadjuvant chemotherapy and 70% had received adjuvant chemotherapy. In all but 11 patients, adjuvant or neoadjuvant chemotherapy was anthracycline-based. Twenty-eight percent of patients had received adjuvant hormonal therapy. Four patients (8%) had been treated with adjuvant trastuzumab. Table 1 summarises clinical features.

All 103 patients received trastuzumab as first-line therapy. This treatment began between the years 1999 and 2007. Ninety-five patients also received concomitant chemotherapy, which included a taxane in 65 (63%) and an anthracycline in 43 (42%). Four patients had to discontinue chemotherapy due to toxic events. Forty-two patients were treated with a hormonal agent, either initially (8 patients) or after the achievement of a complete response with chemotherapy (34 patients). Initial hormonal therapy consisted in letrozol in 4 patients, exemestane in 2 patients and tamoxifen in 2 patients. As inclusion criteria required treatment with chemotherapy, these 8 patients initially treated with a hormonal agent were not accepted for the molecular analysis. Fifty-three patients remain in remission and 48 are still receiving trastuzumab-based therapy; fifty patients have stable disease and 45 of them also continue on trastuzumab. In the whole group of long-term survivors with complete response (n = 71), the liver and the lungs were the most common metastatic sites (25% each), followed by the bones, skin and lymph nodes (23% each). Twenty percent of patients had multiple affected sites. The control group included 18 patients coming from one single centre. These patients had begun first-line therapy with trastuzumab between the years 2005 and 2007. All these patients had clinical data and tumour samples available.

Clinical factors such as grade of differentiation, number of metastatic sites or the location of metastases did not correlate with long-term survival. There were five patients with brain metastasis among survivors: these five patients received local treatment (surgery for isolated lesions plus radiation therapy) in addition to systemic therapy. Only 6 out of 103 patients presented with

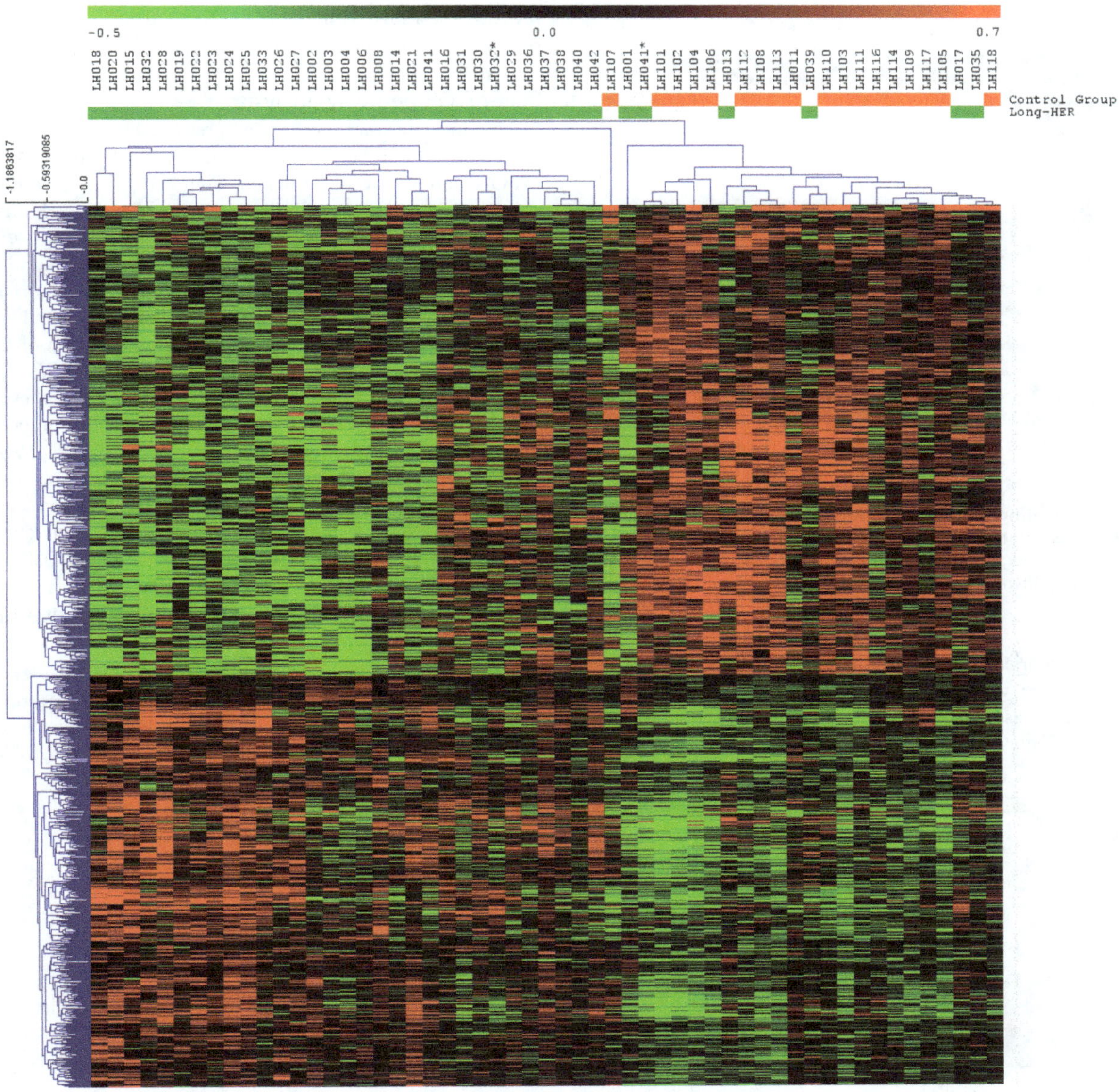

Figure 1. Supervised hierarchical clustering for all samples using 1052 differentially expressed probesets identified using SAM. Each row represents a probeset and each column a sample. Green bars indicate samples from patients in Long-HER group, red bars indicate samples from short-term responders. There are two samples duplicated, * account for metastasis samples.

metastasis in soft-tissues exclusively. Only four of the long-term survivors had received adjuvant trastuzumab. This was the only clinical factor associated with prolonged survival.

Tissue specimens and patients' characteristics for molecular analyses

Samples for the molecular study were selected from the 71 patients achieving a complete response. The molecular study also included a control group coming from patients who had a poor response after trastuzumab-based therapy. In patients with complete response, median duration of response was 62 months (35–127) and the median overall survival 67 months (36–130). In the control group, median duration of response was 6 months (2–12) and the median overall survival 33 months (15–124). Sixty-one FFPE samples with annotated clinical information were selected, 53 of which had enough RNA to perform hybridization. Among these 53 samples, 35 samples corresponded to long-term responders and 18 to the control group. Table 1 shows the clinical features of all Long-HER survivors, Long-HER patients achieving a complete remission, Long-HER patients selected for molecular analysis and the control group. There were no major differences among these categories, although the 71 Long-HER survivors had a lower incidence of liver and lung metastases as compared with the other groups.

Genes related with response to trastuzumab

Comparison of the control group and Long-HER group using SAM showed significant differences in the expression of 1052 probe sets representing 858 genes. 560 probe sets were up-regulated, and 492 probe sets were down-regulated in the control group compared to the Long-HER group (Figure 1 and Table S1). In order to identify those pathways associated with the response to trastuzumab, functional categories of 858 differentially expressed genes were identified using gene ontology analysis. Statistically

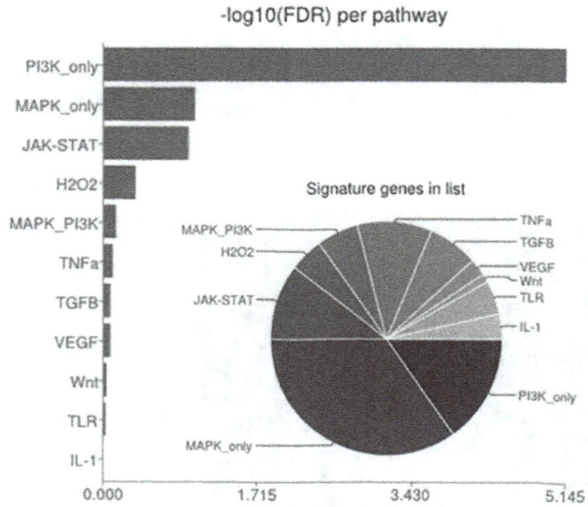

Figure 2. Signaling pathway annotation enrichment analysis for 858 genes related with trastuzumab resistance. This analysis was performed using SPEED software. PI3K pathway appeared as the most relevant pathway in relation with trastuzumab resistance.

significant categories included a large number of genes involved in hypoxia response via HIF activation, EGF receptor signalling pathway, PI3 kinase pathway, apoptosis signalling pathway and p53 pathway (Figure S1). Signalling pathway enrichment analyses revealed the PI3K pathway as the most strongly associated with response to trastuzumab, as shown in Figure 2.

PI3K-mTOR pathway analysis

To elucidate the mechanisms responsible for trastuzumab resistance, 338 probes comprising 97 genes related to the PI3K-mTOR pathway were evaluated. Fourteen genes were differentially expressed between the control group and the Long-HER group (Mann-Whitney $p<0.01$). Five of these genes -*PTEN, AGPAT1, PRKAA1, FKBP8* and *MAP4K3*- were found to act upstream of *mTOR* complexes, and could modulate *mTOR* signalling. Expression values for these genes are shown in Figure 3. Most patients in the control group had low expression of *PTEN, MAP4K3* and *PRKAA1*, and high expression of *AGPAT1* and *FKBP8*. However, these features appeared as isolated events in the Long-HER group (Figure 3). A predictive model for trastuzumab response, including *PTEN, AGPAT1, PRKAA1 FKBP8* and *MAP4K3* gene expression, was built using a discriminant analysis approach. The model classified correctly more than 81% of the samples in the Leave-one-out cross validation and presents an area under the curve of 0.938.

Analysis of the mutational state in HER2-positive breast cancer samples

Using online available data from another study, we assessed the mutational status of the 858 genes related to trastuzumab resistance found in our study, with particular attention to the 97 genes related to the PI3K-mTOR pathway. To do this, online

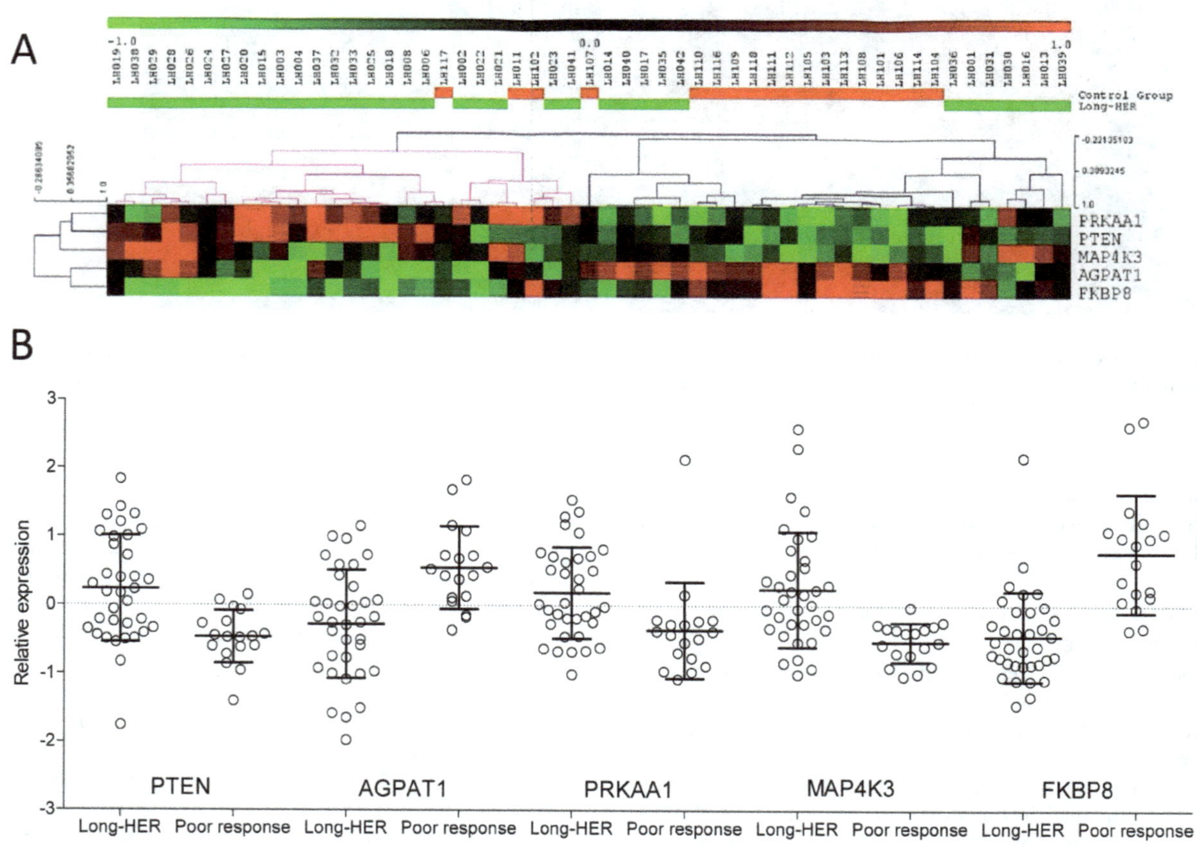

Figure 3. PI3K-mTOR pathway analyses. A) Supervised hierarchical clustering for all samples using five genes from the PI3K-mTOR pathway that are differentially expressed between Long-HER and short-term responders to trastuzumab samples. B) Distribution of the normalized expression of these genes.

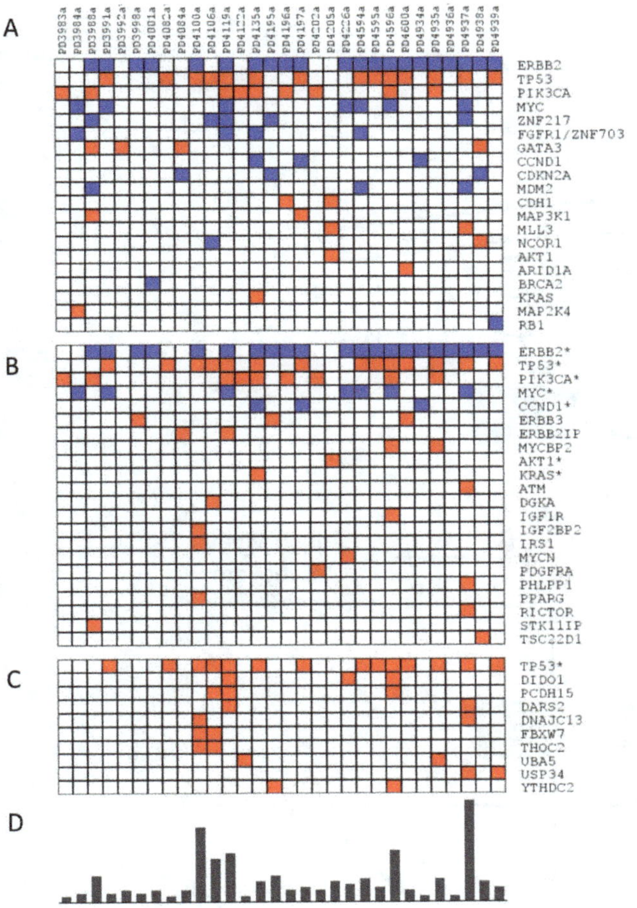

Figure 4. Mutational status of HER2+ patients. Distribution of point mutations (red) and copy number variants (blue) in A) genes considered as carriers of cancer driven mutations by Stephens and co-workers, B) genes from the PI3k-mTOR pathway, and C) genes related with trastuzumab resistance (only genes with two of more mutation events are showed, full report is provided as Additional Figure 1). D) Number of point mutations and copy number variants detected in each patient. *This gene is also considered as carrier of cancer driven mutations.

data from a previously described analysis of mutations and copy number variants in 30 HER2-positive tumours were used [20]. We compiled 2,229 point mutations across the exome and 101 copy number variations considered by the authors as cancer drive mutations. We found 143 point mutations distributed in 114 out of 858 trastuzumab resistance related genes (13%). The number of mutations in each sample varied widely, from 2 to 35 (mean 7.6). Only 10 of these mutations appeared in two of more patients (Figure 4). *TP53* presented the highest mutational rate (14/30 samples, 47%), followed by *PIK3CA* (30%), *ERBB3, DIDO1* and *PCDH15* (10% each). There were also 46 point mutations in 17 out of the 97 genes (17%) in the PI3K-mTOR pathway. Additionally, we found 51 copy number variants in 10 regions containing genes considered as drivers of cancer. *ERBB2* region was amplified in 21 out of the 30 samples (70%), whereas 7/30 (23%) presented MYC amplification (Figure 4). Interestingly, point mutations or copy number variants of *PTEN, AGPAT1, PRKAA1, FKBP8* and *MAP4K3* were not present in these 30 HER2 positive patient samples.

Discussion

Long-term survival without evidence of disease is possible in a small subgroup of patients with metastatic HER2-positive breast cancer. The Long-HER study analysed the clinical and biological characteristics of such patients treated with trastuzumab-based therapy and compared the results with those obtained in a similar series of patients who had experienced disease progression within the first year of treatment.

Clinical factors did not correlate with long-term survival. The presence of brain metastases in five patients with long-term survival implies that central nervous system spread does not preclude long-term survival. Only 6 out of 103 patients presented with metastasis in soft-tissues exclusively, meaning that the vast majority of our study population had visceral dissemination.

Long-term survivors had not received adjuvant trastuzumab because the drug was not used in this indication at the time of initial diagnosis. This was the only clinical factor associated with prolonged survival and suggests the existence of tumours highly sensitive to trastuzumab that could obtain prolonged remissions regardless of the time of drug administration. As trastuzumab is now part of the standard adjuvant therapy for HER2-positive breast cancer, the population analysed in the Long-HER study will be increasingly difficult to find because such patients are cured by adjuvant trastuzumab. An Irish-Italian consortium has recently reported on 13 patients who achieved durable complete responses with trastuzumab-based therapy [21]. These patients had received at least two years of treatment with the monoclonal antibody, whereas many of our patients have continued on therapy beyond 5 years. Other recent studies have reported similar series of long-term survivors among patients treated with trastuzumab [22,23,24].

Tumours in the Long-HER group did not show a uniform expression gene profile. In other words, molecular identification of this subset of patients with excellent prognosis remains an elusive goal. However, tumours in the control group, i.e., those having early progression to trastuzumab-based therapies, were clearly identified in the present study. The Long-HER study serves as a proof-of-principle that whole genome expression analysis on FFPE samples can provide novel mechanistic insights related to drug resistance/sensitivity. Anthracyclines were less used in the control group as compared with the Long-HER in first line, which could have influenced the rate of initial remissions. However, we did not find a significant difference in the Long-HER group according to the type of chemotherapy. Also, the molecular analysis was not influenced by the type of chemotherapy because samples were taken before initiation of first-line therapy.

Mechanisms of resistance to trastuzumab have been categorised in three groups: structural mutations in HER2 protein, increased expression or activation of other tyrosine kinase receptors (such as insulin-like growth factor receptor), or intracellular alterations in HER2 downstream signalling [25,26]. This latter mechanism includes PTEN deficiency [27], SRC activation [28] and PI3K/AKT activation [29]. In our study, genes related to the PI3K pathway appeared most strongly associated with poor response, although other alterations were also found. These results suggest that resistance to trastuzumab does not depend on one or a limited number of mutations, but rather on a variety of changes in involved pathways. A recent review on genomic analysis indicates that the polygenic nature of drug resistance, as well as tumour heterogeneity, constitute important challenges in the development of response predictors [30]. For this reason, gene or protein profiles may provide a more realistic approach than single marker determination to assess resistance.

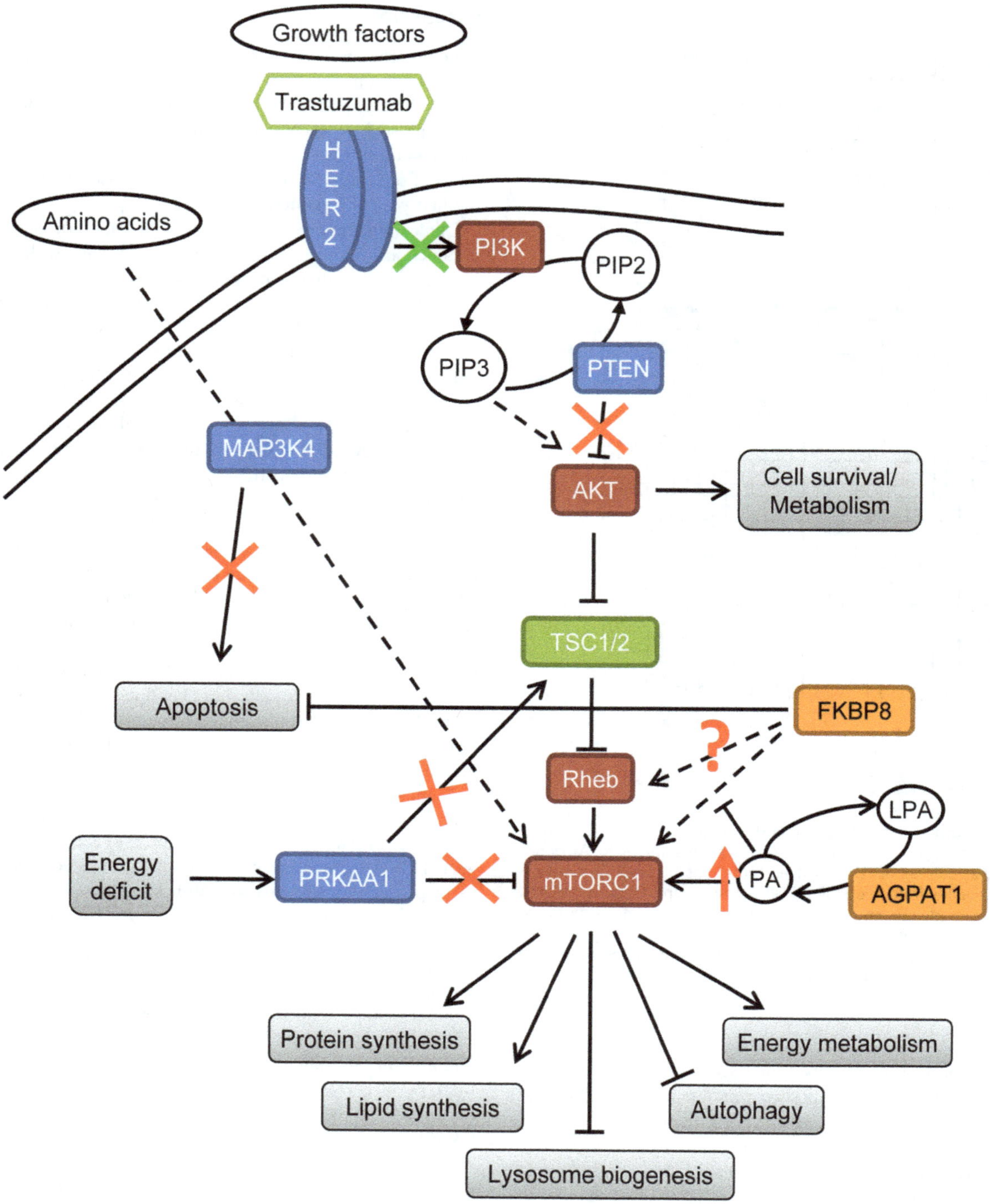

Figure 5. Proposed model of trastuzumab resistance in short-term responders due to Akt/mTOR activation and apoptosis inhibition. Genes in blue are downregulated, genes in orange are upregulated, genes in red favour Akt/mTOR pathway activation and genes in green decrease Akt/mTOR pathway activation. Red signs are new disrupting elements identified. Green arrow indicates the step regulated by trastuzumab.

SAM analyses identified 858 genes related to trastuzumab resistance in our series. Gene ontology and signalling pathway enrichment analyses pointed out the relation between PI3K-mTOR signalling pathway and trastuzumb resistance. PI3K-mTOR signalling pathway analyses showed that tumours from patients who did not obtain prolonged remissions (control group) usually had loss of expression in *PTEN, PRKAA1* and *MAP3K4*, as well as overexpression in *AGPAT1* and *FKBP8*. On the contrary, tumours from the Long-HER group could present with none, one or two of these molecular alterations, which suggests that more than two events (either these or other with similar consequences) are needed to confer resistance to trastuzumab.

Loss of *PTEN* expression has been previously associated with resistance to trastuzumab [31]. Active PRKAA1 directly phosphorylates and enhances the ability of tuberin to inhibit mTOR signalling [32]. Loss of PRKAA1 can lead to an increased mTORC1 activity independently of the energetic status of the cell [33]. MAP4K3 plays an important role in the regulation of mTOR signalling in response to amino acids presence and its loss could disturb cell sensitivity to nutrient absence [34]. MAP4K3 loss can decrease BAX activation, inactivating the apoptosis pathway [35]. AGPAT1 catalyses the conversion of lysophosphatidic acid to phosphatidic acid (PA) [36] and over-expression of AGPAT1 can increase PA in the cell, constitutively activating mTOR [37]. The molecular interaction of Bcl-2 with FKBP8 potentiates the biological function of Bcl-2 and contributes to tumorigenesis and chemoresistance [38]. Additionally, it has been proposed that FKBP8 mediates the activation of mTORC1 by Rheb [39,40,41]. Although recent reports dispute this idea [42,43], it is clear that FKBP8 binds both Rheb and mTORC1, and this interaction is disrupted in the presence of PA [44]. All these gene alterations lead to Akt/mTOR activation and apoptosis inhibition (Figure 5), and could explain the lack of response to trastuzumab in the control group.

Our analysis of 858 genes in a whole-genome mutation database [20] suggests that a common mutation profile does not exist for this population because the incidence of mutations varies widely. Answering clinical questions by performing mutational analysis may be difficult, but expression profiling of either mRNA or proteins could provide useful insights. In our study, the mechanistic analysis of the PI3K-mTOR pathway allowed the identification of some potential key gene expression alterations in a selected population of patients.

Previous studies have shown that PI3K activation and loss of PTEN predict trastuzumab resistance [27,31,45,46]. However, an mTOR inhibitor has recently shown a modest benefit in patients progressing upon trastuzumab, which suggests that further investigation is required before taking these findings to the clinic [47,48]. These trials include patients who have had a progression with trastuzumab-based therapy, but the possibility to identify tumours that will likely be resistant to trastuzumab could be important for the development of therapeutic strategies in earlier stages of disease. Patients less likely to be cured with adjuvant trastuzumab, for instance, would be ideal candidates to participate in clinical trials with new anti-HER2 drugs.

Our study has some limitations. First, patients received a variety of chemotherapy agents along with trastuzumab. A taxane was used in most cases, but no clinical or molecular differences were detected in patients treated with other drugs. This suggests that it is the monoclonal antibody and not its companion what determines prognosis. On the other hand, molecular findings must be interpreted with caution because we analysed many genes and sample size was small. Also, the limited sample size does not allow getting further insight into the molecular pathways involved in the response to trastuzumab. Finally, a proportion of samples in the Long-HER group were not suitable for molecular analysis. We tried to recruit as many patients as possible to gather clinical information, but unfortunately many of corresponding samples were not available or were in poor condition for molecular analysis. This could have produced an uncontrolled bias in the results of the molecular study. On the contrary, patients in the control group were selected from a reference centre with optimal storing conditions and whit the requirement that tumour samples would be available. Validation in an independent series of patients is obviously required. However, very few patients achieve long-term survival, as demonstrated in our series and other published series, so a formal validation may be difficult to perform.

In summary, long-term survival is possible in a selected population of patients with advanced HER2-positive breast cancer. Whole genome expression analysis comparing long-term survivors vs. a control group was able to predict progression to trastuzumab-based therapy. Multiple alterations in genes related to the AKT-mTOR pathway seem to be required to confer resistance to this drug. The validation of a poor-response profile would allow tailoring therapy in future clinical trials.

Supporting Information

Figure S1 Gene Ontology Analyses. Gene ontology analyses including A) pathways, B) biological process and C) molecular functions of the 858 genes related with trastuzumab response were performed using PANTHER. All categories represented are differentially represented when compared with the *Homo sapiens* reference list ($P<0.05$).

Table S1 Expression values of 1052 probe sets differentially expressed between Long-Her and control group. ER: Estrogen receptor status; PGr: Progesterone receptor status; PFS: Progression free survival; M: Metastases; N: lymph node status; T: Tumor size. Clinical criteria are provided according to TNM classification. (http://www.cancer.gov/cancertopics/pdq/treatment/breast/healthprofessional/page3).

Acknowledgments

Dr. Herbert Auer at the Functional Genomics Facility of IRB Barcelona performed sample processing and primary analyses. Control samples came from IdiPAZ Biobank (Spanish Hospital Biobanks Network, www.redbiobancos.es), which is supported by Instituto de Salud Carlos III [RETICC RD09/0076/00073] and Farmaindustria, through the Cooperation Program in Clinical and Translational Research (Comunidad de Madrid). We want to thank Dr. C. Ramírez Medrano for her contribution to data monitoring and collection. We would like to thank our patients for their participation in the Long-HER study.

Author Contributions

Conceived and designed the experiments: AGP EE JAFV PZ. Performed the experiments: AGP RLV JBS. Analyzed the data: AGP JBS EE JAFV PZ. Contributed reagents/materials/analysis tools: RPC LM CC CM IAL MM JLBC XGF AS EMC RA JL GC JVAG JML FJSB MRB EE PZ. Wrote the paper: AGP EE JAFV PZ.

References

1. Gutierrez C, Schiff R (2011) HER2: biology, detection, and clinical implications. Arch Pathol Lab Med 135: 55–62.
2. Slamon DJ, Leyland-Jones B, Shak S, Fuchs H, Paton V, et al. (2001) Use of chemotherapy plus a monoclonal antibody against HER2 for metastatic breast cancer that overexpresses HER2. N Engl J Med 344: 783–792.
3. Burstein HJ, Kuter I, Campos SM, Gelman RS, Tribou L, et al. (2001) Clinical activity of trastuzumab and vinorelbine in women with HER2-overexpressing metastatic breast cancer. J Clin Oncol 19: 2722–2730.
4. Marty M, Cognetti F, Maraninchi D, Snyder R, Mauriac L, et al. (2005) Randomized phase II trial of the efficacy and safety of trastuzumab combined with docetaxel in patients with human epidermal growth factor receptor 2-positive metastatic breast cancer administered as first-line treatment: the M77001 study group. J Clin Oncol 23: 4265–4274.
5. Robert N, Leyland-Jones B, Asmar L, Belt R, Ilegbodu D, et al. (2006) Randomized phase III study of trastuzumab, paclitaxel, and carboplatin compared with trastuzumab and paclitaxel in women with HER-2-overexpressing metastatic breast cancer. J Clin Oncol 24: 2786–2792.
6. Gasparini G, Gion M, Mariani L, Papaldo P, Crivellari D, et al. (2007) Randomized Phase II Trial of weekly paclitaxel alone versus trastuzumab plus weekly paclitaxel as first-line therapy of patients with Her-2 positive advanced breast cancer. Breast Cancer Res Treat 101: 355–365.

7. Valero V, Forbes J, Pegram MD, Pienkowski T, Eiermann W, et al. (2011) Multicenter phase III randomized trial comparing docetaxel and trastuzumab with docetaxel, carboplatin, and trastuzumab as first-line chemotherapy for patients with HER2-gene-amplified metastatic breast cancer (BCIRG 007 study): two highly active therapeutic regimens. J Clin Oncol 29: 149–156.
8. Paik S, Kim CY, Song YK, Kim WS (2005) Technology insight: Application of molecular techniques to formalin-fixed paraffin-embedded tissues from breast cancer. Nat Clin Pract Oncol 2: 246–254.
9. Linton K, Hey Y, Dibben S, Miller C, Freemont A, et al. (2009) Methods comparison for high-resolution transcriptional analysis of archival material on Affymetrix Plus 2.0 and Exon 1.0 microarrays. Biotechniques 47: 587–596.
10. Xie Y, Xiao G, Coombes KR, Behrens C, Solis LM, et al. (2011) Robust gene expression signature from formalin-fixed paraffin-embedded samples predicts prognosis of non-small-cell lung cancer patients. Clin Cancer Res 17: 5705–5714.
11. von Ahlfen S, Missel A, Bendrat K, Schlumpberger M (2007) Determinants of RNA quality from FFPE samples. PLoS One 2: e1261.
12. Gonzalez-Roca E, Garcia-Albeniz X, Rodriguez-Mulero S, Gomis RR, Kornacker K, et al. (2010) Accurate expression profiling of very small cell populations. PLoS One 5: e14418.
13. Tusher VG, Tibshirani R, Chu G (2001) Significance analysis of microarrays applied to the ionizing radiation response. Proc Natl Acad Sci U S A 98: 5116–5121.
14. Saeed AI, Sharov V, White J, Li J, Liang W, et al. (2003) TM4: a free, open-source system for microarray data management and analysis. Biotechniques 34: 374–378.
15. Thomas PD, Campbell MJ, Kejariwal A, Mi H, Karlak B, et al. (2003) PANTHER: a library of protein families and subfamilies indexed by function. Genome Res 13: 2129–2141.
16. Parikh JR, Klinger B, Xia Y, Marto JA, Bluthgen N (2010) Discovering causal signaling pathways through gene-expression patterns. Nucleic Acids Res 38: W109–117.
17. Dowling RJ, Topisirovic I, Fonseca BD, Sonenberg N (2010) Dissecting the role of mTOR: lessons from mTOR inhibitors. Biochim Biophys Acta 1804: 433–439.
18. Laplante M, Sabatini DM (2012) mTOR signaling in growth control and disease. Cell 149: 274–293.
19. Hemmings BA, Restuccia DF (2012) PI3K-PKB/Akt pathway. Cold Spring Harb Perspect Biol 4: a011189.
20. Stephens PJ, Tarpey PS, Davies H, Van Loo P, Greenman C, et al. (2012) The landscape of cancer genes and mutational processes in breast cancer. Nature 486: 400–404.
21. Gullo G, Zuradelli M, Sclafani F, Santoro A, Crown J (2012) Durable complete response following chemotherapy and trastuzumab for metastatic HER2-positive breast cancer. Ann Oncol 23: 2204–2205.
22. Bonifazi M, Franchi M, Rossi M, Zambelli A, Moja L, et al. (2014) Long term survival of HER2-positive early breast cancer treated with trastuzumab-based adjuvant regimen: A large cohort study from clinical practice. Breast.
23. Cortazar P, Zhang L, Untch M, Mehta K, Costantino JP, et al. (2014) Pathological complete response and long-term clinical benefit in breast cancer: the CTNeoBC pooled analysis. Lancet 384: 164–172.
24. Yardley DA, Tripathy D, Brufsky AM, Rugo HS, Kaufman PA, et al. (2014) Long-term survivor characteristics in HER2-positive metastatic breast cancer from registHER. Br J Cancer 110: 2756–2764.
25. Gajria D, Chandarlapaty S (2011) HER2-amplified breast cancer: mechanisms of trastuzumab resistance and novel targeted therapies. Expert Rev Anticancer Ther 11: 263–275.
26. Vu T, Claret FX (2012) Trastuzumab: updated mechanisms of action and resistance in breast cancer. Front Oncol 2: 62.
27. Nagata Y, Lan KH, Zhou X, Tan M, Esteva FJ, et al. (2004) PTEN activation contributes to tumor inhibition by trastuzumab, and loss of PTEN predicts trastuzumab resistance in patients. Cancer Cell 6: 117–127.
28. Zhang S, Huang WC, Li P, Guo H, Poh SB, et al. (2011) Combating trastuzumab resistance by targeting SRC, a common node downstream of multiple resistance pathways. Nat Med 17: 461–469.
29. Kataoka Y, Mukohara T, Shimada H, Saijo N, Hirai M, et al. (2010) Association between gain-of-function mutations in PIK3CA and resistance to HER2-targeted agents in HER2-amplified breast cancer cell lines. Ann Oncol 21: 255–262.
30. Weigelt B, Reis-Filho JS, Swanton C (2012) Genomic analyses to select patients for adjuvant chemotherapy: trials and tribulations. Ann Oncol 23 Suppl 10: x211–x218.
31. Berns K, Horlings HM, Hennessy BT, Madiredjo M, Hijmans EM, et al. (2007) A functional genetic approach identifies the PI3K pathway as a major determinant of trastuzumab resistance in breast cancer. Cancer Cell 12: 395–402.
32. Inoki K, Zhu T, Guan KL (2003) TSC2 mediates cellular energy response to control cell growth and survival. Cell 115: 577–590.
33. Xiao B, Sanders MJ, Underwood E, Heath R, Mayer FV, et al. (2011) Structure of mammalian AMPK and its regulation by ADP. Nature 472: 230–233.
34. Findlay GM, Yan L, Procter J, Mieulet V, Lamb RF (2007) A MAP4 kinase related to Ste20 is a nutrient-sensitive regulator of mTOR signalling. Biochem J 403: 13–20.
35. Lam D, Dickens D, Reid EB, Loh SH, Moisoi N, et al. (2009) MAP4K3 modulates cell death via the post-transcriptional regulation of BH3-only proteins. Proc Natl Acad Sci U S A 106: 11978–11983.
36. Leung DW (2001) The structure and functions of human lysophosphatidic acid acyltransferases. Front Biosci 6: D944–953.
37. Fang Y, Vilella-Bach M, Bachmann R, Flanigan A, Chen J (2001) Phosphatidic acid-mediated mitogenic activation of mTOR signaling. Science 294: 1942–1945.
38. Choi BH, Yoon HS (2011) FKBP38-Bcl-2 interaction: a novel link to chemoresistance. Curr Opin Pharmacol 11: 354–359.
39. Bai X, Ma D, Liu A, Shen X, Wang QJ, et al. (2007) Rheb activates mTOR by antagonizing its endogenous inhibitor, FKBP38. Science 318: 977–980.
40. Ma D, Bai X, Guo S, Jiang Y (2008) The switch I region of Rheb is critical for its interaction with FKBP38. J Biol Chem 283: 25963–25970.
41. Dunlop EA, Dodd KM, Seymour LA, Tee AR (2009) Mammalian target of rapamycin complex 1-mediated phosphorylation of eukaryotic initiation factor 4E-binding protein 1 requires multiple protein-protein interactions for substrate recognition. Cell Signal 21: 1073–1084.
42. Wang X, Fonseca BD, Tang H, Liu R, Elia A, et al. (2008) Re-evaluating the roles of proposed modulators of mammalian target of rapamycin complex 1 (mTORC1) signaling. J Biol Chem 283: 30482–30492.
43. Sato T, Nakashima A, Guo L, Tamanoi F (2009) Specific activation of mTORC1 by Rheb G-protein in vitro involves enhanced recruitment of its substrate protein. J Biol Chem 284: 12783–12791.
44. Yoon MS, Du G, Backer JM, Frohman MA, Chen J (2011) Class III PI-3-kinase activates phospholipase D in an amino acid-sensing mTORC1 pathway. J Cell Biol 195: 435–447.
45. Wang L, Zhang Q, Zhang J, Sun S, Guo H, et al. (2011) PI3K pathway activation results in low efficacy of both trastuzumab and lapatinib. BMC Cancer 11: 248.
46. Razis E, Bobos M, Kotoula V, Eleftheraki AG, Kalofonos HP, et al. (2011) Evaluation of the association of PIK3CA mutations and PTEN loss with efficacy of trastuzumab therapy in metastatic breast cancer. Breast Cancer Res Treat 128: 447–456.
47. O'Regan R, Ozguroglu M, Andre F, Toi M, Jerusalem GHM, et al. (2013) Phase III, randomized, double-blind, placebo-controlled multicenter trial of daily everolimus plus weekly trastuzumab and vinorelbine in trastuzumab-resistant, advanced breast cancer (BOLERO-3). J Clin Oncol 31: abstr 505.
48. O'Brien NA, McDonald K, Tong L, von Euw E, Kalous O, et al. (2014) Targeting PI3K/mTOR overcomes resistance to HER2-targeted therapy independent of feedback activation of AKT. Clin Cancer Res 20: 3507–3520.

10

Upregulation of Autophagy-Related Gene-5 (ATG-5) Is Associated with Chemoresistance in Human Gastric Cancer

Jie Ge[1], Zihua Chen[1], Jin Huang[2], Jinxiang Chen[2], Weijie Yuan[2], Zhenghao Deng[3], Zhikang Chen[1]*

1 Department of Gastrointestinal Surgery, Xiangya Hospital, Central South University, Changsha, Hunan, P. R. China, 2 Department of Oncology, Xiangya Hospital, Central South University, Changsha, Hunan, P. R. China, 3 Department of Pathology, Xiangya Hospital, Central South University, Changsha, Hunan, P. R. China

Abstract

Autophagy-related gene-5 (ATG-5) is one of the key regulators of autophagic cell death. It has been widely regarded as a protective molecular mechanism for tumor cells during the course of chemotherapy. In the present study, we investigated the expression pattern of ATG-5 and multidrug resistance-associated protein-1 (MRP-1) in 135 gastric cancers (GC) patients who were treated with epirubicin, cisplatin and 5-FU adjuvant chemotherapy (ECF) following surgical resection and explored their potential clinical significance. We found that both ATG-5 (77.78%) and MRP-1 (79.26%) were highly expressed in GC patients. ATG-5 expression was significantly associated with depth of wall invasion, TNM stages and distant metastasis of GC ($P<0.05$), whereas MRP-1 expression was significantly linked with tumor size, depth of wall invasion, lymph node metastasis, TNM stages and differentiation status ($P<0.05$). ATG-5 expression was positively correlated with MRP-1 ($r_p = 0.616$, $P<0.01$). Increased expression of ATG-5 and MPR-1 was significantly correlated with poor overall survival (OS; $P<0.01$) and disease free survival (DFS; $P<0.01$) of our GC cohort. Furthermore, we demonstrated that ATG-5 was involved in drug resistant of GC cells, which was mainly through regulating autophagy. Our data suggest that upregulated expression of ATG-5, an important molecular feature of protective autophagy, is associated with chemoresistance in GC. Expression of ATG-5 and MRP-1 may be independent prognostic markers for GC treatment.

Editor: Pankaj K. Singh, University of Nebraska Medical Center, United States of America

Funding: This work was supported by National Natural Science Foundation of Hunan Province, China (No. 2012FJ6088). The funders had no role in study design, data collection and analysis, decision to publish, or preparation of the manuscript.

Competing Interests: The authors have declared that no competing interests exist.

* Email: 4059653@qq.com

Introduction

Despite a considerable decline in its incidence rate in many developed countries, gastric cancer (GC) remains the fourth most commonly diagnosed malignancy, and the second leading cause of cancer-related deaths worldwide [1]. Over the past decades, standard multimodal treatment strategies together with other recommended options (e.g. D2 dissection and adjuvant chemotherapy) have failed to cure a large proportion of patients affected with GC, especially for those with advanced and metastatic diseases, with worse survival rates being seen probably due to the presence of chemoresistance during treatment [2]. Hence, identification of novel molecular events underlying the development of this malignancy and its poor prognosis as well as understanding the mechanisms of GC chemoresistance are urgently required for more effective clinical intervention and better management of patients.

Under physiological conditions, autophagy is a lysosome-dependent self-digesting system primarily responsible for removal and recycling of long-lived proteins and damaged/obsolete intracellularorganelles in order to maintain cell homeostasis [3]. The proteins and organelles destined for destruction are sequestered within "double-membrane" vacuoles (autophagosomes), followed by fusion with lysosomes to build complexes known as autophagosomes, where the contents are degraded by lysosomal hydrolases [4]. It has been documented that autophagy could be induced in response to many unfavorable conditions including nutrient deprivation, oxidative stress or DNA damages and serves as an adaptive cell mechanism, eventually allowing cells to survive and proliferate, while extensive or persistent autophagy results in cell death [5]. Impairments in physiological activation, assembly and function of the autophagic pathway have been increasingly observed in a wide variety of human cancers, although the exact role played by autophagy in cancer genesis and progression is still under controversy. Some data favor the idea that autophagy suppresses tumorigenesis, whereas other evidence suggest that autophagy is able to trigger tumor initiation and protects tumor cells from undergoing apoptosis [6]. Interestingly, inhibition of autophagy was recently found to enhance the anti-tumor activity of several cytotoxic agents. Li and colleagues reported that autophagy was activated as a protective mechanism against the cellular effects of 5-FU-treatment and inhibition of autophagy by 3-methyladenine augmented 5-FU-induced apoptosis in colon cancer cells [7,8]. On the other hand, some anticancer drugs (e.g. cetuximab and dasatinib) were demonstrated to induce autophagic cell death through different mechanisms in some cancer cells [9–

13]. The molecular machinery by which autophagy regulates survival or death of neoplastic cells remains largely obscure hitherto. The autophagy pathway is a highly-modulated dynamic process predominantly executed by the autophagy-related (ATG) family of genes, which is governed by several key kinases including mTOR, PI3k/Akt, AMPK and MAPK [14,15]. ATG-5 is a central regulator necessary for autophagy in terms of its involvement in autophagosome elongation [16]. Enforced expression of ATG-5 sensitized tumor cells to anticancer drug treatment both *in vitro* and *in vivo*; in contrast siRNA-mediated inhibition of ATG-5 led to partial resistance to chemotherapy [17].

Postoperative adjuvant chemotherapy is presently a major treatment for GC; however, the overall efficacy of chemotherapy remains poor possibly as a consequence of the presence of multidrug resistance (MDR) phenotype. Unlike other tumor entities, expression of the classical MDR-mediating molecules such as glutathione S-transferase and multidrug resistance gene 1 is not very prevalent in GC tissues, indicating that there might exist a complicated mechanism for the development of MDR in this malignant disease [18]. As one of the classical drug-resistant mechanisms, multidrug resistance-associated protein 1 (MRP1/ABCC1) has been found to be strongly expressed in GC and thus may exert pivotal roles in mediating MDR in GC [19,20]. However, it remains unknown whether MRP-1 expression is associated with ATG-5 expression. And also whether autophagy is involved in chemoresistence in GC patients is unclear.

In the present study, we first employed immunohistochemistry to investigate the expression profile of ATG-5 and MRP1 in a sum of 135 GC patients who received ECF (epirubicin, cisplatin and 5-FU) adjuvant chemotherapy following surgical resection. The correlations between ATG-5 and MRP-1 expression as well as their expression with various clinicopathological features of GC and clinical outcomes were also assessed.

Materials and Methods

Patients and tissue samples

A total of 135 GC patients consisting of 91 males and 44 females who underwent surgery at the Department of Gastrointestinal Surgery, Xiangya Hospital, Central South University (C.S.U), China, between January 1st 2007 and December 31st 2008 were enrolled in this study. The average age of the cohort was 53.62±9.73 years, with a range of 26 to 72. Theprimary GC tumor tissuesand matched non-cancerous(NC) tissues located at least 5 cm away from the tumor core were obtained after surgical resection and immediately processed and stored until further use. None of the recruited patients had chemotherapy or radiotherapy prior to surgical operation. The histopathological diagnosis was carried out preoperatively and confirmed by surgery. All participants with stage IB to IV tumors received ECF chemotherapy after surgery (Dose: epirubicin 50 mg/m^2 on day 1, cisplatin 60 mg/m^2 on day 1 and continuous intravenous infusion of 5-FU 500 mg/m^2/d for 4 days, repeated every 3 weeks up to 24 weeks). The clinical characteristics of these patients were listed in Table 1.

All cases in this study were reviewed and all specimens were histopathologically re-examined in October, 2012. The depth of wall invasion, regional lymph node metastasis, and histological grade were confirmed by the same group of two experienced senior pathologists. The patients were categorized based on the differentiation status of cancer cells into three histological grades: well, moderate and poor. Based on a combination of loco-regional tumor involvement and the presence of metastasis, all cases were staged according to the TNM Classification of Malignant Tumours (TNM) stage grouping [21]. For the analysis of survival, the date of operation was used to represent the start point of the follow-up visit. Patients who died of other diseases rather than GC or other unexpected events were excluded from the case collection. The cause of death recruited in this study was aggravation of GC. The overall survival (OS) was calculated as a period starting from the date of the initial surgery to the date of death, or the date of the last follow-up as the end point. The disease free survival (DFS) was defined as the time interval from surgery until the date of local relapse or first distant organ metastasis. Informed written consent was obtained from each patient before surgery and this study was approved by the Research Ethics Committee of Central South University, China. All specimens were handled and made anonymous according to the ethical and legal guidelines.

Immunohistochemistry

The fresh specimens were fixed in 10% neutral buffered formalin and subsequently embedded with paraffin. The paraffin-embedded tissues were cut at 4 μm and then deparaffinized with xylene and rehydrated for further H&E or peroxidase immunohistochemistry staining by using the DAKO EnVision System. In brief, following proteolytic digestion and blocking with endogenous peroxidase, tissue slides were incubated with the primary antibodies (ATG5: ab54033; MRP1: ab32574; Abcam Inc., Cambridge, UK) against respective target proteins at a dilution of 1:500 overnight at 4°C. After washing with PBS, peroxidase labeled polymer and substrate-chromogen were then employed in order to visualize the immnohistochemical staining. Finally, sections were counterstained with hematoxylin, cover-slipped with mounting medium, and examined by light microscopy. All the procedures were performed at the Department of Pathology, Xiangya Hospital, C.S.U. Slides were interpreted independently by two experienced pathologists, who were blind to patients' information. We quantified staining intensity and percentage of stained cells using a previously described approach [22,23]: the percentage of positively stained cells (0%–100%) was multiplied by the dominant intensity pattern of staining, considering 1 as negative or trace, 2 as weak, 3 as moderate and 4 as strong. Therefore, the overall score ranged from 0 to 400. Patients were subsequently categorized into four different subgroups: score 0–99, score 100–199, score 200–299 and score 300–400.

Western blot analysis

Whole cell extracts were prepared using 0.14 M NaCl, 0.2 M triethanolamine, 0.2% sodium deoxycholate, 0.5% Nonidet P-40 and supplemented with a protease inhibitor (all of the products were from Sigma, St. Louis, Missouri, USA). Then, protein sample was run through a 12% sodium dodecyl sulfate-polyacrylamide gel electrophoresis (SDS-PAGE) gel and transferred to a membrane. The transferred membranes were subsequently incubated overnight at 4°C with a primary antibody. After washing, the membrane was incubated with a horseradish peroxidase (HRP)-linked secondary antibody for 1 h at room temperature. The primary antibodies were anti-ATG-5 (Santa Cruz, CA, USA), anti-LC3A/B (abcam, Cambridge, UK) and anti- β-Actin (Santa Cruz, CA, USA). All reported results are the average ratios of three different independent experiments.

Cell proliferation assay

Cells were seeded onto 96 well plates (10000 cells/well) for 24 h before treatment. MTT assays were used to assess cell proliferation at different time point after treatment. The MTT assay was performed as follows: MTT was added to each well and the plates were incubated at 37°C for 4 h. The MTT medium mixture was then removed and 150 μL of dimethyl sulfoxide (DMSO) was

Table 1. Association between ATG-5 expression and clinicopathological characteristics of GC patients.

Factors	Patients (n = 135)	ATG-5 expression (%)				P
		0–99	100–199	200–299	300–400	
Gender						0.99
Male	91	21.98	14.29	46.15	17.58	
Female	44	22.73	15.91	45.45	15.91	
Age (years) Mean±SD	135	56.00±9.09	54.5±10.52	53.05±9.13	51.48±11.17	0.370▲
Tumor size (cm)						0.15
<5.0	80	25	18.75	43.75	12.5	
≥5.0	55	18.18	9.09	49.09	23.64	
Location of tumor						0.086
upper	21	19.05	33.33	38.1	9.52	
middle	35	11.43	12.5	54.29	22.86	
low	79	27.85	11.39	44.3	16.46	
H. pylori infection						0.961
Positive	73	23.29	15.07	43.84	17.81	
Negative	62	20.97	14.52	48.39	16.13	
Depth of wall invasion						<0.001
T1	10	50	20	30	0	
T2	15	66.67	13.33	13.33	6.67	
T3	32	25	12.5	43.75	18.75	
T4	78	8.97	15.38	55.13	20.51	
Lymph node metastasis						0.056
N0	18	22.22	33.33	38.89	5.56	
N1	36	33.33	5.56	50	11.11	
N2	44	22.73	9.09	47.73	20.45	
N3	37	10.81	21.62	43.24	24.32	
Distant metastasis						0.018
M0	131	22.9	15.27	46.56	15.27	
M1	4	0	0	25	75	
TNM stages						<0.001
IB	10	70	10	20	0	
II	31	45.16	32.26	22.58	0	
III	90	10	10	57.78	22.22	
IV	4	0	0	25	75	
Differentiation status						0.412
Well	17	41.18	17.65	23.53	17.65	
Moderate	60	20	16.67	48.33	15	
Poor	58	18.97	12.07	50	18.97	

▲Statistical analyses were carried out with the One-Way ANOVA test and others were carried out with the Pearson's χ^2 test.

added to each well. The absorbance was measured at 570 nm using a multiwall spectrophotometer.

RNA interference

siRNA duplexes targeting ATG-5 were synthesized as follows: siRNA-ATG5-486: GACGUUG GUAACUGACAAATT; siRNA-ATG5-695: GUCCAUCUAAGGAUGCAAUTT and siRNA-ATG5-938: GACCUUUCAUUCAGAAGCUTT. siRNA duplexes containing non-specific sequences were used as a negative control (NC): UUCUCCGAACGUGUCACGUTT. Different siRNAs were transfected separately into cells using the Lipofectamine 2000 reagent, and the medium was replaced 6 h after transfection.

Real-time RT-PCR

Total RNA from the cell lines and tissues were extracted using the Trizol reagent (Invitrogen, Carlsbad, USA), following the manufacturer's instructions. The concentration of RNA was measured using a spectrophotometer. A cDNA pool was synthesized using 1 μg of total RNA and TaqMan Reverse Transcription Reagents (Applied Biosystems, Foster City, USA) as described by the manufacturer. The expression of the target gene

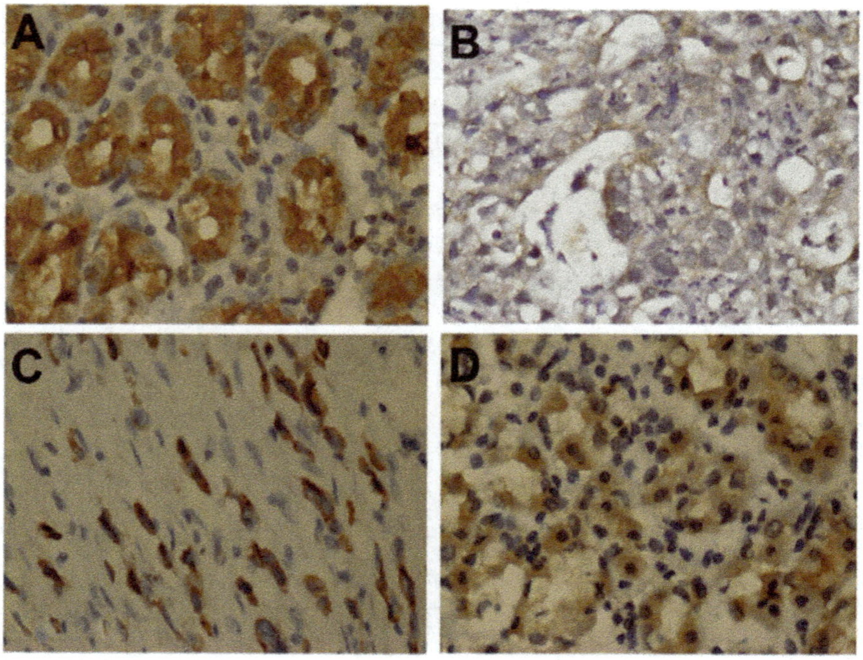

Figure 1. Representative images showing immunohistochemical staining for ATG-5 in non-tumorous and GC tumor tissues. (A) ATG-5 staining in non-cancerous gastric tissues scored 285(×200); (B) ATG-5 staining in GC tumor tissues scored 50(×400); (C) ATG-5 staining in GC tumor tissues scored 270(×400); (D) ATG-5 staining in GC tumor tissues scored 400(×200).

was evaluated using a relative quantification approach ($2^{-\Delta\Delta Ct}$ method) with β-actin as the internal reference.

Immunofluorescence assay

Cells were permeabilized with 0.3% Triton X-100 for 10 min followed by fixation with 2–4% Methanal for 15 min, and blocked with 3% sheep serum at room temperature for 60 min. Then, probed with primary antibodies anti-LC3B (Santa Cruz, CA, USA) overnight at room temperature, and cells were washed three times with PBS. Stained with Alexa Fluor 488 conjugated 488 rabbit anti-goat IgG for 1 h at room temperature, and then the cells were washed three times with PBS. Nuclei were visualized by staining with DAPI (Sigma, USA) for 2 min. The stained cells were observed with inverted fluorescence microscope.

Statistical analysis

All statistical analyses were performed with the SPSS software package 15.0 for Windows (SPSS Inc., Chicago, IL, USA). Quantitative data were presented as Mean ± SD. Pearson's χ^2 test was used to compare the difference among ranked data, while one-Way-ANOVA test was carried out to compare the difference among quantitative data. Survival analyses were carried out by using the Kaplan-Meier method and compared by the log-rank test. The Cox-regression model was performed to evaluate the independent hazard ratio of each variable in the multivariate analysis. The correlation between ATG5 and MRP1 expression was examined using Bivariate Correlation (Pearson) test. Differences were considered as statistically significant when P values were less than 0.05.

Results

Expression of ATG-5 and MRP-1 in GC

The expression pattern and location of ATG-5 and MRP-1 in our GC patients, who were treated with epirubicin, cisplatin and 5-FU adjuvant chemotherapy (ECF) following surgical resection, were examined using immunohistochemical analysis. Among the 135 GC specimens, 105(77.78%) were positive for ATG-5 immunoreactivity, and 107 (79.26%) were MRP-1 positive. As depicted in Figure 1, we found that ATG5 was predominantly expressed in the cytoplasm. Moreover, over-expression of ATG-5 was positively correlated with that of MRP-1 in GC. ($r = 0.616$, $P<0.001$), as revealed by the Bivariate Correlation test. The positive expression in adjacent non-cancerous tissues were 113(83.70%) for ATG-5 and 89(65.93%) for MRP-1. The data showed that both ATG-5 and MRP-1 were positively expressed in cancer and non-cancerous tissues, which suggest that ATG-5 and MRP-1 may be induced by chemotherapy in both tumor and non-tumor tissues. As all our patient samples were treated with ECF chemotherapy, and we found that both ATG-5 and MRP-1 were highly expressed and positively correlated in those samples. Meanwhile, previous study indicates that MRP-1 maybe associated with multi-drug resistance in GC. Together with previous finding, our results suggest that ATG-5 and MRP-1 may be involved in chemoresistance in GC patients.

Associations between expression of ATG-5 or MRP-1 and clinicopathological characteristics of GC

The associations of ATG-5 and MRP1 expression with various clinicopathological parameters of GC are shown in Table 1 and Table 2, respectively. Expression of ATG-5 was significantly associated with depth of wall invasion, distant metastasis and TNM stages of GC ($P<0.001$, $P = 0.018$, $P<0.001$ respectively). MRP-1 expression was significantly associated with increased tumor size, depth of wall invasion, regional lymph nodes metastasis, TNM stages ($P = 0.032$, $P<0.001$, $P = 0.016$, $P<0.001$ respectively) and differentiation status ($P = 0.005$). To further determine the involvement o f ATG-5 and MRP-1 in the GC development, we performed survival analysis within our

Table 2. Association between MRP-1 expression and clinicopathological characteristics of GC patients.

Factors	Patients (n = 135)	ATG-5 expression (%)				P
		0–99	100–199	200–299	300–400	
Gender						0.675
Male	91	19.78	21.98	43.96	14.29	
Female	44	22.73	22.73	34.09	20.45	
Age (years) Mean±SD	135					0.084▲
Tumor size (cm)		54.61±10.31	56.23±8.97	53.31±9.56	49.45±9.61	0.032
<5.0	80					
≥5.0	55	22.5	30	33.75	13.75	
Location of tumor		18.18	10.91	50.91	20	0.15
upper	21					
middle	35	19.05	28.57	38.1	14.29	
low	79	22.86	11.43	40	25.71	
H. pylori infection		20.25	25.32	41.77	12.66	0.51
Positive	73					
Negative	62	16.44	23.29	41.1	19.18	
Depth of wall invasion		25.81	20.97	40.32	12.9	<0.001
T1	10					
T2	15	60	20	20	0	
T3	32	53.33	26.67	20	0	
T4	78	28.13	15.63	37.5	18.75	
Lymph node metastasis		6.41	24.36	48.72	20.51	0.016
N0	18					
N1	36	22.22	44.44	33.33	0	
N2	44	33.33	16.67	36.11	13.89	
N3	37	18.18	22.73	47.73	11.36	
Distant metastasis		10.81	16.22	40.54	32.43	0.193
M0	131	21.37	22.9	40.46	15.27	
M1	4	0	0	50	50	
TNM stages						<0.001
IB	10	70	20	10	0	
II	31	54.84	35.48	9.68	0	
III	90	4.44	18.89	54.44	22.22	
IV	4					
Differentiation status		0	0	50	50	0.005
Well	17	52.94	17.65	23.53	5.88	
Moderate	60	16.67	31.67	36.67	15	
Poor	58	15.52	13.79	50	20.69	

▲Statistical analyses were carried out with the One-Way ANOVA test and others were carried out with the Pearson's χ^2 test.

patient samples. Our survival analyses demonstrated that the total overall survival (OS) rate of our GC cohort was 43.70% with a mean survival of 39.849 months (95% CI, 35.636–44.061 months); whereas the disease free survival (DFS) rate was 34.07% with a mean survival of 35.802 months (95% CI, 31.618–39.986 months). We next classified the patients into four different subgroups according to the scores of immunohistochemistry staining. The Kaplan-Meier survival analysis revealed a higher ATG-5 expression was significantly associated with poorer OS ($P<0.001$) and DFS ($P = 0.003$). Pairwise comparisons indicated that patients carrying the highest ATG-5 expression (scores 300–400) had the poorest survival rates as compared to that of other subgroups (Figure 2A and 2B). Consistently, upregulated MRP-1 expression was found to be significantly associated with poor OS ($P = 0.001$) and DFS ($P = 0.018$) of our GC patients. The subgroup with the highest MRP1 expression scores (0–99) appeared to have the worst prognosis (Figure 2C and 2D) in comparison with other subgroups. Our data also showed that there was a significant correlation between TNM stages and survival of GC patients. Patients with stage III and IV tumors displayed poorer prognosis as compared to those harboring stage IB and II tumors ($P<0.01$) (Figure 2E and 2F). More interestingly, the Cox's multivariate hazard regression model demonstrated that ATG-5 and MRP-1 expression levels and TNM stages were all independent and

Table 3. The multivariate Cox proportional hazard analysis of prognostic factors for OS and DFS rates of 135 GC patients.

Factors	OS				DFS			
	β	Wald	RR# (95.0% CI)	P	β	Wald	RR# (95.0% CI)	P
MRP-1(300–400)		13.035		0.005		11.843		0.008
MRP-1(0–99)	−1.797	9.388	0.166(0.052–0.523)	0.002	−1.785	10.408	0.168(0.0576–0.496)	0.001
MRP-1(100–199)	−1.121	7.799	0.326(0.148–0.716)	0.007	−0.938	6.578	0.391(0.191–0.802)	0.011
MRP-1(200–299)	−0.353	1.373	0.702(0.389–1.268)	0.216	−0.413	2.076	0.662(0.377–1.161)	0.146
ATG-5	0.379	5.538	1.460(1.065–2.002)	0.037	0.486	9.73	1.626 (1.198–2.207)	0.004
TNM stage	1.869	17.151	6.484(2.677–15.705)	<0.001	1.85	18.785	6.362(2.755–14.688)	<0.001
Tumor size	0.109	0.178	0.897(0.542–1.486)	0.673	0.091	0.146	0.913(0.573–1.456)	0.702
Differentiation status	0.177	0.821	1.194(0.814–1.752)	0.365	0.192	1.141	1.212(0.852–1.726)	0.285
Hp infection	−0.115	0.238	0.891(0.560–1.417)	0.626	−0.122	0.307	0.885(0.574–1.364)	0.579
Location	−0.021	0.017	0.979(0.710–1.350)	0.898	−0.091	0.356	0.913(0.677–1.231)	0.551
Gender	0.108	0.44	0.897(0.652–1.236)	0.507	0.187	0.579	0.829(0.512–1.343)	0.447

#Relative Risk; CI: confidence interval.

significant prognostic indicators for predicting the OS ($P = 0.037$, $P = 0.005$, $P<0.001$ respectively) and DFS ($P = 0.004$, $P = 0.008$, $P<0.001$ respectively) of GC (Table 3). Our data indicated the ATG-5 and MRP-1 were closely related with the GC development and may serve as poor prognosis markers in GC treatment.

ATG-5 was significantly upregulated in chemoresistant cells

To further explore the role of ATG-5 in the tumorigenesis and drug resistant. We detected the protein expression in several gastric cancer cell lines (AGS, BGC-832, SGC7901, SGC7901/DPP and MKN45) and in an immortalized human gastric epithelial mucosa cell line (GES). Interestingly, we found that ATG-5 was dramatically overexpressed in DPP resistant cell line, SGC7901/DPP cells, compared with all the other cell lines which include DPP sensitive SGC7901 cells (Figure 3A). We further confirmed that SGC7901/DPP cells are resistant to DPP treatment. The IC 25, IC50 and IC75 were 15.4 μM, 38.7 μM and 93.53 μM in SGC7901 cells. In contrast, The IC 25, IC50 and IC75 were 120.03 μM, 271.9 μM and 423.7 μM in SGC7901/DPP (Figure 3B). It is about 5 to 9 times higher than that in non-drug resistant cells. Our finding strongly suggests that ATG-5 contributes to drug resistant of the GC cells.

Inhibition of ATG-5 sensitized chemoresistant cells to drug treatment

To further prove that ATG-5 contributes to the drug resistant of the GC cells, we used small interfering RNAs (siRNAs) to knockdown the expression of ATG-5. Three siRNAs were designed. Our real time PCR and western blot results showed that all three siRNAs inhibited the expression of ATG-5 at both mRNA and protein level (Figure 4A and 4B). We chose one, siRNA-ATG5-695, with highest knockdown efficiency to perform the following experiment. We knockdown ATG-5 expression and then treated the cells with DPP. Cell proliferation ability was examined at 0, 48 and 72 hours after treatment. Our result showed that knockdowning ATG-5 did not affect cell proliferation in SGC7901/DPP cells compared with control siRNA (siRNA NC). DPP treatment alone slightly inhibited the proliferation of the cells. Interestingly, when we knockdown the expression of ATG-5 and treated the cells with DPP at the same time, the cell proliferation ability was further suppressed compared with cells treated with DPP alone 48 and 72 hours after treatment (Figure 4 C). Our data further support that ATG-5 contributes to the drug resistant of GC cells.

Autophagy was involved in the drug resistant of DC cells

As ATG-5 is a central regulator of autophagy, we speculated that autophagy may be involved in the drug resistant of GC cells. So we used 3MA, which is an autophagy inhibitor, to treat the drug resistant cells. As expected, we found that 3MA together with DPP treatment had a similar effect with ATG-5 kncokdown together with DPP treatment (Figure 4C and 4D). The data demonstrate that autophagy contributes to the drug resistant. Then, we examined whether autophagy was changed during the treatment. We used Immunofluorescence assay to detect LC3B expression level, which is an autophagy marker in the cells. Our data showed that autophagy was suppressed after silencing ATG-5 or treating the cells with 3MA (Figure 5A). And western blot result further confirmed that LC3A/B protein expression was only affected in cells treated with siRNA-ATG5 or 3MA. Accordingly, cell proliferation was further inhibited only when autophagy was inhibited (Figure 4 and figure 5). Therefore, our data revealed that

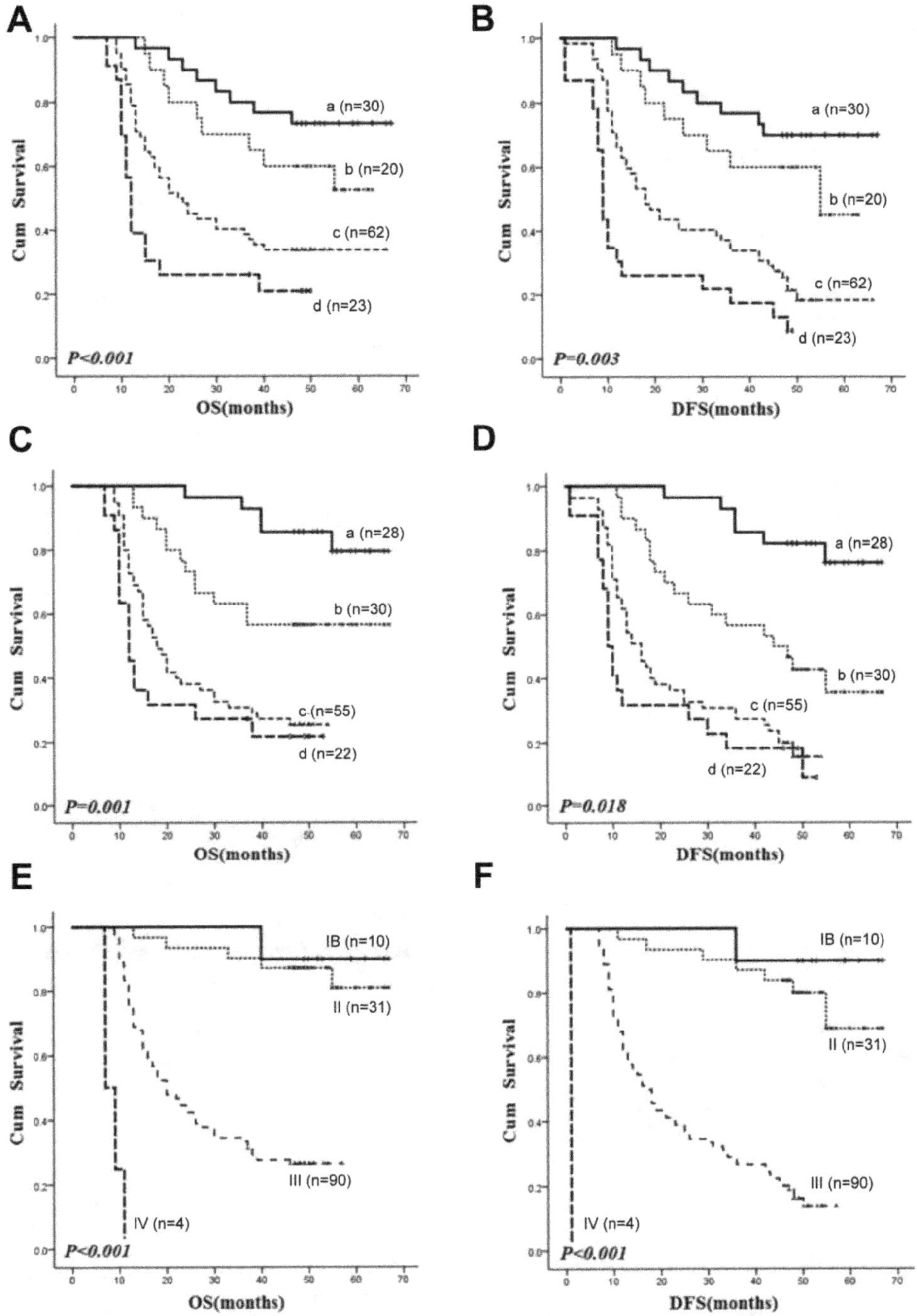

Figure 2. Kaplane-Meier statistical analyses showing OS and DFS in different subgroups of GC patients. (A and B) Patients were divided into four following subgroups based on ATG-5 immunostaining: scored 0–99 (curve a), scored 100–199 (curve b), scored 200–299 (curve c) and scored 300–400 (curve d). The difference among different subgroups was statistically significant as evaluated by overall Log-rank comparisons (OS: $P<0.001$, DFS: $P=0.003$). Pairwise Log-rank comparisons showed that the subgroup D exhibited the poorest survival rates as compared to other subgroups (OS: $P<0.05$, DFS: $P<0.01$). (C and D) Patients were divided into four following subgroups based on MRP-1 immunostaining: scored 0–99 (curve a), scored 100–199 (curve b), scored 200–299 (curve c) and scored 300–400 (curve d). The difference among various subgroups was statistically significant by overall Log-rank comparisons (OS: $P=0.001$, DFS: $P=0.018$). Pairwise Log-rank comparisons showed that the subgroup A had the most favorable prognosis among the four subgroups (OS: $P<0.05$, DFS: $P<0.001$). (E and F) Patients were divided into four subgroups according to different TNM stages. The difference among different subgroups was statistically significant by overall Log-rank comparisons (OS: $P<0.001$, DFS: $P<0.001$). Pairwise Log-rank comparisons showed that subgroups III or IV exhibited poorer survival rates than that of subgroups IB and II (OS: $P<0.01$, DFS: $P<0.001$).

ATG-5 was involved in the drug resistant of DC cells, which was mainly through affect the autophagy of the cancer cells.

Discussion

GC remains one of the most frequent malignant tumors on a global basis in spite of its declining incidence and the total number

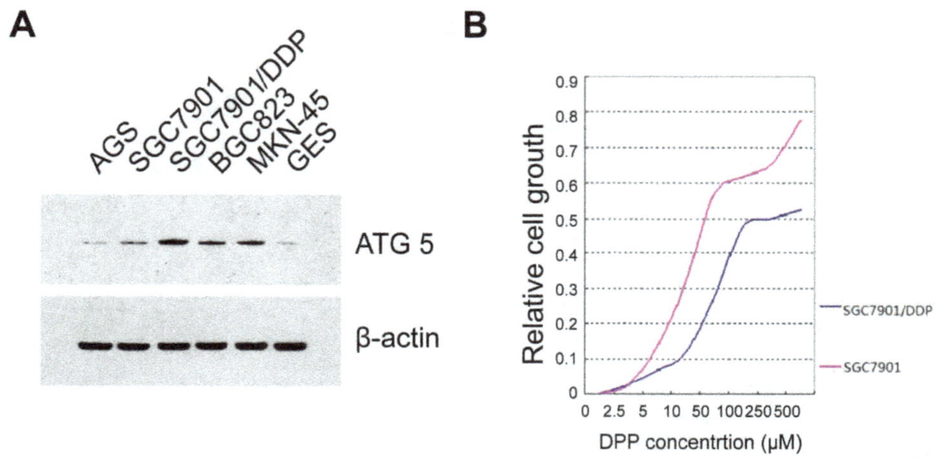

Figure 3. ATG-5 was upregulated in chemoresistant cells. (A) The level of ATG5 was detected in cell lines using western blot analysis. β -actin was used as internal controls.(B) The IC 25, IC50 and IC75 of SGC-7901 and SGC-7901/DDP cells were tested using the MTT assays after DPP treatment.

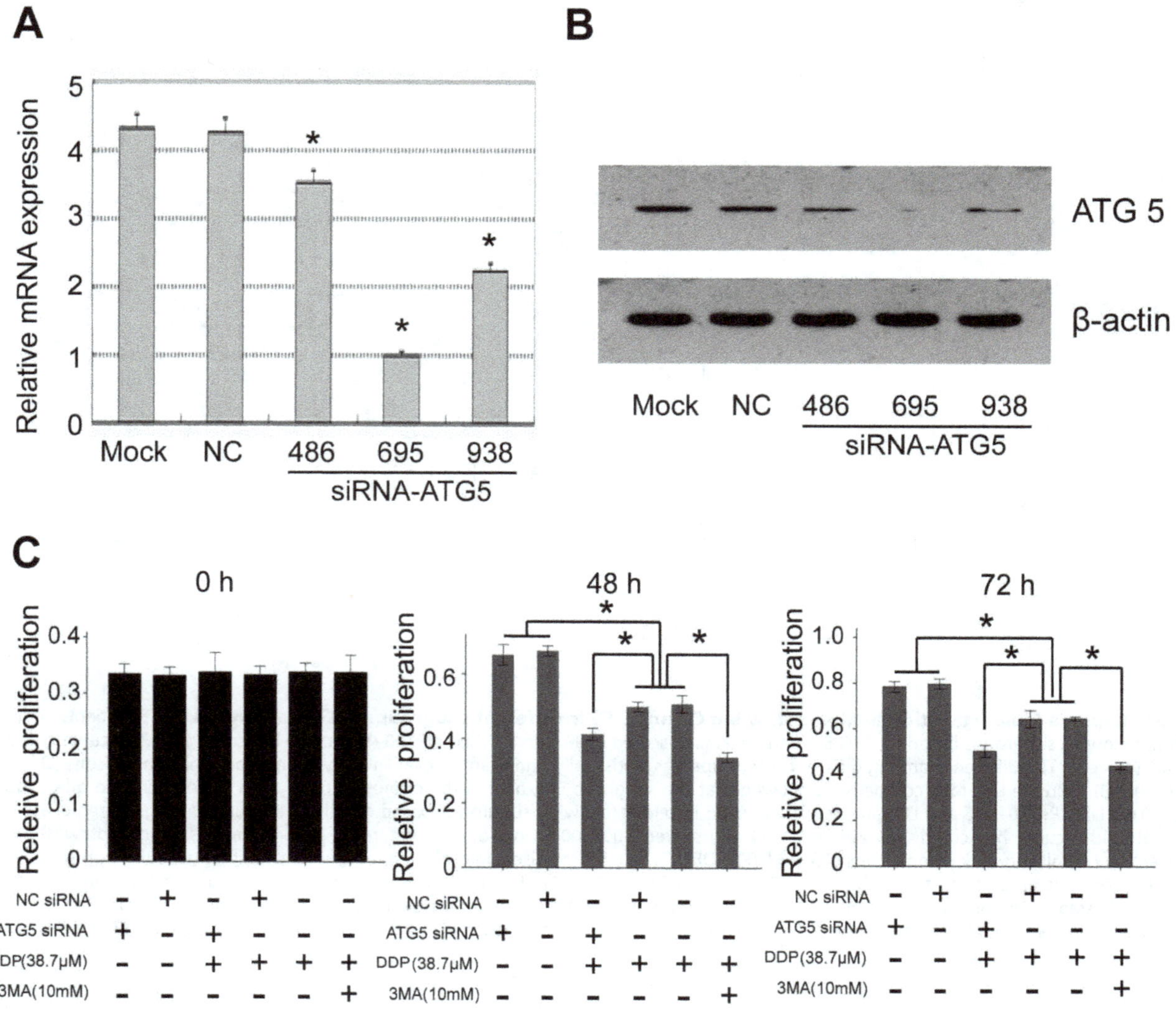

Figure 4. Silencing ATG-5 sensitized chemoresistant cells to drug treatment. (A) The mRNA level of ATG-5 was detected by real time PCR after treatment with siRNAs. GAPDH was used as internal controls. (B) The protein level of ATG-5 was detected by western blot after treatment with siRNAs. β -actin was used as internal controls. (C) The proliferation ability was tested using MTT assay 48 hours or 72 hours after different treatment.

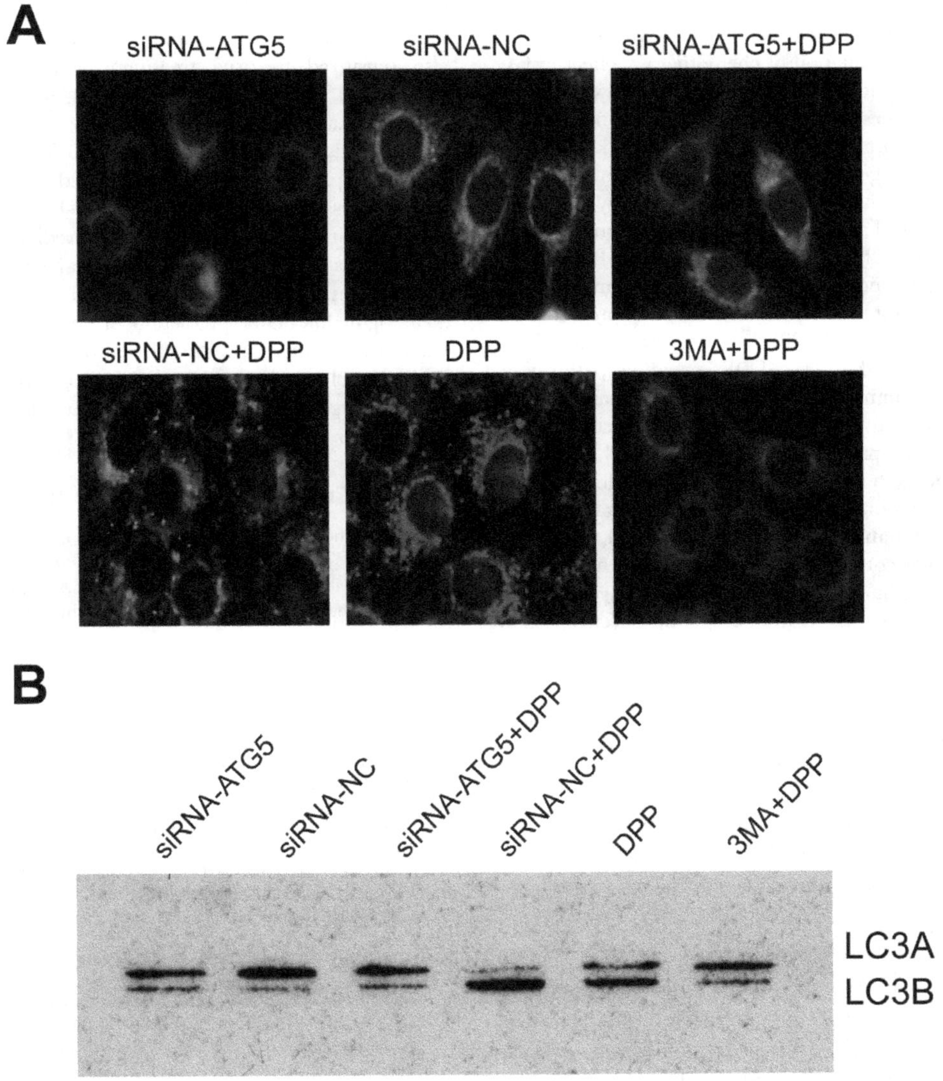

Figure 5. Autophagy was involved in the drug resistant of DC cells. (A) The autophagy was detected by immunofluorescence assay of LC3B in the cells 48 hours after different treatment. (B) The protein levels of LC3A and LC3B were tested by western blot. β-actin was used as internal controls.

is predicted to continuously climb as a result of population growth. In men, GC ranks the second in mortality rate; in women, it is the fourth in mortality [24,25]. The crude mortality rate of GC in China was 25.2 per 100 000 [26]. In our study, we examined the expression of ATG-5 and MRP-1 in a cohort of GC patient after chemotherapy. Then, we demonstrated that ATG-5 was upregulated in cisplatin (DDP) resistant cell line. Furthermore, after ATG-5 expression or aotophogy was inhibited, the cancer cells were sensitized to DPP treatment. Our results provide new insight into the mechanism of chemoresistant in GC progression.

We evaluated the exression profile of ATG-5 and MRP-1 in 135 Chinese GC patients. In an agreement with previous report [22], our results showed that a high percentage of GC tissues expressed ATG-5, and ATG-5 expression was statistically associated with depth of wall invasion, distant metastasis and TNM stages of GC. These findings support a notion that high expression level of ATG5 may contribute to, some extent, a more aggressive and malignant phenotype in GC. This viewpoint is further supported by our finding of the association between higher ATG5 expression in GC and poorer prognosis of patients (see more discussion below). More importantly, we identified a positive correlation between ATG-5 and MRP1 expression in our GC cohort. Considering the fact that MRP1 is an ABC transmembrane transport protein well known to promote the MDR phenotype in GC, it is reasonable to propose that ATG-5 may be also implicated in conferring GC chemoresistance through certain unknown molecular mechanisms.

It is widely accepted that recurrence and metastasis are two major hurdles in our efforts to improve low OS and DFS survival rate of GC. Chemoresistance remains one of the most important reasons leading to tumor repopulation/recurrence following treatment. Appropriate option of individual treatment will be undoubtedly beneficial to improve the clinical outcome; nonetheless, current treatment decision is mostly dependent on the TNM stages [27,28]. Our survival analyses in the 135 GC patients with stage IB to IV tumors revealed that both ATG-5 and MRP-1 expression were able to independently predict the OS and DFS after treatment with adjuvant ECF chemotherapy, suggesting that monitoring their expression levels in combination of conventional prognostic markers may provide us with additional valuable information for a better evaluation of chemotherapy effect in GC patients. Interestingly, we found the ATG-5 was overexpressed in drug resistant GC cell lines. And silencing ATG-5 can sensitized the drug resistant cells to chemotherapy again. Our data suggest that ATG-5 may be a target for chemoresistant paitents.

Accumulating evidence has suggested that autophagy is capable to trigger both cell survival and cell death under different contexts. Liu et al reported that through inhibition of the PI3K/Akt/mTOR pathway, β-elemene could induce protective autophagy to assist GC cells better adapt to stressful conditions and protect them from undergoing apoptosis death [29]. Furthermore, recent studies have shown that the PI3K/Akt/mTOR signaling pathway is frequently activated in human gastrointesti-nal malignancies [30]. The PI3K/Akt signaling also modulates MDR in GC cell through the regulation of p-glycoprotein, Bcl2 and Bax [31]. Likewise, some anticancer agents have been reported to inhibit mTOR signaling and induce autophagy in cancer cells by degrading many major components in the mTOR axis [14,32]. Overall, these data suggest that autophagy could be induced during chemotherapy, and suppression of autophagic pathways using autophagy inhibitor have potential to improve the chemotherapeutic effectiveness in GC patients with ATG-5 high expression. In support, we found that when autophagy was inhibited, the drug resistant cells were also sensitized to drug treatment again as silencing ATG-5 expression. So, our result support that autophagy contributes to chemoresistant in patient.

In summary, over-expression of ATG-5, a key molecular player of the autophagic pathway, is associated with chemoresistance in GC. Expression of ATG-5 and MRP-1 could be considered as independent prognostic markers for predicting OS and DFS of GC patients based on the currently obtained data. On the basis of TNM stages, detection of their expression levels may be clinically meaningful for better prediction of chemotherapeutic treatment outcomes in patients suffering from this malignant disease. Future studies involving assessment of a larger number of cases, ideally from a different ethnic background, are definitely warranted to confirm our findings in this study.

Author Contributions

Conceived and designed the experiments: JG Zihua Chen. Performed the experiments: JG WY JH. Analyzed the data: JG JC WY ZD Zhikang Chen. Contributed reagents/materials/analysis tools: Zihua Chen. Contributed to the writing of the manuscript: Zhikang Chen JG.

References

1. Jemal A, Bray F, Center MM, Ferlay J, Ward E, et al (2011) Global cancer statistics. CA Cancer J Clin 61: 69–90.
2. Zhang D, Fan D (2007) Multidrug resistance in gastric cancer: recent research advances and ongoing therapeutic challenges. Expert Rev Anticancer Ther 7: 1369–78.
3. Levine B (2007) Cell biology: autophagy and cancer. Nature 446: 745–7.
4. Maycotte P, Thorburn A (2011) Autophagy and cancer therapy. Cancer Biol Ther 11: 127–37.
5. Mizushima N (2007) Autophagy: process and function. Genes Dev 21: 2861–73.
6. Marx J (2006) Autophagy: is it cancer's friend or foe? Science 312: 1160–1.
7. Li J, Hou N, Faried A, Tsutsumi S, Kuwano H (2010) Inhibition of autophagy augments 5-fluorouracil chemotherapy in human colon cancer in vitro and in vivo model. Eur J Cancer 46: 1900–9.
8. Li J, Hou N, Faried A, Tsutsumi S, Takeuchi T, et al (2009) Inhibition of autophagy by 3-MA enhances the effect of 5-FU-induced apoptosis in colon cancer cells. Ann Surg Oncol 16: 761–71.
9. Li X, Fan Z (2010) The epidermal growth factor receptor antibody cetuximab induces autophagy in cancer cells by downregulating HIF-1alpha and Bcl-2 and activating the beclin 1/hVps34 complex. Cancer Res 70: 5942–52.
10. Sasaki K, Tsuno NH, Sunami E, Tsurita G, Kawai K, et al (2010) Chloroquine potentiates the anti-cancer effect of 5-fluorouracil on colon cancer cells. BMC Cancer 10: 370.
11. Amaravadi RK, Yu D, Lum JJ, Bui T, Christophorou MA, et al (2007) Autophagy inhibition enhances therapy-induced apoptosis in a Myc-induced model of lymphoma. J Clin Invest 117: 326–36.
12. Hwang MS, Baek WK (2010) Glucosamine induces autophagic cell death through the stimulation of ER stress in human glioma cancer cells. Biochem Biophys Res Commun 399: 111–6.
13. Le XF, Mao W, Lu Z, Carter BZ, Bast RC (2010) Dasatinib induces autophagic cell death in human ovarian cancer. Cancer 116: 4980–90.
14. Jung C, Ro S, Cao J, Otto N, Kim D (2010) mTOR regulation of autophagy. FEBS Lett 584: 1287–95.
15. Mirzoeva OK, Hann B, Hom YK, Debnath J, Aftab D, et al (2011) Autophagy suppression promotes apoptotic cell death in response to inhibition of the PI3K-mTOR pathway in pancreatic adenocarcinoma. J Mol Med (Berl) 89: 877–89.
16. Klionsky DJ (2007) Autophagy: from phenomenology to molecular understanding in less than a decade. Nat Rev Mol Cell Biol 8: 931–7.
17. Yousefi S, Perozzo R, Schmid I, Ziemiecki A, Schaffner T, et al (2006) Calpain-mediated cleavage of Atg5 switches autophagy to apoptosis. Nat Cell Biol 8: 1124–32.
18. Fan K, Fan D, Cheng LF, Li C (2000) Expression of multidrug resistance-related markers in gastric cancer. Anticancer Res 20: 4809–14.
19. Lacueva J, Perez-Ramos M, Soto J, Oliver I, Andrada E, et al (2005) Multidrug resistance-associated protein (MRP1) gene is strongly expressed in gastric carcinomas. Analysis by immunohistochemistry and real-time quantitative RT-PCR. Histopathology 46: 389–95.
20. Zhang D, Fan D (2010) New insights into the mechanisms of gastric cancer multidrug resistance and future perspectives. Future Oncol 6: 527–37.
21. Edge S, Byrd D, Compton C, Fritz A, Greene F, et al (2010) American Joint Committee on Cancer. AJCC cancer staging manual. 7th. New York: Springer.
22. An CH, Kim MS, Yoo NJ, Park SW, Lee SH (2011) Mutational and expressional analyses of ATG5, an autophagy-related gene, in gastrointestinal cancers. Pathol Res Pract 207: 433–7.
23. Ge J, Chen Z, Wu S, Chen J, Li X, et al (2009) Expression levels of insulin-like growth factor-1 and multidrug resistance-associated protein-1 indicate poor prognosis in patients with gastric cancer. Digestion 80: 148–58.
24. Black RJ, Bray F, Ferlay J, Parkin DM (1997) Cancer incidence and mortality in the European Union: cancer registry data and estimates of national incidence for 1990. Eur J Cancer 33: 1075–107.
25. Bray F, Sankila R, Ferlay J, Parkin DM (2002) Estimates of cancer incidence and mortality in Europe in 1995. Eur J Cancer 38: 99–166.
26. Sun XD, Mu R, Zhou YS, Dai XD, Zhang SW, et al (2004) [Analysis of mortality rate of stomach cancer and its trend in twenty years in China]. Zhonghua Zhong Liu Za Zhi 26: 4–9.
27. Cervantes A, Rosello S, Roda D, Rodriguez-Braun E (2008) The treatment of advanced gastric cancer: current strategies and future perspectives. Ann Oncol 19 Suppl 5: v103–7.
28. Suh YS, Lee HJ, Jung EJ, Kim MA, Nam KT, et al (2012) The combined expression of metaplasia biomarkers predicts the prognosis of gastric cancer. Ann Surg Oncol 19: 1240–9.
29. Liu J, Zhang Y, Qu J, Xu L, Hou K, et al (2011) beta-Elemene-induced autophagy protects human gastric cancer cells from undergoing apoptosis. BMC Cancer 11: 183.
30. Ko JK, Auyeung KK (2013) Target-oriented mechanisms of novel herbal therapeutics in the chemotherapy of gastrointestinal cancer and inflammation. Curr Pharm Des 19: 48–66.
31. Han Z, Hong L, Han Y, Wu K, Han S, et al (2007) Phospho Akt mediates multidrug resistance of gastric cancer cells through regulation of P-gp, Bcl-2 and Bax. J Exp Clin Cancer Res 26: 261–8.
32. Fu L, Kim Y, Wang X, Wu X, Yue P, et al (2009) Perifosine inhibits mammalian target of rapamycin signaling through facilitating degradation of major components in the mTOR axis and induces autophagy. Cancer Res 69: 8967–76.

11

Prognostic Value and Staging Classification of Retropharyngeal Lymph Node Metastasis in Nasopharyngeal Carcinoma Patients Treated with Intensity-modulated Radiotherapy

Ling-Long Tang[1], Rui Guo[1], Guanqun Zhou[1], Ying Sun[1], Li-Zhi Liu[2], Ai-Hua Lin[3], Haiqiang Mai[4], Jianyong Shao[5], Li Li[2], Jun Ma[1]*

1 Department of Radiation oncology, Sun Yat-sen University Cancer Center; State Key Laboratory of Oncology in South China; Collaborative Innovation Center for Cancer Medicine, Guangzhou, Guangdong, People's Republic of China, **2** Imaging Diagnosis and Interventional Center, State Key Laboratory of Oncology in South China, Sun Yat-sen University Cancer Center, Collaborative Innovation Center for Cancer Medicine, Guangzhou, Guangdong, People's Republic of China, **3** Department of Medical Statistics and Epidemiology, School of Public Health, Sun Yat-sen University, Guangzhou, Guangdong, People's Republic of China, **4** Department of Nasopharyngeal Carcinoma, Sun Yat-Sen University Cancer Center, Collaborative Innovation Center for Cancer Medicine, Guangzhou, Guangdong, People's Republic of China, **5** Department of Molecular Diagnostics, State Key Laboratory of Oncology in South China, Sun Yat-Sen University Cancer Center, Collaborative Innovation Center for Cancer Medicine, Guangzhou, Guangdong, People's Republic of China

Abstract

Background: The development of intensity-modulated radiotherapy (IMRT) has revolutionized the management of nasopharyngeal carcinoma (NPC). The purpose of this study was to evaluate the prognostic value and classification of TNM stage system for retropharyngeal lymph node (RLN) metastasis in NPC in the IMRT era.

Material and Methods: We retrospectively reviewed data from 749 patients with biopsy-proven, non-metastatic NPC. All patients received IMRT as the primary treatment. Chemotherapy was administered to 86.2% (424/492) of the patients with stage III or IV disease.

Results: The incidence of RLN metastasis was 64.2% (481/749). Significant differences were observed in the 5-year disease-free survival (DFS; 70.6% vs. 85.4%, $P<0.001$) and distant metastasis-free survival (DMFS; 79.2% vs. 90.1%, $P<0.001$) rates of patients with and without RLN metastasis. In multivariate analysis, RLN metastasis was an independent prognostic factor for disease failure and distant failure ($P=0.005$ and $P=0.026$, respectively), but not for locoregional recurrence. Necrotic RLN metastases have a negative effect on disease failure, distant failure and locoregional recurrence in NPC with RLN metastasis ($P=0.003$, $P=0.018$ and $P=0.005$, respectively). Survival curves demonstrated a significant difference in DFS between patients with N0 disease and N1 disease with only RLN metastasis ($P=0.020$), and marginally statistically significant differences in DMFS and DFS between N1 disease with only RLN metastasis and other N1 disease ($P=0.058$ and $P=0.091$, respectively). In N1 disease, no significant differences in DFS were observed between unilateral and bilateral RLN metastasis ($P=0.994$).

Conclusions: In the IMRT era, RLN metastasis remains an independent prognostic factor for DFS and DMFS in NPC. It is still reasonable for RLN metastasis to be classified in the N1 disease, regardless of laterality. However, there is a need to investigate the feasibility of classifying RLN metastasis as N1a disease in future by a larger cohort study.

Editor: Masaru Katoh, National Cancer Center, Japan

Funding: This work was supported by grants from the China Scholarship Council (No. 201308440052, the National Natural Science Foundation of China (No. 81101695 and No. 81071836), the Guangdong Province Universities and Colleges Pearl River Scholar Funded Scheme (2010), and the Innovation Team Development Plan of the Ministry of Education (IRT1297). The funders had no role in study design, data collection and analysis, decision to publish, or preparation of the manuscript.

Competing Interests: The authors have declared that no competing interests exist.

* Email: majun2@mail.sysu.edu.cn

These authors contributed equally to this work.

Introduction

Although nasopharyngeal carcinoma (NPC) is rare in most regions of the world, it is endemic in certain regions, especially Southeast Asia. The incidence of NPC is approximately 30–80 per 100,000 per year in Southern China [1]. The nasopharynx contains a well-developed network of lymph nodes, and the retropharyngeal lymph nodes (RLN) are regarded as one of the key lymph nodes in NPC [2]. Due to the limitations of CT imaging, RLN metastases are isodense and contiguous with the primary tumor, and can be difficult to identify as a separate mass on CT scans; therefore, the true incidence of RLN metastasis was previously underestimated [3–5]. However, due the superior soft tissue contrast and multiplanar capacity of MRI, the incidence of RLN metastasis in NPC is currently approximately 70% [5,6], and RLN metastasis has received increasing attention in recent years.

The recent seventh edition of the International Union against Cancer/American Joint Committee on Cancer (UICC/AJCC) staging system for NPC incorporated RLN metastasis into the tumor-node-metastasis (TNM) classification, and classified it as N1 disease regardless of laterality [7,8]. However, this revision was based on patients treated with a two-dimensional conventional radiotherapy technique. Intensity-modulated radiotherapy (IMRT) offers an improved tumor target conformity, allows safer dose escalations and yields superior results in NPC compared to 2D-CRT, primarily by achieving a higher local tumor control rate [9]. IMRT has gradually replaced two-dimensional conventional radiotherapy as the primary radiotherapy modality for the treatment of NPC; however, the introduction of new therapeutic technologies may require a revaluation of the prognostic value and appropriate classification of TNM staging system for RLN metastasis in NPC.

In this study, we analyzed the outcomes of patients with NPC staged by MRI prior to treatment who subsequently received IMRT and the current standard systemic treatments, to investigate whether it is still reasonable to classify RLN metastasis in NPC as N1 disease in the IMRT era.

Methods and Materials

Patient characteristics

Approval for retrospective analysis of the patient data was obtained from the ethics committee of Sun Yat-sen University Cancer Center. Written consent was waived, while oral consent from the patients was obtained via telephone and documented by telephone recording. All 749 patients with newly diagnosed, biopsy-proven, non-metastatic NPC who were treated at Sun Yat-Sen University Cancer Center using IMRT between January 2003 and December 2007 were retrospectively reviewed. The clinicopathologic characteristics of the patients are shown in Table 1.

All patients completed a pre-treatment evaluation including complete patient history, physical examination, hematology and biochemistry profiles, neck and nasopharyngeal MRI, chest radiography, abdominal sonography and a single photon emission computed tomography (SPECT) whole body bone scan. 18-F-fluorodeoxyglucose (FDG)-positron emission tomography (PET)-CT was performed on 162/749 patients (21.6%). All patients were retrospectively re-staged according to the 7th edition of UICC/AJCC staging system. The distribution of disease stages was: stage I, 10.4%; stage II, 23.9%; stage III, 37.7% and stage IVa–b, 28.0% (Table 1).

MRI techniques and criteria for retropharyngeal lymph node and other cervical lymph node metastasis

All patients underwent MRI scans using a 1.5-T system (Signa, General Electric, CV/i; General Electric Healthcare, Chalfont St. Giles, United Kingdom). The area from the suprasellar cistern to the inferior margin of the sternal end of clavicle was examined with a head and neck combined coil. T1-weighted fast spin-echo images in the axial, coronal and sagittal planes (repetition time of 500–600 ms and echo time of 10–20 ms), and T2-weighted fast spin-echo MR images in the axial plane (repetition time of 4000–6000 ms and echo time of 95–110 ms) were obtained before injection of contrast material. After intravenous injection of Gd-DTPA at a dose of 0.1 mmol/kg body weight, spin-echo T1-weighted axial and sagittal sequences, and spin-echo T1-weighted fat-suppressed coronal sequences were performed sequentially using parameters similar to those used before injection of contrast. The section thickness for the axial plane was 5 mm with a 1 mm interslice gap, and 6 mm with a 1 mm interslice gap for the coronal and sagittal planes.

Two radiologists specializing in head and neck cancers evaluated all of the scans independently. Any disagreements were resolved by consensus. The diagnostic MRI criteria for metastatic lymphadenopathy included: 1) lateral RLN with a minimal axial diameter of ≥5 mm and any node seen in the median retropharyngeal group, or lymph nodes with a minimal axial diameter ≥11 mm in the diagastric region or ≥10 mm for all other cervical nodes except the retropharyngeal group; 2) lymph nodes of any size with central necrosis or a contrast-enhanced rim; and 3) nodal grouping: the presence of three or more contiguous and confluent lymph nodes, each of which should have a minimal axial diameter of 8–10 mm [10–12]. The criteria for extranodal neoplastic spread (ENS) in RLN was the presence of indistinct nodal margins, irregular nodal capsular enhancement or infiltration into the adjacent fat or muscle [13].

Treatment

All patients received IMRT as the primary treatment. The patients were immobilized in supine position by a thermoplastic mask. After administration of intravenous contrast material, 3-mm CT slices, depicting the area of the head until 2 cm below the sterno-clavicular joint, were acquired. The primary tumor and the upper-neck area above the caudal edge of the cricoid cartilage were treated by IMRT. Target volumes were in agreement with the International Commission on Radiation Units and Measurements Reports 50 and 62. The contoured images were transferred to an integrated IMRT planning and delivery system (Peacock, Corvus 3.0, NOMOS Corporation, Sewickley, Pa). The prescribed radiation dose was defined as follows: a total dose of 68 Gy in 30 fractions at 2.27 Gy per fraction to the planning target volume (PTV) of the primary gross tumor volume (GTV-P), 60 to 64 Gy to the PTV of nodal gross tumor volume (GTV-N), 60 Gy to the PTV of CTV-1 (i.e., high-risk regions), and 54 Gy to the PTV of CTV-2 (i.e., low-risk regions) and CTV-N (i.e., neck nodal regions). The treatment was delivered by a dynamic, multileaf, intensitymodulating collimator (called MIMiC). For the lower neck, an anterior cervical field was used. All patients were treated with one fraction daily over 5 days per week.

Chemotherapy was administered to 86.2% (424/492) of the patients with stage III or IV disease. The chemotherapy regimens included concurrent chemotherapy alone, concurrent chemotherapy combined with induction chemotherapy and/or adjuvant chemotherapy in conjunction with a platinum-based therapeutic clinical trial. Reasons for deviation from institutional guidelines included patients' refusal, age (≥70 years), organ severe dysfunc-

Table 1. The clinicpathological characters of 749 patients in this study.

Characteristic	N	Column (%)
Age		
>50	553	73.8
≤50	196	26.2
Gender		
Male	580	77.4
Female	169	22.6
Histologic type		
WHO II/III	744	99.3
WHO I	5	0.7
T category		
T1	177	23.6
T2	140	18.7
T3	264	35.2
T4	168	22.4
N category		
N0	184	24.6
N1	409	54.6
N2	106	14.2
N3	50	6.7
Stage		
I	78	10.4
II	179	23.9
III	282	37.7
Iva-b	210	28.0
Chemotherapy		
No	214	28.6
Concurrent	233	33.5
Concurrent + Induction	246	32.8
Concurrent + Adjuvant	46	6.1
PET-CT		
Yes	162	21.6
No	587	78.4

tion (diabetes, cardiac dysfunction, renal insufficiency, liver insufficiency, et al) that would suggest intolerance to chemotherapy. When possible, salvage treatments such as intracavitary brachytherapy, surgery and chemotherapy were provided in the event of documented relapse or persistent disease.

Follow-up

Median follow-up was 81 months (range, 3–127 months). Each patient was assessed weekly during treatment for treatment response and toxicity, and every 2–3 months during the first 2 years and every 3–6 months during years 3–5 after radiotherapy. Endoscopy, CT or MRI scans of the head and neck were performed every 3 months during the first year and annually during years 2–5. Patients with residual or recurrent local disease underwent biopsy to confirm malignancy. Additional tests were ordered when indicated to evaluate for local or distant failure.

Statistical analysis

All analyses were performed using SPSS version 20.0 (IBM Corporation, Armonk, NY, USA). Actuarial rates were estimated by the Kaplan-Meier method; survival curves were compared using the log-rank test [14]. The following endpoints (measured from the start of treatment to the first defining event) were estimated: locoregional relapse-free survival (LRRFS), local relapse-free survival (LRFS), and nodal relapse-free survival (NRFS), DMFS, disease-free survival (DFS) and overall survival (OS).

Multivariate analyses with the Cox proportional hazards model were used to test for independent significance by backward elimination of insignificant explanatory variables [15]. The Cox proportional hazards model was used to calculate hazard ratios (HRs). Two-tailed P values <0.05 were considered statistically significant.

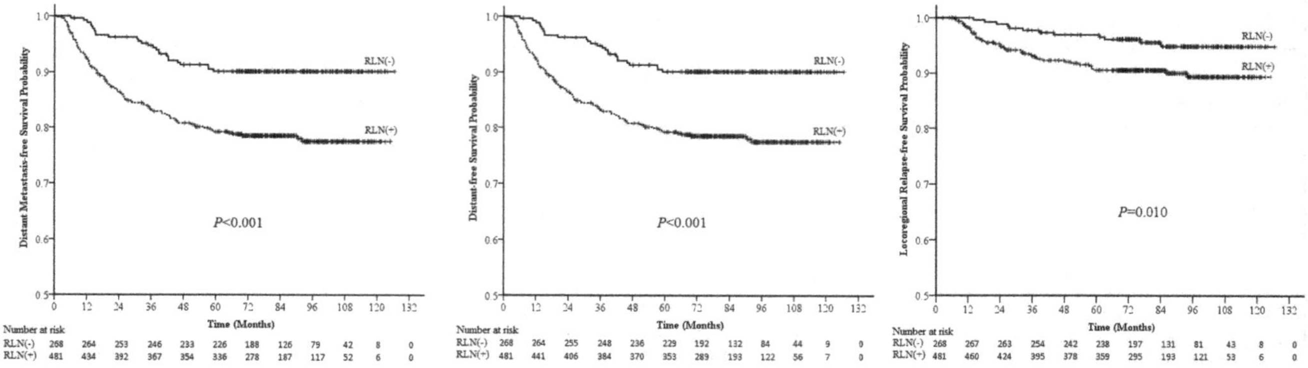

Figure 1. Survival curves for nasopharyngeal carcinoma (NPC) patients with and without retropharyngeal lymph node (RLN) metastasis. RLN (-): NPC patients without RLN metastasis; RLN (+): NPC patients with RLN metastasis.

Results

Incidence of RLN metastasis

In this study, no patient had a metastatic median RLN, and the incidence of lateral RLN metastasis in the current study was 64.2% (481/749 patients). Thirty-two percent (154/481) of patients with RLN metastasis had no evidence of cervical lymph node (CLN) metastasis, and 79.6% (327/411) patients with CLN metastasis had evidence of RLN involvement.

Of 481 the patients with RLN metastasis, 63.2% (304/481) had unilateral RLN involvement, whereas 36.8% (177 of 481) had bilateral involvement. The mean minimal and maximal axial diameters of the RLN metastases were 9.61±4.31 mm (range, 5–28 mm) and 12.66±5.61 mm (range, 5–36 mm). The incidence of RLN necrosis was 13.3% (64/481) and the incidence of ENS was 21.8% (105/481).

Prognostic value of RLN metastasis

There were 56/749 (7.5%) patients developed recurrence, including 34 patients (4.5%) with isolated local recurrences, 15 patients (2.0%) with isolated regional nodal recurrences, and 7 patients (0.9%) with both local and regional nodal recurrence. In addition, there were 129 (17.2%) patients developed distant metastases and 149 (19.9%) died. The 5-year survival rates were: LRRFS, 92.9%; DMFS, 83.1%; DFS, 75.9% and OS, 83.9%.

Significant differences were observed in the 5-year DFS (70.6% vs. 85.4%, $P<0.001$), DMFS (79.2% vs. 90.1%, $P<0.001$) and LRRFS (90.5% vs. 97.0%, $P=0.010$) rates of patients with and without RLN metastasis (Figure 1). Multivariate analysis was performed to adjust for various prognostic factors; the following known important prognostic variables were included in the Cox proportional hazards model: age (≤50 vs.>50 years), gender, T-classification, chemotherapy (yes vs. no), bilateral CLN metastasis (yes vs. no), dimension of CLN metastases (≤6 vs.>6 cm) and the

Table 2. Summary of multivariate analysis of prognostic factors in 749 patients with nasopharyngeal carcinoma.

Endpoint	Variable	B	*P**	HR	95% *CI* for HR
Distant failure	Retropharyngeal lymph node (yes vs. no)	0.520	0.026	1.682	1.065–2.655
	Age (≤50 vs. 50 years)	0.406	0.040	1.501	1.019–2.211
	T-classification	0.451	<0.001	1.570	1.307–1.887
	CLN dimension (≤6 vs. > 6 cm)	1.268	<0.001	3.555	1.965–6.434
	CLN location (with SCLN vs. without SCLN)	0.896	0.003	2.450	1.351–4.443
	Bilateral CLN (yes vs. no)	0.511	0.013	1.668	1.114–2.497
Disease failure	Retropharyngeal lymph node (yes vs. no)	0.509	0.005	1.663	1.169–2.365
	Age (≤50 vs. 50 years)	0.656	<0.001	1.927	1.427–2.602
	T classification	0.435	<0.001	1.544	1.335–1.787
	CLN dimension (≤6 vs. >6 cm)	1.068	<0.001	2.908	1.691–5.001
	CLN location (with SCLN vs. without SCLN)	0.818	0.002	2.266	1.342–3.826
	Bilateral CLN (yes vs. no)	0.362	0.040	1.436	1.016–2.029
Locoregional recurrence	Retropharyngeal lymph node (yes vs. no)	*NS*			
	T-classification	0.438	0.001	1.550	1.183–2.031
	Bilateral CLN (yes vs. no)	0.681	0.022	1.975	1.105–3.530

Abbreviations: CI = confidence interval; HR = hazard ratio; CLN = cervical lymph nodes; NS = not significant; SCLN = Supraclavicular lymph node.
**P* values were calculated using an adjusted Cox proportional-hazards model. The following known important prognostic variables were included in the Cox proportional hazards model: age (≤50 vs. >50 years), gender, T-classification, chemotherapy (yes vs. no), bilateral CLN metastasis (yes vs. no), dimension of CLN metastases (≤6 vs. >6 cm), CLN location (with SCLN vs. without SCLN) and RLN metastasis (yes vs. no).

Table 3. Five-year survival rates for 481 nasopharyngeal carcinoma patients with retropharyngeal lymph nodes metastasis according to the characteristics of retropharyngeal lymph node metastasis.

	Size (minimal axial diameters)			Necrosis			Laterality			Extranodal neoplastic spread		
	<10 mm	≥10 mm	P*	No	Yes	P*	Unilateral	Bilateral	P*	No	Yes	P*
DMFS	86.5	71.9	<0.001	81.6	62.8	<0.001	82.5	73.6	0.032	81.6	70.3	0.001
DFS	78.3	62.9	<0.001	73.3	53.1	<0.001	73.6	65.5	0.054	74.1	58.1	0.002
LRRFS	93.5	87.3	0.017	92.0	80.0	<0.001	91.5	88.9	0.310	92.0	85.2	0.019

Abbreviations: DFS = disease-free survival; DMFS = Distant metastasis-free survival; LRRFS = Locoregional relapse-free survival.
*P values were calculated by the unadjusted log-rank test.

location of CLN metastasis (with supraclavicular lymph nodes metastasis vs. without supraclavicular lymph nodes metastasis). Dimension of CLN metastases (≤6 vs.>6 cm) was measured based on maximal diameter by palpation. RLN metastasis was an independent prognostic factor for disease failure and distant failure (HR = 1.663, 95% CI: 1.169–2.365, $P = 0.005$, and HR = 1.682, 95% CI: 1.065–2.655, $P = 0.026$, respectively), but not for locoregional recurrence (Table 2).

All of the MRI-determined nodal variables were analyzed in the 481 patients with RLN metastasis using univariate analyses and multivariate analyses. The RLN variables were categorized as follows: minimal axial diameters (<10 vs. ≥10 mm MID), necrosis (no vs. yes), laterality (unilateral vs. bilateral) and ENS (no vs. yes). Univariate analysis revealed that necrosis had significant prognostic value for DMFS, DFS and LRRFS ($P<0.001$, $P<0.001$ and $P<0.001$; Table 3). After adjusting for various prognostic factors including age, sex, T-classification, N-classification and chemotherapy, necrosis remained significant for disease failure, distant failure and locoregional recurrence (HR = 1.795, 95%CI: 1.214–2.654, $P = 0.003$; HR = 1.752, 95%CI:1.100–2.790, $P = 0.018$ and HR = 2.614, 95%CI: 1.339–5.103, $P = 0.005$; Table 4).

Survival according to N classification

According to the seventh edition of AJCC staging system, RLN is included as a criterion for N1 disease, and 154 (20.6%) N0 patients would be upgraded to N1 disease (N1 with RLN only). All 749 patients were divided into five groups: N0 disease, N1 disease with retropharyngeal lymph node metastasis and without CLN metastasis (N1 with RLN only), N1 disease with CLN metastasis (N1 with CLN), N2 disease, and N3 disease. The survival curves demonstrated a significant difference in DFS between patients with N0 disease and N1 with RLN only ($P = 0.020$). The differences in DMFS and DFS between N1 with RLN only and N1 with CLN were marginally statistically significant ($P = 0.058$ and $P = 0.091$, respectively; Fig. 2).

In the N1 disease group, no significant differences were observed in the DFS, MDFS, LRFS or NRFS rates of patients with unilateral and bilateral RLN metastasis ($P = 0.994$, $P = 0.752$, $P = 0.398$ and $P = 0.08$ respectively).

Discussion

The TNM staging system is crucial for predicting prognosis, guiding treatment strategy for different risk groups, and facilitating the exchange of information between oncology centers [8,16]. The TNM staging system is continually being modified to account for new developments in diagnostic and therapeutic techniques. There is little controversy that IMRT is the treatment of choice for NPC, as dosimetric studies have demonstrated the clear advantages of IMRT in terms of improving the dose conformity for complex tumor targets and better protecting the adjacent organs at risk [17,18]. This is the first study to demonstrate that it is reasonable for RLN metastasis in NPC to be classified as N1 disease in the IMRT era.

Prognostic value of RLN metastasis

Several studies have reported that neck lymph node involvement in NPC spreads in an orderly manner down the neck [19,20]. RLN metastasis is very common in NPC, as the RLNs are the first echelon lymph node [21]. When treated with two-dimensional conventional radiotherapy, patients with NPC and RLN metastasis had a poor prognosis [7]. In this study of patients treated with IMRT, RLN metastasis remained an independent

Table 4. Summary of multivariate analysis of prognostic factors in 481 nasopharyngeal carcinoma patients with retropharyngeal lymph node metastasis (RLN) metastasis.

Endpoint	Variable	B	P*	HR	95% CI for HR
Disease failure	Age (≤50 vs. 50)	0.659	<0.001	1.933	1.374–2.721
	T-classification	0.330	<0.001	1.391	1.167–1.658
	N-classification	0.349	<0.001	1.417	1.203–1.670
	Necrosis	0.585	0.003	1.795	1.214–2.654
	MID (<10 vs. ≥10 mm)	0.329	0.063	1.389	0.983–1.964
Distant failure	Age (≤50 vs. 50 years)	0.412	0.064	1.510	0.976–2.335
	T-classification	0.318	0.004	1.374	1.107–1.706
	N-classification	0.413	<0.001	1.511	1.249–1.828
	Necrosis	0.561	0.018	1.752	1.100–2.790
	MID (<10 vs. ≥10 mm)	0.490	0.026	1.632	1.059–2.515
Locoregional recurrence	Necrosis	0.961	0.005	2.614	1.339–5.103
	MID (<10 vs. ≥10 mm)	0.570	0.083	1.767	0.929–3.364

Abbreviations: CI = confidence interval, MID = minimal axial diameters.
*P values were calculated using an adjusted Cox proportional-hazards model. The following known important prognostic variables were included in the Cox proportional hazards model: minimal axial diameters of RLN (<10 vs. ≥10 mm MID), necrosis of RLN (no vs. yes), laterality of RLN (unilateral vs. bilateral) and extra nodal neoplastic spread of RLN (no vs. yes), age (≤50 vs. 50), sex, T-classification, N-classification and chemotherapy (no vs. yes).

prognostic factor for DFS and DMFS, even after adjustment for various prognostic factors. It is possible that conventional two-dimensional and three-dimensional conformal radiotherapy and IMRT do not have a significantly different effect on DMFS in patients with RLN metastasis. A number of studies have confirmed that IMRT has improved local control, but not distant control, in NPC [9,17,22]. In this study, the DMFS rate was only 83.1%, indicating that distant failure remains a challenge in patients with RLN metastasis. Therefore, the inclusion of RLN metastasis in the UICC/AJCC staging system would be useful to guide treatment planning, and additional therapeutic improvements are required to achieve a favorable outcome in patients with RLN metastasis.

Central necrosis is considered to be a late event in the biological evolution of tumor metastases within lymph nodes [23]. It has been confirmed that central necrosis primarily occurs in lymph nodes approximately 20.0 mm or larger, and it appears that central necrosis characteristically occurs after massive tumor infiltration [24]. There are few reports about the prognostic value of necrosis in RLN metastases in NPC. In this study, we found that necrosis of RLN metastases had a negative effect on survival in NPC. Tumor necrosis is believed to represent the endpoint of severe, chronic hypoxia in tissues distal to functional blood vessels. Tumor hypoxia may be one factor accounting for the poor prognosis of patients with necrotic RLN metastases [25]. Although IMRT offers improved tumor target coverage, the lack of oxygen

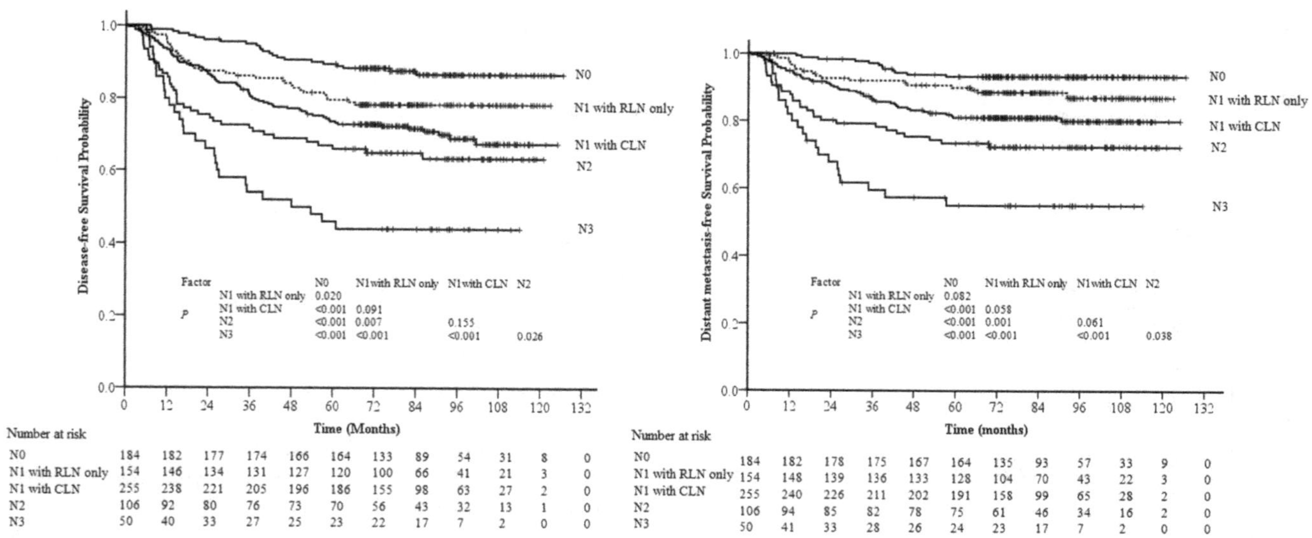

Figure 2. Survival curves for patients with nasopharyngeal carcinoma (NPC) stratified by the N classification of the 7th edition of the UICC/AJCC staging system for NPC. N1 + RLN only: N1 disease with retropharyngeal lymph node metastasis and without cervical lymph node metastasis; N1 + CLN: N1 disease with cervical lymph node metastasis.

in areas of hypoxia not only makes the tissues less susceptible to radiotherapy, but also induces the transcription of a variety of genes which promote tumor progression and increase tumor aggressiveness compared to non-hypoxic tumors [26,27], which may explain why necrosis had significant prognostic value for all endpoints (DFS, DMFS and LRRFS). We propose that RLN necrosis should be adopted as a factor to enhance individualized NPC patient prognostication and clinical decision making, especially as it is simple to assess and could easily be incorporated into routine histopathological examinations.

Classification for RLN metastasis

Due to the limited diagnostic capabilities prior to the era of MRI imaging, consistent guidelines for the designation of RLN metastasis could not be identified in previous TNM staging systems; RLN metastasis was only incorporated into the TNM classification of the most recent 7th edition of the UICC/AJCC staging system for NPC. Evidence from two retrospective studies indicated that patients with RLN alone, regardless of laterality, have a similar risk of distant metastasis (DM) as patients with N1 disease [7,28]. However, all of the patients in one of these studies [7] underwent conventional radiotherapy, and in the other study [28], only 12.7% of the patients underwent IMRT and there were no stratification analyses according to the radiation technique. IMRT achieves a significantly higher survival rate in NPC than CRT [9]; therefore, it was necessary to reevaluate whether it is still reasonable for RLN metastasis to be classified as N1 disease in the IMRT era.

This study, in which all patients received IMRT as the primary treatment, demonstrates that it is still reasonable for RLN metastasis in NPC to be classified as N1 disease, regardless of laterality. There are a number of reasons for this suggestion: Firstly, it is well recognized that the RLNs are the first echelon node in NPC. In most cases, and unlike CT, MRI can discriminate the RLNs from the primary tumor, so RLN metastasis should be classified in the N-classification, not the T-classification. Secondly, the survival curves in this study demonstrated a significant difference in DFS between patients with N0 disease and N1 disease with RLN only; therefore, it is still reasonable for RLN metastasis to be classified as N1 disease in patients treated with IMRT. Lastly, no significant differences were observed in the DFS, MDFS and LRFS rates of patients with unilateral and bilateral RLN metastasis, so RLN laterality does not need to be considered in future revisions of the staging system.

However, it was also observed that the differences in DMFS and DFS between N1 with RLN only and N1 with CLN were marginally statistically significant, and the survival curve could be separated, so there is a need to investigate the feasibility of classifying RLN metastasis as N1a disease in future by a larger cohort study.

It should be emphasized that this study was retrospective, and these results should be confirmed in a prospective study in the future. However, the current analysis of a large number of patients who received a systemic staging workup and were treated at single institution offers valuable information for evaluating appropriate classification of TNM stage for RLN metastasis in the current MRI/IMRT era. More importantly, all patients were treated with IMRT, in compliance with the requirements for studies aimed at formulating improvements in staging systems [16].

In conclusion, in the IMRT era, RLN metastasis remains an independent prognostic factor in NPC, and necrotic RLN metastases have a negative effect on survival in NPC. It is still reasonable for RLN metastasis to be classified in the N1 disease, regardless of laterality. However, there is a need to investigate the feasibility of classifying RLN metastasis as N1a disease in future by a larger cohort study.

Author Contributions

Conceived and designed the experiments: JM LT. Performed the experiments: LT RG GZ YS L. Liu HM JS L. Li. Analyzed the data: AL LT. Contributed reagents/materials/analysis tools: LT RG GZ YS L. Liu L. Li. Wrote the paper: LT JM.

References

1. Parkin DM, Whelan SL, Ferlay J, Raymond L, Young J (1997) Cancer incidence in five continents. IARC, Lyon France, 143: 814–815.
2. Sham JST, Choy D, Wei WI (1990) Nasopharyngeal carcinoma: orderly neck node spread. Int J Radiat Oncol Biol Phys 19: 929–933.
3. Ng SH, Chang TC, Ko SF, Yen PS, Wan YL, et al. (1997) Nasopharyngeal carcinoma: MRI and CT assessment. Neuroradiology 39: 741–746.
4. Olmi P, Fallai C, Colagrande S, Giannardi G (1995) Staging and follow-up of nasopharyngeal carcinoma: magnetic resonance imaging versus computerized tomography. Int J Radiat Oncol Biol Phys 32: 795–800.
5. Liao XB, Mao YP, Liu LZ, Tang LL, Sun Y, et al. (2008) How does magnetic resonance imaging influence staging according to AJCC staging system for nasopharyngeal carcinoma compared with computed tomography? Int J RadiatOncolBiol Phys 72: 1368–1377.
6. Ng SH, Chang JT, Chan SC, Ko SF, Wang HM, et al. (2004) Nodal metastases of nasopharyngeal carcinoma: patterns of disease on MRI and FDG-PET. Eur J Nucl Med Mol Imaging 31: 1073–1080.
7. Ma J, Liu L, Tang L, Zong J, LinA, et al. (2007) Retropharyngeal lymph node metastasis in nasopharyngeal carcinoma: prognostic value and staging categories. Clin Cancer Res 13: 1445–152.
8. Edge SB, Fritz AG, Byrd DR, Greene FL, Compton CC, et al. (2010) AJCC cancer staging manual. Springer, Berlin Heidelberg New York, 41–56.
9. Lai SZ, Li WF, Chen L, Luo W, Chen YY, et al. (2011) How does intensity-modulated radiotherapy versus conventional two-dimensional radiotherapy influence the treatment results in nasopharyngeal carcinoma patients? Int J Radiat Oncol Biol Phys 80: 661–668.
10. Van den Brekel MW, Castelijns JA, Snow GB (1990) Cervical lymph node metastasis: Assessment of radiologic criteria. Radiology 177: 379–384.
11. Lam WW, Chan YL, Leung SF, Metreweli C (1997) Retropharyngeal lymphadenopathy in nasopharyngeal carcinoma. Head Neck 19: 176–181
12. King AD, Tse GM, Ahuja AT, Yuen EH, Vlantis AC, et al. (2004) Necrosis in metastatic neck nodes: Diagnostic accuracy of CT, MR imaging, and US. Radiology 230: 720–726.
13. King AD, Tse GM, Yuen EH, To EW, Vlantis AC, et al.(2004) Comparison of CT and MR imaging for the detection of extranodal neoplastic spread in metastatic neck nodes. Eur J Radiol 52: 264–70.
14. Kaplan EL, Meier P (1958) Nonparametric Estimation from Incomplete Observations. Journal of the American Statistical Association. 53: 457–481.
15. Cox DR (1972) Regression Models and Life-Tables. Journal of the Royal Statistical Society. Series B (Methodological). 34: 187–220.
16. Groome PA, Schulze K, Boysen M, Hall SF, Mackillop WJ (2001) A comparison of published head and neck stage groupings in carcinomas of the oral cavity. Head Neck 23: 613–624.
17. Ng WT, Lee MC, Hung WM, Choi CW, Lee KC, et al. (2011) Clinical outcomes and patterns of failure after intensity-modulated radiotherapy for nasopharyngeal carcinoma. Int J Radiat Oncol Biol Phys 79: 420–428.
18. Xia P, Fu KK, Wong GW, Akazawa C, Verhey LJ (2000) Comparison of treatment plans involving intensity-modulated radiotherapy for nasopharyngeal carcinoma. Int J Radiat Oncol Biol Phys 48: 329–337.
19. Sham JST, Choy D, Wei WI (1990) Nasopharyngeal carcinoma: orderly neck node spread. Int J Radiat Oncol Biol Phys 19: 929–933.
20. Tang L, Mao Y, Liu L, Liang SB, Chen Y, et al. (2009) The volume to be irradiated during selective neck irradiation in nasopharyngeal carcinoma: analysis of the spread patterns in lymph nodes by magnetic resonance imaging. Cancer 115: 680–688.
21. King AD, Ahuja AT, Leung SF, Lam WW, Teo P, et al. (2000) Neck node metastases from nasopharyngeal carcinoma: MR imaging of patterns of disease. Head Neck 22: 275–281.
22. Kong F, Ying H, Huang S, Du C, Zhou J, et al. (2014) Preliminary results of nasopharyngeal carcinoma treated with intensity-modulated radiotherapy: a retrospective study of 364 patients. Eur Arch Otorhinolaryngol DOI 10.1007/s00405-014-2900-2. In press.
23. Som P (1987) Lymph nodes of the neck. Radiology 165: 593–600.
24. Don DM, Anzai Y, Lufkin RB, Fu YS, Calcaterra TC (1995) Evaluation of cervical lymph node metastases in squamous cell carcinoma of the head and neck. Laryngoscope 105: 669–674.

25. Rischin D, Hicks RJ, Fisher R, Binns D, Corry J, et al. (2006) Prognostic significance of [18F]-misonidazole positron emission tomography-detected tumor hypoxia in patients with advanced head and neck cancer randomly assigned to chemoradiation with or without tirapazamine: a substudy of Trans-Tasman Radiation Oncology Group Study 98.02. J Clin Oncol 24: 2098–2104.
26. Toustrup K, Sorensen BS, Lassen P, Wiuf C, Alsner J, et al. (2012) Gene expression classifier predicts for hypoxic modification of radiotherapy with nimorazole in squamous cell carcinomas of the head and neck. Radiother Oncol 102: 122–129.
27. Toustrup K, Sorensen BS, Nordsmark M, Busk M, Wiuf C, et al. (2011) Development of a hypoxia gene expression classifier with predictive impact for hypoxic modification of radiotherapy in head and neck cancer. Cancer Res 71: 5923–5931.
28. Tang L, Li L, Mao Y, Liu LZ, Liang SB, et al. (2008) Retropharyngeal lymph node metastasis in nasopharyngeal carcinoma detected by magnetic resonance imaging: prognostic value and staging categories. Cancer 113: 347–354.

12

In Vitro and *In Vivo* Anti-Schistosomal Activity of the Alkylphospholipid Analog Edelfosine

Edward Yepes[1,2], Rubén E. Varela-M[2], Julio López-Abán[1], E L Habib Dakir[2], Faustino Mollinedo[2], Antonio Muro[1]*

1 IBSAL-CIETUS (Instituto de Investigación Biomédica de Salamanca-Centro de Investigación de Enfermedades Tropicales de la Universidad de Salamanca), Facultad de Farmacia, Universidad de Salamanca, Salamanca, Spain, **2** Instituto de Biología Molecular y Celular del Cáncer, Centro de Investigación del Cáncer, CSIC-Universidad de Salamanca, Campus Miguel de Unamuno, Salamanca, Spain

Abstract

Background: Schistosomiasis is a parasitic disease caused by trematodes of the genus *Schistosoma*. Five species of *Schistosoma* are known to infect humans, out of which *S. haematobium* is the most prevalent, causing the chronic parasitic disease schistosomiasis that still represents a major problem of public health in many regions of the world and especially in tropical areas, leading to serious manifestations and mortality in developing countries. Since the 1970s, praziquantel (PZQ) is the drug of choice for the treatment of schistosomiasis, but concerns about relying on a single drug to treat millions of people, and the potential appearance of drug resistance, make identification of alternative schistosomiasis chemotherapies a high priority. Alkylphospholipid analogs (APLs), together with their prototypic molecule edelfosine (EDLF), are a family of synthetic antineoplastic compounds that show additional pharmacological actions, including antiparasitic activities against several protozoan parasites.

Methodology/Principal Findings: We found APLs ranked edelfosine> perifosine> erucylphosphocholine> miltefosine for their *in vitro* schistosomicidal activity against adult *S. mansoni* worms. Edelfosine accumulated mainly in the worm tegument, and led to tegumental alterations, membrane permeabilization, motility impairment, blockade of male-female pairing as well as induction of apoptosis-like processes in cells in the close vicinity to the tegument. Edelfosine oral treatment also showed *in vivo* schistosomicidal activity and decreased significantly the egg burden in the liver, a key event in schistosomiasis.

Conclusions/Significance: Our data show that edelfosine is the most potent APL in killing *S. mansoni* adult worms *in vitro*. Edelfosine schistosomicidal activity seems to depend on its action on the tegumental structure, leading to tegumental damage, membrane permeabilization and apoptosis-like cell death. Oral administration of edelfosine diminished worm and egg burdens in *S. mansoni*-infected CD1 mice. Here we report that edelfosine showed promising antischistosomal properties *in vitro* and *in vivo*.

Editor: Henk D. F. H. Schallig, Royal Tropical Institute, Netherlands

Funding: This work was supported by the Spanish Ministerio de Ciencia e Innovación (SAF2011-30518, and RD12/0036/0065 from Red Temática de Investigación Cooperativa en Cáncer, Instituto de Salud Carlos III, cofunded by the Fondo Europeo de Desarrollo Regional of the European Union), European Community's Seventh Framework Programme FP7-2007-2013 (grant HEALTH-F2-2011-256986, PANACREAS), Junta de Castilla y León (CSI052A11-2and SA342U13), Sociedad Española de Medicina Tropical y Salud Internacional (RFEF-SEMTSI 2013) and the Universidad de Salamanca (USAL17008). The funders had no role in study design, data collection and analysis, decision to publish, or preparation of the manuscript.

Competing Interests: The authors have declared that no competing interests exist.

* Email: ama@usal.es

Introduction

Schistosomiasis is a parasitic disease caused by trematodes of the genus *Schistosoma*, being a major problem of public health. The genus *Schistosoma* contains 21 species, which are classified into four groups according to the geographic distribution, morphology of the parasite's eggs, and the intermediate host. Five major schistosome species are able to infect humans: *S. haematobium*, *S. mansoni*, *S. intercalatum*, *S. japonicum*, and *S. mekongi*, although human infections by *S. malayensis*, *S. mattheei*, and *S. guineensis* have also been described. Schistosomiasis is acquired by contact with freshwater contaminated with cercariae larvae, which actively penetrate mammal skin and transform into the schistosomula phase, migrating toward the lungs and then re-entering the venous circulation [1]. Both male and female schistosome parasites achieve sexual maturity in the bloodstream, then sexual reproduction occurs with the deposition of hundreds to thousands of eggs per day. Deposition of *Schistosome* eggs in the tissues is a stimulus to the influx of immune cells that leads to the development of a granulomatous reaction. This immunological reaction protects the host by neutralizing the schistosome egg antigens and destroying eggs. However, the granulomas are the

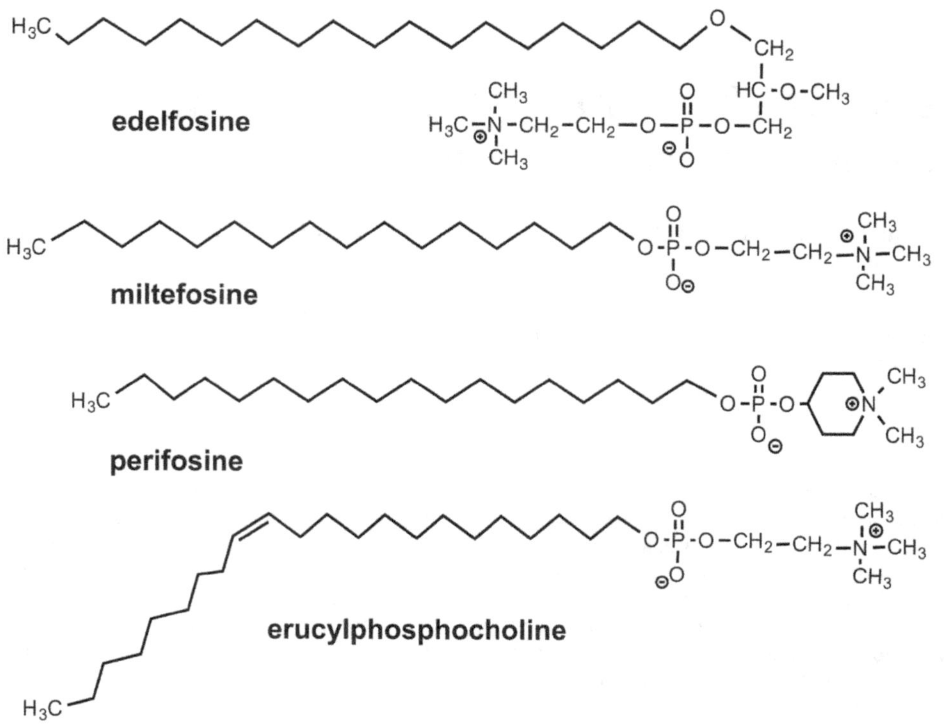

Figure 1. Chemical structures of edelfosine, miltefosine, perifosine and erucylphosphocholine.

most important pathogenic event in schistosomiasis since the deposition of collagen and the development of fibrosis cause the fibro-obstructive disease. Nevertheless, paradoxically, the development of granulomatous inflammation around parasite eggs has an essential host-protective and facilitates the successful excretion of the eggs from the host [2–4]. The World Health Organization (WHO) announced in October 2001 that schistosomiasis epidemiology should be recalculated. It is estimated more than 700 million people in 78 countries endemic for schistosomiasis are at risk of this disease. Furthermore, 240 million people are infected (80% in sub-Saharan Africa), 120 million have symptoms, and 20 million have severe disease, which results in approximately 280,000 deaths annually [2,5,6]. An additional report even increases the estimate of infected people to 391–597 million [7]. Some authors report the significant impact of the morbidity caused by schistosomiasis, as reflected in the loss of 1.53 million disability-adjusted life years [1]. The disease is among the Neglected Tropical Diseases catalogued by the Global Plan to combat Neglected Tropical Diseases 2008–2015, and is considered to be the second most socioeconomically devastating parasitic disease by the WHO, immediately after malaria [8].

Praziquantel is the main drug for the treatment of schistosomiasis, since oxamniquine and metrifonate are not currently available [9,10]. However, praziquantel does not prevent reinfection and its administration requires taking into consideration the stage of the disease. Praziquantel is highly efficient against adult worms, being less effective against juvenile parasites (7–35 days) [11]. In the chronic phase, the dose of praziquantel depends on the species involved [2,12]. The fact that schistosomiasis treatment is limited to one single pharmaceutical presents the risk associated with the appearance of resistances. The WHO has recognized the necessity of identifying new compounds as alternatives to praziquantel. In the last decade, only derivatives of artemisinin have appeared as a complement to the therapy against schistosomiasis. The use of these derivatives in combination with praziquantel can be a good strategy of control, since the artemisinin derivatives are effective against the juvenile phases of the parasite [9]. In addition, the activity of the artemisinin derivatives as antiparasitic chemotherapy has been demonstrated in numerous clinical trials [13–15]. However, the use of these antimalarial drugs in the treatment and/or control of schistosomiasis might lead to the appearance of malaria resistance to these compounds. Several experts are warning about the putative emergence of resistance to praziquantel, due to its massive use in schistosomiasis control campaigns, and the existence of drug resistant parasites in laboratory isolates [16]. This makes it necessary to find new molecules or therapeutic targets for schistosomiasis control.

Alkylphospholipid analogs (APLs) are a class of structurally related synthetic lipid compounds, including edelfosine, miltefosine, perifosine, and erucylphosphocholine (Figure 1), that act on cell membranes rather than on DNA [17–19]. Edelfosine (1-*O*-octadecyl-2-*O*-methyl-*rac*-glycero-3-phosphocholine), considered as the prototype APL molecule, is a promising antitumor ether phospholipid drug [20–22], which acts by activating apoptosis through its interaction with cell membranes [19,23–25]. In addition to its antitumor activity, edelfosine has been shown to exert *in vitro* and *in vivo* antiparasitic activity against different species of *Leishmania* parasites [26]. Miltefosine has also been shown to exert activity against leishmaniasis and schistosomiasis [27,28]. Both *Leishmania* and *Schistosoma* parasites share geographic areas in tropical and subtropical countries [29,30]. Here we have investigated the putative anti-schistosomal properties of edelfosine, as compared to other APLs, by *in vitro* and *in vivo* approaches, using an experimental mouse model of *S. mansoni* infection.

Materials and Methods

Ethics statement

Animal procedures in this study complied with the Spanish (Ley 32/2007, Ley 6/2013 and Real Decreto 53/2013) and the European Union (European Directive 2010/63/EU) regulations on animal experimentation for the protection and humane use of laboratory animals, and were conducted at the accredited Animal Experimentation Facility of the University of Salamanca (Register number: PAE/SA/001). Procedures were approved by the Ethics Committee of the University of Salamanca (protocol approval number 48531). The animals' health status was monitored throughout the experiments by a health surveillance program according to Federation of European Laboratory Animal Science Associations (FELASA) guidelines.

Drugs

Edelfosine (1-*O*-octadecyl-2-*O*-methyl-*rac*-glycero-3-phosphocoline) was obtained from R. Berchtold (Biochemisches Labor, Bern, Switzerland). Miltefosine (hexadecylphosphocholine) was from Calbiochem (Cambridge, MA). Perifosine (octadecyl-(1,1-dimethyl-piperidinio-4-yl)-phosphate) and erucylphosphocholine ((13Z)-docos-13-en-1-yl 2-(trimethylammonio)ethyl phosphate) were from Zentaris (Frankfurt, Germany). Stock sterile solutions of the distinct APLs (2 mM) were prepared in RPMI-1640 culture medium (Invitrogen, Carlsbad, CA), supplemented with 10% heat-inactivated fetal bovine serum (FBS), 2 mM glutamine, 100 IU/mL penicillin, and 100 µg/mL streptomycin, as previously described [20]. Praziquantel (PZQ) was obtained as Biltricide tablets (Bayer Vital, Leverkusen, Germany) and was dispersed in water with 2–2.5% Cremophor A6 oil-in-water emulsifier (Sigma, MO).

Parasite maintenance, recovery and culture

Cercariae of *Schistosoma mansoni* (LE strain) were maintained routinely in *Biomphalaria glabrata* snails and female CD1 mice (Charles River, Criffa S.A., Barcelona, Spain) at University of Salamanca. Mice were maintained in polycarbonate and wire standard cages for 10 mice with food and water *ad libitum* in an environment under an alternating 12/12-h light-dark cycle at 20°C. Six-week-old females weighing 23–26 g were percutaneously infected with 150 *S. mansoni* cercariae per animal after being restrained with a mixture of ketamine 50 mg/kg of body weight, diazepam 5 mg/kg and atropine 1 mg/kg injected intraperitoneally. After 7–8 weeks, mice were killed with a lethal dose of 60 mg/kg of pentobarbital plus heparin (2 IU/mL) and then perfused aseptically with PBS and heparin (500 IU/L) to obtain couples, males and females from the portal and mesenteric veins [31,32]. The worms were washed in RPMI-1640 culture medium (Invitrogen, Carlsbad, CA), kept at pH 7.5 with 20 mM HEPES and supplemented with 10% heat-inactivated fetal bovine serum (FBS), 2 mM L-glutamine, 100 IU/mL penicillin, and 100 µg/mL streptomycin, as previously described [31]. All mice were monitored daily by the staff from Animal Experimentation facility and after day 42 post-infection by a member of the research group qualified in animal welfare. Animals presenting any deterioration of the health status were killed with a lethal dose of pentobarbital 60 mg/kg.

In vitro antischistosomal activity

Adult worms washed in RPMI-1640 were collected, counted, and transferred to RPMI-1640 medium (supplemented with 20 mM HEPES, 100 IU/mL penicillin, 100 µg/mL streptomycin and 2 mM L-glutamine). The worms were rinsed twice with this medium and distributed one pair of adult worms per well in 24-well culture plates. FBS was added to a final concentration of 10%, and the cultures were incubated at 37°C in a 5% CO_2 atmosphere. After 2 h of culture to allow for adaptation, APLs were added to a final concentration of 1 to 80 µM (from a stock solution of 2 mM in RPMI-1640). The effects of APLs on *S. mansoni* adult worms were monitored every 24 h during 168 h for control groups and APL treatments. A number of parameters were evaluated to assess worm general condition, including: motility, alterations in the tegument, mortality rate, and changes in pairing [33]. The worms were considered dead when no movement was detected for at least 2 min of examination [34]. Additional criteria for viability were the MTT assay (see below), as well as pairing, egg production, and video-imaging to record morphological alterations and dead worms [35]. Worms were observed under a Nikon eclipse Ti inverted research microscope (Nikon Instruments, Amstelveen, The Netherlands). Video recordings were taken using a ProgRes C3 camera and a ProgRes MAC CapturePro software version 2.7 (JENOPTIK Optical Systems, Jena, Germany). As controls, pairs of *S. mansoni* adult worms were incubated in the presence RPMI-1640 (negative control) or were killed by heating at 56°C or treatment with 10 µM PZQ (positive control). All experiments were carried in quadruplicate.

Assay for parasite viability

A three-step colorimetric quantitative assay based on 3-(4,5-dimethylthiazol-2-yl)-2,5-diphenyl tetrazolium bromide (MTT) was used to assess parasite viability [36]. The MTT assay is based on the uptake of the tetrazolium salt by viable/living cells followed by its reduction in the mitochondria to purple formazan, the colored product. The amount of formazan produced is proportional to the number of living cells, giving a measure of viability. In this study, worms were distributed (one pair of adult worms per well) in 96-well culture plates, containing 100 µL of phosphate buffered saline (PBS) with 0.5 mg MTT/mL for 30 min at 37°C. The solution was carefully removed and replaced with 200 µL dimethylsulfoxide (DMSO). Worms incubated in drug-free RPMI-1640 medium (negative control group) were allowed to stand in DMSO at room temperature for 1 h, and absorbance was read at 550 nm using an ELISA reader (Anthos 2010; Anthos Labtec Instruments, Wals, Austria). Heat-killed worms at 56°C and worms treated with 10 µM PZQ were used as positive control groups. APLs were added to a final concentration of 1 to 80 µM (from a stock solution of 2 mM in RPMI-1640) for up to 168 h incubation.

We studied the incorporation of propidium iodide (PI) in adult worms to assess the differential membrane permeability to this dye. The effect of edelfosine (1–80 µM) was analyzed following incubation for 24 h. After washing the parasites, PI was simultaneously added to each well of the microtiter plate to obtain a final concentration of 2.0 mg/mL in 96-well microtiter plates. Fluorescently labeled parasites were subsequently detected using a BioTek Synergy 2 (BioTek Instruments, Winooski, VT) fluorescent plate reader containing appropriate filters (485/20 nm excitation, 645/20 nm emission). All experiments were carried in quadruplicate.

Distribution of fluorescent edelfosine analog in *S. mansoni*

Four couples of adult worms were transferred and maintained in RPMI-1640 medium supplemented with 20 mM HEPES, 100 IU/mL penicillin, 100 µg/mL streptomycin. Each well of a 24-well culture plate containing 2 mL of RPMI-1640 culture medium and two parasitic couples was incubated for 1 h with 10 µM of the

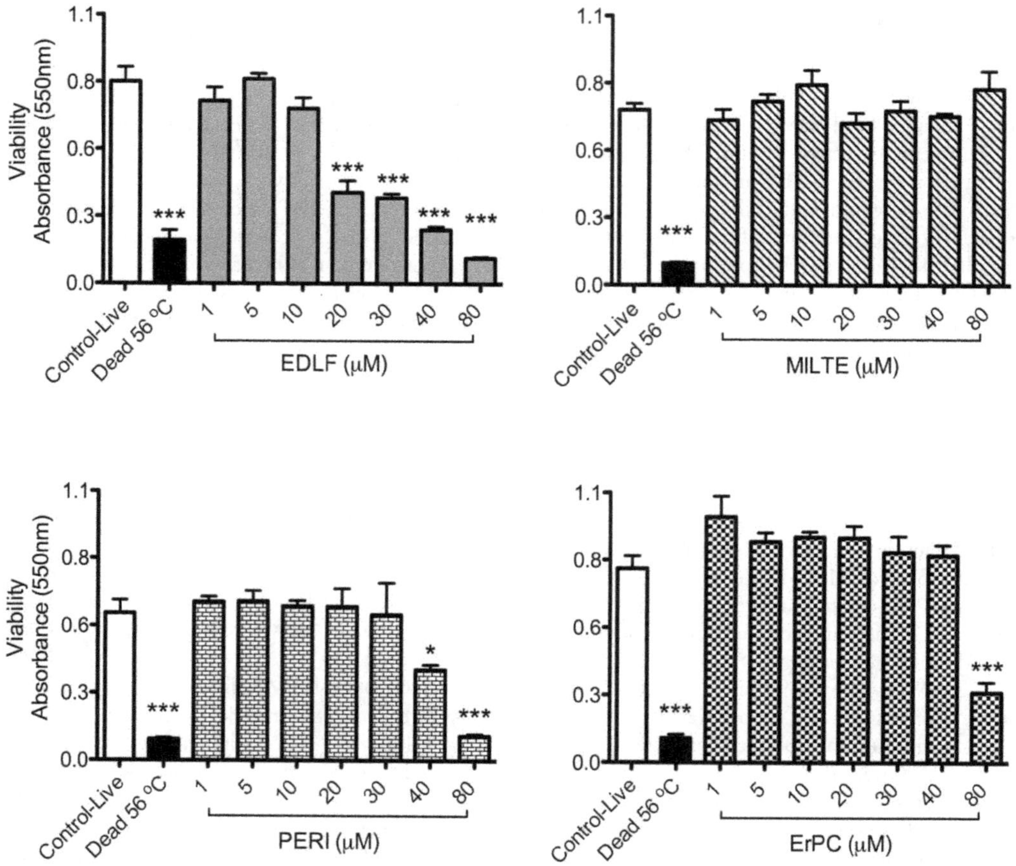

Figure 2. *In vitro* effects of APLs on the viability of *S. mansoni* adult worms measured by MTT assay. Couples of adult worms were treated with edelfosine (EDLF), miltefosine (MILTE), perifosine (PERI) or erucylphosphocholine (ErPC) at the indicated concentrations for 168 h. Data are means ± SEM of three separate experiments. Asterisks represent statistical significance with respect to control-live group. (*) P<0.05; (***) P<0.001.

fluorescent edelfosine 1-*O*-[11′-(6″-ethyl-1″,3″,5″,7″-tetramethyl-4″, 4″-difluoro-4″-bora-3a″,4a″-diaza-s-indacen-2″-yl)undecyl]-2-*O*-methyl-*rac*-glycero-3-phosphocholine [37,38]. In addition, two parasitic couples were incubated in RPMI-1640 only (control of autofluorescence). Parasites were analyzed with a Zeiss Axioplan 2 fluorescence microscope (Carl Zeiss, Oberkochen, Germany). All experiments were performed in quadruplicate.

Assessment of apoptosis by TUNEL Assay

The DeadEnd Fluorometric TUNEL System (Promega, Madison, WI) was used to detect apoptosis. Parasite sections (4 μm) were deparaffinized in xylene, and rehydrated in graded ethanol and distilled water. After being rinsed three time with PBS, the slides were permeabilized with proteinase K (20 μg/mL) in proteinase K buffer (100 mM Tris-HCl, pH 8.0, 50 mM EDTA) for 15 min at room temperature. The slides were incubated with equilibrium buffer [200 mM potassium cacodylate, 25 mM Tris-HCl, pH 6.6, 0.2 mM dithiothreitol (DTT), 0.25 mg/mL bovine serum albumin, 2.5 mM cobalt chloride] at room temperature for 30 min, followed by assessment of cell apoptosis with a terminal deoxynucleotidyl transferase dUTP nick end labeling kit according to the manufacturer's instructions, and using fluorescence microscopy (Carl Zeiss). In histological sections, the apoptotic index, defined as the percentage of apoptotic cells, was used as a quantitative measure of apoptosis. The apoptotic index was determined as follows: (number of TUNEL-positive cells/total number of cells) x 100.

Histopathological analysis

Parasites were fixed in 4% buffered paraformaldehyde and embedded in paraffin. The tissue sections of schistosomes (4 μm) were deparaffinized and hydrated in graded ethanol and PBS, and stained with hematoxylin and eosin (H&E). Histopathological evaluation was done under microscope analysis. The slides were viewed using an Olympus BX51 microscope coupled with Olympus DP Controller software to capture images [39,40].

In vivo study of antischistosomal activity

Six-week-old female CD1 mice (Charles River), weighing 23–26 g, were kept in the Animal Experimentation Facility. Mice were randomly allocated into three experimental groups and all were chemically restrained and percutaneously exposed to 150 *S. mansoni* cercariae per animal [32]. Group 1 received the vehicle solution (water) via oral administration from day 42 to day 52 post-infection (p.i.) (n = 7); group 2 were orally treated with 500 mg/kg/day of PZQ on days 47 and 48 p.i. (n = 7); and group 3 were orally treated with 45 mg/kg/day of edelfosine from day 42 and 52 p.i. (n = 7). Mice were euthanized at week 9 p.i. with a lethal dose of pentobarbital (60 mg/kg), and then perfused to recover adult worms from portal and mesenteric veins [31,32]. The number of parasite eggs per gram (epg) in liver was counted after digestion with 25 mL 5% KOH (16 h at 37°C with gentle shaking) [41].

Table 1. *In vitro* effects of APLs on 56-day-old *S. mansoni* worms upon 168 h of culture.

Samples	Number of worms	Number of separated worms	Number of dead worm	Motor activity reduction		Number of worms with tegumental alterations	
				Slight	Significant	Partial	Extensive
Control-Live [a]	8	-	-	-	-		-
Dead 56°C [b]	8	-	8	-	8	4	4
PZQ [c]	8	-	8	-	8	-	8
Edelfosine							
1 µM	8	-	-	2	-	4	-
5 µM	8	6	-	2	6	4	4
10 µM	8	8	4	4	4	2	6
20 µM	8	8	8	-	8	-	8
30 µM	8	8	8	-	8	-	8
40 µM	8	8	8	-	8	-	8
80 µM	8	8	8	-	8		8
Miltefosine							
1 µM	8	-	-	-	-	-	-
5 µM	8	-	-	-	-	-	-
10 µM	8	-	-	-	-	-	-
20 µM	8	-	-	-	-	-	-
30 µM	8	-	-	-	-	-	-
40 µM	8	-	-	4	-	-	-
80 µM	8	4	-	6	-	-	4
Perifosine							
1 µM	8	2	-	-		-	-
5 µM	8	-	-	-		-	-
10 µM	8	2	-	4	-	6	-
20 µM	8	8	2	6	2	6	2
30 µM	8	8	2	-	8	2	8
40 µM	8	8	6	2	6	-	8
80 µM	8	8	8	-	8	-	8
Erucylphosphocholine							
1 µM	8	-	-	-	-	-	
5 µM	8	-	-	-	-	-	
10 µM	8	-	-	-	-	-	

Table 1. Cont.

Samples	Number of worms	Number of separated worms	Number of dead worm	Motor activity reduction		Number of worms with tegumental alterations	
				Slight	Significant	Partial	Extensive
20 μM	8	-	-	-	-	-	
30 μM	8	4	-	-	-	-	
40 μM	8	8	-	2	6	2	2
80 μM	8	8	8	-	8	-	8

[a]RPMI 1640.
[b]Control – positive.
[c]Tested at concentration of 10 μM.

Statistical analysis

Results were analyzed in GraphPad Prism Version 5 (Graphpad Software Inc.) and are expressed as mean ± SEM. Test for normality was performed by Kolmogorov-Smirnov, and then one-way ANOVA analysis of variance, followed by Dunnett's or Kruskall Wallis comparison test, were performed to determine any statistical differences between treated groups and untreated controls. The data were considered significant if P-value was < 0.05.

Results

In vitro schistosomicidal activity of APLs

First we analyzed the schistosomicidal activity of the four most clinically relevant APLs, namely edelfosine, perifosine, miltefosine and erucylphosphocholine, used at the range of 1–80 μM, against adult worms. By testing parasite viability using the MTT assay after 168 h incubation, we found that edelfosine was the most active APL in killing *S. mansoni* adult worms, being effective at 20 μM, whereas miltefosine was inactive even at the highest concentration used (80 μM) (Figure 2). Perifosine decreased parasite viability at 40 μM and erucylphosphocholine at 80 μM (Figure 2). The differential schistosomicidal activity of the above APLs was further supported by the microscopic observation of *S. mansoni* adult worms incubated as above with the four APLs at a concentration range of 1–80 μM to examine separation of coupled pairs, mortality, decrease in motor activity, and tegumental alterations as shown in Table 1 and Tables S1–S3. Again, edelfosine was the most potent APL in promoting parasite death (50% at 10 μM and 100% at 20 μM) in *S. mansoni* adult forms after 168 h treatment (Table 1). Incubations with 1 and 5 μM edelfosine resulted in effects on motor activity and tegumental alterations (Table 1), indicating that *S. mansoni* adult forms were very sensitive to edelfosine treatment. Perifosine also showed significant schistosomicidal activity, but higher drug concentrations were required to achieve similar effects to those exerted by edelfosine (Table 1; Tables S1–S3). In contrast, erucylphosphocholine (erucyl-PC) and miltefosine required very high doses of> 40 μM to elicit some effects on the parasites (Table 1). On the basis of these morphological observations, erucylphosphocholine was only able to kill parasites at 80 μM, whereas miltefosine was unable to promote parasite death even at that concentration (Table 1), thus further supporting the above MTT data.

Dose- and time-dependent effects of edelfosine on *S. mansoni* adult worms

Because edelfosine was the most potent APL against *S. mansoni* adults, we further analyzed the effects of this drug on these worms. A time-course analysis of the effect of different concentrations of edelfosine showed that this drug could kill *S. mansoni* adult worms when incubated at 20 μM for 72 h (Figure 3) and at 30 μM for 48 h incubation (Figure 3). This is of interest as this concentration range was similar to that found as steady-state concentration of edelfosine in plasma (10–20 μM) in animal model *in vivo* assays [21,22,42]. The induction of structural damage and death in *S. mansoni* adult parasites by edelfosine was further supported by time-lapse videomicroscopy (Video S1), showing an increased intestinal lumen and oral as well as ventral sucker paralysis. In addition, membrane permeabilization was detected by incorporation of propidium iodide (PI) into dead parasites (Figure 4A). Parasite motility was also observed and measured under an inverted light microscope, as lack of motility represents the death of the parasite. We found that low concentrations of edelfosine (5–10 μM) were enough to promote structural changes in the

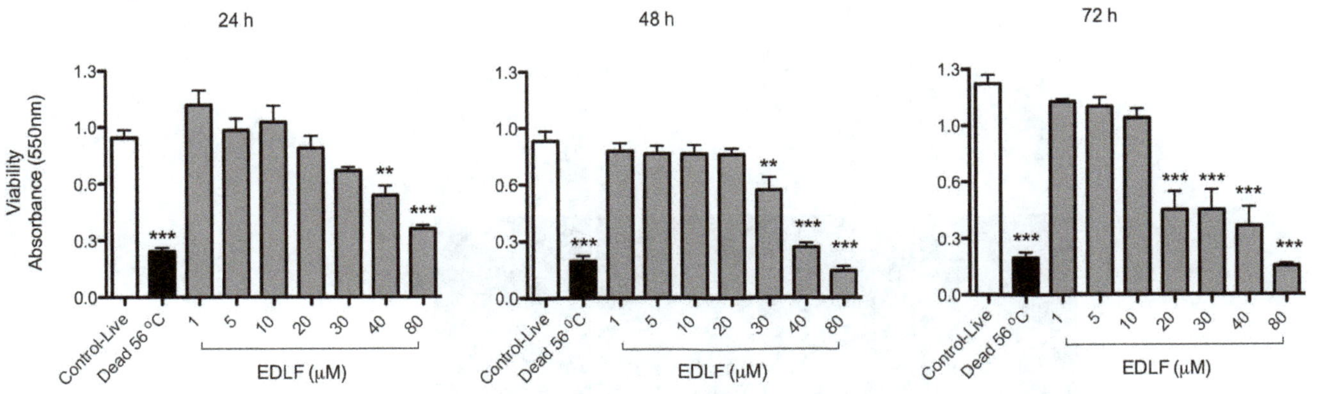

Figure 3. *In vitro* effects of edelfosine (EDLF) on the viability of *S. mansoni* adult worms measured by MTT assay. Couples of adult worms were treated with EDLF at the indicated concentrations for 24 h, 48 h and 74 h. Data are means ± SEM of three separate experiments. Asterisks represent statistical significance with respect to control-live group. (**) P<0.01; (***) P<0.001.

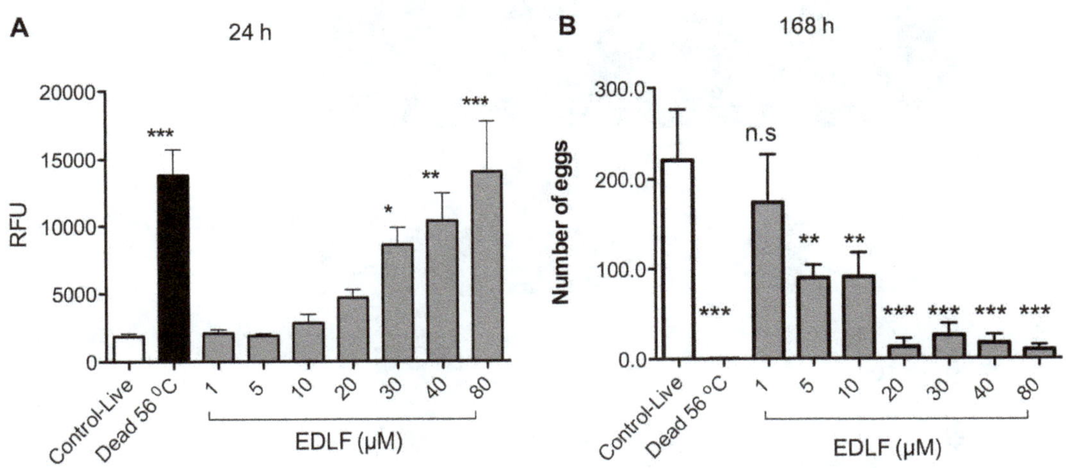

Figure 4. *In vitro* effects of edelfosine (EDLF) on the viability of *S. mansoni* adult worms measured by propidium iodide (PI) permeabilization and *in vitro* effects of edelfosine on egg production. Couples of adult worms were treated with EDLF at the indicated concentrations for 24 h (A) or 168 h (B), and then analyzed for membrane permeabilization using PI staining (A) and for the number of laid eggs, monitored using an inverted microscope (B). RFU, relative fluorescence units. Data are means ± SEM of three separate experiments. Asterisks represent statistical significance with respect to control-live group. (**) P<0.01; (***) P<0.001.

parasite, both in motor activity reduction and in the tegument, as well as to split the pairs of coupled adult worms into individual female and male worms (Table 1 and Video S1), the latter being more affected than the former following incubation with 10 μM edelfosine.

Effect of edelfosine on the egg production of *S. mansoni* adult worms

Schistosome eggs are considered a major cause of liver injury and illness. About half of the laid eggs lodge in the liver sinusoids, where they are trapped acting as granulomatogenic triggers, granuloma formation being strictly dependent on viable mature eggs [43]. In order to evaluate the action of edelfosine on egg production by adult worms of *S. mansoni*, edelfosine was incubated at different concentrations for 168 h. As shown in Fig. 4B, edelfosine (5–80 μM) treatment showed a significant decrease in the number of eggs after 168 h of incubation. The effect of edelfosine on the separation of the coupled adult worms could be related to this decrease on egg production.

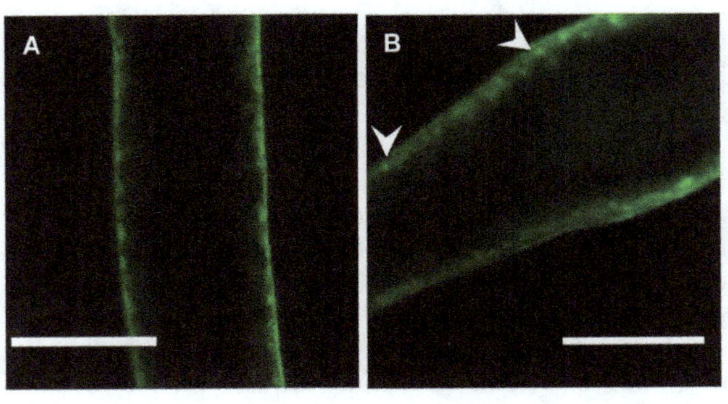

Figure 5. Distribution of the fluorescent edelfosine analog in *S. mansoni* adult female worms. A) Control of autofluorescence in a female cultured in RPMI-1640 only. B) Female incubated with the fluorescent edelfosine analog. Arrows show a slightly increased staining at the tegument. Scale bar, 0.2 mm.

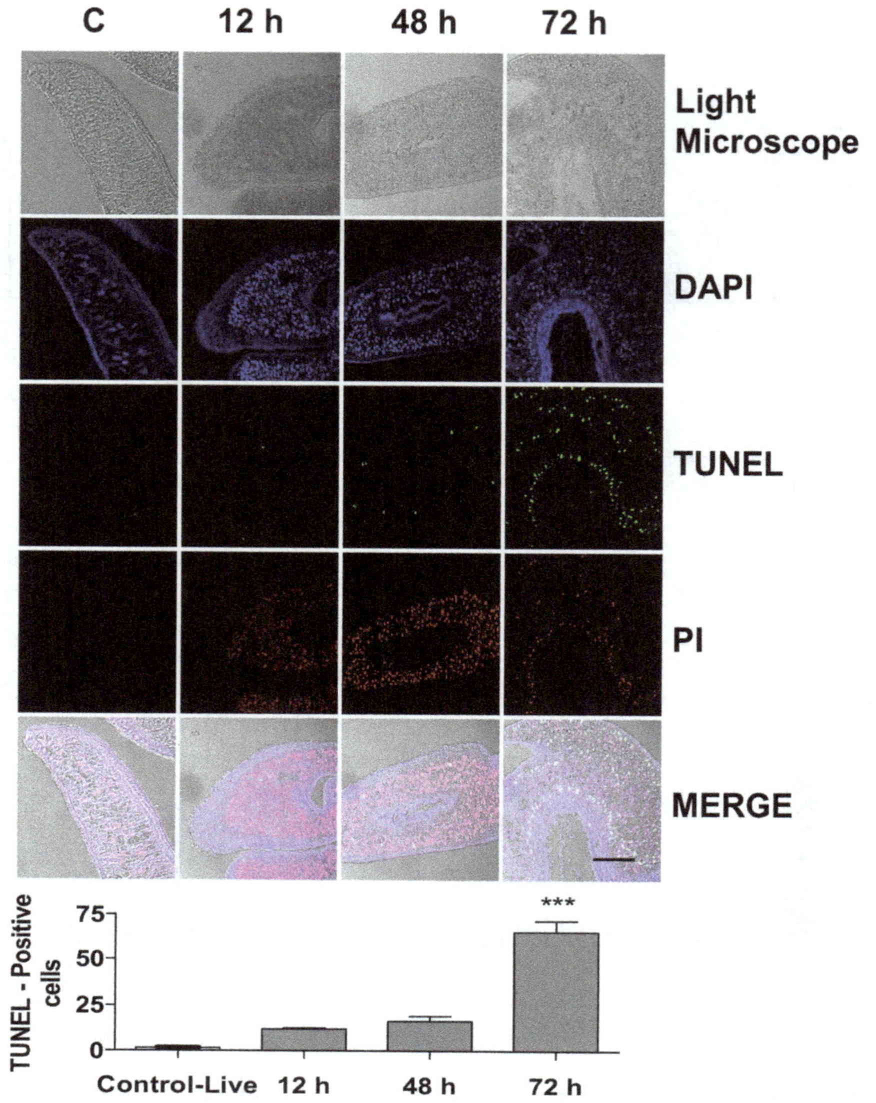

Figure 6. Edelfosine-induced apoptosis-like death as assessed by TUNEL assay. Adult worms were untreated (Control) or treated with 20 μM edelfosine (EDLF) for 12 h, 48 h and 72 h. Worms were analyzed by fluorescence microscopy for propidium iodide (PI) staining and TUNEL assay, as well as for DAPI staining (nuclei) and light microscopy morphology. Merging of PI and TUNEL panels (Merge) shows the apoptotic nuclei in yellow. Data shown are representative of four independent experiments. Histograms indicate the percentage of TUNEL-positive cells, as an estimate of cells undergoing apoptosis. For each experiment, at least 100 cells were analyzed. Data are means ± SEM of three separate experiments. Asterisks represent statistical significance with respect to control-live group. (***) $P<0.001$. Scale bar, 100 μm.

Distribution of fluorescent edelfosine analog in pairs of adult *S. mansoni* worms

The major interface and physical barrier between the schistosome and its external environment is through the tegument, consisting of a syncytium enclosed by a double outer tegumental membrane made up of two apposed lipid bilayers, which coats the worm and is a prime site of intimate host-parasite interaction. It performs vital functions and is of crucial importance for modulation of the host response and parasite survival [28]. By using the fluorescent edelfosine analog 1-*O*-[11′-(6″-ethyl-1″,3″,5″,7″-tetramethyl-4″,4″-difluoro-4″-bora-3a″,4a″-diaza-s-indacen-2″-yl)undecyl]-2-*O*-methyl-*rac*-glycero-3-phosphocholine, which has been previously used as a reliable analog of edelfosine to analyze its subcellular localization in single cells [37,38], we found that adult *S. mansoni* worms took up the fluorescent analog, showing a rather diffuse staining in the whole worm, although it appeared to be most concentrated at the tegument (Figure 5). Thus, these data indicate that edelfosine is incorporated at the adult worm with a major tegumental location.

Edelfosine induces apoptosis-like death in *S. mansoni* adult worms and changes at the tegument

Induction of apoptotic cell death is one of the main mechanisms by which edelfosine exerts its antitumor action [20,24,25]. On these grounds, we analyzed whether edelfosine could promote apoptosis in *S. mansoni* adult worms, by using the terminal deoxynucleotidyl transferase-mediated dUTP nick-end labeling (TUNEL) technique for detecting DNA damage. Labeling of the 3′-OH ends of DNA, generated by DNA fragmentation, through incorporation of fluorescein-12-dUTP allowed visualization of apoptotic cells as green fluorescent cells. Worms were permeabilized and stained with 4′,6-diamidino-2-phenylindole (DAPI) and

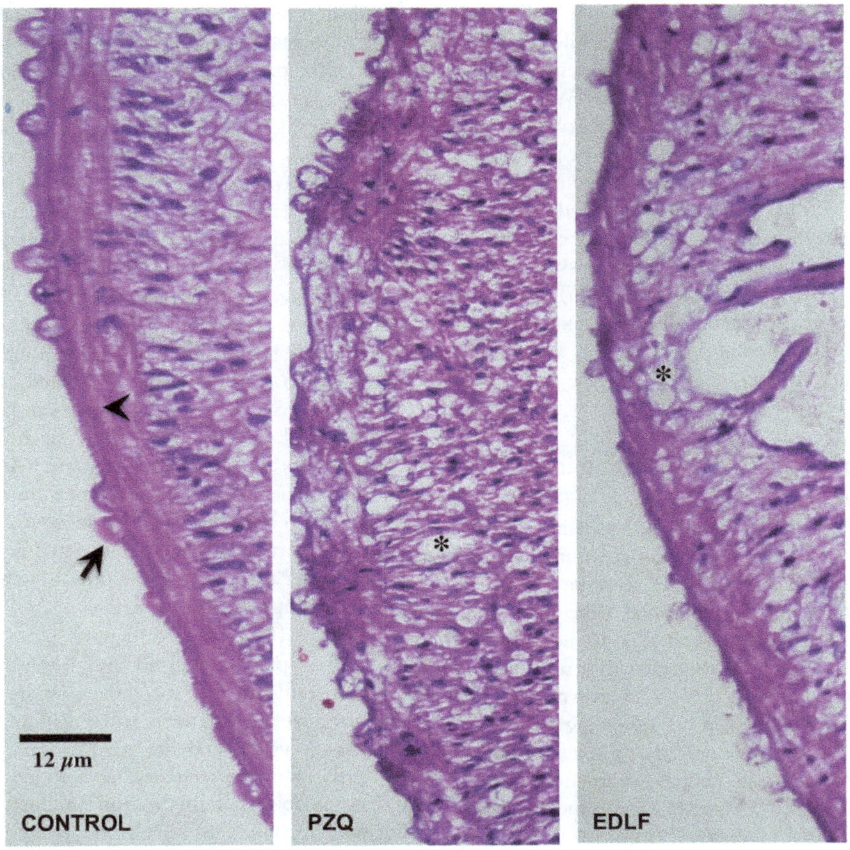

Figure 7. Morphological changes in *S. mansoni* adult worms following praziquantel or edelfosine treatments. H&E stained sections of freshly recovered male parasites that were untreated (Control) or treated with 10 μM praziquantel (PZQ) or 20 μM edelfosine (EDLF) for 2 days. Tubercle collapse (arrow), damages of the tegument surface, vacuolization of the subtegumental cells (asterisk) and destruction of muscle layers (arrowhead) were observed after treatment with PZQ or EDLF.

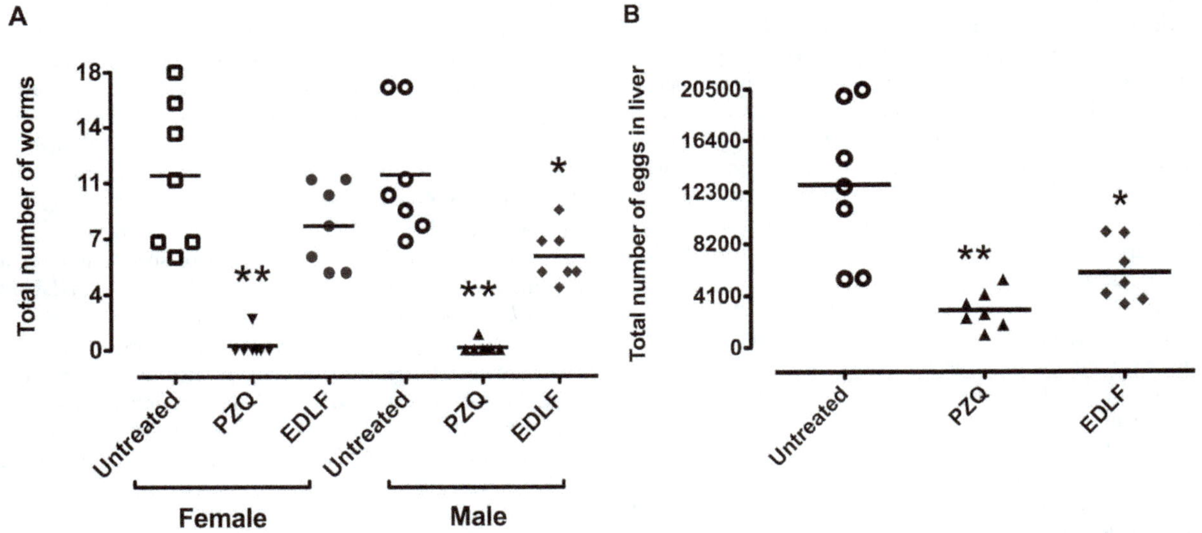

Figure 8. Effect on adult worm and egg burdens after treatment of *S. mansoni*-infected mice with praziquantel (PZQ) or edelfosine (EDLF). (A) male and female worm burdens. (B) egg burden in liver. Infected mice were treated with 500 mg/kg (x2) PZQ or 45 mg/kg (x10) EDLF. Each point represents data from an individual mouse. Horizontal bars indicate average values. (*) $P<0.05$. (**) $P<0.01$.

propidium iodide (PI) to visualize all nuclei from both non-apoptotic and apoptotic cells in blue and red, while TUNEL-positive cells were stained yellow in the row of the merged images and non apoptotic cells as pink fluorescent cells. We found a potent apoptosis-like response in edelfosine-treated *S. mansoni* adult worms, this apoptotic-like response being particularly abundant in cells close to the tegument (Figure 6). This edelfosine-induced apoptosis-like response increased with the incubation time (Figure 6). In addition, edelfosine treatment led to severe lesions of the tegument and subtegument tissues in both male and female worms, such as: *i)* tubercle collapse; *ii)* exfoliation and erosion of the tegument surface together with exposure and vacuolization of the subtegumental cells in the perinuclear cytoplasm of syncytium and epithelium; *iii)* extensive destruction of muscle layers (Figure 7 and Video S1).

In vivo schistosomicidal activity of edelfosine in mice infected by *S. mansoni*

Daily oral administration of 15 or 30 mg/kg edelfosine was well tolerated by CD1 mice, 45 mg/kg being the maximum tolerated dose, following toxicity analyses, where animals were monitored for body weight loss or any appreciable side effect, including changes in strength and general condition. We found that oral treatment of mice infected with *S. mansoni* led to a reduction in the male (46.84 %) and female (29.1 %) worm burdens (Figure 8A), the decrease in male worm burden being statistically significant. PZQ treatment led to a practically complete depletion of adult worms (Figure 8A), so praziquantel treatment was more potent than that of edelfosine. Interestingly, edelfosine treatment dramatically decreased the total number of eggs recovered in livers (54.2% reduction), this inhibition in egg production being statistically significant as was the corresponding reduction (77%) exerted by praziquantel (Figure 8B).

Discussion

Our results show the first evidence for the *in vitro* and *in vivo* schistosomicidal activity of the ether phospholipid edelfosine. This ether lipid is considered as the prototype of APLs, a family of compounds that act as promising drugs for diverse biomedical applications, including the treatment of parasitic diseases [19,44]. Two previous reports have shown *in vivo* [28] and *in vitro* [45]. schistosomicidal activity of the APL miltefosine. However, here we found that edelfosine showed a more potent schistosomicidal activity, and APLs ranked edelfosine> perifosine> erucylphosphocholine> miltefosine for their *in vitro* activity against *S. mansoni* adult worms. Edelfosine shows also *in vivo* schistosomicidal activity, and although its activity is not as potent as that of praziquantel, the current drug of choice for schistosomiasis treatment, our data indicate that oral treatment with edelfosine decreases significantly the egg burden in liver, a key event in schistosomiasis. Our present data suggest that edelfosine is incorporated mainly in the worm tegument, promoting tegumental alterations, membrane permeabilization, motility impairment, blockade of male-female pairing and additional structural changes, which eventually lead to parasite death. In addition, we showed the induction of apoptosis-like cell death in cells apposed to the tegument, as visualized by TUNEL assays.

The integrity and function of the surface tegumental membrane are critical to the survival and proliferation of *Schistosoma*. The tegument, a syncytium covered by two lipid bilayers that is a unique structure to all trematodes [46–49]. In fact the two lipid bilayer structure pertains only to trematodes that live within blood vessels [50], plays vital roles like evasion of the immune system, acquisition of nutrients, excretion of catabolic products, targeted drug absorption and other physiological processes [47,49,51–54]. Most of the drugs active against schistosomiasis damage the worm tegument, including praziquantel [55], oxamniquine [56], artemether [57], mefloquine [34,58], atorvastatin alone or in combination with medroxyprogesterone acetate [59], and thioxo-imidazoline compounds [60]. Scanning electron microscopy studies have recently shown that miltefosine induces severe tegumental damage in adult schistosomes [28,45,61]. In this regard, our present data on the tegumental damage elicited by edelfosine agree with those previously reported with miltefosine [28,45], thus suggesting that APLs could be promising drugs for schistosomiasis. Furthermore, miltefosine has been reported to have *in vitro* ovicidal, larvicidal as well as lethal activity on adult worms of *S. mansoni* and *S. haematobium*, and displays molluscicidal activity on their snail hosts [61]. Miltefosine is approved for use in humans against leishmaniasis [27,62], and pharmacokinetic as well as different studies on animal models have shown the relative lack of significant toxicity of edelfosine when used at pharmacologically relevant doses [21,22,38,42,63]. On these grounds, APLs might be promising and rather safe drugs for the treatment of schistosomiasis.

Since the 1970s the treatment of schistosomiasis has relied on a single drug, praziquantel, [8,64,65], that is considered as the gold standard and the drug of choice, having been successfully used over the past 35 years to control schistosomiasis in many countries. This exclusive dependency on praziquantel is alarming, raising concerns about the reliance on a single drug to treat over 200 million people that might lead to the potential appearance of massive resistance to the drug [10,11,16,65–68]. As a result, identification of alternative schistosomiasis chemotherapies is a high priority issue.

The results shown here indicate that edelfosine significantly decreases egg burden *in vitro* and *in vivo*. This effect could be due, at least in part, to the separation of male and female schistosomes parasites induced by edelfosine, since female schistosomes produce eggs only when they are in intimate association with a male [69]. Edelfosine kills mainly adult male worms through an apoptosis-like cell death mechanism. In this regard, it is worth mentioning that edelfosine is a proapoptotic agent in cancer cells [20,24,25], and it seems to promote an apoptosis-like process in *Leishmania* parasites [26]. The likely involvement of different mechanisms of action for the schistomicidal activities of praziquantel and edelfosine might suggest that the combination of these two drugs could promote a synergistic action and/or minimize the possibility of drug resistance, as has been proposed for the combined use of praziquantel and artemisinin derivatives or mefloquine [70,71]. Taking together the results herein reported as well as our previous studies showing the leishmanicidal activity of edelfosine, it might be envisaged that this drug could be of special interest in the treatment of patients that are co-infected with both *Leishmania* and *Schistosoma* parasites [29,30,72–74].

The studies reported here provide for the first time compelling evidence for schistomicidal activity of edelfosine, which, together with the low toxicity profile and the anti-inflammatory activity shown by this APL [21,22,38,63], warrant further studies for the putative use of edelfosine as a possible treatment against schistosomiasis.

Supporting Information

Table S1 *In vitro* effects of edelfosine and perifosine on 56-day-old *S. mansoni* worms upon 24 h of culture.

Table S2 ***In vitro*** **effects of edelfosine and perifosine on 56-day-old** ***S. mansoni*** **worms upon 48 h of culture.**

Table S3 ***In vitro*** **effects of edelfosine and perifosine on 56-day-old** ***S. mansoni*** **worms upon 72 h of culture.**

Video S1 ***In vitro*** **effects following edelfosine treatment on** ***S. mansoni*** **adult worms.** Untreated control group (Live) shows no alteration in morphology and was able to produce eggs. Dead worms following heating at 56°C or treatment with 10 μM praziquantel (PZQ) (positive controls) showed no motility and became nontranslucent. Worms treated with the indicated concentrations of edelfosine (EDLF) for 48 h, 72 h and 168 h showed toxic actions when used ≥ 10 μM. In the video one arrow shows severely dilated gut of a female worm and two arrows show extensive damage on the tegument of a male worm following treatment with 30 μM of EDLF for 48 h. After the 4:30 min, another arrow shows extensive peeling in the tegument of a female worm treated with 10 μM EDLF for 168 h.

Acknowledgments

We thank Belén Vicente for excellent technical assistance and Dr. Felipe Castro for reviewing the manuscript.

Author Contributions

Conceived and designed the experiments: AM EY REV FM. Performed the experiments: EY REV JL-A EHD. Analyzed the data: EY REV FM JL-A AM. Contributed reagents/materials/analysis tools: FM JL-A AM. Wrote the paper: EY FM AM. Animal welfare: EY JL-A.

References

1. Muro A, Pérez del Villar L (2012) Schistosoma and Schistosomiasis. In: Liu D, editor. Molecular Detection of Human Parasitic Pathogens: CRC Press. pp.441–454.
2. Ross AG, Bartley PB, Sleigh AC, Olds GR, Li Y, et al. (2002) Schistosomiasis. N Engl J Med 346: 1212–1220.
3. Pearce EJ, MacDonald AS (2002) The immunobiology of schistosomiasis. Nat Rev Immunol 2: 499–511.
4. Hams E, Aviello G, Fallon PG (2013) The schistosoma granuloma: friend or foe? Front Immunol 4: 89.
5. WHO: Schistosomiasis. Available: http://www.who.int/schistosomiasis/en/. Accessed 24 April, 2014.
6. WHO: Schistosomiasis, Fact sheet N° 115, Update February 2014. Available: http://www.who.int/mediacentre/factsheets/fs115/en/. Accessed 24 April, 2014.
7. King CH (2010) Parasites and poverty: the case of schistosomiasis. Acta Trop 113: 95–104.
8. Rokni MB (2012) Schistosomiasis. In: Rokni MB, editor. Schistosomiasis: InTech. pp.310.
9. Fenwick A, Savioli L, Engels D, Robert Bergquist N, Todd MH (2003) Drugs for the control of parasitic diseases: current status and development in schistosomiasis. Trends Parasitol 19: 509–515.
10. Doenhoff MJ, Cioli D, Utzinger J (2008) Praziquantel: mechanisms of action, resistance and new derivatives for schistosomiasis. Curr Opin Infect Dis 21: 659–667.
11. Pica-Mattoccia L, Cioli D (2012) Praziquantel: Too Good to be Replaced? Parasitic Helminths: Wiley-VCH Verlag GmbH & Co. KGaA. C.R. . Caffrey, ed. pp.309–321.
12. Gryseels B, Polman K, Clerinx J, Kestens L (2006) Human schistosomiasis. Lancet 368: 1106–1118.
13. Perez del Villar L, Burguillo FJ, Lopez-Aban J, Muro A (2012) Systematic review and meta-analysis of artemisinin based therapies for the treatment and prevention of schistosomiasis. PLoS One 7: e45867.
14. Danso-Appiah A, Olliaro PL, Donegan S, Sinclair D, Utzinger J (2013) Drugs for treating Schistosoma mansoni infection. Cochrane Database Syst Rev 2: CD000528.
15. Liu R, Dong HF, Guo Y, Zhao QP, Jiang MS (2011) Efficacy of praziquantel and artemisinin derivatives for the treatment and prevention of human schistosomiasis: a systematic review and meta-analysis. Parasit Vectors 4: 201.
16. Melman SD, Steinauer ML, Cunningham C, Kubatko LS, Mwangi IN, et al. (2009) Reduced susceptibility to praziquantel among naturally occurring Kenyan isolates of Schistosoma mansoni. PLoS Negl Trop Dis 3: e504.
17. Danker K, Reutter W, Semini G (2010) Glycosidated phospholipids: uncoupling of signalling pathways at the plasma membrane. Br J Pharmacol 160: 36–47.
18. van Blitterswijk WJ, Verheij M (2013) Anticancer mechanisms and clinical application of alkylphospholipids. Biochim Biophys Acta 1831: 663–674.
19. Gajate C, Mollinedo F (2002) Biological activities, mechanisms of action and biomedical prospect of the antitumor ether phospholipid ET-18-OCH_3 (edelfosine), a proapoptotic agent in tumor cells. Curr Drug Metab 3: 491–525.
20. Mollinedo F, Fernandez-Luna JL, Gajate C, Martin-Martin B, Benito A, et al. (1997) Selective induction of apoptosis in cancer cells by the ether lipid ET-18-OCH_3 (Edelfosine): molecular structure requirements, cellular uptake, and protection by Bcl-2 and Bcl-X_L. Cancer Res 57: 1320–1328.
21. Mollinedo F, de la Iglesia-Vicente J, Gajate C, Estella-Hermoso de Mendoza A, Villa-Pulgarin JA, et al. (2010) *In vitro* and *In vivo* selective antitumor activity of Edelfosine against mantle cell lymphoma and chronic lymphocytic leukemia involving lipid rafts. Clin Cancer Res 16: 2046–2054.
22. Mollinedo F, de la Iglesia-Vicente J, Gajate C, Estella-Hermoso de Mendoza A, Villa-Pulgarin JA, et al. (2010) Lipid raft-targeted therapy in multiple myeloma. Oncogene 29: 3748–3757.
23. Gajate C, Mollinedo F (2001) The antitumor ether lipid ET-18-OCH_3 induces apoptosis through translocation and capping of Fas/CD95 into membrane rafts in human leukemic cells. Blood 98: 3860–3863.
24. Gajate C, Mollinedo F (2007) Edelfosine and perifosine induce selective apoptosis in multiple myeloma by recruitment of death receptors and downstream signaling molecules into lipid rafts. Blood 109: 711–719.
25. Gajate C, Del Canto-Janez E, Acuna AU, Amat-Guerri F, Geijo E, et al. (2004) Intracellular triggering of Fas aggregation and recruitment of apoptotic molecules into Fas-enriched rafts in selective tumor cell apoptosis. J Exp Med 200: 353–365.
26. Varela MR, Villa-Pulgarin JA, Yepes E, Muller I, Modolell M, et al. (2012) *In vitro* and *in vivo* efficacy of ether lipid edelfosine against Leishmania spp. and SbV-resistant parasites. PLoS Negl Trop Dis 6: e1612.
27. Sundar S, Jha TK, Thakur CP, Bhattacharya SK, Rai M (2006) Oral miltefosine for the treatment of Indian visceral leishmaniasis. Trans R Soc Trop Med Hyg 100 Suppl 1: S26–33.
28. Eissa MM, El-Azzouni MZ, Amer EI, Baddour NM (2011) Miltefosine, a promising novel agent for schistosomiasis mansoni. Int J Parasitol 41: 235–242.
29. Cota GF, Gomes LI, Pinto BF, Santos-Oliveira JR, Da-Cruz AM, et al. (2012) Dyarrheal Syndrome in a Patient Co-Infected with Leishmania infantum and Schistosoma mansoni. Case Rep Med 2012: 240512.
30. Abruzzi A, Fried B (2011) Coinfection of Schistosoma (Trematoda) with bacteria, protozoa and helminths. Adv Parasitol 77: 1–85.
31. Lewis F (2001) Schistosomiasis. Curr Protoc Immunol Chapter 19: Unit 19 11.
32. Mann VH, Morales ME, Rinaldi G, Brindley PJ (2010) Culture for genetic manipulation of developmental stages of Schistosoma mansoni. Parasitology 137: 451–462.
33. Xiao SH, Keiser J, Chollet J, Utzinger J, Dong Y, et al. (2007) *In vitro* and *in vivo* activities of synthetic trioxolanes against major human schistosome species. Antimicrob Agents Chemother 51: 1440–1445.
34. Manneck T, Haggenmuller Y, Keiser J (2010) Morphological effects and tegumental alterations induced by mefloquine on schistosomula and adult flukes of Schistosoma mansoni. Parasitology 137: 85–98.
35. Peak E, Hoffmann KF (2011) Cross-disciplinary approaches for measuring parasitic helminth viability and phenotype. An Acad Bras Cienc 83: 649–662.
36. Nare B, Smith JM, Prichard RK (1991) Differential effects of oltipraz and its oxy-analogue on the viability of Schistosoma mansoni and the activity of glutathione S-transferase. Biochem Pharmacol 42: 1287–1292.
37. Mollinedo F, Fernandez M, Hornillos V, Delgado J, Amat-Guerri F, et al. (2011) Involvement of lipid rafts in the localization and dysfunction effect of the antitumor ether phospholipid edelfosine in mitochondria. Cell Death Dis 2: e158.
38. Gajate C, Matos-da-Silva M, Dakir el H, Fonteriz RI, Alvarez J, et al. (2012) Antitumor alkyl-lysophospholipid analog edelfosine induces apoptosis in pancreatic cancer by targeting endoplasmic reticulum. Oncogene 31: 2627–2639.
39. Galanti SE, Huang SC, Pearce EJ (2012) Cell death and reproductive regression in female Schistosoma mansoni. PLoS Negl Trop Dis 6: e1509.
40. Zhang CW, Xiao SH, Utzinger J, Chollet J, Keiser J, et al. (2009) Histopathological changes in adult Schistosoma japonicum harbored in mice treated with a single dose of mefloquine. Parasitol Res 104: 1407–1416.
41. Cheever AW (1970) Relative resistance of the eggs of human schistosomes to digestion in potassium hydroxide. Bull World Health Organ 43: 601–603.
42. Estella-Hermoso de Mendoza A, Campanero MA, de la Iglesia-Vicente J, Gajate C, Mollinedo F, et al. (2009) Antitumor alkyl ether lipid edelfosine: tissue distribution and pharmacokinetic behavior in healthy and tumor-bearing immunosuppressed mice. Clin Cancer Res 15: 858–864.
43. Jurberg AD, Goncalves T, Costa TA, de Mattos AC, Pascarelli BM, et al. (2009) The embryonic development of Schistosoma mansoni eggs: proposal for a new staging system. Dev Genes Evol 219: 219–234.

44. Mollinedo F (2007) Antitumour ether lipids: proapoptotic agents with multiple therapeutic indications. Expert Opinion on Therapeutic Patents 17: 385–405.
45. Bertao HG, da Silva RA, Padilha RJ, de Azevedo Albuquerque MC, Radis-Baptista G (2012) Ultrastructural analysis of miltefosine-induced surface membrane damage in adult Schistosoma mansoni BH strain worms. Parasitol Res 110: 2465–2473.
46. Marr JJ, Nilsen TW, Komuniecki R (2003) Molecular medical parasitology. Amsterdam; Boston: Academic Press. xii, 488 p.
47. Jones MK, Gobert GN, Zhang L, Sunderland P, McManus DP (2004) The cytoskeleton and motor proteins of human schistosomes and their roles in surface maintenance and host-parasite interactions. Bioessays 26: 752–765.
48. Skelly PJ (2005) The surface of schistosomes within the vertebrate host. In: Secor WE, Colley, Daniel G., editor. Schistosomiasis. pp.82–100.
49. Wilson RA (2012) The cell biology of schistosomes: a window on the evolution of the early metazoa. Protoplasma 249: 503–518.
50. McLaren DJ, Hockley DJ (1977) Blood flukes have a double outer membrane. Nature 269: 147–149.
51. Ruppel A, McLaren DJ (1986) Schistosoma mansoni: surface membrane stability *in vitro* and *in vivo*. Exp Parasitol 62: 223–236.
52. Van Hellemond JJ, Retra K, Brouwers JF, van Balkom BW, Yazdanbakhsh M, et al. (2006) Functions of the tegument of schistosomes: clues from the proteome and lipidome. Int J Parasitol 36: 691–699.
53. Faghiri Z, Skelly PJ (2009) The role of tegumental aquaporin from the human parasitic worm, Schistosoma mansoni, in osmoregulation and drug uptake. FASEB J 23: 2780–2789.
54. Pereira AS, Padilha RJ, Lima-Filho JL, Chaves ME (2011) Scanning electron microscopy of the human low-density lipoprotein interaction with the tegument of Schistosoma mansoni. Parasitol Res 109: 1395–1402.
55. Shaw MK, Erasmus DA (1983) Schistosoma mansoni: dose-related tegumental surface changes after in vivo treatment with praziquantel. Z Parasitenkd 69: 643–653.
56. Fallon PG, Fookes RE, Wharton GA (1996) Temporal differences in praziquantel- and oxamniquine-induced tegumental damage to adult Schistosoma mansoni: implications for drug-antibody synergy. Parasitology 112 (Pt 1): 47–58.
57. Xiao S, Binggui S, Chollet J, Tanner M (2000) Tegumental changes in 21-day-old Schistosoma mansoni harboured in mice treated with artemether. Acta Trop 75: 341–348.
58. Xiao SH, Xue J, Shen B (2010) Transmission electron microscopic observation on ultrastructural alterations in Schistosoma japonicum caused by mefloquine. Parasitol Res 106: 1179–1187.
59. Soliman MF, Ibrahim MM (2005) Antischistosomal action of atorvastatin alone and concurrently with medroxyprogesterone acetate on Schistosoma haematobium harboured in hamster: surface ultrastructure and parasitological study. Acta Trop 93: 1–9.
60. Neves JK, de Lima Mdo C, Pereira VR, de Melo CM, Peixoto CA, et al. (2011) Antischistosomal action of thioxo-imidazolidine compounds: an ultrastructural and cytotoxicity study. Exp Parasitol 128: 82–90.
61. Eissa MM, El Bardicy S, Tadros M (2011) Bioactivity of miltefosine against aquatic stages of Schistosoma mansoni, Schistosoma haematobium and their snail hosts, supported by scanning electron microscopy. Parasit Vectors 4: 73.
62. Dorlo TP, Balasegaram M, Beijnen JH, de Vries PJ (2012) Miltefosine: a review of its pharmacology and therapeutic efficacy in the treatment of leishmaniasis. J Antimicrob Chemother 67: 2576–2597.
63. Mollinedo F, Gajate C, Morales AI, del Canto-Janez E, Justies N, et al. (2009) Novel anti-inflammatory action of edelfosine lacking toxicity with protective effect in experimental colitis. J Pharmacol Exp Ther 329: 439–449.
64. Gonnert R, Andrews P (1977) Praziquantel, a new board-spectrum antischistosomal agent. Z Parasitenkd 52: 129–150.
65. Cioli D, Pica-Mattoccia L (2003) Praziquantel. Parasitol Res 90 Supp 1: S3–9.
66. King CH, Muchiri EM, Ouma JH (2000) Evidence against rapid emergence of praziquantel resistance in Schistosoma haematobium, Kenya. Emerg Infect Dis 6: 585–594.
67. Fenwick A, Webster JP (2006) Schistosomiasis: challenges for control, treatment and drug resistance. Curr Opin Infect Dis 19: 577–582.
68. Norton AJ, Gower CM, Lamberton PH, Webster BL, Lwambo NJ, et al. (2010) Genetic consequences of mass human chemotherapy for Schistosoma mansoni: population structure pre- and post-praziquantel treatment in Tanzania. Am J Trop Med Hyg 83: 951–957.
69. Kunz W (2001) Schistosome male-female interaction: induction of germ-cell differentiation. Trends Parasitol 17: 227–231.
70. Utzinger J, Chollet J, You J, Mei J, Tanner M, et al. (2001) Effect of combined treatment with praziquantel and artemether on Schistosoma japonicum and Schistosoma mansoni in experimentally infected animals. Acta Trop 80: 9–18.
71. Keiser J, Manneck T, Vargas M (2011) Interactions of mefloquine with praziquantel in the Schistosoma mansoni mouse model and *in vitro*. J Antimicrob Chemother 66: 1791–1797.
72. O'Neal SE, Guimaraes LH, Machado PR, Alcantara L, Morgan DJ, et al. (2007) Influence of helminth infections on the clinical course of and immune response to Leishmania braziliensis cutaneous leishmaniasis. J Infect Dis 195: 142–148.
73. Hassan MF, Zhang Y, Engwerda CR, Kaye PM, Sharp H, et al. (2006) The Schistosoma mansoni hepatic egg granuloma provides a favorable microenvironment for sustained growth of Leishmania donovani. Am J Pathol 169: 943–953.
74. La Flamme AC, Scott P, Pearce EJ (2002) Schistosomiasis delays lesion resolution during Leishmania major infection by impairing parasite killing by macrophages. Parasite Immunol 24: 339–345.

13

Regulation of Nitric Oxide Production by δ-Opioid Receptors during Glaucomatous Injury

Shahid Husain*, Yasir Abdul, Sudha Singh, Anis Ahmad, Mahvash Husain

Hewitt Laboratory of the Ola B. Williams Glaucoma Center, Department of Ophthalmology, Storm Eye Institute, Medical University of South Carolina, Charleston, South Carolina, United States of America

Abstract

To determine the roles of nitric oxide in glaucomatous injury and its regulation by δ-opioid-receptor activation, animals were treated with: 1) a selective inducible nitric oxide synthase (iNOS) inhibitor (aminoguanidine; AG; 25 mg/kg, i.p.); 2) δ-opioid-receptor agonist (SNC-121; 1 mg/kg, i.p.); or 3) with both drugs simultaneously for 7 days, once daily. The loss in retinal ganglion cell (RGC) numbers and their function in glaucomatous eyes were significantly improved in the presence of AG or SNC-121; however, we did not see any significant additive or synergistic effects when animals were treated with both drugs simultaneously. The levels of nitrate-nitrite were significantly increased in the glaucomatous retina when compared with normal retina (normal retina 86±9 vs. glaucomatous retina 174±10 mM/mg protein), which was reduced significantly when animals were treated either with SNC-121 (121±7 mM/mg protein; $P<0.05$) or AG (128±10 mM/mg protein; $P<0.05$). Additionally, SNC-121-mediated reduction in nitrate-nitrite levels was not only blocked by naltrindole (a δ-opioid-receptor antagonist), but naltrindole treatment potentiated the nitrate-nitrite production in glaucomatous retina (235±4 mM/mg protein; $P<0.001$). As expected, naltrindole treatment also fully-blocked SNC-121-mediated retina neuroprotection. The nitrotyrosine level in the glaucomatous retina was also increased, which was significantly reduced in the SNC-121-treated animals. Additionally, the expression level of iNOS was clearly increased over the control levels in the glaucomatous retina and optic nerves, which was also reduced by SNC-121 treatment. In conclusion, our data support the notion that nitric oxide plays a detrimental role during glaucomatous injury and inhibition of nitric oxide production provided RGC neuroprotection. Furthermore, δ-opioid receptor activation regulates the production of nitric oxide via inhibiting the activity of iNOS in the retina and optic nerve.

Editor: Steven Barnes, Dalhousie University, Canada

Funding: Supported in part by National Institutes of Health/National Eye Institute grant EY019081 (SH), and an unrestricted grant to MUSC-SEI from Research to Prevent Blindness, New York, New York. This work was conducted in a facility constructed with support from the National Institutes of Health, Grant Number C06 RR015455 from the Extramural Research Facilities Program of the National Center for Research Resources. The funders had no role in study design, data collection and analysis, decision to publish, or preparation of the manuscript.

Competing Interests: The authors have declared that no competing interests exist.

* Email: Husain@musc.edu

Introduction

Glaucoma is a slowly progressing optic neuropathy that causes loss of retinal ganglion cells (RGCs), optic disc changes, and visual-field loss [1,2]. Currently, intraocular pressure (IOP) lowering strategies are the only effective way to control the disease progression. However, reduction in IOP is not always successful and many patients continue to experience the progressive loss of vision [3,4]. The mechanisms that lead to the RGC death during disease progression are unclear. However, accumulating literature suggests that multiple mechanisms are involved in RGC death in glaucoma including inflammation [5–8], apoptosis [9–11], neurotrophic factor deprivation [12,13], and nitric oxide production [14–16]. During the progression of glaucoma, glial cells, mainly astrocytes within the optic nerve head (ONH) [17], also play key roles in the initiation of lesions in glaucomatous optic neuropathy [18]. While astrocytes play a vital role in maintaining a normal physiological state in RGCs, they become activated in response to glaucomatous injury and produce neurotoxic substances like proinflammatory cytokines [7,8] and nitric oxide which ultimately leads to axonal and RGC loss [14,15,19].

Nitric oxide is an important signaling molecule, which regulates various physiological processes in numerous tissues. In the eye it regulates IOP [20,21], and small quantities could be beneficial to maintain metabolites and blood circulation [22]. However, sustained levels of nitric oxide production may result in direct tissue toxicity and contribute to neuronal degeneration [23]. Nitric oxide is produced by nitric oxide synthase (NOS); three isoforms of NOS have been cloned: constitutive (NOS-1 or nNOS), endothelial (NOS-3 or eNOS), and inducible (iNOS or NOS-2). Inducible NOS has been implicated in several neurodegenerative human diseases including Parkinson and stroke [24]. However, conflicting data have been reported for the role of nitric oxide and nitric oxide synthase in glaucoma-induced retina degeneration and RGC loss [14–16,25,26].

To clarify the role of nitric oxide in glaucoma pathology we have used a chronic ocular-hypertensive rat glaucoma model [27] and determined if δ-opioid-receptor activation regulates nitric oxide production. Additionally, we determined if δ-opioid-receptor-mediated retina neuroprotection is partly via nitric-oxide-dependent pathways. The data we provide herein support the idea that nitric oxide, mainly produced by iNOS, played a detrimental role during glaucomatous injury, and its inhibition either by its selective inhibitor, aminoguanidine (AG), or by δ-opioid-receptor agonist (SNC-121), provided retina neuroprotection against glaucomatous injury.

Materials and Methods

Animals

Adult female Brown Norway rats (3–5 months of age; 150–200 grams; Harlan Laboratories, Inc., Indianapolis, IN, and Charles River laboratory, San Diego, CA) were used in this study. Female rats were chosen because they are calm and easy to handle when measuring IOP in conscious rats. Rats were kept under a cycle of 12-hours light and 12-hours dark for all the studies. Animal handling was performed in accordance with the ARVO Statement for the Use of Animals in Ophthalmic and Vision Research; and the study protocol was approved by the Animal Care and Use Committee at the Medical University of South Carolina.

Drug Preparation

Delta (δ)-opioid-receptor agonist, SNC-121 (Santa Cruz Biotechnology, Dallas, TX), was dissolved in normal saline (0.9%). SNC-121 (1 mg/kg) was injected intraperitoneally (i.p.) into Brown Norway rats 30 minutes after glaucomatous injury, and treatment was continued for 7 days, once daily. Inducible nitric oxide synthase (iNOS or NOS-2) inhibitor, 25 mg/kg aminoguanidine hydrochloride (AG; Sigma-Aldrich, St. Louis, MO) was also intraperitoneally (i.p.) injected 30 minutes after glaucoma surgery. The AG treatment was continued for 7 days, once daily. In a separate group, animals were treated with both AG and SNC-121 simultaneously for 7 days, once daily. In this group, animals were first treated with AG (25 mg/kg, i.p.) 30 minutes after glaucomatous injury, followed by SNC-121 (1 mg/kg, i.p.) treatment at an interval of 15 minutes. A group of animals was also treated with a selective δ-opioid-receptor antagonist, naltrindole (3 mg/kg; i.p.), 30 minutes after glaucomatous injury, followed by SNC-121 treatment for 7 days, once daily. Drug administration (150–200 μL) was performed daily at the same time between 9 am-11 am. The control group was handled

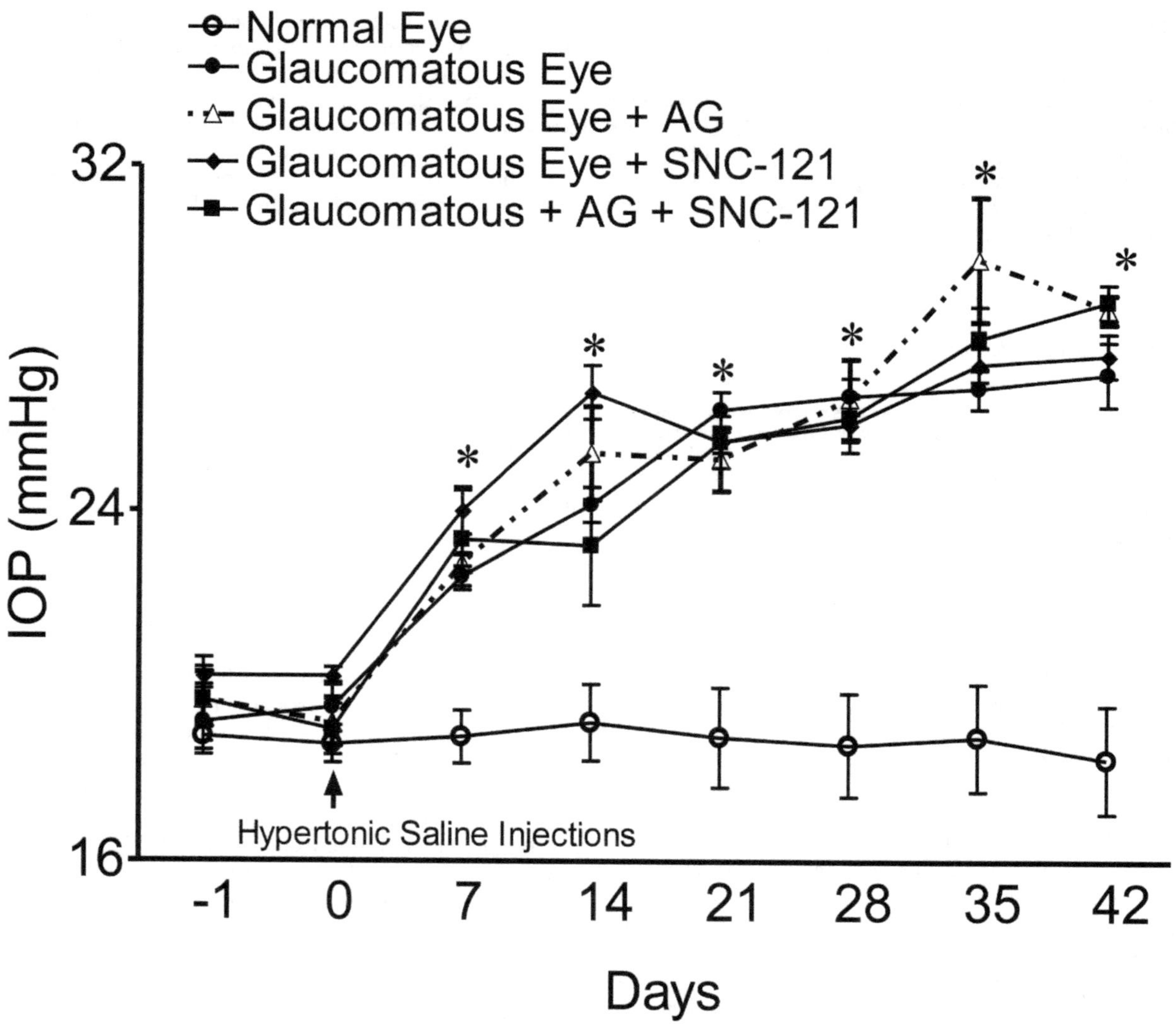

Figure 1. Intraocular pressure (IOP) measurements in normal and glaucomatous eyes. IOP of normal eyes and eyes from a chronic glaucoma model with and without AG (25 mg/kg; i.p.) and SNC-121 (1 mg/kg) treatment for 7 days (once daily) was measured as described in the Methods. IOP was elevated in one eye of Brown Norway rats by injecting approximately 50 μL of 2.0 M hypertonic saline, while the contralateral eye served as the control. Rats were maintained for up to 6 weeks post-surgery. Data are mean ± SE. *$P<0.05$; n = 6–8 for each group.

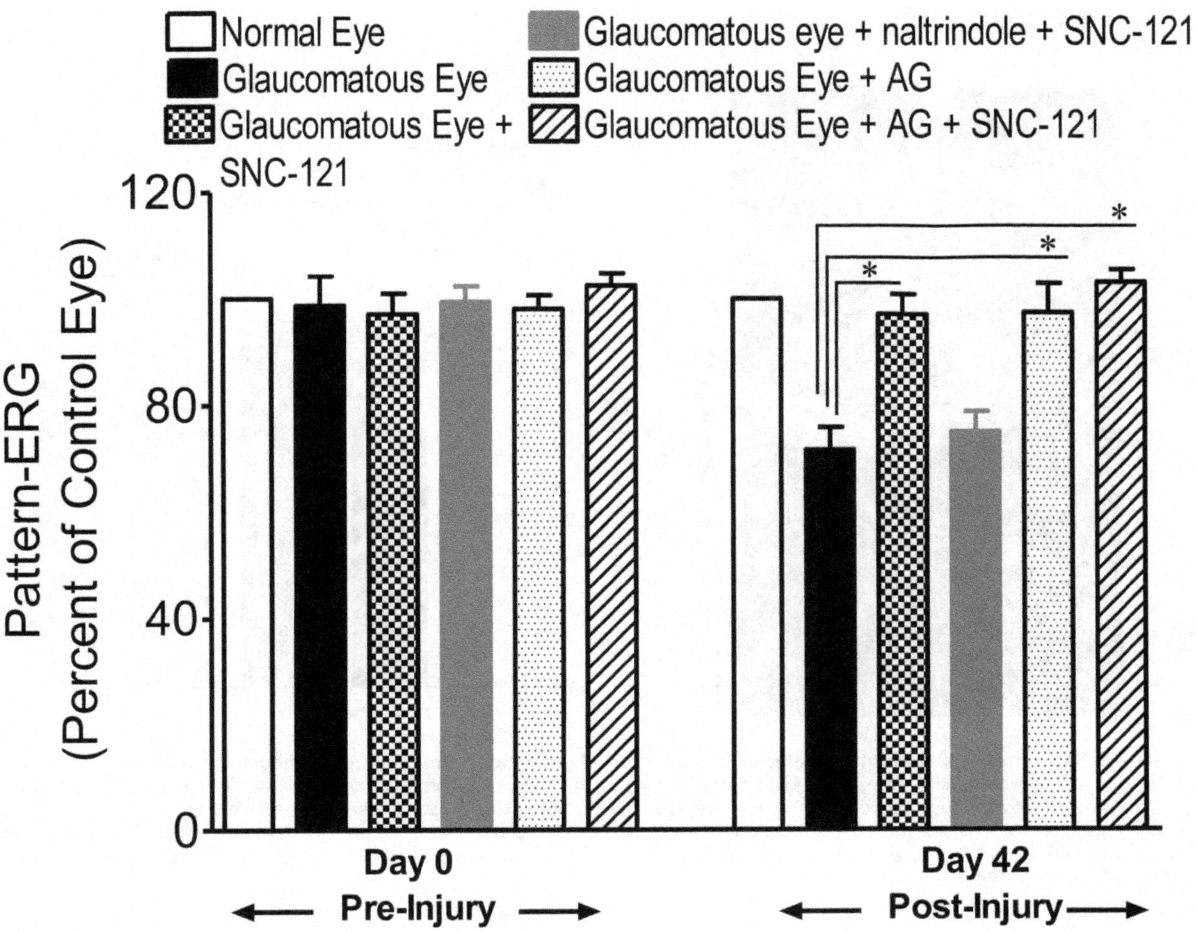

Figure 2. Pattern ERG recordings in normal and glaucomatous eyes. Changes observed in Pattern ERGs of untreated, AG or SNC-121-treated glaucomatous rat eyes are shown as a percentage of the contralateral control eye. In these experiments, Brown Norway rats were treated with AG (25 mg/kg, i.p.) or SNC-121 (1 mg/kg, i.p.), individually or together simultaneously, 30 minutes after hypertonic saline injections. Animals were treated with naltrindole 30 minutes after glaucomatous injury followed by SNC-121 treatment. The drug treatment was continued once daily for 7 days in all groups. Data are mean ± SE; *$P<0.05$; n = 7–8.

in a similar fashion except that normal saline was injected without SNC-121 or AG.

Development of Glaucoma Model by Hypertonic Saline Injection

Brown Norway rats (150–200 gm body weight) were housed under a standard 12:12 (light:dark) cycle. A stable baseline IOP was documented prior to hypertonic saline injection. Rats were anesthetized with ketamine (75 mg/kg) and xylazine (8 mg/kg) and body temperature was maintained at 37°C with a heating pad. Topical proparacaine (0.5%) was applied to the cornea. IOP was elevated using 50 μL of 2 M hypertonic saline into the circumferential limbal vein near the cornea as described earlier [7,27]. After surgery, an antibacterial ointment (neomycin) was applied at the injection site of each animal to prevent infections. As inclusion criteria following hypertonic saline injection, only animals with an elevated IOP that was at least 25% over baseline were included in the study.

Pattern Electroretinogram (Pattern-ERG) Recordings

Rats were anesthetized with ketamine (75 mg/kg) and xylazine (8 mg/kg) and body temperature was maintained at 37°C with a heating pad. Pattern-ERG recordings (without dark adaptation) were conducted in both eyes (sequentially) 3 days prior to IOP elevation by hypertonic saline injection, and then weekly post-surgery as described earlier [7,27]. For the Pattern-ERG amplitudes, measurements were made between a peak and adjacent trough of the waveform as described earlier [27]. Pattern-ERG amplitudes were obtained for each eye by collecting 300 sweeps at an interval of 1 second. The final pattern-ERG amplitude was an average of 300 sweeps for each eye.

Retinal Ganglion Cell (RGC) Counting

RGCs were visualized and counted by retrograde-labeling using fluorogold as described earlier [7,27]. Briefly, animals were anesthetized with ketamine (75 mg/kg, i.p.) and xylazine (8 mg/kg, i.p.), and 5% Fluorogold (Fluorochrome, LLC; Denver, CO) was injected into the superior colliculus in animals immobilized in a stereotaxic apparatus. Seven days after injection, animals were euthanized and their eyes were enucleated and fixed in 4% paraformaldehyde for 24 hours at 4°C. After rinsing with PBS, each retina was detached from the eyecup and prepared as a flatmount by mounting with the vitreous side-up. RGCs were counted and averaged per 8 microscopic fields of identical size (150 μm^2; 20x magnification) per retina by using Image J software (NIH, Bethesda, MD). The automated RGC numbers generated

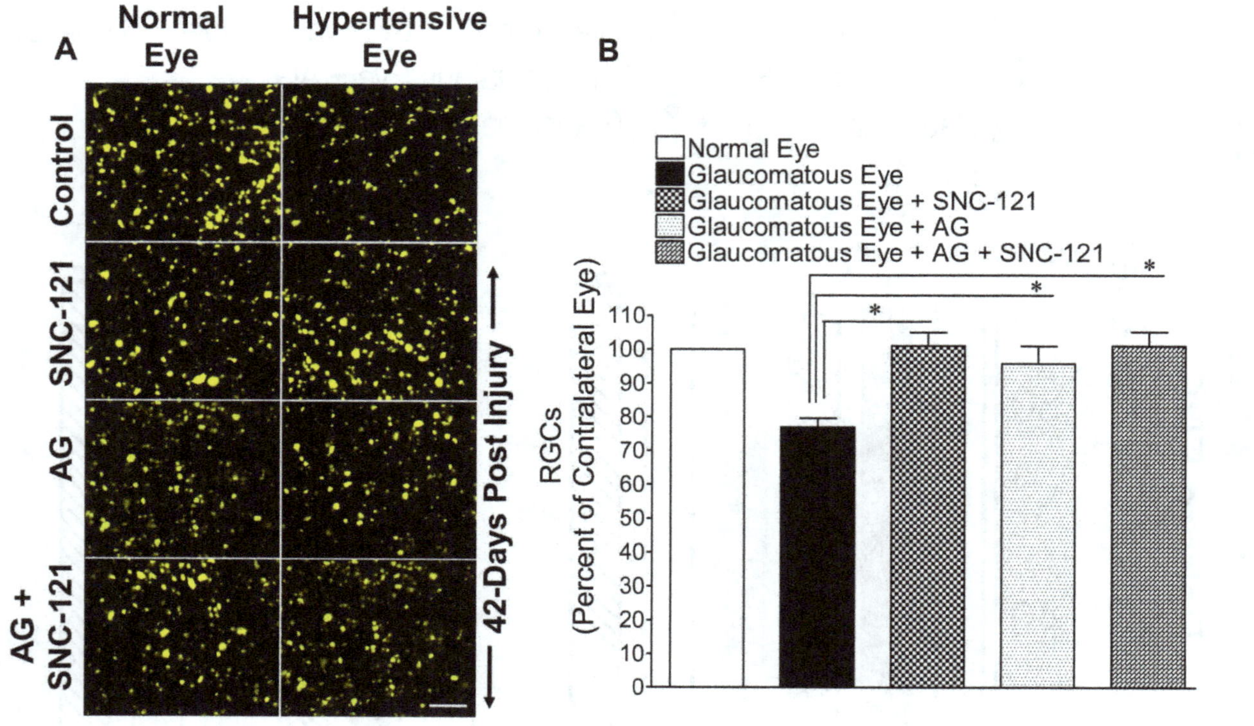

Figure 3. Retina flat mounts of normal and glaucomatous eyes. Fluorescence micrographs of flatmounted retinas depicting Fluorogold-labeled retina ganglion cells (RGCs) in normal and glaucomatous eyes in the absence or presence of drugs (**A**). Briefly, 3 μL of a 5% solution of Fluorogold was injected into the superior colliculus of anesthetized animals. Seven days post injection, animals were euthanized and retinas were prepared as flatmounts, vitreous-side facing up. Fluorescent RGCs were visualized under Zeiss microscopy. Bar = 20 μm. Total RGC tallies in glaucomatous eyes in the absence or presence of drugs. RGCs were counted in 8 microscopic fields of identical size (150 μm^2 area) for each retina, using Image J software (**B**). *$P<0.05$; n = 6 for each group.

by Image J software were comparable when RGCs were counted manually by two operators in a masked fashion.

Immunohistochemistry

Optic nerves and eyes of normal and glaucomatous animals were collected at the 7th and 42nd day post glaucomatous injury, as described earlier [7,27]. Optic nerves and eyes were fixed in paraformaldehyde (4%) overnight at 4°C, then cryoprotected in a 30% sucrose solution overnight at 4°C. Optic nerves and eyes were washed with cold PBS and embedded in OCT compound embedding medium over dry ice. Cryosections of optic nerve and retina were cut in a cryostat at −20°C and tissues were incubated with primary antibody (anti iNOS at 1:100 dilution; BD BioSciences, San Jose, CA) followed by incubation with FITC-conjugated secondary antibody (1:400 dilutions; Jackson Immuno Research Laboratories, Inc., West Grove, PA). Negative control slides were incubated with 0.5% BSA instead of primary antibodies. Tissue sections were viewed under a fluorescent microscope and digitized images were captured by a digital camera (Zeiss).

Western Blotting

An equivalent amount of retina lysate (15 μg/lane) was loaded onto 10% SDS-PAGE. Proteins were separated and transferred to nitrocellulose membrane. The membranes were blocked with 5% nonfat dry milk, and then incubated with appropriate primary antibody (anti-Nitrotyrosine at a 1:1000 dilution; anti-iNOS at a 1:1000 dilution; or anti-β-actin at a 1:3000 dilution) for 12 hours at 4°C. After washing, membranes were incubated with appropriate secondary antibodies (HRP-conjugated at 1:3000 dilution). The membranes were treated with enhanced chemiluminescent reagent to detect the signals using a Biorad Versadoc imaging system (Biorad, Hercules, CA).

Measurements of Nitrate-Nitrite in Retina Extracts

Nitrate-nitrite was estimated by using "Cayman's Assay Kit" (Cayman, Item number-780001, Ann Arbor, MI). This method involves a two-step process. Briefly, the retinas were homogenized and centrifuged at 10,000 *g* for 10 minutes. The supernatant was collected to measure nitrates-nitrites. The reaction was started by adding 80 μL of retina samples, 10 μL of enzyme cofactor, and 10 μL nitrate reductase in a 96-well plate. After 1 hour, 50 μL Greiss reagents were added and allowed to incubate for 30 minutes. The changes in absorbance were measured at 550 nm. The amount of nitrate-nitrite was expressed as mM of nitrate-nitrite per milligram protein.

Statistical Analysis

The data are expressed as mean ± SEM. The comparisons were made using Student *t* test for paired samples or ANOVA with Bonferroni post test for multiple comparisons (Graph Pad Software, Inc., San Diego, CA). A *P* value of <0.05 is considered significant.

Results

Intraocular pressure (IOP) was raised by injecting 2 M hypertonic saline into limbal veins and IOP was measured up to 42 days at an interval of 7 days, as described earlier [7]. A significant elevation in IOP was seen as early as 7 days post

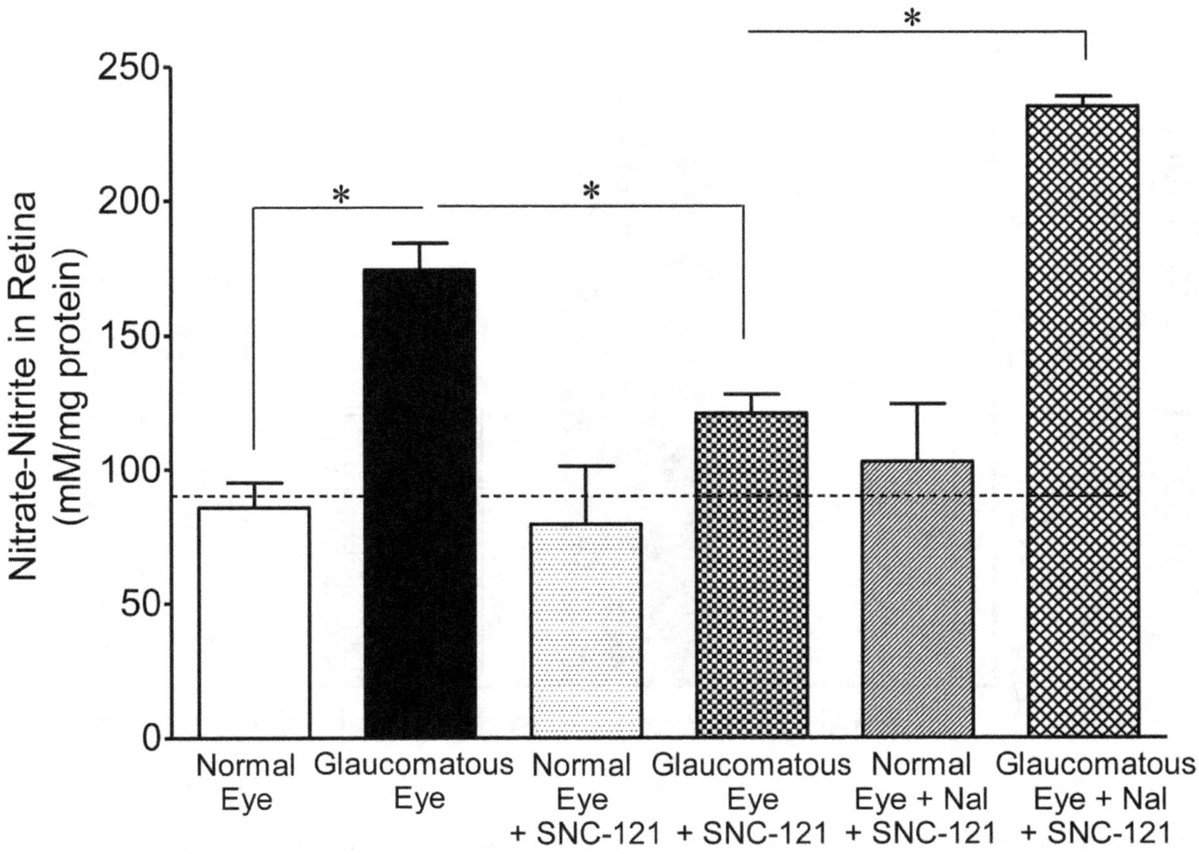

Figure 4. Measurements of nitrate-nitrite in normal and glaucomatous eyes in the presence of SNC-121. Animals were treated with SNC-121 (1 mg/kg, i.p.) 30 minutes after glaucomatous injury, and continued once daily for 7 days. A separate group of animals was pretreated with naltrindole (Nal; 3 mg/kg, i.p.) followed by SNC-121 (1 mg/kg, i.p.) treatment 30 minutes after glaucomatous injury, and continued for 7 days, once daily. The absorbance was read at 550 nm and absorbance was plotted against the nitrate standards. The amount of nitrate-nitrite is expressed as millimolar nitrates-nitrites per milligram protein. Data are expressed as mean ± SEM, (*$P<0.05$; n = 4–7).

surgery and was maintained up to 42 days following IOP elevation. Similar to our previous studies, we did not see any significant changes in IOP of normal and glaucomatous eyes when animals were treated with a selective δ-opioid-receptor agonist, SNC-121 (1 mg/Kg, i.p.), for 7 days [7] (**Figure 1**). To determine the effects of aminoguanidine (AG) alone or in combination with SNC-121 on IOP, animals were either treated with AG (25 mg/kg, i.p.) alone for 7 days, once daily, or with AG (25 mg/kg, i.p.) and SNC-121 (1 mg/Kg, i.p.) simultaneously for 7 days, once daily. As shown in **Figure 1**, elevated IOP in glaucomatous animals was not changed significantly when animals were treated either with AG or AG plus SNC-121 simultaneously. The functional response of retinal ganglion cells (RGCs) in normal and glaucomatous eyes was measured by pattern-electroretinogram (Pattern-ERG) at 42nd day, post glaucomatous injury. To determine if δ-opioid-receptor-mediated retina neuroprotection was partly mediated via nitric oxide-dependent pathways, animals were treated with a selective iNOS inhibitor (AG; 25 mg/kg, i.p.), a selective δ-opioid-receptor agonist (SNC-121; 1 mg/kg, i.p.) individually or with both drugs simultaneously for 7 days, once daily. As shown in **Figure 2**, the Pattern-ERG amplitudes were reduced by 35% in glaucomatous animals (control eyes 100±00% vs. glaucomatous eyes 65±6%; $P<0.05$). Treatment of animals with AG for 7 days provided retina neuroprotection against glaucomatous injury (glaucomatous eyes, 65±6% vs. glaucomatous eyes + AG, 93±6%; $P<0.05$). Similar to our previous findings [7], SNC-121 treatment also provided a significant amount of retina neuroprotection; however, we did not see any significant additive or synergistic effects when animals were treated with both drugs (e.g., AG and SNC-121) simultaneously (glaucomatous eyes, 65±6% vs. glaucomatous eyes + AG + SNC-121, 110±8%; $P<0.05$). As expected, SNC-121-mediated retina neuroprotection was fully-blocked by pretreatment with δ-opioid-receptor antagonist, naltrindole (**Fig. 2**).

To confirm that declines in Pattern-ERG amplitudes were due to the loss of RGCs, they were visualized by retrograde-labeling with bilateral injections of fluorogold into the superior colliculus (**Fig. 3A**). The loss of RGCs in the glaucomatous eyes was reduced when animals were treated either with AG (25 mg/kg; i.p.) or SNC-121 (1 mg/kg; i.p.) for 7 days; however, we did not see any further decline in the rate of RGC loss when animals were treated with both drugs simultaneously. Quantification of RGCs in normal eyes, glaucomatous eyes, AG-treated glaucomatous eyes, SNC-121-treated glaucomatous eyes, or both drug-treated glaucomatous eyes are shown in **Figure 3B**. The mean number (± SE) of fluorogold-positive RGCs were: normal eyes, 2150±99 RGCs/mm^2; glaucomatous eyes, 1666±105 RGCs/mm^2 (23% less than normal eyes; $P<0.05$); AG-treated glaucomatous eyes, 2012±108.1 RGCs/mm^2 (21% greater than the glaucomatous eyes; $P<0.05$), SNC-121-treated glaucomatous eyes, 2223±75 RGCs/mm^2 (33% greater than the glaucomatous eyes; $P<0.05$),

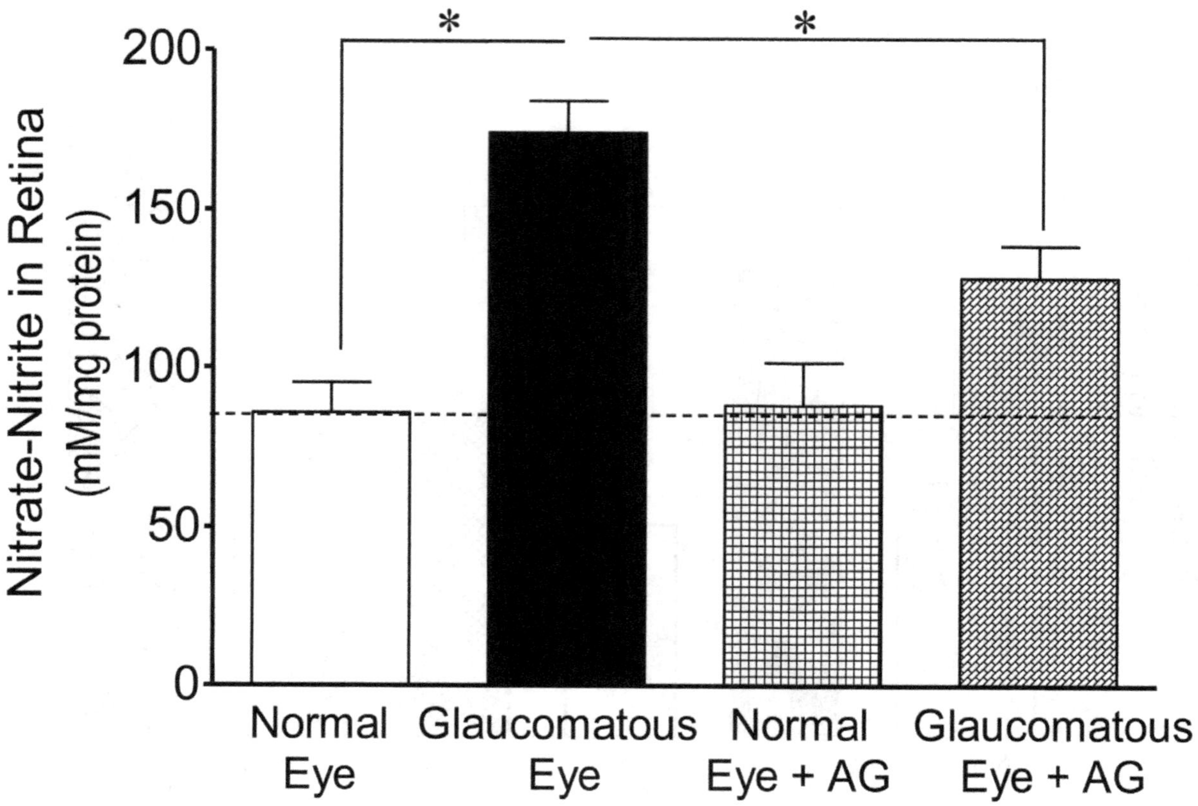

Figure 5. Measurements of nitrate-nitrite in normal and glaucomatous eyes in the presence of AG. Animals were treated with AG (25 mg/kg, i.p.) 30 minutes after glaucomatous injury and continued for 7 days, once daily. The absorbance was measured at 550 nm and absorbance was plotted against the nitrate standards. The amount of nitrate-nitrite is expressed as millimolar nitrates-nitrites per milligram protein. Data are expressed as mean ± SEM, (*$P<0.05$; n = 4–6).

and AG + SNC-121-treated glaucomatous eyes, 2181±94.59 RGCs/mm^2 (31% greater than the glaucomatous eyes; $P<0.05$).

To dissect out the molecular mechanisms, we measured the nitrate and nitrite levels, which are the end products of nitric oxide metabolism. We believe that nitric oxide is produced in an early stage of glaucoma; so we collected whole retina extracts to measure nitrates and nitrites at the 7th day, post glaucomatous injury. The levels of nitrate-nitrite were significantly increased in the retina sample of glaucomatous eyes when compared with normal eyes (normal eyes, 86±9 vs. glaucomatous eyes, 174±10 mM/mg protein; $P<0.001$; **Figs. 4–5**). The levels of nitrate-nitrite were significantly reduced in glaucomatous eyes when animals were treated either with SNC-121 (121±7 mM/mg protein; $P<0.05$; **Fig. 4**) or AG (128±10 mM/mg protein; $P<0.05$; **Fig. 5**) for 7 days, once a day. To confirm that SNC-121-mediated reduction in nitrate-nitrite levels was via activation of δ-opioid receptors, animals were treated with a selective δ-opioid-receptor antagonist, naltrindole. As shown in **Figure 4**, SNC-121-mediated reduction in nitrate-nitrite levels was not only blocked, but naltrindole treatment potentiated the nitrate-nitrite production in glaucomatous eyes (235±4 mM/mg protein; $P<0.001$; **Fig. 4**). Surprisingly, naltrindole increased the basal levels of nitrate-nitrite in normal eyes, although this change was not statistically significant. Nitric oxide is a versatile free-radical that mediates numerous biological functions. Although nitric oxide can modify numerous signaling pathways, the reaction of nitric oxide with cysteine residues in proteins, a process known as nitrosylation, is emerging as one of the most important mechanisms. This post-translational modification, *S*-nitrosylation, is a physiologically-important event that affects a wide variety of proteins involved in a number of cellular processes. As shown in **Figure 6**, an increase in the nitrotyrosine level in the retina sample of glaucomatous eyes was seen when compared with the normal eye on the 7th day, post injury. Interestingly, the nitrotyrosine levels were reduced in SNC-121-treated animals (**Fig. 6**).

To further confirm that elevation in nitric oxide production during glaucomatous injury is due to iNOS up-regulation and/or activation**,** we measured the iNOS levels in optic nerve at 7 and 42 days, post injury. As shown in **Figures 7–8**, the expression levels of iNOS were clearly increased over control levels in glaucomatous optic nerves, which was fully-attenuated in SNC-121-treated glaucomatous optic nerve. However, the iNOS expression pattern was not changed by SNC-121 treatment in normal optic nerves. Additionally, expression of iNOS was increased in the retina on day 7th and 42nd, post glaucomatous injury; which was significantly reduced by SNC-121 treatment (**Fig. 9**).

Discussion

We determined that activation of δ-opioid receptors by exogenous ligand (SNC-121) blocked nitric oxide production and subsequently rescued retinal ganglion cells (RGCs) from glaucomatous injury. Nitric oxide at physiological concentrations controls vascular inflammation and vascular injury by inhibiting the proinflammatory gene expression, but excessive production of nitric oxide can cause tissue toxicity and cell death [24]. Although the pathological role of nitric oxide in several neurodegenerative human diseases is somewhat clear, the pathological role of nitric

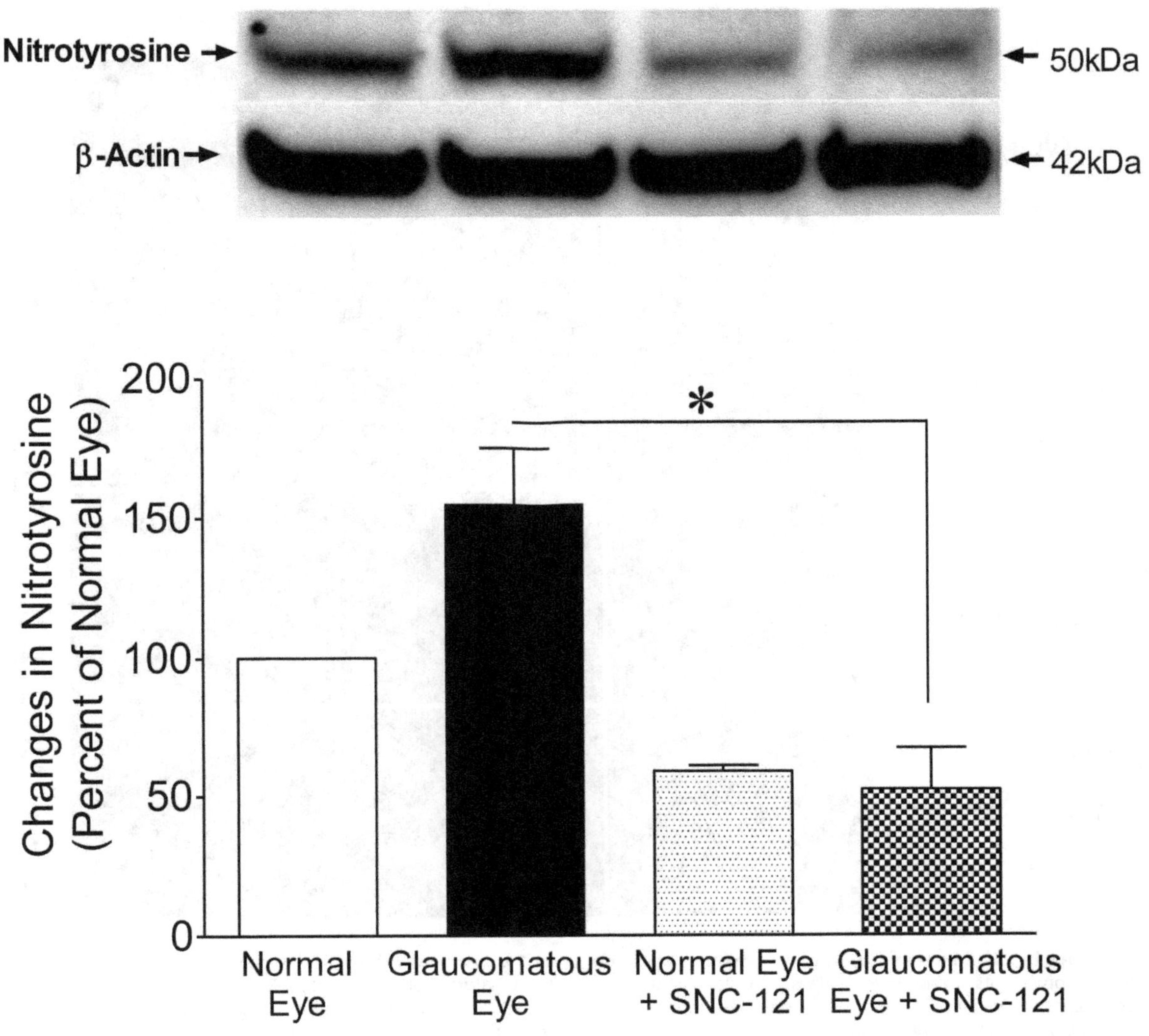

Figure 6. Measurement of protein nitrosylation in retina by Western blotting using nitrotyrosine antibodies in response to glaucomatous injury. Animals were treated with SNC-121 (1 mg/kg, i.p.) 30 minutes after glaucomatous injury and continued for 7 days, once daily. Retina extracts were collected at the 7th day, post injury, and analyzed using anti-nitrotyrosine antibodies and appropriate secondary antibodies (HRP-conjugated; dilution 1:3000). The signal was captured using enhanced chemiluminescent reagent and the Biorad Versadoc imaging system. Data shown are representative of four independent experiments. Data are expressed as mean ± SEM. $^{*}P<0.05$; n = 4.

oxide in glaucoma remains in question. For example: an increase in the inducible nitric oxide synthase (iNOS) has been reported in astrocytes and the optic nerve head of primary open-angle glaucoma (POAG) patients [14,16,28]. Furthermore, aminoguanidine (AG), a selective iNOS inhibitor, treatment provides RGC neuroprotection in an extraocular vein cauterization glaucoma model [15]. There was a 36% loss in RGCs in this cautery glaucoma model which was reduced to 9.6% by 60 mg/kg AG treatment. In non-glaucoma models, nitric oxide is produced mainly by iNOS that has been implicated in ischemia-induced retinal degeneration [29,30]. The iNOS inhibition resulted in the RGC neuroprotection against ischemia [31] and axotomy [32]. In contrast, studies also have shown that iNOS levels are not changed in POAG patients [26] and iNOS does not play a detrimental role in glaucomatous injury in chronically-elevated IOP glaucoma model (i.e., a model of aqueous humor outflow obstruction). Moreover, iNOS expression was not correlated with the severity of optic nerve damage [26]. Additional studies have shown that iNOS does not play a detrimental role in optic neuropathy in the DBA/2J glaucoma model [25]. In view of these conflicting results obtained from different laboratories using different experimental glaucoma models, we decided to further test the potential involvement of nitric oxide and inducible NOS (iNOS) in glaucomatous injury. Additionally, we determined if δ-opioid-receptor activation regulates the nitric oxide production.

Although, contradictory reports have been presented in the literature for RGC and optic nerve neuroprotection by iNOS inhibitor (e.g., AG), but all the studies were agreed that AG treatment does not change IOP in normal and glaucomatous animals [15,26]. Our data is in agreement with previous reports showing that AG treatment had no significant effect on IOP (**Fig. 1**). Additionally, our data presented herein clearly demonstrated that blocking nitric oxide either directly by AG or indirectly via activating δ-opioid-receptors by SNC-121, provided RGC neuroprotection. The functional outcome (Pattern-ERG) of the retina is also changed in the δ-opioid-receptor agonist-treated animals, suggesting that SNC-121 possibly crosses the blood retinal barrier. The most striking findings were that iNOS

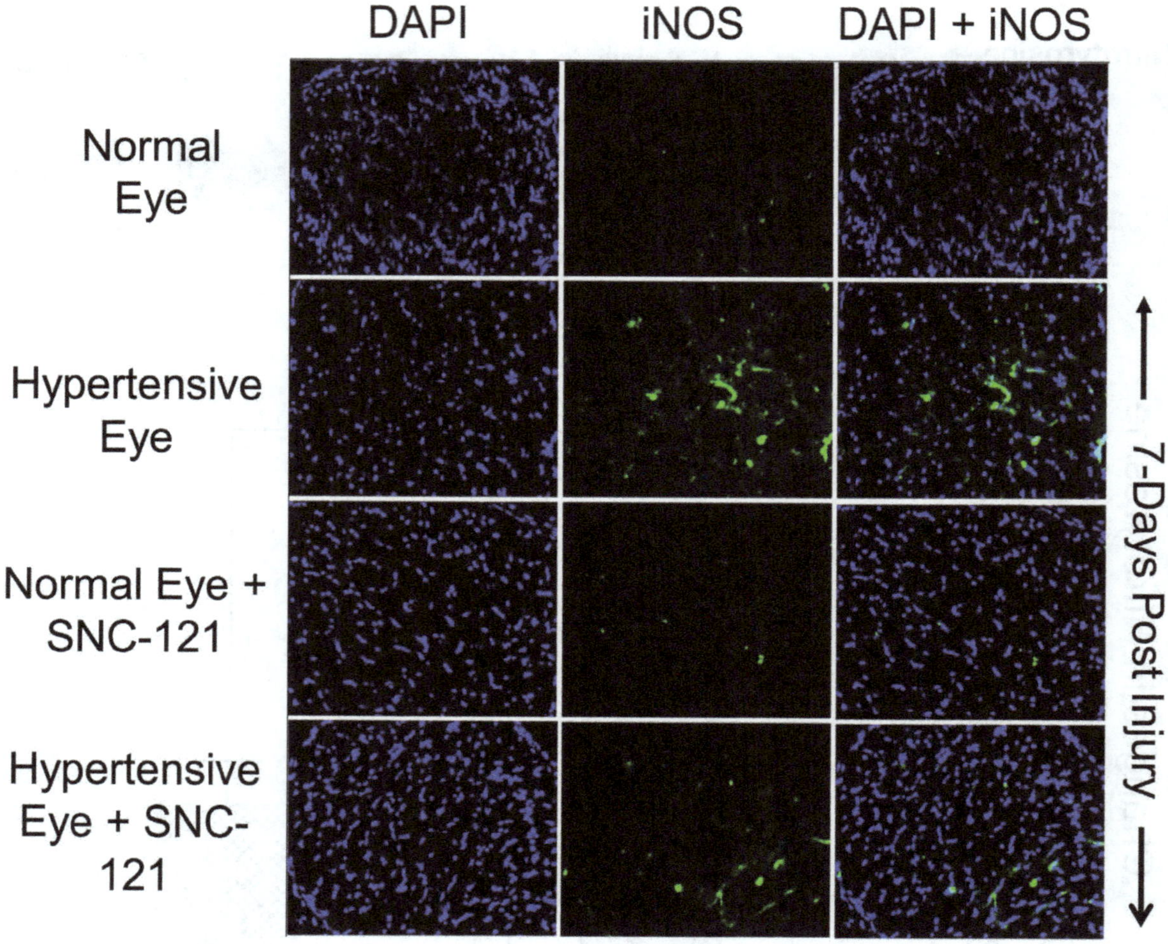

Figure 7. Changes in iNOS expression in glaucomatous optic nerve at 7 days, post injury. The optic nerve (non-myelinated; 2 mm post globe) of Brown Norway rats was removed 7-days post glaucomatous injury. Contralateral optic nerve was used as the normal control. Cryosections were immunostained by anti-iNOS antibodies as indicated horizontally. Ocular treatments are indicated vertically. Green color indicates staining for iNOS and blue nuclei for DAPI. There was no positive staining when primary antibodies were omitted (data not shown). Data shown here are representations of at least four independent experiments. A total of 10 animals were used in this experiment. Comparable staining for iNOS was seen in at least 4 animals in each treatment group.

production was not only elevated in the retina, but also increased in the optic nerve in response to glaucomatous injury, which was attenuated in the presence of SNC-121. Additionally, we have shown that changes in iNOS expression are occurring at an early stage of glaucoma progression (day 7), while other studies [15,26] have measured such changes in iNOS expression at 6–9 months, post glaucomatous injury. Our results confirmed that the enhanced levels of nitric oxide seen in glaucomatous eyes were due to up-regulation of iNOS not only in the retina, but also in the optic nerve, which may be playing a crucial role in orchestrating RGC death in a paracrine fashion during the pathogenesis of glaucoma.

Our findings are consistent with Shareef and Neufeld [15,16] who reported that treatment of glaucomatous rats with AG provide retina neuroprotection. However, our results do not agree with Pang and colleagues [26] while both studies have used a similar glaucoma rat model. However, there were numerous procedural differences in the two studies (e.g., Pang [26] and current study) and the discrepancies seen in these studies could be related to such variation in the protocols. For example: 1) normal and glaucomatous animals were kept under constant dim light that resulted in a higher baseline IOP (28 mmHg) versus dark-light cycle with baseline IOP (18–21 mmHg) in our studies; 2) pretreatment of animals with AG for 7 days prior to glaucomatous injury versus treatment of animals 30 minutes post glaucomatous injury in our studies; 3) duration of AG treatment in drinking water for 42 days versus AG treatment (intraperitoneally) for 7 days in our studies, 4) dosage differences of AG; and 5) the lack of RGC function measurement versus Pattern-ERG measurements in our studies. At this time, we cannot explain why genetic ablation of iNOS is not neuroprotective in the DBA/2J model. We believe, this area of research is still not fully-developed and more work is needed to understand a broader role of nitric oxide in general, and iNOS in particular for glaucoma pathology. Overall, our IHC data in retina and optic nerve, Western blotting data, and functional data (Pattern-ERG) support a neurodegenerative role of iNOS during glaucomatous injury.

Recently, we have shown that activation of δ-opioid receptors by a selective agonist (SNC-121) provides retina neuroprotection against glaucomatous injury via attenuation of p38 MAP kinase activity and TNF-α production [7]. Studies have shown that δ- and κ-opioid-receptor-activation provides brain neuroprotection via nitric oxide regulation [33,34]. The role of nitric oxide in δ-opioid-mediated retinal neuroprotection against glaucomatous

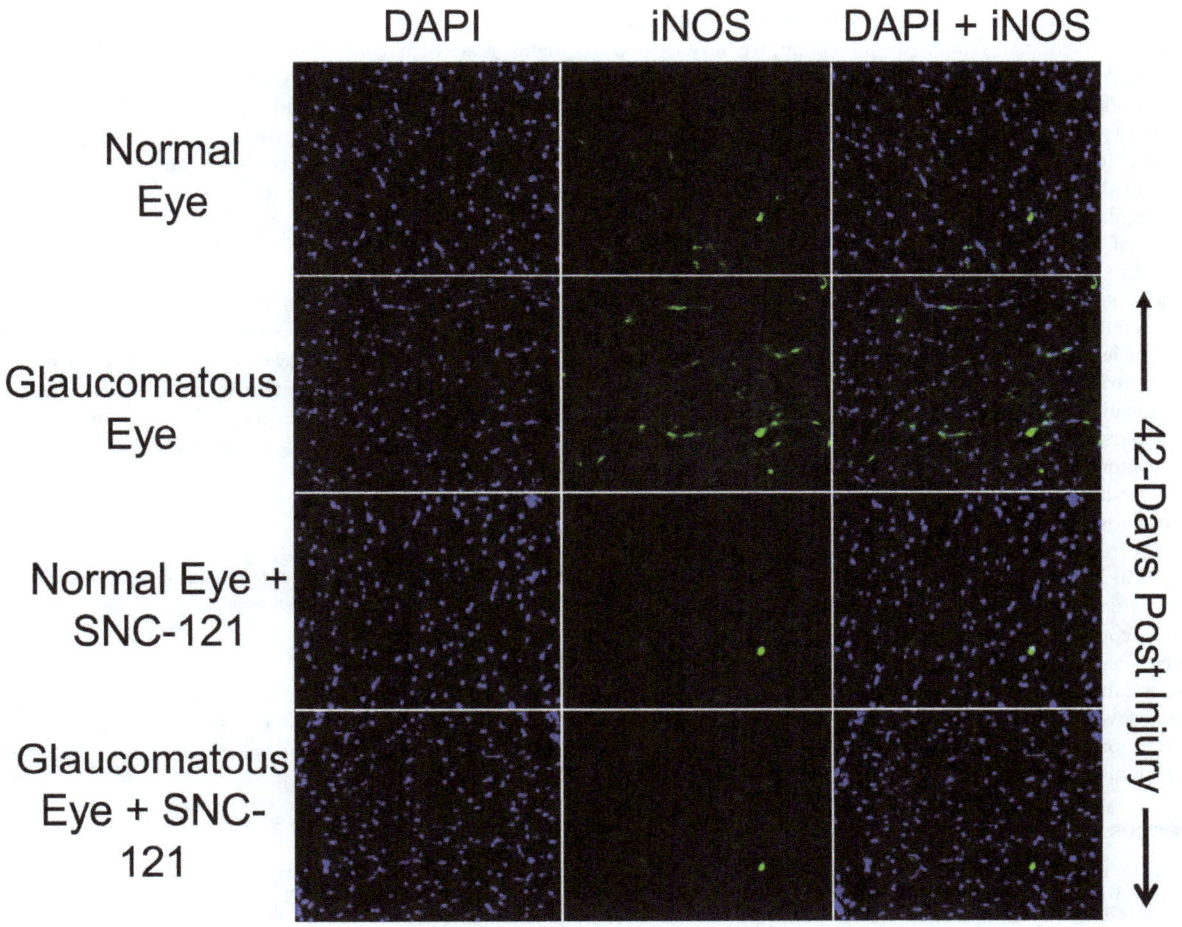

Figure 8. Changes in iNOS expression in glaucomatous optic nerve at 42 days, post injury. The optic nerve (non-myelinated; 2 mm post globe) of Brown Norway rats was removed 42-days post glaucomatous injury. Contralateral optic nerve was used as the normal control. Cryosections were immunostained by anti-iNOS antibodies as indicated horizontally. Ocular treatments are indicated vertically. Data shown in this Figure are a representation of at least four independent experiments. A total of 10 animals were used in this experiment. Comparable staining for iNOS was seen in at least 4 animals in each treatment group.

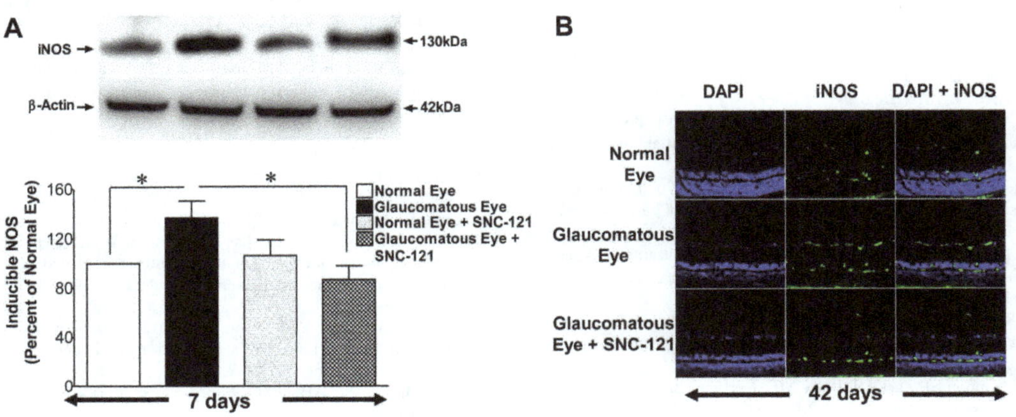

Figure 9. Changes in iNOS expression in glaucomatous retina at 7 and 42 days, post injury. (A) Brown Norway rats were treated with SNC-121 (1 mg/kg, i.p.) 30 minutes after glaucomatous injury and continued for 7 days, once daily. Retina extracts were collected at the 7th day, post injury, and analyzed using anti-iNOS antibodies and appropriate secondary antibodies (HRP-conjugated; dilution 1:3000). The signal was captured using enhanced chemiluminescent reagent and the Biorad Versadoc imaging system. Data are expressed as mean ± SEM. $^{*}P<0.05$; n = 4. (B) The eyes of Brown Norway rats were removed 42-days post glaucomatous injury. Cryosections of retina were immunostained by anti-iNOS antibodies as indicated horizontally. Ocular treatments are indicated vertically. Data shown in this Figure are a representation of at least four independent experiments.

injury has not been defined. To determine the roles of iNOS in δ-opioid-receptor-mediated retina neuroprotection, we have treated animals with AG and SNC-121 after glaucomatous injury. We did not see any additional beneficial effects on RGC neuroprotection when animals were simultaneously-treated with AG and SNC-121, suggesting that SNC-121 treatment fully blocked the activity of iNOS. To further confirm the roles of δ-opioid-receptor-activation in iNOS regulation during glaucomatous injury, we measured the production of nitrates and nitrites in the presence or absence of SNC-121. It is very difficult to measure appreciable levels of nitric oxide due to its short life; however nitrites are the stable reservoir that can reduced to bioactive nitric oxide and other nitrogen reactive species during hypoxic conditions [35]. Both AG and SNC-121 treatment reduced the amount of nitrates-nitrites significantly in the glaucomatous eyes. As expected, SNC-121-mediated reduction in nitrates-nitrites was reversed by the δ-opioid-receptor antagonist, naltrindole. These data suggested that SNC-121-mediated reduction in nitrates-nitrites was due to δ-opioid-receptor-activation. It is important to emphasize that naltrindole treatment potentiated the levels of nitrate-nitrite production in both normal and glaucomatous retinas, suggesting that an endogenous tone of δ-opioid-receptor-activation is required to control endogenous levels of nitric oxide.

Nitrotyrosine is identified as an indicator or marker of cell damage, inflammation, and nitric oxide production. In general, oxidative stress increases the production of superoxide (O_2^-) and nitric oxide forming $ONOO^-$ (peroxynitrite). Under pathophysiological conditions, iNOS synthesizes excessive quantities of nitric oxide, which combines chemically with superoxide to form the highly reactive and destructive peroxynitrite [36]. Peroxynitrite causes the nitrosylation of cellular proteins, lipids, and DNA, which triggers apoptosis and ultimately cell death [37]. It is difficult to determine the production of peroxynitrite, usually nitrotyrosination of proteins is a detectable marker for peroxynitrite$^-$. Our data demonstrate that nitrotyrosination was increased in response to glaucomatous injury and δ-opioid-receptor-activation significantly reduced the nitrotyrosination in glaucomatous eyes.

In summary, the findings of the present study support the notion that nitric oxide plays a detrimental role during glaucomatous injury and inhibition of nitric oxide provides RGC neuroprotection. Furthermore, the activation of δ-opioid receptors regulates the iNOS activity/expression that will lead to the attenuation of nitric oxide production and rescue RGCs from glaucomatous injury.

Acknowledgments

The authors thankfully acknowledge Dr. Luanna Bartholomew (MUSC-SEI) for critical review of the manuscript.

Author Contributions

Conceived and designed the experiments: SH. Performed the experiments: SH YA SS AA MH. Analyzed the data: SH. Contributed reagents/materials/analysis tools: SH. Contributed to the writing of the manuscript: SH.

References

1. Quigley HA (1999) Neuronal death in glaucoma. Prog Retin Eye Res 18: 39–57.
2. Gupta N, Weinreb RN (1997) New definitions of glaucoma. Curr Opin Ophthalmol 8: 38–41.
3. Kass MA, Heuer DK, Higginbotham EJ, Johnson CA, Keltner JL, et al. (2002) The Ocular Hypertension Treatment Study: a randomized trial determines that topical ocular hypotensive medication delays or prevents the onset of primary open-angle glaucoma. Arch Ophthalmol 120: 701–713; discussion 829–730.
4. Lichter PR, Musch DC, Gillespie BW, Guire KE, Janz NK, et al. (2001) Interim clinical outcomes in the Collaborative Initial Glaucoma Treatment Study comparing initial treatment randomized to medications or surgery. Ophthalmology 108: 1943–1953.
5. Nakazawa T, Nakazawa C, Matsubara A, Noda K, Hisatomi T, et al. (2006) Tumor necrosis factor-alpha mediates oligodendrocyte death and delayed retinal ganglion cell loss in a mouse model of glaucoma. J Neurosci 26: 12633–12641.
6. Zhou H, Li XM, Meinkoth J, Pittman RN (2000) Akt regulates cell survival and apoptosis at a postmitochondrial level. J Cell Biol 151: 483–494.
7. Abdul Y, Akhter N, Husain S (2013) Delta-opioid agonist SNC-121 protects retinal ganglion cell function in a chronic ocular hypertensive rat model. Invest Ophthalmol Vis Sci 54: 1816–1828.
8. Tezel G, Li LY, Patil RV, Wax MB (2001) TNF-alpha and TNF-alpha receptor-1 in the retina of normal and glaucomatous eyes. Invest Ophthalmol Vis Sci 42: 1787–1794.
9. Fuchs C, Forster V, Balse E, Sahel JA, Picaud S, et al. (2005) Retinal-cell-conditioned medium prevents TNF-alpha-induced apoptosis of purified ganglion cells. Invest Ophthalmol Vis Sci 46: 2983–2991.
10. McKinnon SJ, Lehman DM, Tahzib NG, Ransom NL, Reitsamer HA, et al. (2002) Baculoviral IAP repeat-containing-4 protects optic nerve axons in a rat glaucoma model. Mol Ther 5: 780–787.
11. Reichstein D, Ren L, Filippopoulos T, Mittag T, Danias J (2007) Apoptotic retinal ganglion cell death in the DBA/2 mouse model of glaucoma. Exp Eye Res 84: 13–21.
12. Quigley HA, McKinnon SJ, Zack DJ, Pease ME, Kerrigan-Baumrind LA, et al. (2000) Retrograde axonal transport of BDNF in retinal ganglion cells is blocked by acute IOP elevation in rats. Invest Ophthalmol Vis Sci 41: 3460–3466.
13. Pease ME, McKinnon SJ, Quigley HA, Kerrigan-Baumrind LA, Zack DJ (2000) Obstructed axonal transport of BDNF and its receptor TrkB in experimental glaucoma. Invest Ophthalmol Vis Sci 41: 764–774.
14. Neufeld AH, Hernandez MR, Gonzalez M (1997) Nitric oxide synthase in the human glaucomatous optic nerve head. Arch Ophthalmol 115: 497–503.
15. Neufeld AH, Sawada A, Becker B (1999) Inhibition of nitric-oxide synthase 2 by aminoguanidine provides neuroprotection of retinal ganglion cells in a rat model of chronic glaucoma. Proc Natl Acad Sci U S A 96: 9944–9948.
16. Shareef S, Sawada A, Neufeld AH (1999) Isoforms of nitric oxide synthase in the optic nerves of rat eyes with chronic moderately elevated intraocular pressure. Invest Ophthalmol Vis Sci 40: 2884–2891.
17. Anderson DR (1969) Ultrastructure of human and monkey lamina cribrosa and optic nerve head. Arch Ophthalmol 82: 800–814.
18. Varela HJ, Hernandez MR (1997) Astrocyte responses in human optic nerve head with primary open-angle glaucoma. J Glaucoma 6: 303–313.
19. Neufeld AH, Shareef S, Pena J (2000) Cellular localization of neuronal nitric oxide synthase (NOS-1) in the human and rat retina. J Comp Neurol 416: 269–275.
20. Dortch-Carnes J, Russell K (2007) Morphine-stimulated nitric oxide release in rabbit aqueous humor. Exp Eye Res 84: 185–190.
21. Dortch-Carnes J, Russell KR (2006) Morphine-induced reduction of intraocular pressure and pupil diameter: role of nitric oxide. Pharmacology 77: 17–24.
22. Sugiyama T, Oku H, Ikari S, Ikeda T (2000) Effect of nitric oxide synthase inhibitor on optic nerve head circulation in conscious rabbits. Invest Ophthalmol Vis Sci 41: 1149–1152.
23. Dawson VL, Dawson TM, Bartley DA, Uhl GR, Snyder SH (1993) Mechanisms of nitric oxide-mediated neurotoxicity in primary brain cultures. J Neurosci 13: 2651–2661.
24. Dawson VL, Dawson TM (1998) Nitric oxide in neurodegeneration. Prog Brain Res 118: 215–229.
25. Libby RT, Howell GR, Pang IH, Savinova OV, Mehalow AK, et al. (2007) Inducible nitric oxide synthase, Nos2, does not mediate optic neuropathy and retinopathy in the DBA/2J glaucoma model. BMC Neurosci 8: 108.
26. Pang IH, Johnson EC, Jia L, Cepurna WO, Shepard AR, et al. (2005) Evaluation of inducible nitric oxide synthase in glaucomatous optic neuropathy and pressure-induced optic nerve damage. Invest Ophthalmol Vis Sci 46: 1313–1321.
27. Husain S, Abdul Y, Crosson CE (2012) Preservation of retina ganglion cell function by morphine in a chronic ocular-hypertensive rat model. Invest Ophthalmol Vis Sci 53: 4289–4298.
28. Liu B, Neufeld AH (2000) Expression of nitric oxide synthase-2 (NOS-2) in reactive astrocytes of the human glaucomatous optic nerve head. Glia 30: 178–186.
29. Sennlaub F, Courtois Y, Goureau O (2002) Inducible nitric oxide synthase mediates retinal apoptosis in ischemic proliferative retinopathy. J Neurosci 22: 3987–3993.
30. Neufeld AH, Kawai S, Das S, Vora S, Gachie E, et al. (2002) Loss of retinal ganglion cells following retinal ischemia: the role of inducible nitric oxide synthase. Exp Eye Res 75: 521–528.
31. Geyer O, Almog J, Lupu-Meiri M, Lazar M, Oron Y (1995) Nitric oxide synthase inhibitors protect rat retina against ischemic injury. FEBS Lett 374: 399–402.

32. Koeberle PD, Ball AK (1999) Nitric oxide synthase inhibition delays axonal degeneration and promotes the survival of axotomized retinal ganglion cells. Exp Neurol 158: 366–381.
33. Yang Y, Xia X, Zhang Y, Wang Q, Li L, et al. (2009) delta-Opioid receptor activation attenuates oxidative injury in the ischemic rat brain. BMC Biol 7: 55.
34. Goyagi T, Toung TJ, Kirsch JR, Traystman RJ, Koehler RC, et al. (2003) Neuroprotective kappa-opioid receptor agonist BRL 52537 attenuates ischemia-evoked nitric oxide production in vivo in rats. Stroke 34: 1533–1538.
35. Lundberg JO, Weitzberg E, Gladwin MT (2008) The nitrate-nitrite-nitric oxide pathway in physiology and therapeutics. Nat Rev Drug Discov 7: 156–167.
36. Beckman JS, Koppenol WH (1996) Nitric oxide, superoxide, and peroxynitrite: the good, the bad, and ugly. Am J Physiol 271: C1424–1437.
37. Muijsers RB, Folkerts G, Henricks PA, Sadeghi-Hashjin G, Nijkamp FP (1997) Peroxynitrite: a two-faced metabolite of nitric oxide. Life Sci 60: 1833–1845.

14

Valproic Acid and Fatalities in Children: A Review of Individual Case Safety Reports in VigiBase

Kristina Star[1]*, I. Ralph Edwards[1], Imti Choonara[2]

1 Uppsala Monitoring Centre, WHO Collaborating Centre for International Drug Monitoring, Uppsala, Sweden, 2 Academic Division of Child Health, University of Nottingham, Derbyshire Children's Hospital, Nottingham, United Kingdom

Abstract

Introduction: Valproic acid is an effective first line drug for the treatment of epilepsy. Hepatotoxicity is a rare and potentially fatal adverse reaction for this medicine.

Objective: Firstly to characterise valproic acid reports on children with fatal outcome and secondly to determine reporting over time of hepatotoxicity with fatal outcome.

Methods: Individual case safety reports (ICSRs) for children ≤17 years with valproic acid and fatal outcome were retrieved from the WHO Global ICSR database, VigiBase, in June 2013. Reports were classified into hepatotoxic reactions or other reactions. Shrinkage observed-to-expected ratios were used to explore the relative reporting trend over time and for patient age. The frequency of polytherapy, i.e. reports with more than one antiepileptic medicine, was investigated.

Results: There have been 268 ICSRs with valproic acid and fatal outcome in children, reported from 25 countries since 1977. A total of 156 fatalities were reported with hepatotoxicity, which has been continuously and disproportionally reported over time. There were 31 fatalities with pancreatitis. Other frequently reported events were coma/encephalopathy, seizures, respiratory disorders and coagulopathy. Hepatotoxicity was disproportionally and most commonly reported in children aged 6 years and under (104/156 reports) but affected children of all ages. Polytherapy was significantly more frequently reported for valproic acid with fatal outcome (58%) compared with non-fatal outcome (34%).

Conclusion: Hepatotoxicity remains a considerable problem. The risk appears to be greatest in young children (6 years and below) but can occur at any age. Polytherapy is commonly reported and seems to be a risk factor for hepatotoxicity, pancreatitis and other serious adverse drug reactions with valproic acid.

Editor: Hari K Koul, Louisiana State University Health Sciences center, United States of America

Funding: The authors have no support or funding to report.

Competing Interests: Kristina Star and Imti Choonara have declared that no competing interests exist relevant for this study. I. Ralph Edwards has provided expert testimony relating to valproic acid and fetal damage.

* Email: Kristina.Star@who-umc.org

Introduction

Valproic acid is a widely used antiepileptic drug (AED) that is highly effective both in adults and children. It is one of the first line drugs for the treatment of epilepsy. It was first used in Europe in 1968 and in the USA in 1978 [1]. The most frequent adverse drug reactions (ADRs) of valproic acid include somnolence, weight gain, fatigue and headache [2]. The most serious ADRs include hepatotoxicity and pancreatitis, both of which can be fatal.

The first case reports of hepatotoxicity following the use of valproic acid were in the late seventies [3,4]. In 1987 a comprehensive review of 37 cases of fatal hepatotoxicity in the USA occurring in patients receiving valproic acid between 1978 and 1984 was carried out [5]. This comprehensive review by Dreifuss identified three major risk factors. The risk was greatest in children under the age of three years, in patients on polytherapy and those with signs of developmental delay [5]. A year later, Scheffner described the deaths of 16 children in Germany [6]. Eleven of these children were on polytherapy and 11 had developmental delay. Only two of the 16 children, however, were under the age of three years. In 1989 Dreifuss again reviewed the US data and described a significant reduction in mortality associated with valproic acid in the USA and suggested that more rational prescribing in terms of using valproic acid as monotherapy had resulted in decreased mortality [7]. Other rare ADRs of valproic acid that may result in death include pancreatitis [8].

In a British review of suspected ADRs and fatalities in children, valproic acid was the AED most frequently reported with a fatality [9]. We were therefore interested in characterising suspected ADRs with fatal outcome for valproic acid reported worldwide and to determine whether hepatotoxicity with fatal outcome was still reported as a considerable problem following the guidance suggested by Dreifuss.

Methods

The WHO Collaborating Centre for International Drug Monitoring in Uppsala, Sweden, i.e. the Uppsala Monitoring

Centre (UMC), receives individual case safety reports (ICSRs) of suspected ADRs from national pharmacovigilance centres around the world. The reports are stored in the WHO Global ICSR database, VigiBase [10]. The database is an appropriate source to retrieve information on rare ADRs particularly in subpopulations such as in children because of its worldwide coverage [11]. More than 8 million ICSRs from more than 100 countries had been compiled in VigiBase up to June 2013.

ICSRs for children (age 1 month to 17 years) recorded with valproic acid (suspected or interacting), according to the preferred base in the WHO Drug Dictionary Enhanced, were extracted from VigiBase containing data up to June 2013. Fatalities were defined as reports with adverse reactions recorded with outcome 'died', or reports coded with a term indicating death (e.g. 'Sudden death' or 'Death'), or with the seriousness criteria classified as 'death', or recorded with a post-mortem code.

Suspected duplicate reports were excluded by using an automated screening method applied to VigiBase data and previously described in detail [12]. A manual screening for additional duplicates was subsequently performed. However, duplicate reports could still remain, especially when containing very little data. Reports specified as being sent by lawyers or recorded as originating from published literature cases were excluded from the analysis. Reports originating from the US are not coded to be literature reports or not, therefore these types of reports could still remain in the data retrieved for this study. The restriction of using reports 1 month of age and above was applied to reduce the number of reports relating to maternal exposure. A manual review to remove reports with congenital anomalies resulting from maternal exposure to valproic acid was also performed. Reports with reactions that were most unlikely to be the cause of death were also excluded.

Reports were grouped into being related to hepatotoxicity or not. Several suspected ADRs can be listed on a report and when any of the reported terms was subordinated to the Medical Dictionary for Regulatory Activities (MedDRA) 'Hepatic and hepatobiliary disorders' (High-level group term), 'Liver function analyses' (High-level term), 'Coma hepatic', 'Hepatic encephalopathy' (Preferred terms), the report was classified as related to hepatotoxicity. A manual review of all terms for each report was also performed resulting in three additional reports with hyperammonaemia and encephalopathy to be classified to the group of hepatotoxic reports.

The case series considered in this study with valproic acid and fatal outcome in the child age group were:

- All fatal reports with and without hepatotoxic events.
- Fatal reports with hepatotoxic events (as previously defined).
- Fatal reports without hepatotoxic events.

To define the timing of an event in this study, the onset date of the event was used if completed on the report. If this was not available the date was estimated, using firstly the suspected drug stop date, or otherwise the date of when the national centre received the report, or lastly the date of first VigiBase entry. Reporting by time of the event (or estimated as described previously) was investigated. The first time period encompassed

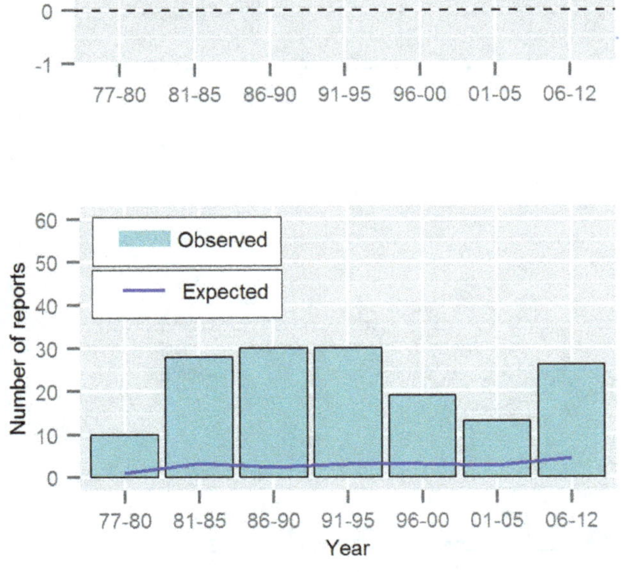

Figure 1. Reporting over time for valproic acid and fatalities *with* hepatotoxicity; displaying the Information Component (IC) and its 95% credibility interval, observed and expected number of reports from VigiBase. The timing of the report is based on the estimated onset date of the event.

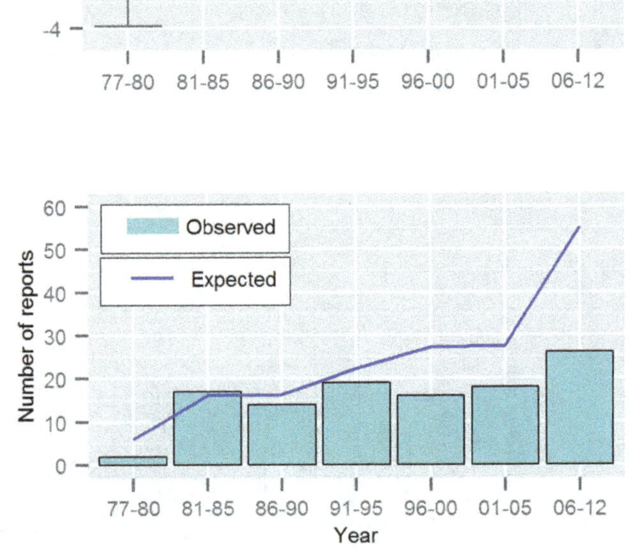

Figure 2. Reporting over time for valproic acid and fatalities *without* hepatotoxicity; displaying the Information Component (IC) and its 95% credibility interval, observed and expected number of reports from VigiBase. The timing of the report is based on the estimated onset date of the event.

Table 1. Overall reporting of valproic acid with fatal outcome in children before and after 1990.

Year of reaction	No. reports with valproic acid and fatal outcome	Mean No. reports with valproic acid and fatal outcome per year	No. reports with valproic acid	Mean No. reports with valproic acid per year
1977–1990	101	7.2	1702	122
1991–2012	167	7.6	5058	230
1977–2012	**268**	**7.4**	**6760**	**188**

the period 1977–1990 when hepatotoxicity was first recognised and three key reviews describing risk factors of hepatotoxicity were published [5–7]. The second time period was 1991 up to June 2013.

Relative reporting trends were graphically displayed by using shrinkage observed-to-expected ratios on a logarithmic scale [13,14]. The observed value consisted of the number of reports within each case series as defined above and grouped by year of age or time period. The expected number was computed based on the total number of reports for valproic acid, the total number of the event; i.e. fatalities with hepatotoxicity or fatalities without hepatotoxicity; and the total number of reports for the children (any drug or event), by year of age or time period. The measure is referred to as the Information Component (IC), which is given with its 95% credibility interval (IC025), where the lower positive value is used to highlight disproportional reporting. The observed and expected numbers are also included in the graphs. Non-cumulative reporting for 5-year time periods and for each yearly patient age is displayed.

Reports with more than one reported AED (i.e., reports listing AEDs in addition to valproic acid) were considered cases of polytherapy in this study. The co-reported drugs could be assigned by the original reporter to be suspect, interacting or concomitant. Reporting of polytherapy for the three case series with fatal outcome were compared with corresponding groups of non-fatal reports for valproic acid using log shrinkage odds ratios.

Ethics statement

De-identified individual case safety reports have been routinely collected as a public health service internationally since 1968, through the WHO Programme for International Drug Monitoring. The protection of the identity of the patient and the reporter has been routine from the outset.

Results

After exclusion of literature reports (n = 42), reports concerning lawyers (n = 1), suspected duplicates (n = 63), maternal exposure (n = 8) and non-fatal events (n = 5), 268 reports remained and were analysed. Reports had been received from 25 countries worldwide from 1977 until the end of 2012. Ages ranged from 2 months to 17 years, and 54% of the reports with a recorded patient sex

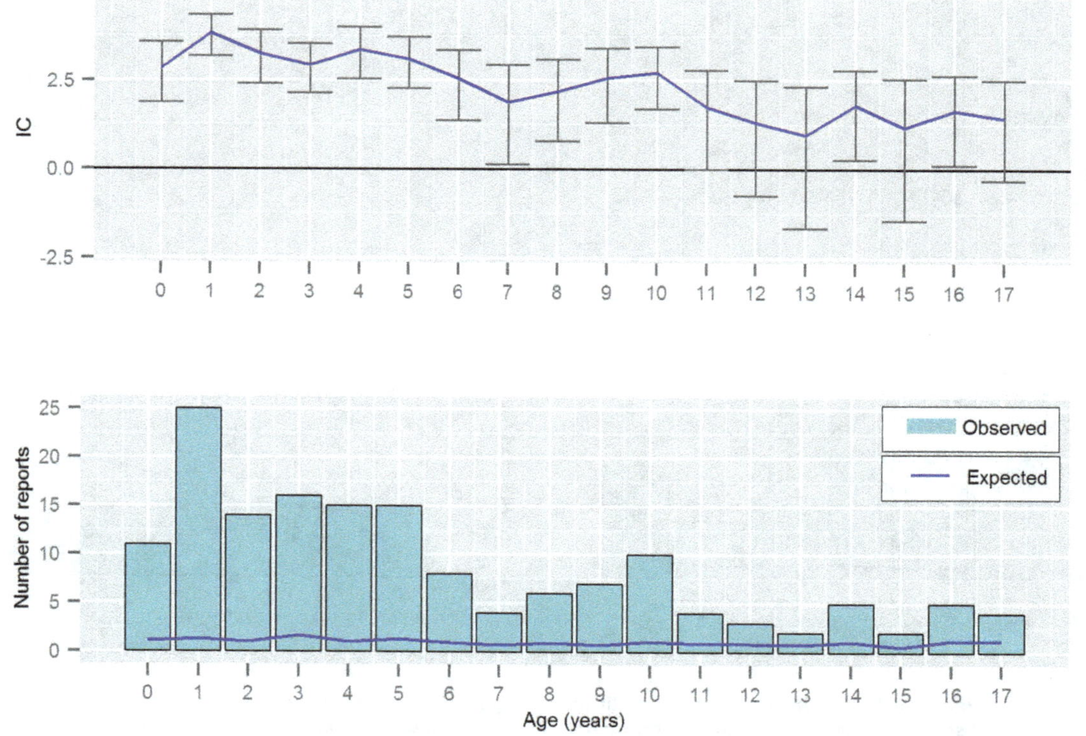

Figure 3. Reporting by patient age in years for valproic acid and fatalities *with* hepatotoxicity; displaying the Information Component (IC) and its 95% credibility interval, observed and expected number of reports from VigiBase.

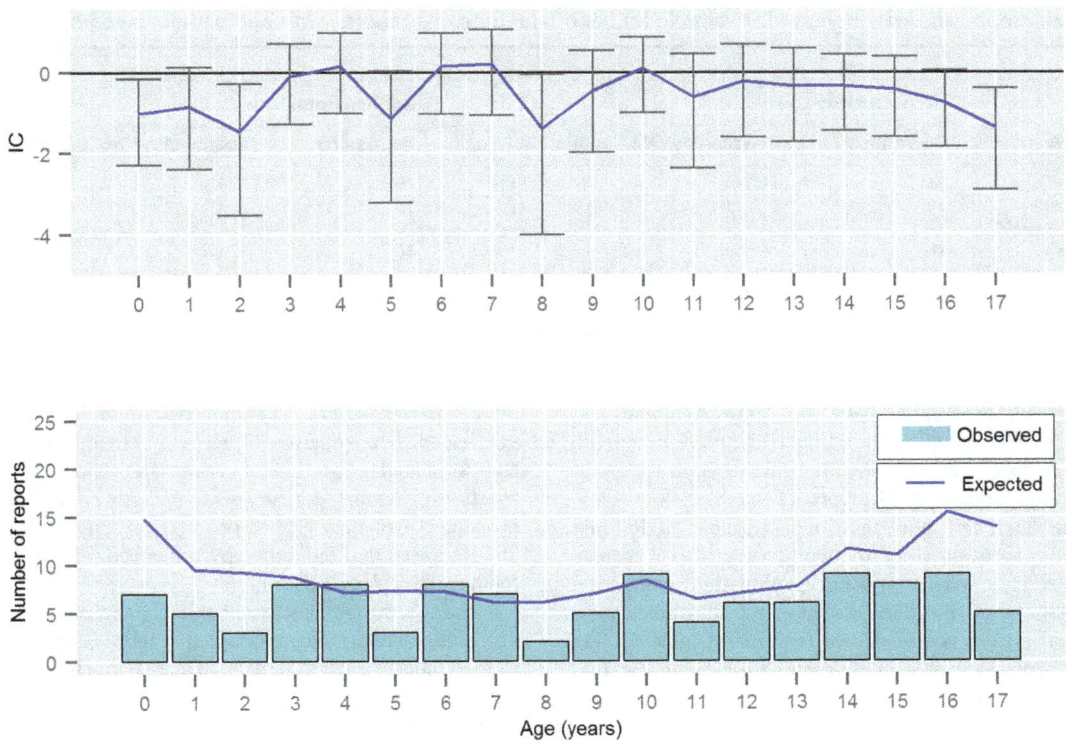

Figure 4. Reporting by patient age in years for valproic acid and fatalities *without* hepatotoxicity; displaying the Information Component (IC) and its 95% credibility interval, observed and expected number of reports from VigiBase.

concerned boys. In 156 reports the fatalities were recorded with hepatotoxicity, of which hepatic failure, hepatic necrosis, abnormal hepatic function and hepatocellular injury were most frequently reported. The median number of days from start of valproic acid to onset of reaction (time-to-onset) for the group with hepatotoxic reactions was 66 days (IQR: 38.75–121.5) and for the group without hepatotoxic reactions specified, the median time-to-onset was 130 days (IQR: 54–478). The median time-to-onset is based on reports where dates needed for the calculation had been recorded.

The number of fatalities each year has ranged from one to 24 reports. The greatest number of reported fatalities occurred in 1983 (16 cases of hepatotoxicity and eight others). The mean number of fatalities reported per year was 7.4 reports (Table 1) with little change before and after 1990. Between 1977 and 1990, 68 fatalities with hepatotoxicity were reported. There were 88 fatalities reported with hepatotoxicity in the second time period (1991–2012). However, the overall mean reporting of valproic acid had increased from 122 per year to 230 after 1990 (Table 1). Fatalities with hepatotoxicity have been disproportionally reported throughout the complete time period (Figure 1). Non-hepatotoxic fatalities have been evenly reported over time, although less frequently than what was expected in VigiBase (Figure 2).

Hepatotoxicity was disproportionally reported for almost all ages included in this study (Figure 3), whilst reports without hepatotoxicity were not (Figure 4). Hepatotoxicity was most commonly reported in children aged 6 years and under (104/156 reports). The median ages and frequency of AED polytherapy before and after 1990 are illustrated in Table 2. The table includes both fatalities with hepatotoxicity and those without hepatotoxicity. The relationship between polytherapy and age is shown more completely in Table 3.

In 155 (58%) reports, one or more AEDs were reported alongside valproic acid. A total of 28 different AEDs were reported and the ten most frequently reported AEDs in the hepatotoxic and non-hepatotoxic groups are listed in Table 4. Phenobarbital,

Table 2. Overall reporting of valproic acid and fatal outcome reports in children with and without hepatotoxicity before and after 1990.

Type of reaction	Year of reaction	No. reports	Mean No. reports per year	Median age (years)	IQR age (years)	Polytherapy* No. reports (%)
Hepatotoxicity	1977–1990	68	4.9	4	2–8	45 (66)
	1991–2012	88	4.0	5	2–9.25	48 (55)
Not hepatotoxicity	1977–1990	33	2.4	6	2–7	20 (61)
	1991–2012	79	3.6	11	6.5–14.5	42 (53)

*Reports recorded with more than one suspected, interacting or concomitant antiepileptic medicine.

Table 3. Age groups and polytherapy* for valproic acid and fatal outcome reports, with and without hepatoxicity.

	Hepatotoxicity		Not hepatotoxicity	
Age groups (years)	**No. reports**	**Polytherapy* No. reports (%)**	**No. reports**	**Polytherapy* No. reports (%)**
0 to 2	50	34 (68)	15	7 (47)
3 to 6	54	34 (63)	27	17 (63)
7 to 11	31	14 (45)	27	17 (63)
12 to 17	21	11 (52)	43	21 (49)

*Reports recorded with more than one suspected, interacting or concomitant antiepileptic drug.

phenytoin and carbamazepine were the most frequently co-reported AEDs. Polytherapy was significantly more frequently reported for the three case series with fatalities contrasted with corresponding non-fatal group of reports (Table 5).

Many of the cases had more than one suspected ADR listed. Among the 268 reports, the most frequently reported events (apart from hepatotoxicity) were coma/encephalopathy, convulsion, pancreatitis, respiratory disorders, coagulopathy, thrombocytopenia and cardiac arrest/ventricular arrhythmias (Table 6). The second largest group consisted of children who were in a coma/ encephalopathy, of which 35 of the 49 reports were co-reported with a hepatotoxic reaction. A large group of reports involved children who died in status epilepticus or following a seizure. It is unlikely that these were ADRs as such, but rather that the drug was ineffective. A number of events, not usually associated with valproic acid were reported: metabolic acidosis, disseminated intravascular coagulation, hyperammonaemia, apnoea, toxic epidermal necrolysis (TEN) and aplastic anaemia. Apart from the last two, the others seemed to be events complicating seriously ill patients.

Discussion

Valproic acid with fatal outcome and hepatotoxicity has continuously been reported disproportionally since 1977. Polytherapy was significantly more frequently reported in fatalities than for non-fatalities and appears to remain as a considerable risk factor for serious ADRs, including hepatotoxicity. The younger age groups reported with hepatotoxicity had the highest proportions of co-reported AEDs, suggesting that these ages are particularly vulnerable to polytherapy. This is in keeping with the previous reviews of fatal hepatotoxicity in association with valproic acid [5,6]. In the 70s, many patients with epilepsy (adults and children) received polytherapy [15]. A prospective study in adults in the late 1970s showed that monotherapy was effective for epilepsy and also reduced the risk of ADRs [15].

Although the greatest number of fatal cases of hepatotoxicity occurred in children aged between 1 and 2 years (Figure 1), there were a considerable number of cases in children of all ages, especially in children aged six years and below. It has been suggested that young children (less than 7.5 years) have an increased risk of hepatotoxicity due to their abnormal metabolism of valproic acid [16]. Clinicians need to be aware that the risk of fatal hepatotoxicity appears to be greatest in young children (six years and below) but that it can occur at any age. This corresponds with two recent reviews of German fatal and non-fatal cases where the risk of valproic acid associated hepatotoxicity was not restricted to infants [17,18].

Unfortunately, for many reports there was insufficient information to be certain of the full nature of the suspected ADR (coma, convulsion and cardiac/respiratory arrest). Fatalities reported with pancreatitis occurred in 31 reports. Pancreatitis was first reported in 1979 and subsequently there have been several reviews and case series [19,20]. One study, in a single hospital, identified 22 children with pancreatitis (diagnosed by using strict criteria) over a 10-year period [21]. This suggests that many cases of valproic toxicity resulting in pancreatitis are not reported. Polytherapy was not identified as a risk factor in any of the previous case series or

Table 4. The ten most frequently co-reported antiepileptic drugs with valproic acid and fatal outcome in children.*

Drug	Total No. reports	No. reports with hepatotoxicity	No. reports *without* hepatotoxicity
Phenobarbital	54	44	10
Phenytoin	50	38	12
Carbamazepine	45	28	17
Clonazepam	26	17	9
Diazepam	19	7	12
Lamotrigine	11	6	5
Clobazam	7	3	4
Lorazepam	7	6	1
Topiramate	6	3	3
Levetiracetam	5	2	3

*Numbers do not add up, since more than one antiepileptic drug (AED) could be recorded on one report. AEDs could have been recorded as suspected, interacting or concomitant medicines on the reports.

Table 5. Valproic acid reports with polytherapy* and fatal outcome were contrasted with non-fatal outcome reports in children, grouped by reports with or without hepatotoxicity, or with any event.

	Valproic acid and fatal outcome		Valproic acid *without* fatal outcome		Log shrinkage odds ratios (OR)**	
	No. reports	Polytherapy* No. reports (%)	No. reports	Polytherapy* No. reports (%)	OR	OR005
Hepatotoxicity	156	93 (60)	695	323 (46)	0.76	0.35
Not hepatotoxicity	112	62 (55)	5755	1892 (33)	1.32	0.81
Any event	268	155 (58)	6450	2215 (34)	1.38	1.07

*Reports recorded with more than one suspected, interacting or concomitant antiepileptic drug.
**The lower level of the 99% credibility interval for the log shrinkage odds ratio (OR005) was considered significant when above zero.

reviews. The majority of patients with pancreatitis in a review of the literature, however, were receiving polytherapy [19]. In relation to reports in VigiBase, polytherapy could be a risk factor for pancreatitis.

Coagulopathies secondary to valproic acid are thought to occur in up to 4% of children [22]. Thrombocytopenia is thought to occur in between 5 and 40% of children receiving valproate [23,24]. In the vast majority of cases, the coagulopathies are minor and result in no clinical problems. Factors associated with increased clinical severity of the coagulopathies are undetermined and needs further investigation.

Both aplastic anaemia and TEN are extremely rare ADRs in patients receiving AEDs. Aplastic anaemia has been reported in adults receiving valproic acid [25]. It has only previously been reported in paediatric patients in isolated case reports [23,26,27]. Similarly, Stevens-Johnson syndrome (SJS) and TEN have predominantly been reported in adults [28] with only isolated cases described in children on valproic acid [29]. The six cases with SJS or TEN in our study originated from six separate countries and were co-reported with phenobarbital (n = 2); carbamazepine; lamotrigine plus acetazolamide; paroxetine; and carbamazepine plus phenytoin. In an overall review of VigiBase reports (any age and with any outcome), a disproportionally higher reporting frequency was noted for children compared with adults for valproic acid and aplastic anaemia. A higher number of reports for aplastic anaemia in children with fatal outcome were also noted (5/8 cases were children).

Table 6. The most frequently reported adverse reactions for valproic acid with fatal outcome in children.

Adverse reaction	No. reports			Median age (years)	Polytherapy** No. reports (%)
	Total	Hep*	Non-Hep*		
Hepatotoxicity	156	156	0	4	93 (60)
Coma states/Disturbances in consciousness/Encephalopathies	49	35	14	5	31 (63)
Seizures	42	28	14	7.5	27 (64)
Pancreatitis	31	11	20	9	16 (52)
Respiratory disorders (apnoea, respiratory depression/failure/arrest)	27	10	17	7	17 (63)
Coagulopathy/Disseminated intravascular coagulation	25	19	6	7	19 (76)
Thrombocytopenias	21	10	11	4	14 (67)
Cardiac arrest/Ventricular arrhythmias	18	5	13	11.5	8 (44)
Infections (sepsis, pneumonia)	18	10	8	8	14 (78)
Anaemias (incl. aplastic) and marrow depression	13	3	10	5	10 (77)
Renal disorders (excl nephropathies)	12	7	5	7	9 (75)
Overdose (intentional/accidental/suicide)	11	0	11	12	2 (18)
Acidosis/Metabolic acidosis/Lactic acidosis	10	6	4	6	7 (70)
Brain oedema/Increased intracranial pressure	10	6	4	7	4 (40)
Haemorrhages (incl. cerebral)	7	3	4	7	3 (43)
Gastrointestinal haemorrhages	6	4	2	8	3 (50)
Toxic epidermal necrolysis/Stevens-Johnson syndrome	6	0	6	10	5 (83)
Hyperammonaemia	4	4	0	3.5	2 (50)

Numbers do not add up, since one report can be recorded with more than one reaction.
*'Hep' are reports with hepatotoxicity events recorded and 'Non-Hep' reports are without hepatotoxicity events recorded.
**Reports recorded with more than one suspected, interacting or concomitant antiepileptic drug.

This study presents the *reporting* patterns with its caveat for valproic acid and children with fatal outcome, see further Appendix S1 [30]. Reports in VigiBase come from a variety of sources and the likelihood that the reported suspected adverse reaction is drug-related is not the same in all cases. VigiBase reports are stored in structured format with basic information about the patient, the drug and adverse reaction. Narratives describing the case in more detail are rarely available electronically. In this study we only used the VigiBase data available in structured format, therefore case details to confirm a diagnosis or to assess the likelihood of a causal relationship between a drug and event was limited.

Several of the most commonly co-reported AEDs in this study can in themselves be associated with liver damage. As a consequence, there is uncertainty as to whether it was valproic acid or the co-reported drug that induced the reaction. To reduce this uncertainty, our report extraction generated only reports where valproic acid had been considered the suspected drug by the reporter.

Another limitation of the data is that co-reported AEDs may have been omitted on the report, which could have resulted in an underestimation of polytherapy in this study. However, we also made an assumption that the recorded AEDs with missing treatment dates had been used concomitantly with valproic acid so we may have overestimated the frequency of polytherapy.

There may have been a reporting bias towards reporting more young children with hepatotoxicity as their susceptibility to hepatotoxicity had been reported previously [5]. The problem of valproic acid and hepatotoxicity were introduced in the scientific literature towards the end of 1980. This might have introduced a bias of increased reporting around this time. The decreased relative reporting after 1996 might therefore be an artefact explained by unusually higher reporting before this time period. The decreased relative reporting frequency could also reflect that the problem is occurring less because of more careful prescribing.

We are unable to comment on the relative risk of specific ADRs or fatalities in relation to valproic acid use because we do not have information regarding the denominator, i.e. the number of prescriptions for valproic acid for children with epilepsy worldwide. Instead we used the overall reporting in VigiBase to generate a relative frequency for our report series. Even if we could have accessed number of the worldwide use of valproic acid in the child population, we still would not have been able to generate a reliable risk estimate using our data because of the known problem of underreporting of spontaneous reports [31,32]. We know that valproic acid is the most frequently prescribed AED for children in several countries in Europe [33,34] and the second most frequently prescribed AED for children in the USA, Cuba and Egypt [35-37]. Although the number of fatalities reported is small in relation to the number of likely prescriptions, one again needs to recognise that the vast majority of ADRs are unreported or unsuspected [31,32]. This, unfortunately, includes serious as well as minor ADRs.

Risk factors for hepatotoxicity, pancreatitis and other serious ADRs in association with valproic acid apart from polytherapy, young age and metabolic disorders (not considered in this study) need to be further explored. Is there for example a genetic disposition in children and adults that make them more vulnerable for hepatotoxicity. Until we know more, clinicians need to be aware of the risk of rare, serious ADRs, and identify and act on early signs of hepatotoxicity [38]. They also need to recognise that polytherapy appears to be a major risk factor for many of the serious ADRs in association with valproic acid.

Epilogue

As parents ourselves, we can understand that this paper might cause concerns in parents of children, or children themselves, using valproic acid. However, serious adverse reactions are rare, especially those leading to fatalities, and the benefit of using an antiepileptic medicine (to prevent seizures with their own risk) almost certainly outweighs the risk of serious adverse reactions that we discuss here. **If you perceive unexpected changes in your child's health, particularly those symptoms noted in the product information leaflet/package insert, we encourage you to report these to your family physician.**

Supporting Information

Appendix S1 Caveat document: Accompanying statement to data released from the Uppsala Monitoring Centre, WHO Collaborating Centre for International Drug Monitoring.

Acknowledgments

The authors are indebted to the National Pharmacovigilance Centres that contribute data to VigiBase. The opinions and conclusions in this study are not necessarily those of the various centres or of the WHO. The authors give special thanks to Kristina Juhlin at the Uppsala Monitoring Centre for the computational support given to this study.

Author Contributions

Conceived and designed the experiments: IC KS. Performed the experiments: KS. Analyzed the data: KS IC IRE. Contributed reagents/materials/analysis tools: KS. Wrote the paper: KS IC IRE.

References

1. Colletti RB, Trainer TD, Krawisz BR (1986) Reversible valproate fulminant hepatic failure. J Pediatr Gastroenterol Nutr 5: 990–4.
2. Anderson M, Choonara I (2010) A systematic review of safety monitoring and drug toxicity in published randomised controlled trials of antiepileptic drugs in children over a 10-year period. Arch Dis Child 95: 731–8.
3. Donat JF, Bocchini JA Jr, Gonzalez E, Schwendimann RN (1979) Valproic acid and fatal hepatitis. Neurology 29: 273–4.
4. Suchy FJ, Balistreri WF, Buchino JJ, Sondheimer JM, Bates SR, et al. (1979) Acute hepatic failure associated with the use of sodium valproate. N Engl J Med 300: 962–6.
5. Dreifuss FE, Santilli N, Langer DH, Sweeney KP, Moline KA, et al. (1987) Valproic acid hepatic fatalities: a retrospective review. Neurology 37: 379–85.
6. Scheffner D, Konig S, Rauterberg-Ruland I, Kochen W, Hofmann WJ, et al. (1988) Fatal liver failure in 16 children with valproate therapy. Epilepsia 29: 530–42.
7. Dreifuss FE, Langer DH, Moline KA, Maxwell JE (1989) Valproic acid hepatic fatalities. II. US experience since 1984. Neurology 39: 201–7.
8. Grauso-Eby NL, Goldfarb O, Feldman-Winter LB, McAbee GN (2003) Acute pancreatitis in children from Valproic acid: case series and review. Pediatr Neurol 28: 145–8.
9. Clarkson A, Choonara I (2002) Surveillance for fatal suspected adverse drug reactions in the UK. Arch Dis Child 87: 462–6.
10. Lindquist M (2008) Vigibase, the WHO Global ICSR Database System: Basic Facts. Drug Information Journal 42: 409–19.
11. Star K, Noren GN, Nordin K, Edwards IR (2011) Suspected adverse drug reactions reported for children worldwide: an exploratory study using VigiBase. Drug Saf 34: 415–28.
12. Norén GN, Orre R, Bate A, Edwards IR (2007) Duplicate detection in adverse drug reaction surveillance. Data Mining and Knowledge Discovery 14: 305–28.
13. Norén GN, Hopstadius J, Bate A (2013) Shrinkage observed-to-expected ratios for robust and transparent large-scale pattern discovery. Stat Methods Med Res 22: 57–69.
14. Bate A, Lindquist M, Edwards IR, Olsson S, Orre R, et al. (1998) A Bayesian neural network method for adverse drug reaction signal generation. Eur J Clin Pharmacol 54: 315–21.

15. Shorvon SD, Chadwick D, Galbraith AW, Reynolds EH (1978) One drug for epilepsy. BMJ 1: 474–6.
16. Gopaul S, Farrell K, Abbott F (2003) Effects of age and polytherapy, risk factors of valproic acid (VPA) hepatotoxicity, on the excretion of thiol conjugates of (E)-2,4-diene VPA in people with epilepsy taking VPA. Epilepsia 44: 322–8.
17. Koenig SA, Buesing D, Longin E, Oehring R, Häussermann P, et al. (2006) Valproic acid-induced hepatopathy: Nine new fatalities in Germany from 1994 to 2003. Epilepsia 47: 2027–31.
18. Schmid MM, Freudenmann RW, Keller F, Connemann BJ, Hiemke C, et al. (2013) Non-fatal and fatal liver failure associated with valproic acid. Pharmacopsychiatry 46: 63–8.
19. Chapman SA, Wacksman GP, Patterson BD (2001) Pancreatitis associated with valproic acid: a review of the literature. Pharmacotherapy 21: 1549–60.
20. Sinclair DB, Berg M, Breault R (2004) Valproic acid-induced pancreatitis in childhood epilepsy: case series and review. J Child Neurol 19: 498–502.
21. Werlin SL, Fish DL (2006) The spectrum of valproic acid-associated pancreatitis. Pediatrics 118: 1660–3.
22. Gerstner T, Teich M, Bell N, Longin E, Dempfle CE, et al. (2006) Valproate-associated coagulopathies are frequent and variable in children. Epilepsia 47: 1136–43.
23. Acharya S, Bussel JB (2000) Hematologic toxicity of sodium valproate. J Pediatr Hematol Oncol 22: 62–5.
24. Kose G, Arhan E, Unal B, Ozaydin E, Guven A, et al. (2009) Valproate-associated coagulopathies in children during short-term treatment. J Child Neurol 24: 1493–8.
25. Handoko KB, Souverein PC, van Staa TP, Meyboom RH, Leufkens HG, et al. (2006) Risk of aplastic anemia in patients using antiepileptic drugs. Epilepsia 47: 1232–6.
26. Kishi T, Fujita N, Kawaguchi H, Ishimae M, Watanabe K, et al. (1994) Bone marrow suppression induced by high dose valproic acid. Arch Dis Child 71: 153–5.
27. Rajantie J, Kajosaari M, Ylitalo V (1992) Fatal pancytopenia during high-dose valproate monotherapy. Eur J Pediatr 151: 619.
28. Rzany B, Correia O, Kelly JP, Naldi L, Auquier A, et al. (1999) Risk of Stevens-Johnson syndrome and toxic epidermal necrolysis during first weeks of antiepileptic therapy: a case-control study. Study Group of the International Case Control Study on Severe Cutaneous Adverse Reactions. Lancet 353: 2190-4.
29. Koh MJ-A, Tay Y-K (2010) Stevens-Johnson syndrome and toxic epidermal necrolysis in Asian children. J AM ACAD DERMATOL 62: 54–60.
30. Uppsala Monitoring Centre. WHO Collaborating Centre for International Drug Monitoring. Caveat document. http://www.who-umc.org/graphics/25300.pdf. Accessed 26 Sep 2013.
31. Fletcher AP (1991) Spontaneous adverse drug reaction reporting vs event monitoring: a comparison. J R Soc Med 84: 341–4.
32. Hazell L, Shakir SA (2006) Under-reporting of adverse drug reactions: a systematic review. Drug Saf 29: 385–96.
33. Cvitanovic-Sojat L, Bielen I, Sruk A, Kosicek M, Planjar-Prvan M, et al. (2010) Social and medical care of preschool children with epilepsy in Croatia: population-based survey. Eur J Paediatr Neurol 14: 73–7.
34. Hsia Y, Neubert A, Sturkenboom MC, Murray ML, Verhamme KM, et al. (2010) Comparison of antiepileptic drug prescribing in children in three European countries. Epilepsia 51: 789–96.
35. Arencibia ZB, Leyva AL, Pena YM, Reyes AR, Napolez MA, et al. (2012) Access to antiepileptic drug therapy in children in Camaguey Province, Cuba. Int J Pharm Pract 20: 390–4.
36. Berg AT, Levy SR, Testa FM, Shinnar S (1999) Treatment of newly diagnosed pediatric epilepsy: a community-based study. Arch Pediatr Adolesc Med 153: 1267–71.
37. Talaat F, El-Rabbat M, Atef M, Shaker E, Mohammed H (2009) Prevalence of epilepsy in school children in El-Manyal Island. Egypt J Neurol Psychiatr Neurosurg 46: 19–32.
38. Electronic Medicines Compendium. Summary of Product Characteristics for Epilim Chronosphere. 2014; http://www.medicines.org.uk/emc/medicine/26144. Accessed July 09 2014.

15

Tissue MicroRNAs as Predictors of Outcome in Patients with Metastatic Colorectal Cancer Treated with First Line Capecitabine and Oxaliplatin with or without Bevacizumab

Mogens K. Boisen[1*], Christian Dehlendorff[2], Dorte Linnemann[3], Boye S. Nielsen[4], Jim S. Larsen[5], Kell Østerlind[6], Svend E. Nielsen[7], Line S. Tarpgaard[8], Camilla Qvortrup[8], Per Pfeiffer[8], Niels H. Holländer[9], Nina Keldsen[10], Torben F. Hansen[11], Brita B. Jensen[12,13], Estrid V. S. Høgdall[3], Benny V. Jensen[1], Julia S. Johansen[1,14]

1 Department of Oncology, Herlev University Hospital, Herlev, Denmark, 2 Statistics, Bioinformatics and Registry, Danish Cancer Society Research Center, Copenhagen, Denmark, 3 Department of Pathology, Herlev University Hospital, Herlev, Denmark, 4 Bioneer, Hørsholm, Denmark, 5 Department of Oncology, Roskilde Hospital, Roskilde, Denmark, 6 Department of Oncology, Rigshospitalet, Copenhagen, Denmark, 7 Department of Oncology and Palliation, Hillerød Hospital, Hillerød, Denmark, 8 Department of Oncology, Odense University Hospital, Odense, Denmark, 9 Department of Oncology, Næstved Hospital, Næstved, Denmark, 10 Department of Oncology, Herning Hospital, Herning, Denmark, 11 Department of Oncology, Vejle Hospital, Vejle, Denmark, 12 Department of Medicine, Queen Ingrid Hospital, Nuuk, Greenland, 13 Department of Oncology, Sydvestjysk Hospital, Esbjerg, Denmark, 14 Department of Medicine, Herlev University Hospital, Herlev, Denmark

Abstract

Purpose: We tested the hypothesis that expression of microRNAs (miRNAs) in cancer tissue can predict effectiveness of bevacizumab added to capecitabine and oxaliplatin (CAPEOX) in patients with metastatic colorectal cancer (mCRC).

Experimental Design: Patients with mCRC treated with first line CAPEOX and bevacizumab (CAPEOXBEV): screening (n = 212) and validation (n = 121) cohorts, or CAPEOX alone: control cohort (n = 127), were identified retrospectively and archival primary tumor samples were collected. Expression of 754 miRNAs was analyzed in the screening cohort using polymerase chain reaction (PCR) arrays and expression levels were related to time to disease progression (TTP) and overall survival (OS). Significant miRNAs from the screening study were analyzed in all three cohorts using custom PCR arrays. *In situ* hybridization (ISH) was done for selected miRNAs.

Results: In the screening study, 26 miRNAs were significantly correlated with outcome in multivariate analyses. Twenty-two miRNAs were selected for further study. Higher miR-664-3p expression and lower miR-455-5p expression were predictive of improved outcome in the CAPEOXBEV cohorts and showed a significant interaction with bevacizumab effectiveness. The effects were strongest for OS. Both miRNAs showed high expression in stromal cells. Higher expression of miR-196b-5p and miR-592 predicted improved outcome regardless of bevacizumab treatment, with similar effect estimates in all three cohorts.

Conclusions: We have identified potentially predictive miRNAs for bevacizumab effectiveness and additional miRNAs that could be related to chemotherapy effectiveness or prognosis in patients with mCRC. Our findings need further validation in large cohorts, preferably from completed randomized trials.

Editor: Ratna B. Ray, Saint Louis University, United States of America

Funding: This study was supported by an unrestricted grant from Roche Denmark (www.roche.dk), the Herlev Hospital Research Foundation (www.herlevhospital.dk), and a proof-of-concept grant from the Technical University of Denmark (www.dtu.dk). All grants were given to MKB alone, or to both MKB and JSJ. The funders had no role in study design, data collection and analysis, decision to publish, or preparation of the manuscript.

Competing Interests: The authors have read the journal's policy and the authors of this manuscript have the following competing interests: BVJ: Roche, consultant/advisory role; SEN: Roche, consultant/advisory role; PP: Roche, consultant/advisory role; JSJ: Roche, honoraria and research funding; MKB: Roche, research funding. JSJ and MKB are co-inventors on a patent-application related to the mentioned miRNAs. Patent application info: Name "Micrornas for prediction of treatment efficacy and prognosis of cancer patients"; Application number "PCT/DK2013/050015". BSN is employed by a commercial company (Bioneer).

* Email: mogens.karsboel.boisen@regionh.dk

Introduction

Colorectal cancer (CRC) is a leading cause of cancer-related mortality worldwide [1]. Most deaths occur as a result of the development of metastatic CRC (mCRC). Standard of care for patients with mCRC who cannot undergo radical resection of metastases is system chemotherapy with or without a targeted agent [2]. Bevacizumab is a monoclonal antibody that binds the ligand 'vascular endothelial growth factor' (VEGF-A) and thereby inhibits the ability of cancers to produce new blood vessels from existing vessels, a process called angiogenesis. Bevacizumab has demonstrated efficacy in patients with mCRC when used in combination with standard chemotherapy but the benefit is modest when used unselectively and bevacizumab adds significant toxicity and cost to the treatment [3–7]. Therefore, the identification of predictive biomarkers for bevacizumab has become a major goal of biomarker research in patients with mCRC. Due to its widespread adoption as a standard first- or second line treatment [8], the ability to individualize bevacizumab treatment would have a great impact on clinical practice. Numerous studies have investigated potential biomarkers in the form of RNA, DNA, or protein [9,10]. None has made it into the clinic. Currently, no commercially available test can identify patients who will benefit from bevacizumab.

MicroRNAs (miRNAs) are small, ~22 nucleotides long, non-coding RNAs involved in post-transcriptional regulation of gene expression. They have been intensely investigated as biomarkers in patients with cancer because their expression levels are dysregulated in cancer cells, they can influence cancer behavior, and they are relatively resistant to degradation in commonly used sampling media [11–16]. Several studies have identified dysregulation of miRNAs in CRC tumor tissue and in blood samples from patients with CRC; and some of the identified miRNAs were also associated with prognostic factors like depth of invasion, stage, and lymph node metastases [17]. Furthermore, important molecular features in CRC such as micro-satellite instability (MSI) and *BRAF* mutational status have been shown to be associated with distinct miRNA expression patterns [18]. Hence, there is a strong rationale for investigating the potential utility of miRNA expression as a predictive or prognostic biomarker in patients with CRC. To date, no published study has explored the predictive value of miRNA expression for bevacizumab effectiveness in a comprehensive manner.

We aimed to identify miRNAs that were predictive of outcome in patients with mCRC treated with first line capecitabine and oxaliplatin with and without bevacizumab (CAPEOXBEV/CAPEOX) and to identify which of these miRNAs could be predictive for the effect of bevacizumab-addition to chemotherapy.

Methods

Study design

A screening study using an array approach was performed on primary CRC tissue samples from patients treated with CAPEOXBEV (screening cohort) to identify candidate miRNAs with expression levels related to outcome. Thereafter, the expression levels of the identified candidate miRNAs were measured using a more precise method with duplicate determinations in three cohorts: a subgroup of the screening cohort; a validation cohort, which was an independent group of patients treated with CAPEOXBEV; and a control cohort, consisting of patients treated with CAPEOX alone.

Patients, data extraction, and end points

The BETmiRC (Bevacizumab Tissue microRNAs in Colorectal cancer) study retrospectively included patients with mCRC treated with first line CAPEOXBEV in 10 Danish hospitals from 2006 to 2011,and patients treated with first line CAPEOX at Herlev Hospital or in a randomized study from 2003 to 2006 [19], before bevacizumab was approved, as previously described [20].The end points time to disease progression (TTP) and overall survival (OS) were measured from initiation of treatment to disease progression or death from any cause, respectively (detailed definition in File S1). Vital status was updated July 5, 2013.

Tissue samples

Formalin-fixed paraffin-embedded (FFPE) tissue blocks containing samples from primary tumors were retrieved using the National Pathology Registry. Control samples from patients resected for inflammatory bowel disease were also included. An experienced gastro-intestinal pathologist (DL) selected which tissue blocks to retrieve and scored the blocks for tumor cell percentage. Three 10-µm sections were cut from each block without micro- or macro-dissection and the sections were placed in sterile Eppendorf tubes. All tissue samples were collected prior to any systemic treatment or radiotherapy.

MiRNA expression analysis

RNA was purified using the miRNeasy FFPE Kit (Qiagen, Hilden, Germany) using the manufacturer's instructions. The purification order was randomized for the validation and control cohort samples. The non-human miRNA ath-miR-159a was added to each sample before cDNA synthesis as a spike-in control.

The TaqMan Human MicroRNA array A and B Cards Set v3.0 (Applied Biosystems) was used to quantify expression of 754 human miRNAs with single determinations in the screening study. In the subsequent study of the reduced screening-, validation-, and control cohorts, miRNA expression was measured using TaqMan Custom LDA cards (Applied Biosystems) profiling 22 selected miRNAs in duplicate with 8 samples on each card. The 22 miRNAs were selected from the screening study and the microfluidic cards were pre-configured from the manufacturer according to our specifications. Samples were analyzed in a randomized order on the Custom LDA cards.

The instructions and reagents from the manufacturer were used in all steps (https://www.products.appliedbiosystems.com). All RNA purification- and miRNA expression studies were performed by AROS Applied Biotechnology (Aarhus, Denmark). The company was blinded to all clinical information.

MiRNA *in situ* hybridization

In situ hybridization (ISH) was performed using double-FAM (carboxyfluorescein) labeled locked nucleic acid (LNA [21]) probes (Exiqon, Vedbæk, Denmark) for miR-185-5p, miR-455-5p, miR-592, miR-664-3p, miR-21-5p, and miR-126-3p, as previously described [22]. All ISH studies were performed by Bioneer (Hørsholm, Denmark).

Statistical analysis

No sample size calculation was done prior to study initiation. We aimed for the greatest sample size possible and equal sizes of the three cohorts.

MiRNA expression analyses – screening study. Raw cycle threshold (C_t) for each miRNA was checked for outliers and data were corrected using spike-in values. In a univariate selection method, the expression of each miRNA was related to TTP and

Table 1. Patient and sample characteristics.

	Clinical CAPEOXBEV cohort	Clinical CAPEOX cohort	Screening cohort (LDA A+B card)	Screening cohort (cLDA)	Validation cohort (cLDA)	CAPEOXBEV included vs. not-included *P*	CAPEOX cohort (cLDA)	CAPEOX included vs. not-included *P*
Treatment start years, range	2006–2011	2003–2006	2006–2010	2006–2010	2007–2011		2003–2006	
Number of patients	623	211	203	155	121		127	
Age, median (range)	65 (22–84)	63 (36–85)	65 (37–84)	65 (40–84)	67 (22–82)	0.27	62 (36–82)	0.24
Sex, female (%)	281 (45%)	77 (36%)	111 (55%)	83 (54%)	40 (33%)	0.75	45 (35%)	0.66
Primary tumor location						0.15		0.45
Cecum, ascending colon	133 (21%)	37 (18%)	52 (26%)	38 (25%)	23 (19%)		26 (20%)	
Right flexure, transverse colon	60 (10%)	16 (8%)	15 (7%)	11 (7%)	7 (6%)		8 (6%)	
Left flexure, descending colon	33 (5%)	12 (6%)	9 (4%)	6 (4%)	7 (6%)		9 (7%)	
Sigmoid colon	192 (31%)	62 (29%)	70 (34%)	56 (36%)	38 (31%)		37 (29%)	
Rectum	205 (33%)	84 (40%)	57 (28%)	44 (28%)	46 (38%)		47 (37%)	
Primary tumor resected	319 (51%)	157 (74%)	186 (92%)	148 (95%)	84 (69%)	**<0.0001**	116 (91%)	**<0.0001**
Number of metastatic sites						**0.004**		1.00
1	198 (32%)	71 (34%)	74 (36%)	63 (41%)	42 (35%)		42 (33%)	
>1	425 (68%)	140 (66%)	129 (64%)	92 (59%)	79 (65%)		85 (67%)	
No. of first line cycles, median (range)	7 (1–46)	6 (1–16)*	7 (1–46)	7 (1–46)	7 (1–23)	0.25	6 (1–15)*	0.92
Treated with irinotecan	357 (58%)*	105 (64%)*	117 (58%)	95 (61%)	76 (63%)	0.05	64 (72%)	0.29
Performance status						**0.04**		0.32
0	260 (61%)	81 (50%)	93 (61%)	75 (65%)	60 (71%)		48 (48%)	
1	138 (32%)	66 (41%)	52 (34%)	37 (32%)	19 (22%)		39 (39%)	
≥2	27 (6%)	15 (9%)	8 (5%)	3 (3%)	6 (7%)		12 (12%)	
Missing	198	49	50	40	36		28	
Prior adjuvant treatment, no. (%)	57 (9%)	37 (18%)	28 (14%)	22 (14%)	13 (11%)	**0.008**	26 (20%)	0.20
TTP events				130 (84%)	98 (81%)		115 (91%)	
Median time to disease progression	8.6 mo	7.6 mo	9.2 mo	9.5 mo	8.3 mo	**0.04**	8.4 mo	0.27
OS events				130 (84%)	93 (77%)		125 (98%)	
Median overall survival	16.1 mo	15.2 mo	19.0 mo	25.0 mo	21.9 mo	**<0.0001**	16.4 mo	0.12
Sample type								
Resection	–	–	–	146 (94%)	83 (69%)		115 (91%)	
Biopsy	–	–	–	9 (6%)	38 (31%)		12 (9%)	
Tumor cell percentage, median (range)	–	–	–	30 (2–70)	30 (5–70)		30 (5–70)	

Table 1. Cont.

	Clinical CAPEOXBEV cohort	Clinical CAPEOX cohort	Screening cohort (LDA A+B card)	Screening cohort (cLDA)	Validation cohort (cLDA)	CAPEOXBEV included vs. not-included *P*	CAPEOX cohort (cLDA)	CAPEOX included vs. not-included *P*
cLDA mean C_t, median (1./3. quartile)	-	-	-	19.9 (19.5/20.9)	20.8 (20.0/22.0)		20.7 (20.3/21.7)	

* Data were missing for some patients; ranges and percentages are based on the patients with available data.

OS using a Cox proportional hazards (CPH) model [23,24]. Candidate miRNAs were included in a multivariate CPH model adjusted for age, sex, histology, number of metastatic sites, primary tumor location, and prior adjuvant treatment, which was simplified using a backwards elimination procedure based upon Akaike's Information Criterion [25]. The analysis was then repeated for data sets normalized using quantile- and mean normalization. Finally, 22 miRNAs were selected for further study based primarily on their performance in the multivariate analyses. The number of miRNAs to include in the second study was chosen pragmatically as it allowed for duplicate measurements on the custom platform.

MiRNA expression analyses – screening-, validation-, and control cohorts. Mean C_t of the duplicate measurements was calculated and transformed to 40-C_t. If one of the two measurements was undetermined, the C_t of the other measurement was used. In each of the three cohorts, expression of the 22 miRNAs was related to TTP and OS using CPH models with adjustment for age, sex, primary tumor location, prior adjuvant treatment, and number of metastatic sites. Results were reported as hazard ratios (HR) per inter-quartile range increase in expression level with 95% confidence intervals (CI).The possible interaction between miRNA expression level and bevacizumab treatment effect was tested in the three cohorts combined using a likelihood ratio test.

Since outcome for the patients treated with bevacizumab differed greatly depending on primary tumor location [20], we also performed the interaction analyses for proximal and distal primary cancers separately.

$P<0.05$ was considered statistically significant and no formal corrections for multiple comparisons were made. The statistical software packages R [26] (www.r-project.org) and GraphPad Prism 5 (GraphPad Software, Inc) were used for all analyses.

Target prediction

In silico predicted gene targets for selected miRNAs were identified using the open-access DIANA-microT-CDS tool (http://www.microrna.gr/microT-CDS) [27].

Ethics

The study was approved by the Regional Scientific Ethics Committee of the Capital Region of Denmark (http://www.regionh.dk/vek, approval number: H-1-2010-081). Since this retrospective study would not have any influence on treatment and since most of the participants were deceased, written consent was not obtained, and this was approved by the ethics committee.

Reporting of the results was prepared according to the REMARK guidelines [28,29].

Further details are described in File S1.

Results

MiRNA expression was measured in 460 FFPE samples. The number of samples in each cohort was: screening cohort = 212, reduced screening cohort = 155, validation cohort = 121, and control cohort = 127 (Figure S1 in File S1).

The patients included in the reduced screening- and the validation miRNA cohorts differed from the patients not included. They were more likely to have: resected primary tumor, a single metastatic site, performance status 0, and prior adjuvant therapy. They also experienced a longer TTP and OS (Table 1). The patients in the control cohort were similar to the patients not included except for them being more likely to have had the primary tumor resected.

Table 2. Focused miRNA panel – miRNAs significantly associated with time to disease progression.

	Screening CAPEOXBEV cohort			Validation CAPEOXBEV cohort			Combined CAPEOXBEV cohort			Control CAPEOX cohort			Interaction[a]		
	n = 155			n = 121			n = 276			n = 127			all	distal	proximal
miRNA	**HR[b]**	**95% CI**	***P***	**HR**	**95% CI**	***P***	**HR**	**95% CI**	***P***	**HR**	**95% CI**	***P***	***P***	***P***	***P***
Raw expression values															
miR-15a-5p	0.88	0.73–1.06	0.19	0.73	0.54–0.98	**0.04**	0.86	0.73–1.00	0.05	1.03	0.80–1.31	0.84	0.14	0.25	0.15
miR-17-3p	0.68	0.54–0.84	**0.0005**	0.92	0.68–1.23	0.57	0.77	0.64–0.91	**0.003**	1.01	0.78–1.31	0.92	0.16	0.11	0.67
miR-193b-5p	0.82	0.70–0.95	**0.01**	0.74	0.54–1.01	0.06	0.82	0.72–0.94	**0.004**	0.92	0.77–1.10	0.34	–[c]	–	–
miR-204-5p	0.83	0.71–0.96	**0.02**	0.92	0.68–1.23	0.56	0.83	0.71–0.97	**0.02**	0.90	0.71–1.14	0.38	0.86	0.60	0.25
miR-501-5p	0.78	0.63–0.97	**0.03**	0.88	0.63–1.23	0.46	0.81	0.66–0.99	**0.04**	0.96	0.69–1.32	0.78	0.48	0.47	0.84
miR-545-3p	0.87	0.77–1.00	**0.04**	0.87	0.73–1.05	0.15	0.86	0.77–0.96	**0.005**	1.00	0.88–1.14	0.97	0.11	0.17	0.29
miR-592	0.71	0.54–0.93	**0.01**	0.80	0.62–1.01	0.06	0.77	0.67–0.90	**0.0007**	0.81	0.58–1.12	0.21	0.14	0.11	0.82
miR-664-3p	0.87	0.66–1.15	0.32	0.60	0.41–0.87	**0.007**	0.80	0.65–0.99	**0.04**	0.81	0.58–1.13	0.21	0.10	**0.04**	0.31
Mean-normalized expression values															
miR-17-3p	0.78	0.63–0.98	**0.03**	1.05	0.83–1.34	0.68	0.89	0.76–1.05	0.16	1.10	0.82–1.48	0.52	0.22	0.09	0.26
miR-155-5p	1.36	1.07–1.71	**0.01**	1.33	1.00–1.77	0.05	1.38	1.15–1.64	**0.0005**	1.05	0.79–1.38	0.74	0.05	0.18	0.18
miR-185-5p	1.45	1.17–1.80	**0.0008**	1.23	0.87–1.74	0.24	1.30	1.10–1.54	**0.003**	0.89	0.67–1.19	0.44	0.06	0.20	0.43
miR-204-5p	0.82	0.68–0.98	**0.03**	1.13	0.87–1.46	0.38	0.90	0.78–1.03	0.13	0.95	0.79–1.13	0.54	0.15	0.07	0.14
miR-449a	1.25	1.03–1.52	**0.02**	0.97	0.73–1.28	0.81	1.15	0.99–1.35	0.07	1.00	0.80–1.26	0.96	0.55	0.89	0.74

[a] Interaction tests were performed for all patients and for patients with distal (sigmoid and rectum) and proximal (cecum to descending) primary tumor location, separately.
[b] Hazard ratio is per inter-quartile range expression increase and is adjusted for age, sex, number of metastatic sites, prior adjuvant treatment and primary tumor location.
[c] miRNA was missing in >10% of samples so interaction was not tested.
Abbreviations: HR, hazard ratio; CI, confidence interval.

Table 3. Focused miRNA panel – miRNAs significantly associated with overall survival.

	Screening CAPEOXBEV cohort			Validation CAPEOXBEV cohort			Combined CAPEOXBEV cohort			Control CAPEOX cohort			Interaction[a]		
	n = 155			n = 121			n = 276			n = 127			all	distal	proximal
miRNA	HR[b]	95% CI	*P*	HR	95% CI	*P*	HR	95% CI	*P*	HR	95% CI	*P*	*P*	*P*	*P*
Raw expression values															
miR-15a-5p	0.80	0.65–0.99	**0.04**	0.87	0.66–1.16	0.34	0.81	0.69–0.97	**0.02**	1.05	0.83–1.34	0.68	0.31	0.41	0.74
miR-196b-5p	0.83	0.69–1.01	0.06	0.66	0.50–0.87	**0.003**	0.77	0.66–0.90	**0.0008**	0.78	0.62–0.98	**0.04**	0.20	0.06	0.23
miR-204-5p	0.76	0.64–0.91	**0.003**	0.88	0.66–1.18	0.38	0.77	0.64–0.93	**0.005**	1.02	0.81–1.28	0.87	0.94	0.80	0.54
miR-338-3p	0.81	0.65–1.00	**0.045**	0.93	0.70–1.24	0.63	0.85	0.72–1.01	0.07	1.01	0.80–1.27	0.92	0.52	0.40	0.68
miR-545-3p	0.85	0.74–0.98	**0.03**	0.95	0.80–1.12	0.53	0.90	0.81–1.01	0.06	1.06	0.95–1.19	0.30	0.39	0.39	0.45
miR-552	0.77	0.61–0.96	**0.02**	0.93	0.68–1.27	0.63	0.77	0.63–0.95	**0.01**	1.02	0.80–1.31	0.85	0.44	0.29	0.76
miR-592	0.69	0.69–0.92	**0.01**	0.76	0.60–0.95	**0.01**	0.73	0.62–0.86	**0.0001**	0.76	0.55–1.05	0.10	0.31	0.33	0.85
miR-664-3p	0.64	0.48–0.86	**0.003**	0.60	0.44–0.82	**0.002**	0.61	0.49–0.75	**<0.0001**	0.85	0.61–1.17	0.31	**0.02**	**0.03**	0.50
Mean-normalized expression values															
miR-1	1.01	0.77–1.32	0.96	1.19	0.84–1.69	0.32	1.08	0.87–1.32	0.49	1.36	1.02–1.82	**0.04**	0.98	0.82	0.75
miR-155-5p	1.31	1.03–1.67	**0.03**	1.21	0.91–1.61	0.19	1.23	1.03–1.47	**0.03**	0.96	0.75–1.23	0.76	0.38	0.70	0.30
miR-185-5p	1.49	1.18–1.88	**0.0008**	1.23	0.89–1.72	0.21	1.34	1.12–1.60	**0.001**	0.91	0.70–1.18	0.46	0.09	0.23	0.57
miR-196b-5p	0.89	0.67–1.18	0.43	0.70	0.51–0.96	**0.03**	0.79	0.64–0.97	**0.03**	0.73	0.58–0.93	**0.01**	0.99	0.43	0.09
miR-204-5p	0.75	0.61–0.93	**0.009**	0.95	0.70–1.28	0.71	0.85	0.72–1.01	0.06	1.01	0.85–1.21	0.89	0.43	0.61	0.40
miR-455-5p	1.19	0.95–1.49	0.14	1.27	1.03–1.56	**0.03**	1.24	1.06–1.45	**0.007**	0.99	0.85–1.15	0.91	**0.02**	0.19	0.38
miR-592	0.77	0.59–1.00	0.05	0.76	0.63–0.93	**0.007**	0.77	0.66–0.89	**0.0004**	0.71	0.53–0.96	**0.03**	0.52	0.21	0.35
miR-664-3p	0.66	0.49–0.91	**0.01**	0.55	0.39–0.79	**0.001**	0.60	0.48–0.76	**<0.0001**	0.81	0.59–1.11	0.18	**0.02**	**0.02**	0.45

[a] Interaction was tested for all patients and for patients with distal (sigmoid to rectum) and proximal (cecum to descending colon) primary tumor location separately.
[b] Hazard ratio is per inter-quartile range expression increase and is adjusted for age, sex, number of metastatic sites, prior adjuvant treatment and primary tumor location.
Abbreviations: HR, hazard ratio; CI, confidence interval.

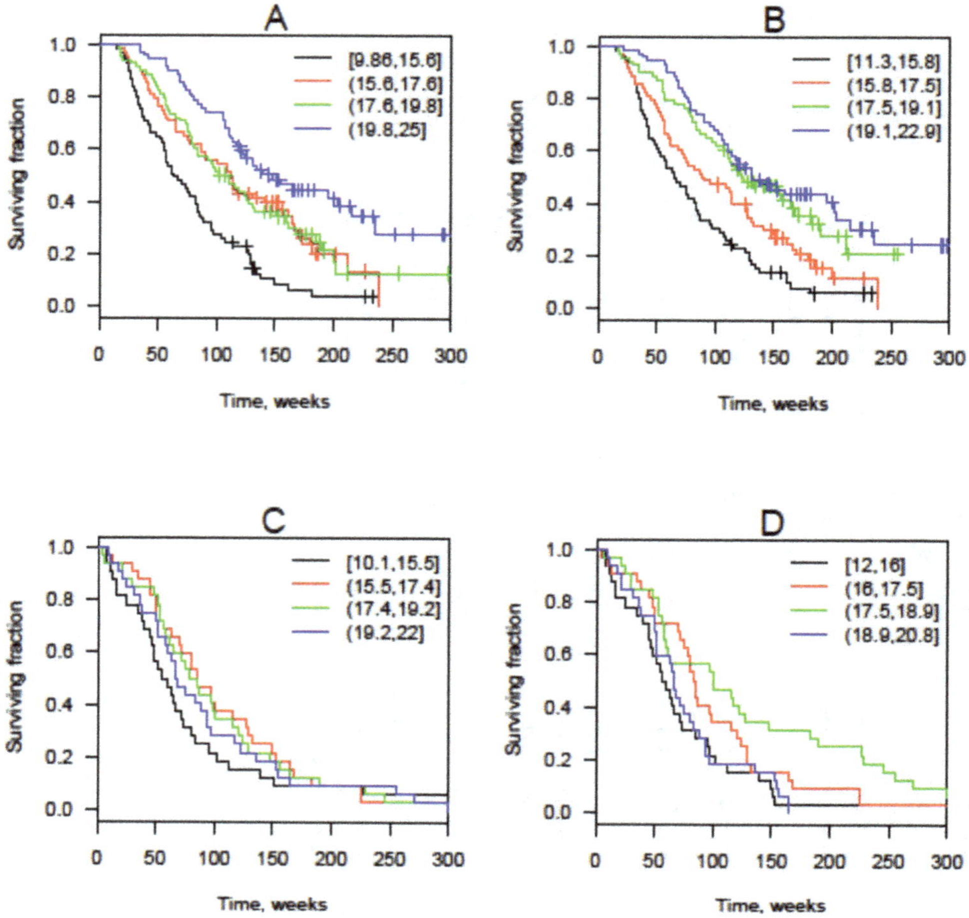

		Raw expression		Mean-normalized expression	
Cohort	Quartile	HR	95% CI	HR	95% CI
CAPEOXBEV	1	1	[reference]	1	[reference]
	2	0.50	0.34 – 0.74	0.66	0.45 – 0.98
	3	0.50	0.34 – 0.76	0.41	0.27 – 0.63
	4	0.30	0.20 – 0.46	0.34	0.23 – 0.54
CAPEOX	1	1	[reference]	1	[reference]
	2	0.75	0.42 – 1.53	0.68	0.38 – 1.25
	3	0.76	0.41 – 1.61	0.49	0.26 – 0.92
	4	0.86	0.46 – 1.70	0.98	0.59 – 1.89

Figure 1. Overall survival according to quartiles of mir-664-3p expression. Kaplan-Meier plots are shown for patients treated with CAPEOXBEV using raw (A) or mean-normalized (B) expression and patients treated with CAPEOX alone using raw (C) and mean-normalized (D) expression. Hazard ratios (HR) are unadjusted and confidence intervals (CI) are calculated using bootstrapping. The expression intervals shown in the upper right-hand corner are 40-C_t, so higher values correspond to higher expression. Black line = lowest quartile; red line = second quartile; green line = third quartile; blue line = highest quartile.

Screening study

Nine samples were identified as outliers based on a low number of miRNAs detected and these were excluded, leaving 203 samples for outcome calculations. Twenty-six miRNAs were associated with TTP or OS in multivariate analysis using raw-, quantile-normalized, or mean-normalized expression data (Table S1 in File S1). Twenty-two of these were selected for further study: miR-1, miR-15a-5p, miR-17-3p, miR-22-3p, miR-29b-3p, miR-145-3p, miR-155-5p, miR-185-5p, miR-193b-5p, miR-196b-5p, miR-204-5p, miR-214-5p, miR-338-3p, miR-382-5p, miR-449a, miR-455-5p, miR-497-5p, miR-501-5p, miR-545-3p, miR-552-3p, miR-592 and miR-664-3p.

Focused miRNA panel – miRNAs associated with TTP

Eleven miRNAs were significantly associated with TTP in either the screening- or the validation cohort, but not in both cohorts and no significant interactions were found between miRNA expression and bevacizumab effect (Table 2).

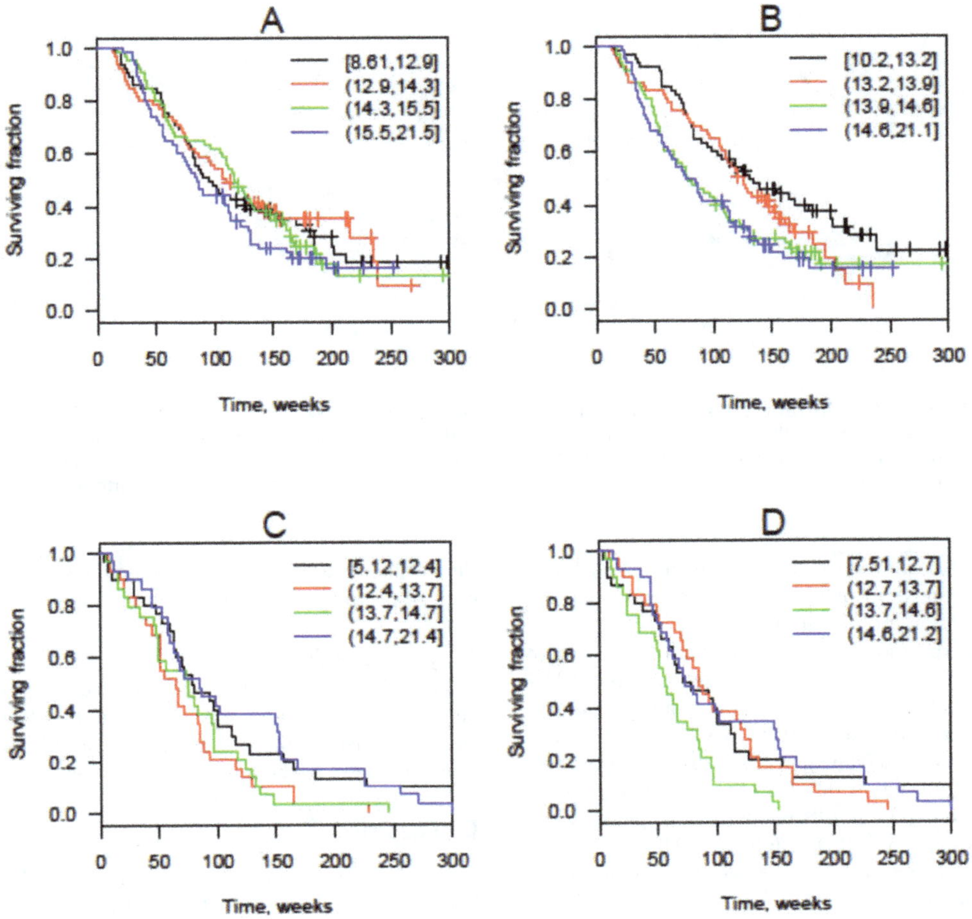

		Raw expression		Mean-normalized expression	
Cohort	Quartile	HR	95% CI	HR	95% CI
CAPEOXBEV	1	1	[reference]	1	[reference]
	2	0.89	0.59 – 1.36	1.19	0.83 – 1.70
	3	0.97	0.68 – 1.36	1.61	1.09 – 2.41
	4	1.22	0.81 – 1.75	1.71	1.13 – 2.55
CAPEOX	1	1	[reference]	1	[reference]
	2	1.70	1.01 – 2.89	1.12	0.69 – 1.79
	3	1.61	0.96 – 2.56	2.07	1.26 – 3.56
	4	1.01	0.62 – 1.65	1.01	0.62 – 1.62

Figure 2. Overall survival according to quartiles of mir-455-5p expression. Kaplan-Meier plots are shown for patients treated with CAPEOXBEV using raw (A) or mean-normalized (B) expression and patients treated with CAPEOX alone using raw (C) and mean-normalized (D) expression. Hazard ratios (HR) are unadjusted and confidence intervals (CI) are calculated using bootstrapping. The expression intervals shown in the upper right-hand corner are 40-C_t, so higher values correspond to higher expression. Black line = lowest quartile; red line = second quartile; green line = third quartile; blue line = highest quartile.

Kaplan-Meier curves for TTP according to quartiles of miR-664-3p- and miR-455-5p expression are shown in Figure S2 and S3 in File S1.

Focused miRNA panel – miRNAs associated with OS

Twelve miRNAs were significantly associated with OS in one or more of the screening-, validation- and control cohorts (Table 3). Higher miR-664-3p expression was associated with longer OS in the screening and validation cohorts using raw expression: HR 0.64 (CI 0.48–0.86) and 0.60 (CI 0.44–0.82); and normalized expression: HR 0.66 (CI 0.49–0.91) and 0.55 (CI 0.39–0.79). No association between miR-664-3p expression and OS was found in the control cohort. A significant interaction between miR-664-3p expression and bevacizumab effect was observed using both raw- and normalized expression ($P = 0.02$ and $P = 0.02$). Kaplan-Meier plots for OS according to quartiles of miR-664-3p expression are shown in Figure 1.

Higher miR-455-5p expression was associated with shorter OS in the combined bevacizumab-treated cohort when using normalized expression: HR 1.24 (CI 1.06–1.45), but not in the control

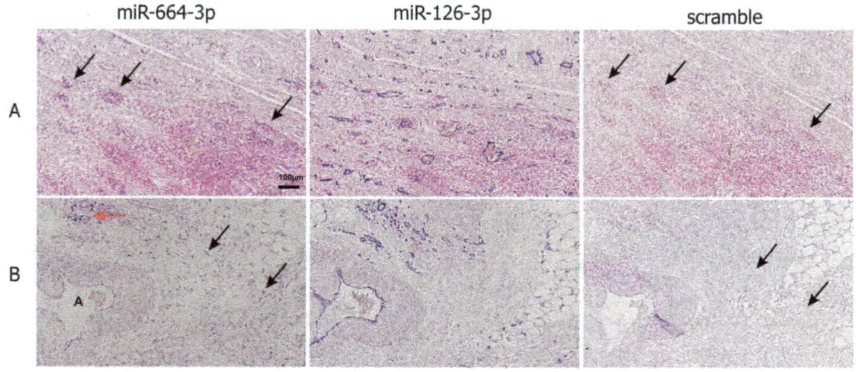

Figure 3. MiR-664-3p *in situ* hybridization (ISH). Panels A and B show examples of miR-664-3p ISH in infiltrating lymphocytes (A) and fibroblasts (B). Consecutive sections were stained with LNA probes against miR-664-3p, miR-126-3p and a scramble sequence. MiR-664-3p ISH signal is seen in infiltrating lymphocytes (A, arrows; B, red arrow) and in fibroblasts (B, black arrows), whereas no ISH signal is obtained with scramble probe. A strong ISH signal is seen in endothelial cells with the positive control probe miR-126-3p. The "A" in panel B indicates an artery.

cohort. There was a significant interaction with bevacizumab effect ($P = 0.02$). Kaplan-Meier plots for OS according to quartiles of miR-455-5p expression are shown in Figure 2.

Higher miR-592 expression was associated with longer OS in the screening- and validation cohorts using raw expression: HR 0.69 (CI 0.69–0.92) and 0.76 (CI 0.60–0.95); and in the validation cohort using normalized expression: HR 0.76 (CI 0.63–0.93), with a similar trend in the screening cohort using normalized expression: HR 0.77 (CI 0.59–1.00). Higher miR-592 expression was also associated with longer OS in the control group when using normalized expression: HR 0.71 (CI 0.53–0.96).

Higher miR-196b-5p expression was associated with longer OS using raw- and normalized expression both in the combined bevacizumab-treated cohort: HR 0.77 (CI 0.66–0.90) and 0.79 (CI 0.64–0.97); and in the control group: HR 0.78 (CI 0.62–0.98) and 0.73 (CI 0.58–0.93).

Focused miRNA panel – primary tumor location and second line outcome

In analyses stratified for primary tumor location, a significant interaction with bevacizumab effect was seen for miR-664-3p expression in the sigmoid colon and rectum group for both TTP using raw expression and for OS using raw- and normalized expression. Expression levels of all miRNAs according to primary tumor location are shown in Figure S4 in File S1.

In patients continuing bevacizumab in second line, high miR-664-3p expression was associated with longer TTP (HR 0.30, $P = 0.04$) and high miR-455-5p expression was associated with a trend towards shorter TTP (HR 2.72, $P = 0.09$), while no such associations were seen in patients that did not continue bevacizumab (Figure S5 in File S1).

MiRNA *in situ* hybridization

An intense miR-664-3p ISH signal, primarily with a cytoplasmic localization, was seen in subpopulations of tumor-infiltrating lymphocytes, fibroblasts, and endothelial cells located at the invasive border (Figure 3). A weak miR-664-3p ISH signal was seen in tumor epithelial cells, but a similar staining was observed with the scramble probe, suggesting an unspecific binding of the probe to these cells. MiR-455-5p ISH signal was found in some lymphocyte-like stromal cells in half of the samples, while tumor epithelial cells were negative (Figure S6 in File S1). No ISH signal was obtained with the probes against miR-185, miR-449a or miR-592. Positive control probes for miR-21-5p and miR-126-3p showed moderate to intense staining in fibroblasts and endothelial cells, respectively, in all cases.

Target prediction

Table S2 in File S1 shows the 20 highest ranked predicted gene targets for miR-196b-5p, miR-455-5p, miR-592, and miR-664-3p, and references published articles regarding the function and expression level of these miRNAs in cancer.

Discussion

This is the first comprehensive study of miRNAs as predictive biomarkers for bevacizumab effectiveness in CRC. Of the 22 miRNAs selected from the screening study, miR-664-3p and miR-455-5p showed the greatest potential as predictive biomarkers for bevacizumab effectiveness.

The association between miR-664-3p and OS differed significantly between patients treated with bevacizumab and patients treated with chemotherapy alone: Increasing miR-664-3p expression in primary CRC tissue was associated with longer OS in both cohorts of patients treated with bevacizumab combined with CAPEOX but not in the cohort treated with chemotherapy alone. Increasing miR-664-3p expression was also associated with longer TTP in patients treated with bevacizumab, but the interaction test was only significant in the subgroup of patients with sigmoid colon- and rectal primary tumors. We previously hypothesized that this subgroup of patients could be more likely to derive benefit from treatment with bevacizumab than patients with more proximal primary tumors [20]. MiR-664-3p expression was also higher in these patients than in patients with more proximal primary tumors (Figure S4 in File S1). In the small cohort of patients with available second line outcome data, high miR-664-3p expression was also associated with a longer TTP only in patients continuing bevacizumab, supporting a connection between miR-664-3p expression and bevacizumab effectiveness.

We observed high expression of miR-664-3p in stromal cells, including endothelial cells, which is in accordance with a role for miR-664-3p in angiogenesis. Very little data have been published about this miRNA (Table S2 in File S1). Interestingly, among the top predicted targets of miR-664-3p are neuroligin 1 (NLGN1), MDGA2, and gephyrin, which are all involved in the same synaptogenic process in the nervous system [30,31]. Recently, neuroligin and its binding partner neurexin have been shown to be widely expressed in the vascular system and involved in angiogenesis [30]. Overexpression of neuroligin 1 in endothelial cells grown in a tumorigenic environment increased angiogenesis, and knockdown of neurexin reduced fibroblast growth factor 2-induced angiogenesis [32]. In a zebra fish embryo model of angiogenesis, inhibition of VEGF-A or neuroligin caused similar magnitudes of vascular defects, but inhibition of both resulted in a more than additive anti-angiogenic effect [33]. Hypothetically, the impact of miR-664-3p expression on outcome may thus be explained by its downregulation of the neuroligin system and the resulting synergy with VEGF-A inhibition by bevacizumab.

Increasing miR-455-5p expression was associated with shorter OS in the combined bevacizumab treated cohort while no such association was observed in the cohort treated with chemotherapy alone. We identified high expression of this miRNA in lymphocyte-like cells located in the stroma around the cancer cells. MiR-455-5p has been reported to be dysregulated in cancer; however, no validated targets have been identified (Table S2 in File S1).

Increasing expression of both miR-196b-5p and miR-592 was associated with longer OS in all three cohorts, with similar effect estimates. Both these miRNAs have been shown to be downregulated in CRCs with deficient mismatch repair (dMMR) [34]. Higher miR-592 expression has been shown to be associated with improved OS in patients receiving salvage anti-EGFR treatment and higher miR-196b-5p expression has been linked to response to neo-adjuvant 5-FU and radiotherapy in patients with locally advanced rectal cancer [35,36]. MiR-592 expression has been reported to be higher in left-sided compared to right-sided CRCs [37], which we also found in our study. We could not stain our tissue sections for miR-592, but expression of both miR-592 and miR-196b-5p has previously been shown to be 2.5–3.7 fold higher in CRC epithelium than in CRC stroma [38]. The function of miR-592 has not been described. MiR-196b-5p is dysregulated in many malignancies, has been related to cancer prognosis, and targets c-myc, ERG, MEIS1, FAS, ABL1, BCL-2 and several HOX genes (Table S2 in File S1).

There are important limitations to consider regarding our results. We studied retrospectively identified cohorts from different time periods, which increases the risk of bias, since differences other than the treatments used could exist between the cohorts. We used mean expression for normalization, but since the miRNAs used for calculating the mean were related to outcome, this is sub-optimal. Even though the association with outcome for some of the miRNAs was identified in two or three independent cohorts, the predictive effect related to bevacizumab remains unvalidated. We did not correct for multiple testing, but miR-664-3p would still be significantly associated with OS in the validation cohort, even after correcting for the 22 miRNAs tested. Also, effect estimates were similar in the cohorts, indicating a non-random association. Among the strengths of our study are the large sample size, the initial comprehensive screening study, the use of three independent cohorts, and randomization of purification- and miRNA expression analysis order.

In conclusion, this is the first study to examine the potential for miRNA expression in primary tumors to predict benefit of bevacizumab in patients with mCRC. We have identified miR-664-3p and miR-455-5p as possible predictive biomarkers for bevacizumab. MiR-592 and miR-196b-5p were predictive of outcome both with and without bevacizumab and these could be prognostic biomarkers or biomarkers related to chemotherapy effectiveness. These findings need validation in independent cohorts – preferably from randomized trials and using stable miRNA normalizers –before they can be implemented in clinical decision making. Elucidation of the cellular origins and biological functions of these miRNAs is warranted.

Supporting Information

File S1 This file contains supplementary methods, supplementary Table S1 and S2, and supplementary Figure S1–S6.

Acknowledgments

We would like to thank: Jørgen Hansen, MD from the Department of Oncology at Aalborg Hospital, Denmark for help regarding acquisition of patient data; Mel Heeran, PhD for excellent technical assistance with the sectioning of the FFPE tissue samples; Jakob Z. Johansen, MD for inputting clinical data in the BETmiRC database; Mogens Kruhøffer, PhD, from AROS Applied Biotechnology A/S, Denmark for help with the miRNA analyses, and the Danish CancerBiobank (DCB) for biological material and for the data regarding handling and storage.

Author Contributions

Conceived and designed the experiments: MKB CD DL BSN EVSH BVJ JSJ. Analyzed the data: MKB CD DL BSN JSL KØ SEN LST CQ PP NHH NK TFH BBJ EVSH BVJ JSJ. Contributed reagents/materials/analysis tools: MKB CD DL BSN JSL KØ SEN LST CQ PP NHH NK TFH BBJ EVSH BVJ JSJ. Wrote the paper: MKB CD DL BSN JSL KØ SEN LST CQ PP NHH NK TFH BBJ EVSH BVJ JSJ.

References

1. Ferlay J, Soerjomataram I, Ervik M, Dikshit R, Eser S, et al. (2013) GLOBOCAN 2012 v1.0, Cancer Incidence and Mortality Worldwide: IARC CancerBase No. 11 [Internet]. Lyon, France: International Agency for Research on Cancer.
2. Van Cutsem E, Nordlinger B, Cervantes A, Group EGW (2010) Advanced colorectal cancer: ESMO Clinical Practice Guidelines for treatment. Ann Oncol 21 Suppl 5: v93–97.
3. Bennouna J, Sastre J, Arnold D, Osterlund P, Greil R, et al. (2013) Continuation of bevacizumab after first progression in metastatic colorectal cancer (ML18147): a randomised phase 3 trial. Lancet Oncol 14: 29–37.
4. Giantonio BJ, Catalano PJ, Meropol NJ, O'Dwyer PJ, Mitchell EP, et al. (2007) Bevacizumab in combination with oxaliplatin, fluorouracil, and leucovorin (FOLFOX4) for previously treated metastatic colorectal cancer: results from the Eastern Cooperative Oncology Group Study E3200. J Clin Oncol 25: 1539–1544.
5. Hurwitz H, Fehrenbacher L, Novotny W, Cartwright T, Hainsworth J, et al. (2004) Bevacizumab plus irinotecan, fluorouracil, and leucovorin for metastatic colorectal cancer. N Engl J Med 350: 2335–2342.
6. Hurwitz HI, Tebbutt NC, Kabbinavar F, Giantonio BJ, Guan ZZ, et al. (2013) Efficacy and safety of bevacizumab in metastatic colorectal cancer: pooled analysis from seven randomized controlled trials. Oncologist 18: 1004–1012.
7. Saltz LB, Clarke S, Diaz-Rubio E, Scheithauer W, Figer A, et al. (2008) Bevacizumab in combination with oxaliplatin-based chemotherapy as first-line therapy in metastatic colorectal cancer: a randomized phase III study. J Clin Oncol 26: 2013–2019.
8. Kopetz S, Chang GJ, Overman MJ, Eng C, Sargent DJ, et al. (2009) Improved survival in metastatic colorectal cancer is associated with adoption of hepatic resection and improved chemotherapy. J Clin Oncol 27: 3677–3683.
9. Jubb AM, Harris AL (2010) Biomarkers to predict the clinical efficacy of bevacizumab in cancer. Lancet Oncol 11: 1172–1183.
10. Lambrechts D, Lenz HJ, de Haas S, Carmeliet P, Scherer SJ (2013) Markers of response for the antiangiogenic agent bevacizumab. J Clin Oncol 31: 1219–1230.
11. Cortez MA, Bueso-Ramos C, Ferdin J, Lopez-Berestein G, Sood AK, et al. (2011) MicroRNAs in body fluids–the mix of hormones and biomarkers. Nat Rev Clin Oncol 8: 467–477.
12. Farazi TA, Spitzer JI, Morozov P, Tuschl T (2011) miRNAs in human cancer. J Pathol 223: 102–115.
13. Kong YW, Ferland-McCollough D, Jackson TJ, Bushell M (2012) microRNAs in cancer management. Lancet Oncol 13: e249–258.
14. Nana-Sinkam SP, Fabbri M, Croce CM (2010) MicroRNAs in cancer: personalizing diagnosis and therapy. Ann N Y Acad Sci 1210: 25–33.
15. Xi Y, Nakajima G, Gavin E, Morris CG, Kudo K, et al. (2007) Systematic analysis of microRNA expression of RNA extracted from fresh frozen and formalin-fixed paraffin-embedded samples. RNA 13: 1668–1674.

16. Schwarzenbach H, Nishida N, Calin GA, Pantel K (2014) Clinical relevance of circulating cell-free microRNAs in cancer. Nat Rev Clin Oncol 11: 145–156.
17. Mazeh H, Mizrahi I, Ilyayev N, Halle D, Brucher B, et al. (2013) The Diagnostic and Prognostic Role of microRNA in Colorectal Cancer - a Comprehensive review. J Cancer 4: 281–295.
18. Nosho K, Igarashi H, Nojima M, Ito M, Maruyama R, et al. (2014) Association of microRNA-31 with BRAF mutation, colorectal cancer survival and serrated pathway. Carcinogenesis 35: 776–783.
19. Qvortrup C, Jensen BV, Fokstuen T, Nielsen SE, Keldsen N, et al. (2010) A randomized study comparing short-time infusion of oxaliplatin in combination with capecitabine XELOX(30) and chronomodulated XELOX(30) as first-line therapy in patients with advanced colorectal cancer. Ann Oncol 21: 87–91.
20. Boisen MK, Johansen JS, Dehlendorff C, Larsen JS, Osterlind K, et al. (2013) Primary tumor location and bevacizumab effectiveness in patients with metastatic colorectal cancer. Ann Oncol 24: 2554–2559.
21. Braasch DA, Corey DR (2001) Locked nucleic acid (LNA): fine-tuning the recognition of DNA and RNA. Chem Biol 8: 1–7.
22. Nielsen BS, Jorgensen S, Fog JU, Sokilde R, Christensen IJ, et al. (2011) High levels of microRNA-21 in the stroma of colorectal cancers predict short disease-free survival in stage II colon cancer patients. Clin Exp Metastasis 28: 27–38.
23. Andersen PK, Gill RD (1982) Cox Regression-Model for Counting-Processes - a Large Sample Study. Annals of Statistics 10: 1100–1120.
24. Cox DR (1972) Regression Models and Life-Tables. Journal of the Royal Statistical Society Series B-Statistical Methodology 34: 187–220.
25. Sakamoto MIGKY (1986) Akaike Information Criterion Statistics: D. Reidel Publishing Company.
26. R Core Team (2013) R: A Language and Environment for Statistical Computing. R Foundation for Statistical Computing.
27. Paraskevopoulou MD, Georgakilas G, Kostoulas N, Vlachos IS, Vergoulis T, et al. (2013) DIANA-microT web server v5.0: service integration into miRNA functional analysis workflows. Nucleic Acids Res 41: W169–173.
28. McShane LM, Altman DG, Sauerbrei W, Taube SE, Gion M, et al. (2005) Reporting recommendations for tumor marker prognostic studies. J Clin Oncol 23: 9067–9072.
29. Altman DG, McShane LM, Sauerbrei W, Taube SE (2012) Reporting recommendations for tumor marker prognostic studies (REMARK): explanation and elaboration. BMC Med 10: 51.
30. Bottos A, Rissone A, Bussolino F, Arese M (2011) Neurexins and neuroligins: synapses look out of the nervous system. Cell Mol Life Sci 68: 2655–2666.
31. Lee K, Kim Y, Lee SJ, Qiang Y, Lee D, et al. (2013) MDGAs interact selectively with neuroligin-2 but not other neuroligins to regulate inhibitory synapse development. Proc Natl Acad Sci U S A 110: 336–341.
32. Bottos A, Destro E, Rissone A, Graziano S, Cordara G, et al. (2009) The synaptic proteins neurexins and neuroligins are widely expressed in the vascular system and contribute to its functions. Proc Natl Acad Sci U S A 106: 20782–20787.
33. Rissone A, Foglia E, Sangiorgio L, Cermenati S, Nicoli S, et al. (2012) The synaptic proteins beta-neurexin and neuroligin synergize with extracellular matrix-binding vascular endothelial growth factor a during zebrafish vascular development. Arterioscler Thromb Vasc Biol 32: 1563–1572.
34. Sarver AL, French AJ, Borralho PM, Thayanithy V, Oberg AL, et al. (2009) Human colon cancer profiles show differential microRNA expression depending on mismatch repair status and are characteristic of undifferentiated proliferative states. BMC Cancer 9: 401.
35. Mosakhani N, Lahti L, Borze I, Karjalainen-Lindsberg ML, Sundstrom J, et al. (2012) MicroRNA profiling predicts survival in anti-EGFR treated chemorefractory metastatic colorectal cancer patients with wild-type KRAS and BRAF. Cancer Genet 205: 545–551.
36. Svoboda M, Sana J, Fabian P, Kocakova I, Gombosova J, et al. (2012) MicroRNA expression profile associated with response to neoadjuvant chemoradiotherapy in locally advanced rectal cancer patients. Radiat Oncol 7: 195.
37. Schee K, Lorenz S, Worren MM, Gunther CC, Holden M, et al. (2013) Deep Sequencing the MicroRNA Transcriptome in Colorectal Cancer. PLoS One 8: e66165.
38. Nishida N, Nagahara M, Sato T, Mimori K, Sudo T, et al. (2012) Microarray analysis of colorectal cancer stromal tissue reveals upregulation of two oncogenic miRNA clusters. Clin Cancer Res 18: 3054–3070.

16

Whole Brain Radiotherapy Plus Concurrent Chemotherapy in Non-Small Cell Lung Cancer Patients with Brain Metastases

Hong Qin, Feng Pan, Jianjun Li, Xiaoli Zhang, Houjie Liang*, Zhihua Ruan*

Department of Oncology, Southwest Hospital, the Third Military Medical University, Chongqing, PR China

Abstract

Objective: The aim of the present meta-analysis is to evaluate the response rate, median survival time (MST) and toxicity in patients with brain metastases (BM) originating from non-small cell lung cancer (NSCLC) and who were treated using either whole brain radiotherapy (WBRT) plus concurrent chemotherapy or WBRT alone.

Methods: PubMed, EMBASE, Web of Science, The Cochrane Library, clinical trials and current controlled trials were searched to identify any relevant publications. After screening the literature and undertaking quality assessment and data extraction, the meta-analysis was performed using Stata11.0 software.

Results: In total, six randomized controlled trials (RCT) involving 910 participants were included in the meta-analysis. The results of the analysis indicate that WBRT plus concurrent chemotherapy was more effective at improving response rate (RR = 2.06, 95% CI [1.13, 3.77]; P = 0.019) than WBRT alone. However, WBRT plus concurrent chemotherapy did not improve median survival time (MST) (HR = 1.09, 95%CI [0.94, 1.26]; P = 0.233) or time of neurological progression (CNS-TTP) (HR = 0.93, 95%CI [0.75, 1.16]; P = 0.543), and increased adverse events (Grade≥3) (RR = 2.59, 95% CI [1.88, 3.58]; P = 0.000). There were no significant differences in Grade 3–5 neurological or hematological toxicity between two patient groups (RR = 1.08, 95%CI [0.23, 5.1]; P = 0.92).

Conclusion: The combination of chemotherapy plus WBRT in patients with BM originating from NSCLC may increase treatment response rates of brain metastases with limited toxicity. Although the therapy schedule did not prolong MST or CNS-TTP, further assessment is warranted.

Editor: Matthew B. Schabath, H. Lee Moffitt Cancer Center, United States of America

Funding: These authors have no support or funding to report.

Competing Interests: The authors have declared that no competing interests exist.

* Email: zhihuaruan@gmail.com (ZR); lianghoujie@sina.com (HL)

Introduction

Approximately 20% to 40% of patients with cancer develop brain metastases (BM) during their disease course. Patients with solid tumors, such as lung and, breast cancer or melanoma, are at high risk for BM. In particular, it has been estimated that approximately 50% of primary lung cancers develop into BM [1]. Furthermore, non-small cell lung cancer (NSCLC) accounts a large percentage of lung cancer cases. It has also been estimated that 25% to 30% of newly diagnosed NSCLC patients also suffer from brain metastases [2]. NSCLC patients who develop BM often have poor prognoses, severe neurological symptoms, poor quality of life and dismal survival rates. The overall survival time (OS) for NSCLC patients with BM is less than 3–6 months when left untreated [3]; effective treatment options for NSCLC patients with BM are needed urgently.

Whole brain radiotherapy (WBRT) has been the standard therapy for most patients with multiple BM.WBRT can palliate neurological symptoms and control the local disease. However, it has been difficult to eradicate the tumors due to the limitations of radiation therapy. One study reported that one-third of included patients had uncontrollable localized tumors following WBRT treatment and that 50% of patients died of intracranial tumor progression [4]. Systemic chemotherapy has also been used to reduce tumor burden in patients with BM originating from NSCLC. However, the treatment's effectiveness is limited due to the brain-blood barrier (BBB). Clinical doctors, therefore, faced a dilemma when treating NSLCL patients with BM. Some researchers have suggested that chemical drugs can infiltrate the brain tissue when radiation destroys the BBB, and several clinical trials have indicated that WBRT combined with chemotherapy is not only more effective than WBRT alone, but also improves the response rate and prolongs survival [5–7]. Other studies have failed to confirm the efficacy of chemotherapy and suggest that chemotherapy concurrent with WBRT increases the incidence of adverse events and does not benefit NSCLC patients with BM [8–10]. The role of chemotherapy concurrent with WBRT for the treatment of patients with BM originating from NSCLC is controversial. We have therefore conducted a meta-analysis assessing the efficacy and safety of chemotherapy combined with WBRT versus treatment with WBRT alone.

Materials and Methods

Search strategy

PubMed, EMBASE, the Cochrane Library, Web of Science, clinical trials and current controlled trials were searched to identify relevant studies in the published literature. The search was performed on September 25, 2013, using both Mesh and free text words. The following basic search terms were used: lung neoplasms, lung tumor, lung cancer, brain metastasis, brain neoplasms, radiotherapy and chemotherapy. The search was performed without any language limitations.

Inclusion criteria

All articles which met the following criteria were eligible: (1) randomized controlled trials (RCT) with voluntarily enrolled patients; (2) patients had histologically or cytologically confirmed NSCLC and had been diagnosed with multiple brain metastases using CT or MRI; (3) the trials compared WBRT plus chemotherapy with WBRT alone; (4) trials did not include patients with chemotherapy contraindications or serious vital organ dysfunction and Karnofsky performance status (KPS) scores ≥70; (5) the analyses included response rate, median survival time (MST), the time to neurological progression (CNS-TTP), adverse events (Grade≥3) or hematological toxicity (Grade≥3); (6) response rate was determined using the Response Evaluation Criteria in Solid Tumors (RECIST) or WHO evaluation criteria on solid tumors. complete remission (CR) was defined as tumor completely disappearing for at least four weeks without any new lesions, partial response (PR) was defined as more than 50% tumor regression for at least for four weeks without new lesions, Progressive disease (PD) was defined as an increase in the sum of the longest diameters (LD) of the target lesions by 25% or higher, using as reference the smallest sum LD recorded since treatment started or the appearance of one or more new lesions. Stabilized disease (SD) was defined as a ≤50% tumor regression or an increase ≤25%. (7) Toxicity was evaluated according to the National Cancer Institute Common Terminology Criteria for Adverse Events.

Study selection

The eligibility assessment was first performed by screening titles and abstracts and subsequently reviewing the full text of articles. The selection of all studies was performed independently, according to the inclusion criteria, by two reviewers. Disagreement on whether an article should be included was resolved using a third reviewer.

Data extraction

Two authors independently extracted data from all the eligible studies. When the extracted data were not uniform, consultation was needed to make a final determination. All of the studies included in the analysis contain the following data: first author's name, published year, type of study, trial phase, country of origin study, percentage of men, performance status, number of patients, average ages, interventions and outcomes.

Quality assessment

All of the selected studies were evaluated by two reviewers according to the Cochrane Handbook for RCT, based on the following criteria: (1) randomized method; (2) allocation concealment; (3) blinding of participants, personnel and outcome assessment; and (4) intention-to-treat analysis if the trials lost participants to follow-up or if participants quit. Each trial for bias based on the criteria listed above was marked as 'low risk', 'high risk' or 'unclear risk'. Trials judged as low risk of bias (i.e. A rating) when all criteria are assessed as low risk; Trials judged as moderate risk of bias (i.e. B rating) when one or more criteria are assessed as unclear risk; Trials judged as high risk of bias (i.e. C rating) when one or more criteria are assessed as high risk.

Statistical analysis

Statistical analyses were performed using Stata software11.0. Chi-square and I-square tests were used to test the heterogeneity of different studies [11]; no heterogeneity was considered to exist when P>0.1 and I^2<50%. A fixed-effect model was applied to pool the study results. Significant heterogeneity was found if P< 0.1 and I^2>50%, and a random-effects statistical model was used [12]. Response rate, severe hematological toxicity and advent events were analyzed using dichotomous variables. MST and CNS-TTP were calculated using effect variables.

Results

Selection of studies

In total, we identified 2104 studies that met our selection criteria after searching the relevant databases; 236 of these studies were excluded due to duplication. By verifying related terms in the titles and abstracts, we excluded 1847 irrelevant articles, and another 15 articles were excluded after the full text was read. Finally, six RCTs [10,13–17] were selected for the present meta-analysis. A flowchart depicting the study selection is shown in figure 1.

General characteristics of included studies

There were 910 patients with BM originating from NSCLC in the six selected RCT trials, with 478 patients having received WBRT concurrent with chemotherapy and 432 patients having received only WBRT; these results are summarized in table 1. Of the six RCTs, three were phase III clinical trials [10,14,16], two were phase II studies [15,17], and one was a study [13] that did not mention a trial phase. The analyzed interventions were WBRT plus chemotherapy and WBRT alone, except in the case

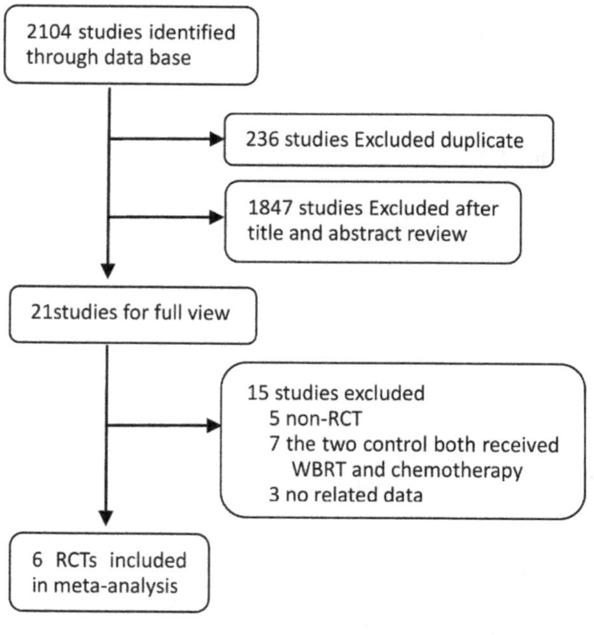

Figure 1. A flow chart on selection included of trials in the Meta-analysis.

of Sperduto, P. W.2013, which compared the combination treatment WBRT, stereotactic radiotherapy (SRS) and chemotherapy with WBRT+SRS treatment. Among all of the included studies, chemotherapy drugs included temozolomide (TMZ), carboplatin, motexafin gadolinium (MGD), chloroethylnitrosoureas and tegafur. TMZ was used in three of the trials. Outcomes included response rate, adverse events, hematological toxicity, median survival time (MST) and time to central nervous system progression (CNS-TTP).

Methodological quality

In accordance with the recommendations of the Cochrane Handbook for Systematic Reviews, two authors evaluated the eligible studies using the four aspects mentioned above. Four studies [10,15–17] mentioned the use of random allocation, but only two articles discussed the methods [13,14]. None of the studies performed or reported their allocation concealment and blinding methods. The Hassler, M.R.2013 [15] trial reported follow-up information, but the other studies did not. All of the articles applied the intent-to-treat analysis. The six eligible studies all received B quality scores, as shown in table 1.

Response rate

Three of the included studies [13,15,16] reported the efficacy of treatment using WBRT plus concurrent chemotherapy and WBRT alone. Ushio, Y.1991 [13] reported tumor response rates in the WBRT and WBRT plus chemotherapy groups were 36% and 71%, respectively. Hassler, M.R.2013 [15] reported two cases of PR in the WBRT arm, and two CR and three PR cases in the WBRT plus chemotherapy arm. Guerrieri, M.2004 [16] reported response rates were 10% and 29% in the WBRT and WBRT plus carboplatin arms, respectively. There was no heterogeneity ($P = 0.801$, $I^2 = 0.0\%$) among the three studies, and as a result, the fixed effect model was used for the meta-analysis. The results indicate that WBRT plus concurrent chemotherapy resulted in superior response rates when compared with WBRT alone ($RR = 2.06$, 95%CI [1.13, 3.77]; $P = 0.019$) (figure 2).

Adverse events

Three studies [10,15,17] reported the occurrence of drug-related hematological toxicity (Grade≥3). A random effects model was used for the meta-analysis of these studies based on the heterogeneity values ($P = 0.041$, $I^2 = 68.8\%$). The results indicate no significant difference in hematological toxicity between WBRT plus chemotherapy and WBRT alone ($RR = 1.08$, 95% CI [0.23, 5.1]; $P = 0.92$) (figure 3). However, another four studies [10,14,15,17] described adverse events (Grade≥3) and included both hematological and non-hematological toxicity. A fixed effect model was used for the meta-analysis of these studies because heterogeneity did not exist ($P = 0.500$, $I^2 = 0.0\%$). The results indicate that the incidence of severe adverse events was higher in the group treated using WBRT concurrent with chemotherapy ($RR = 2.59$, 95% CI [1.88, 3.58]; $P = 0.000$) (figure 4).

Survival

Five of the studies [10,14–17] reported MST for both patient groups; the studies were not heterogeneous ($P = 0.425$, $I^2 = 0.0\%$). Analysis using a fixed effect model suggests that in NSCLC patients diagnosed with BM, there was no significant MST difference between those who were treated with chemotherapy and those who were not ($HR = 1.09$, 95% CI [0.94, 1.26]; $P = 0.233$) (figure 5). The most meaningful outcome was the time to neurological progression (CNS-TTP). Three studies [10,14,17]

Table 1. Characteristics of trials included in the Meta-analysis.

Studies	Country	Trial phase	N (T/C)	Male (T/C,%)	Ages (T/C, years)	ECOG	Interventions T	Interventions C	Outcomes	Study quality
Ushio, Y.1991	Japan	NM	69/31	80/87	57/63	NM	WBRT+methyl-CCNU/ACNU/tegafur	WBRT	Response rate	B
Sperduto, P.W.2013	American	3	40/44	NM	63/64	0–1	WBRT+SRS+TMZ	WBRT+SRS	MST, OS, CNS-TTP, toxicity	B
Mehta, M.P.2009	France	3	279/275	59/55	59/59	0–2	WBRT+MGD	WBRT	MST, CNS-TTP, Adverse event	B
Hassler, M.R.2013	Austria	2	22/13	59/62	69/64	0–2	WBRT+TMZ	WBRT	Response rate, MST, Toxicity, Adverse events	B
Guerrieri, M.2004	Australia	3	21/21	71/71	60/63	0–2	WBRT+ carboplatin	WBRT	MST, Response rate	B
Chua, D.2010	China	2	47/48	64/67	59/62	0–2	WBRT+TMZ	WBRT	MST, CNS-TTP, Toxicity, Adverse event	B

T: treatment group (chemotherapy plus WBRT group); C: control group (WBRT group); NM: not mentioned; ECOG: ECOG/WHO performance status WBRT: Whole brain radiotherapy; TMZ: temozolomide; MST: median survival time; OS: overall survival; CNS: central nervous system; MGD: motexafin gadolinium; TTP: time to progression.

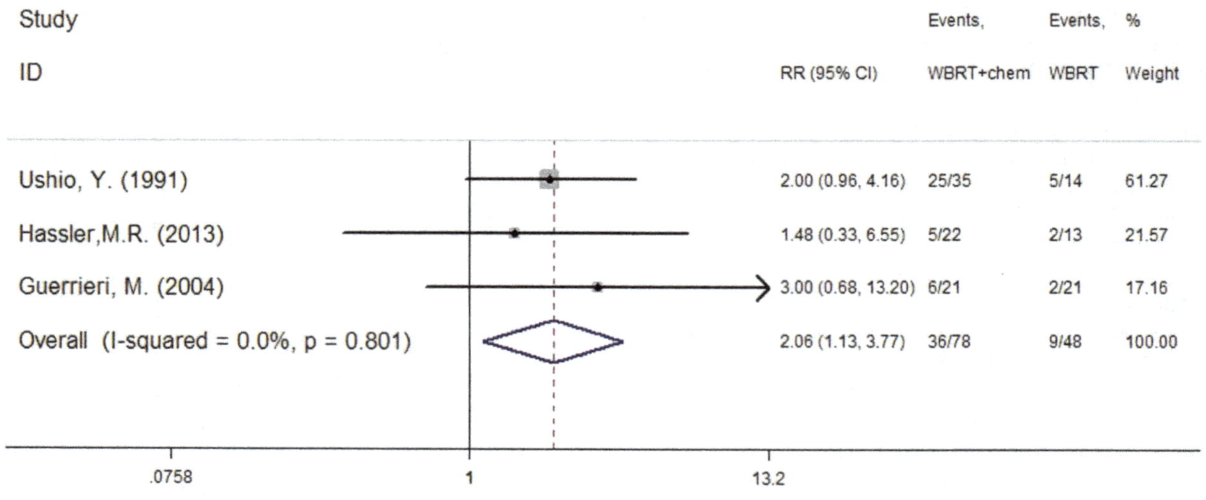

Figure 2. Response rate (P = 0.019).

reported CNS-TTP, and there was no significant heterogeneity between them (P = 0.186, $I^2 = 40.5\%$); accordingly, a fixed effect model was used for the meta-analysis of CNS-TTP. The results suggest that combining chemotherapy with WBRT could prolong the time of neurological progression (HR = 0.93, 95% CI [0.75, 1.16]; P = 0.543) (figure 6). In conclusion, this meta-analysis suggests that WBRT concurrent with chemoradiotherapy significantly increased response rate and potentially prolonged the time of neurologic progression for patients with BM originating from NSCLC. However, more hypotoxic chemotherapy drugs still need to be explored in future clinical research.

Discussion

Currently, WBRT is the standard therapy for NSCLC patients whose disease has metastasized to the brain. Several studies have verified that WBRT palliates the neurological symptom associated with BM. However, because radiotherapy doses are limited, the treatment has been unsuccessful at curing malignant lesions. Furthermore, the brain-blood barrier (BBB) prevents the transport of most anticancer agents to the central nervous system and restricts the delivery of drugs to infiltrating BM. These additional barriers restrict the use of chemotherapy for patients with BM. Results of several trails have indicated that chemotherapy combined with WBRT benefits NSCLC patients with BM. Some clinicians found that WBRT could allow chemotherapy drugs to pass through the BBB. Additionally, chemotherapy had the potential to make brain tumor cells more sensitive to radiotherapy. Several studies have indicated that WBRT plus concurrent chemotherapy is playing an increasing role in the treatment of BM. Mehta, M. P. 2009 [14] reported that treatment using motexafin gadolinium (MGd) improved the neurologic progression interval when compared with WBRT alone (15 months vs.10 months). Verger, E. 2005 [18] reported results of patients who received the combination treatment of WBRT with TMZ, noting that they exhibited good tolerance and significantly better progression-free survival of BM at 90 days (54% vs. 72%; P = 0.03). Nonetheless, some studies have suggested that WBRT had a minor effect on promoting chemotherapy drugs across the BBB. Adding chemotherapy to WBRT treatment did not confer any benefits to the patients, but did increase the incidence of adverse events. For instance, Neuhaus, T.2009 [19] reported that concurrent radiochemotherapy (WBRT+topotecan) did not achieve significant curative effects in patients with lung cancer.

A total of six RCTs were included in present meta-analysis. The response rate was significantly improved in patients treated with

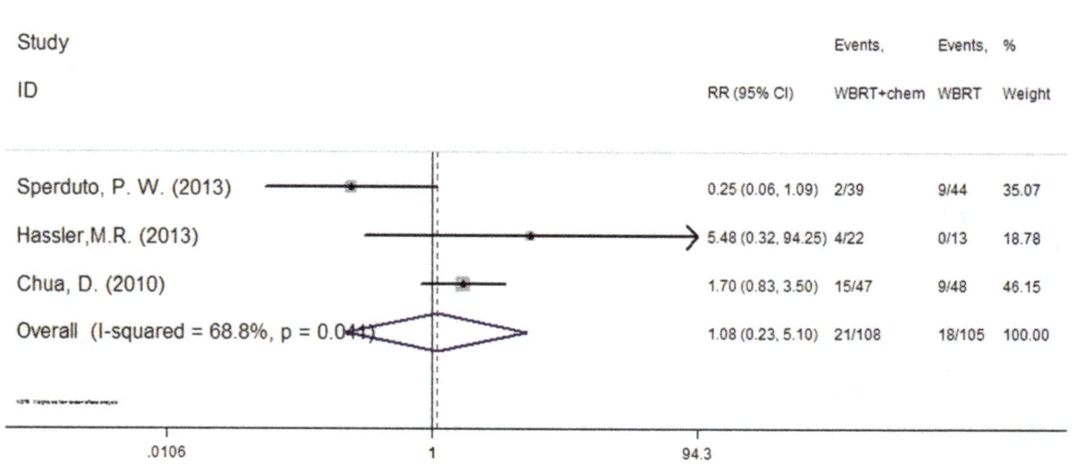

Figure 3. Severe haematological toxicity (P = 0.92).

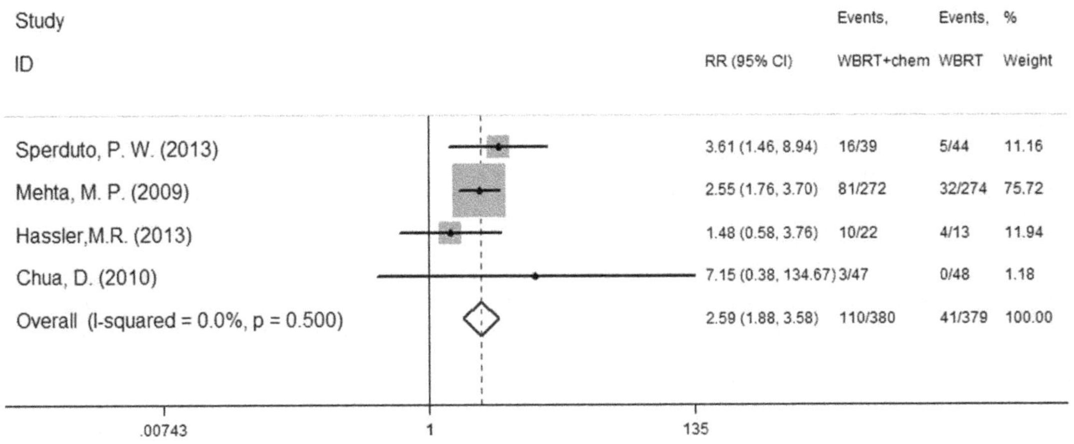

Figure 4. Severe adverse event (P = 0.000).

WBRT plus chemotherapy. However, WBRT plus chemotherapy did not improve MST and CNS-TTP for patients with malignant lesions. WBRT plus chemotherapy increased the incidence of adverse reactions, such as asthenia, fatigue, nausea, vomiting, infection, thrombocytopenia, anemia and neutropenia, but there were no significant differences in the rates of severe hematological toxicity. Each group of patients in the Sperduto, P. W.2013 study received SRS, which might have influenced the final outcomes of the meta-analysis; therefore, we extracted these data and re-analyzed MST and CNS-TTP. Although no significant statistical differences were found, treatment with both WBRT with concurrent chemotherapy tended to prolong MST and CNS-TTP (MST: HR = 1.06, 95% CI [0.91, 1.23], P = 0.462; CNS-TTP: HR = 0.84, 95% CI [0.65, 1.08], P = 0.183).

Researchers hold the opinion that the favorable therapeutic effects of combining chemotherapy with WBRT depend on the drugs crossing the BBB [20]. Temozolomide (TMZ) protocols have been recommended for the favorable distribution of the chemotherapy drug through the BBB and to achieve an effective concentration in the brain tissue [21]. A number of trials have shown that TMZ was well tolerated by patients with BM and achieved high release rates [22,23]. By contrast, some chemotherapy drugs, such as etoposide and cisplatin, had difficulty reaching the intracranial environment because of the BBB. Those agents did not improve response rates and only increased the incidence of neurological toxicity [8]. Due to a lack of response rates and CNS-TTP data, we did not analyze the differences between TMZ and non-TMZ treatments.

Our present systematic review suggests that the combination of chemotherapy and WBRT does not obviously improve MST and CNS-TTP. Moreover, we found a tendency toward prolonged CNS-TTP intervals in the concurrent chemoradiotherapy group.

Our results suggest that the combination of chemotherapy and WBRT significantly increased adverse events of Grade 3 or higher, although there was insufficient evidence to indicate that the treatment resulted in severe nervous-system toxicity. Sperduto, P. W.2013 [10] reported that rates of Grade 3–5 toxicity for WBRT/SRS and WBRT/SRS/TMZ were 11% and 41%, respectively. However, most of the adverse events were fatigue, dehydration and other aspecific symptoms. Chua, D.2010 [17] reported that three patients suffered adverse events (≥Grade 3), and none of these events were related to neurologic toxicity.

Meta-analysis is based on the results of published articles and several steps of integration; thus, certain biases are inevitable. Also, 6 studies included in the meta-analysis were published in the period 1991–2013. Although the dose of WBRT for the treatment of multiple brain metastases did not change during this 22-year period, more precisely delineated target regional and advanced equipment would affect the effectiveness of treatment as technology advances. In addition, as more and more researchers focused their attention on the investigation of targeted drug combine with WBRT in the treatment of multiple brain metastases, and many chemoradiotherapy-related studies were retrospective study and single-arm study, limited RCT were included in this study. Furthermore, the methods of randomization, allocation concealment, and blinding in most of the included studies are not clear. As

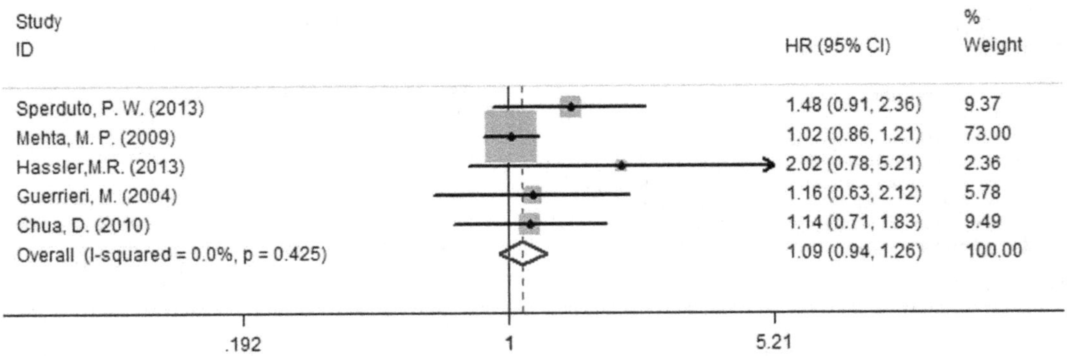

Figure 5. Median survival time (MST) (P = 0.233).

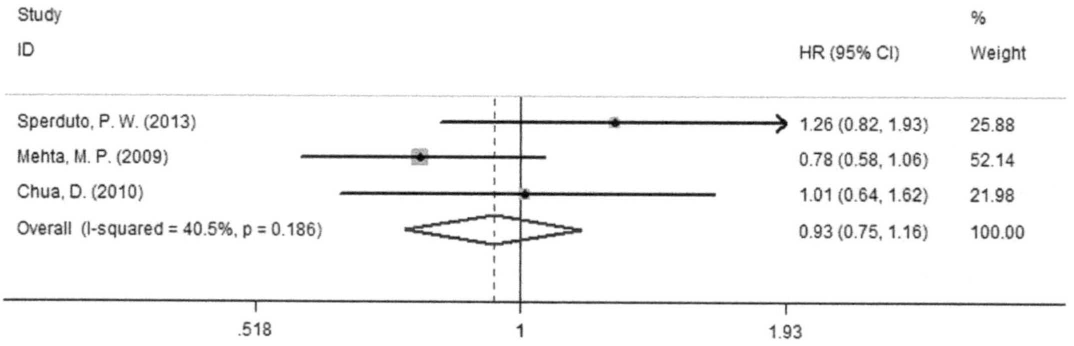

Figure 6. The time to CNS-progression (P = 0.543).

a result, the quality of the 6 RCTs was not high. The different strategies used to divide groups and the dose of WBRT and chemotherapy drugs were not clear; these procedures may have influenced the final outcomes. More high quality and large scale trials are necessary to confirm the efficacy and safety of WBRT plus concurrent chemotherapy for the treatment of patients with BM originating from NSCLC.

In conclusion, this meta-analysis reports that concurrent chemoradiotherapy significantly increased response rates and had the potential to prolong neurologic progression time NSCLC patients with BM. However, additional future clinical research is needed to explore the use of more hypotoxic chemotherapy drugs.

(DOC)

Figure S1 PRISMA Flow Diagram.
(DOC)

Acknowledgments

The authors thank all the participants in this study.

Author Contributions

Conceived and designed the experiments: HQ HL ZR. Performed the experiments: HQ FP JL XZ. Analyzed the data: HQ ZR. Wrote the paper: HQ FP.

References

1. Seoane J and De Mattos-Arruda L (2014) Brain metastasis: New opportunities to tackle therapeutic resistance. Mol Oncol 8: 1120–1131.
2. Berger LA, Riesenberg H, Bokemeyer C and Atanackovic D (2013) CNS metastases in non-small-cell lung cancer: Current role of EGFR-TKI therapy and future perspectives. Lung Cancer 80: 242–248.
3. Sperduto PW, Kased N, Roberge D, Xu Z, Shanley R, et al. (2012) Summary report on the graded prognostic assessment: an accurate and facile diagnosis-specific tool to estimate survival for patients with brain metastases. J Clin Oncol 30: 419–425.
4. Gijtenbeek JM, Ho VK, Heesters MA, Lagerwaard FJ, de Graeff A, et al. (2011) [Practice guideline Brain metastases' (revision)]. Ned Tijdschr Geneeskd 155: A4141.
5. Siu TL, Jeffree RL and Fuller JW (2011) Current strategies in the surgical management of cerebral metastases: an evidence-based review. J Clin Neurosci 18: 1429–1434.
6. Bailon O, Chouahnia K, Augier A, Bouillet T, Billot S, et al. (2012) Upfront association of carboplatin plus pemetrexed in patients with brain metastases of lung adenocarcinoma. Neuro-Oncology 14: 491–495.
7. Barlesi F, Gervais R, Lena H, Hureaux J, Berard H, et al. (2011) Pemetrexed and cisplatin as first-line chemotherapy for advanced non-small-cell lung cancer (NSCLC) with asymptomatic inoperable brain metastases: a multicenter phase II trial (GFPC 07-01). Ann Oncol 22: 2466–2470.
8. Kaba SE, Kyritsis AP, Hess K, Yung WK, Mercier R, et al. (1997) TPDC-FuHu chemotherapy for the treatment of recurrent metastatic brain tumors. J Clin Oncol 15: 1063–1070.
9. Nieder C (1999) Front-line chemotherapy with cisplatin and etoposide for patients with brain metastases from breast carcinoma, nonsmall cell lung carcinoma, or malignant melanoma. A prospective study. Cancer 86: 900–903.
10. Sperduto PW, Wang M, Robins HI, Schell MC, Werner-Wasik M, et al. (2013) A phase 3 trial of whole brain radiation therapy and stereotactic radiosurgery alone versus WBRT and SRS with temozolomide or erlotinib for non-small cell lung cancer and 1 to 3 brain metastases: Radiation Therapy Oncology Group 0320. Int J Radiat Oncol Biol Phys 85: 1312–1318.
11. Higgins JPT, Thompson SG, Deeks JJ and Altman DG (2003) Measuring inconsistency in meta-analyses. BMJ (Clinical research ed) 327: 557–560.
12. Ford AC, Forman D, Hunt RH, Yuan Y and Moayyedi P (2014) Helicobacter pylori eradication therapy to prevent gastric cancer in healthy asymptomatic infected individuals: systematic review and meta-analysis of randomised controlled trials. BMJ (Clinical research ed) 348: g3174.
13. Ushio Y, Arita N, Hayakawa T, Mogami H, Hasegawa H, et al. (1991) Chemotherapy of brain metastases from lung carcinoma: a controlled randomized study. Neurosurgery 28: 201–205.
14. Mehta MP, Shapiro WR, Phan SC, Gervais R, Carrie C, et al. (2009) Motexafin gadolinium combined with prompt whole brain radiotherapy prolongs time to neurologic progression in non-small-cell lung cancer patients with brain metastases: results of a phase III trial. Int J Radiat Oncol Biol Phys 73: 1069–1076.
15. Hassler MR, Pfeifer W, Knocke-Abulesz TH, Geissler K, Altorjai G, et al. (2013) Temozolomide added to whole brain radiotherapy in patients with multiple brain metastases of non-small-cell lung cancer: a multicentric Austrian phase II study. Wien Klin Wochenschr 125: 481–6.
16. Guerrieri M, Wong K, Ryan G, Millward M, Quong G, et al. (2004) A randomised phase III study of palliative radiation with concomitant carboplatin for brain metastases from non-small cell carcinoma of the lung. Lung Cancer 46: 107–111.
17. Chua D, Krzakowski M, Chouaid C, Pallotta MG, Martinez JI, et al. (2010) Whole-brain radiation therapy plus concomitant temozolomide for the treatment of brain metastases from non-small-cell lung cancer: a randomized, open-label phase II study. Clin Lung Cancer 11: 176–181.
18. Verger E, Gil M, Yaya R, Vinolas N, Villa S, et al. (2005) Temozolomide and concomitant whole brain radiotherapy in patients with brain metastases: a phase II randomized trial. Int J Radiat Oncol Biol Phys 61: 185–191.
19. Neuhaus T, Ko Y, Muller RP, Grabenbauer GG, Hedde JP, et al. (2009) A phase III trial of topotecan and whole brain radiation therapy for patients with CNS-metastases due to lung cancer. Br J Cancer 100: 291–297.
20. Biswas G, Bhagwat R, Khurana R, Menon H, Prasad N, et al. (2006) Brain metastasis-evidence based management. J Cancer Res Ther 2: 5–13.
21. Addeo R and Caraglia M (2011) Combining temozolomide with other antitumor drugs and target-based agents in the treatment of brain metastases: An unending quest or chasing a chimera? Expert Opin Investig Drugs 20: 881–895.
22. Adonizio CS, Babb JS, Maiale C, Huang C, Donahue J, et al. (2002) Temozolomide in non-small-cell lung cancer: preliminary results of a phase II trial in previously treated patients. Clin Lung Cancer 3: 254–258.
23. Addeo R, Caraglia M, Faiola V, Capasso E, Vincenzi B, et al. (2007) Concomitant treatment of brain metastasis with Whole Brain Radiotherapy WBRT and Temozolomide TMZ is active and improves Quality of Life. BMC cancer 7: doi: 10.1186/1471-2407-7-18.

17

Characterization of Ring-Like F-Actin Structure as a Mechanical Partner for Spindle Positioning in Mitosis

Huan Lu[1], Qun Zhao[1], Hao Jiang[1], Tongge Zhu[1,2], Peng Xia[1], William Seffens[2], Felix Aikhionbare[2], Dongmei Wang[1], Zhen Dou[1], Xuebiao Yao[1]*

1 Anhui Key Laboratory of Cellular Dynamics and Chemical Biology, University of Science and Technology of China, Hefei, Anhui, China, 2 Department of Physiology, Morehouse School of Medicine, Atlanta, Georgia, United States of America

Abstract

Proper spindle positioning and orientation are essential for accurate mitosis which requires dynamic interactions between microtubule and actin filament (F-actin). Although mounting evidence demonstrates the role of F-actin in cortical cytoskeleton dynamics, it remains elusive as to the structure and function of F-actin-based networks in spindle geometry. Here we showed a ring-like F-actin structure surrounding the mitotic spindle which forms since metaphase and maintains in MG132-arrested metaphase HeLa cells. This cytoplasmic F-actin structure is relatively isotropic and less dynamic. Our computational modeling of spindle position process suggests a possible mechanism by which the ring-like F-actin structure can regulate astral microtubule dynamics and thus mitotic spindle orientation. We further demonstrated that inhibiting Plk1, Mps1 or Myosin, and disruption of microtubules or F-actin polymerization perturbs the formation of the ring-like F-actin structure and alters spindle position and symmetric division. These findings reveal a previously unrecognized but important link between mitotic spindle and ring-like F-actin network in accurate mitosis and enables the development of a method to theoretically illustrate the relationship between mitotic spindle and cytoplasmic F-actin.

Editor: Quansheng Du, Georgia Regents University, United States of America

Funding: This work was supported, in whole or in part, by National Institutes of Health Grants DK56292, CA164133, and G12RR03034. This project was also supported by Chinese 973 Project Grants 2010CB912103, 2012CB917204, and 2014CB964800; Anhui Province Key Project Grant 08040102005; International Collaboration Grant 2009DFA31010; Chinese Natural Science Foundation Grants 91313303, 91129714, 81270466, 90913016, 31000602, 31071184, 31171300, 31271439; and MOE grants (20113402130010, PCSIRT-CDCB, WK2060190018, and WK2340000021). The funders had no role in study design, data collection and analysis, decision to publish, or preparation of the manuscript.

Competing Interests: The authors have declared that no competing interests exist.

* Email: yaoxb@ustc.edu.cn

These authors contributed equally to this work.

Introduction

For the past decades, our understanding on molecular components, assembly and function of mitotic spindle has achieved great advance [1]. Comparing the biochemical mechanism of mitotic spindle, the biophysical mechanism, especially a mechanical force chain stretching across the mitotic cell, remains elusive. This force chain starts in the region of extracellular substrate-cell cortex fringe with adhesion proteins and actin filaments [2,3,4,5]. As the second part of the force chain, astral microtubules stretch from spindle pole to cell cortex. Astral microtubules conduct the pulling force mainly produced by cortical dynein and regulate spindle positioning and orientation [6,7,8,9,10,11]. Spindle positioning, orientation and chromosome segregation are also mechanically orchestrated by mutual motion of Myosin and F-actin around spindle pole [12,13]. Finally, the pulling and pushing force on spindle microtubules is regulated by motor proteins and mitotic signals [14,15,16,17]. This part is involved in the spindle assembly checkpoint (SAC), which precludes anaphase entry until all chromosomes achieve bi-orientation [18,19,20].

Microtubules and F-actin are key players of many biological processes including cell division and embryonic morphogenesis [21,22]. The cooperation between microtubules and F-actin in regulating the second part of the force chain may be one of the most fascinating and significant events. It is required for spindle positioning in yeast [22,23,24] and asymmetrical cell division in polarized epithelial cells [25]. It has been shown that mitotic spindle adapts its orientation by sensing the matrix geometry [22]. The statistics on spindle orientation of the HeLa cells cultured in various shaped matrix substantiates the conclusion that the metaphase spindle angle is influenced by the distribution of cortical F-actin [2,3]. The main opinion on such influence of matrix towards spindle orientation is that the dynein-mediated astral microtubule-cortex interactions provide the pulling force to dynamically regulate mitotic spindle positioning and orientation [8,9,18,26,27]. Knockdown of some proteins participating in this process such as MISP, results in more randomized spindle angles as the result of uncontrolled spindle orientation [28]. Inhibiting the polymerization of tubulin or actin by the treatment with Nocodazole or Latrunculin B (Lat B) results in metaphase arrest and abnormally rotated spindles [4]. Collectively, these studies suggest a unique role of microtubule-F-actin interaction in spindle positioning and orientation. However, it remains elusive on how the cytoplasmic force rather than the cortical affects the spindle.

One recent work suggests that Myosin 10 and cytoplasmic actin filaments in *Xenopus Laevis* embryos control spindle length and orientation [13]. Persistently stabilized actin filaments may attenuate the connection between astral microtubules and cell cortex [29]. But it becomes controversial that the reported cytoplasmic actin structure revolving around the spindle has a unique organization and motile pattern [30]. Additionally, a ring-like actin structure related to spindle position and symmetric division is found in mouse zygote, but the dynamic of this structure remains unclear [31]. Mathematical model drawing on the experimental data and model of previous works have been established to deal with the calculation of spindle-cytoskeleton dynamics [2,10,32].

We inferred that actin filaments, together with Myosin play a pivotal role in the force chain, and inhibiting Myosin would weaken the interactions between mitotic spindle and cytoplasmic actin filament. In our experiment, we used specific chemical compounds to harness the enzymatic activities of kinases such as Plk1 and Mps1, motility of Myosin, and polymerization of F-actin. We observed that a ring-like F-actin structure forms in metaphase cells or maintains in MG132-arrested cells. Then we presented a model raising possible mechanism underlying the function of cytoplasmic actin filaments. We observed that the drugs perturb the formation of the ring-like F-actin structure, coupled with translated spindles and altered symmetric division. In summary, we characterized the formation of the ring-like F-actin structure as a mitotic event and developed a method to theoretically describe the relationships between mitotic spindle and cytoplasmic F-actin.

Materials and Methods

Plasmids and antibodies

The cDNA sequence of human Utrophin (RP11-352E13.1) was obtained from NCBI database and the DNA fragment of UtroCH [30] was synthesized by BGI and cloned into pUC118. We sub-cloned UtroCH into pcDNA-mCherry-N via HindIII and BamHI sites and pEGFP-C2 via EcoRI and BamHI sites. A Kozak-sequence was added on the N-terminal of UtroCH to enhance the expression.

Anti-α-tubulin (DM1A, Sigma Chemical), Secondary antibodies such as FITC-conjugated goat-anti-mouse (Pierce) and Rhodamine-Phalloidin (Invitrogen) were obtained commercially.

Cell culture and transfection

HeLa cells from American Type Culture Collection (Manassas, VA, USA) were cultured as sub-confluent monolayers in DMEM (Invitrogen) with 10% fetal bovine serum (FBS, Hyclone, Logan, UT) and penicillin-streptomycin (100 international units/ml and 100 mg/ml, respectively, GIBCO) at 37°C with 10% CO_2. The coverslips were pretreated with collagen (Sigma) according to the manufacturer's instructions.

HeLa cells were double blocked by Thymidine at the concentration of 2 mM to synchronize them at G1/S, then washed with PBS three times and cultured in Thymidine-free medium for at least 8 hours to release. After the first release, mCherry-UtroCH and GFP-tubulin were transfected into cells using Lipofectamine 2000 (Invitrogen) in Opti-MEM (Invitrogen) according to the manufacturer's instructions. When the second block was over, cells were released about 8 hr for immunofluorescence and live-cell imaging.

Drug Treatments

HeLa cells were grown on coverslips in 24-well plates (Corning, New York). For each drug treatment, we prepared 6 wells of cells. After the second release from Thymidine for 8 hours, cells were treated with aliquots of MG132, 10 minutes later, the first well of cells were collected, labeled as " 0' " and fixed for appropriate examination. Remaining wells of cells were exposed to DMSO, BI2536, Blebbistatin, Reversine and Lat B. We collected and fixed these cells every 10 minutes in a row. To collect anaphase cells for analysis of symmetric division, drugs were added 8 hours after release from Thymidine without MG132.

Reversine was used at 0.3 μM, Blebbistatin at 100 μM, BI2536 at 100 nM, Lat B at 10 μM, Nocodazole at 100 ng/ml and MG132 at 20 μM.

Immunofluorescence microscopy, image processing and quantification

Cells were seeded onto sterile, collagen-treated 12-mm coverslips in 24-well plates (Corning Glass Works, Coring, NY) for transfection or drug treatment, HeLa cells grown on coverslips were rinsed for 1 minute with PHEM buffer (100 mM PIPES, 20 mM HEPES, pH 6.9, 5 mM EGTA, 2 mM $MgCl_2$ and 4 M glycerol) and permeabilized for 1 minute with PHEM buffer plus 0.1% Triton X-100. And then extracted HeLa cells were fixed in freshly prepared 3.7% formaldehyde in PHEM buffer and rinsed three times in 1× PBS. HeLa cells seeded on coverslips were blocked with 0.05% Tween-20 in 1× PBS (1× TPBS) with 1% bovine serum albumin (Sigma) for 45~60 minutes. Then they were incubated with primary antibodies in a humidified chamber for 1 hour and with FITC-conjugated secondary antibodies for 1 hour at room temperature. Phalloidin-Texas was incubated with the secondary antibodies. DNA was stained with 4′-6-diamidino-2-phenylindole (DAPI, Sigma). Samples were examined with a DeltaVision wide-field deconvolution microscope (Applied Precision Inc., WA, USA). Z-stacks were taken at an interval of 0.2 μm. Images were deconvoluted using Softworx (Applied Precision). Measurements of intensities were performed using Image-J (http://rsb.info.nih.gov/ij/) software on un-deconvoluted images. Images were also processed by Image-J.

Quantification of the intensity of F-actin in mitotic cells was conducted as previously described [33]. A specific description of the approach is provided in the article. To be consistent with the statistical diagrams in the figures, all quantified experimental data were displayed in Table S1 and Table S2.

Live cell imaging

Cells were cultured in a glass-bottomed culture dish (MatTek, MA) pretreated with collagen. Then, the cells were transfected with mCherry-UtroCH/GFP- tubulin and double blocked by Thymidine as described previously. About 8 hours after release, DME medium was replaced with CO_2- independent medium (Invitrogen) containing 10% FBS and 1% glutamine in a sealed chamber at 37°C. FBS was added according to drug property, as Lat B is unstable in medium with FBS. MG132 was added 5 minutes before the addition of drugs when the cells entered metaphase. We acquired each image every 1 minute over a timeframe of 1 hour or 1.5 hours with Delta-Vision Real Time System built on an Olympus IX-70 inverted microscope base. The live-cell images were also processed with Image-J.

Results

Identification of a ring-like F-actin structure during mitosis

It is generally believed that mitotic spindle governs chromosome partitioning and segregation in eukaryotes. However, several lines of recent evidence suggest the role of F-actin-based structure in spindle assembly and positioning [2,3,6,13,30,31]. To validate if there are any cytoplasmic F-actin structures in mitotic cells, we carried out immunofluorescence analyses on F-actin and spindle of mitotic cells. To this end, asynchronized HeLa cells were fixed and stained with Rhodamine-Phalloidin and anti-tubulin antibody (DM1A) to visualize F-actin and microtubule, respectively. As shown in Fig. 1A, F-actin staining is mainly distributed on the cortex and retraction fibers through mitosis. Careful examination revealed that the F-actin staining is organized around the spindle poles in prophase cells (Fig. 1A; ***a***, arrow). As the cell goes through metaphase, F-actin staining becomes apparent around the entire spindle (Fig. 1A; ***b***, arrow). In the anaphase A cell, the F-actin staining appears more recognizable (Fig. 1A; ***c***, arrow). Once cells enter into anaphase B, F-actin staining becomes concentrated to contractile ring. During the course of telophase and cytokinesis, the intensity of the F-actin staining in cytoplasm is as low as its intensity in prophase.

The cytoplasmic F-actin is a large collection of bundled actin filaments (Fig. 1B; [34]). It is practically a continuous structure stretching from spindle to cell cortex as well as the astral microtubule. By convention, we defined an X-axis through the spindle poles when spindle is at the equilibrium position, and a Z-axis perpendicular to the imaging plane at the center of the cell. We chose the axis perpendicular simultaneously to X-axis and Z-axis as Y-axis (Fig. 2A). We imaged cells at different layers with an interval of 0.2 μm. The cytoplasmic F-actin changes only slightly along the Z-axis (Fig. 1C, yellow arrows) no matter how much the spindle is rotated. We found that the relative intensity of the cytoplasmic F-actin in different regions varies slightly compared with the $Z=0$ plane. Thus we concluded the distribution of cytoplasmic F-actin is isotropic (Fig. S3C, Table for Fig. S3C in Table S1). Compared to the distribution of astral microtubule (Fig. 1D, yellow arrows), the cytoplasmic F-actin structure distributes around the spindle continuously.

To examine this ring-like structure in metaphase arrested cells, an aliquot of HeLa cells was synchronized by a double-Thymidine treatment followed by release into MG132-containing DMEM to prevent anaphase onset. As predicted, treatment of Lat B perturbed the ring-like F-actin structure. These cells treated with other drugs except for Lat B exhibit a distinct actin filament ring (Fig. S3B).

Unlike previous publication [29], F-actin bundling exists during mitosis in normal HeLa cells with considerable intensity. Comparing with the revolving network [30], the cytoplasmic F-actin we found around the mitotic spindle is relatively more relaxed and smooth. The kymograph of the real-time images (Movie S1 and Movie S2) of metaphase arrested cells indicates that the ring-like F-actin structure is relatively less dynamic and cytoplasmic actin filaments have a random motile pattern (Fig. S3E, the teeth appear in a different pattern from reported [30,44]). Thus, we reasoned that a ring-like cytoplasmic F-actin structure is present around the mitotic spindle in normal HeLa cells during mitosis (Fig. 1C, yellow arrows) and maintains in metaphase arrested cells. This ring-like F-actin staining was mainly observed in metaphase or anaphase of asynchronized cells, and it was observed in all MG132-synchronized cells.

Modeling of spindle positioning and hypothesis of the function of ring-like F-actin structure

First, we established a 3D-coordinate to localize the point inside the cell. When the spindle is at the equilibrium state during metaphase, the axis vertical to the medium plane is Z-axis, and the axis linking two spindle poles is X-axis, and Y-axis is vertical to X-axis and Z-axis (Fig. 2A). Then we can get an equation to describe the hypothetical ellipsoidal surface of the cell (Fig. 2B), and we used a vector $\vec{\mathbf{D}}$ to mark the vector from the center of the cell to the surface. Supposing the translation and rotation simultaneously exist, the distance from spindle pole to equate plate is **A**. The coordinate of the geometrical center of spindle and the rotation angle of spindle in cell coordinate are marked by parameters Θ,Φ on Z-X and X-Y sections (Fig. 2C).

Then we introduced a 1-D spring oscillator to simulate the motion of microtubule-motor protein complex (Fig. 2D, [35]). Here, K is the elastic modulus, μ is the frictional coefficient, $\vec{\mathbf{D}}_{-c}$ is the vector from one spindle pole to the cortex and $\vec{\mathbf{D}}_{-c0}$ is the similar vector as $\vec{\mathbf{D}}_{-c}$ when the oscillator is at the equilibrium position [35].

Supposing all the mass of spindle is concentrated on the spindle pole regardless of the structural dynamics near the equate plate, the force acting on the oscillators is not conservative, and the motion of each spindle pole is independent to each other, we can get the simplified mechanical equation:

$$\vec{\mathbf{F}} = -K\left(\vec{\mathbf{D}} - \vec{\mathbf{D}}_0\right) - \mu \frac{d\vec{\mathbf{D}}_{-c}}{dt} \quad (1)$$

Then we introduced the offset to the equilibrium position ($D = |\vec{\mathbf{D}}| - |\vec{\mathbf{D}}_0|$), the velocity ($v = \frac{dD}{dt}$) and the momentum ($p = mv$, m is the equivalent mass of the oscillator). The potential and kinetic energy of each oscillator is:

$$E_j = E_k + E_p = \frac{p^2}{2m} + \frac{KD^2}{2} \quad (2)$$

The distribution function of the oscillators statistically follows an 1-D Maxwell-Boltzmann distribution with its partition function Z, and $k_B T$ is a modified form of inner energy of the oscillator:

$$f(D,p) = \frac{1}{2\pi k_B T}\left(\frac{K}{m}\right)^{\frac{1}{2}} \exp\left(-\frac{p^2 + KmD^2}{2mk_B T}\right) \quad (3)$$

Supposing the oscillators with D in the interval $[D_1, D_2]$ and a positive momentum form effective connections, the number of effective connections is $N_e(t_0)$ and the number of ineffective connections is $N_i(t_0)$ at the initial time point. Moreover, a dynamic transition between $N_e(t_0)$ and $N_i(t_0)$ exists during a short period Δt, and we supposed the transition rate from $N_e(t_0)$ to $N_i(t_0)$ is $\omega_{e \to i}$ and the transition rate from $N_i(t_0)$ to $N_e(t_0)$ is $\omega_{i \to e}$ (Fig. 2E).

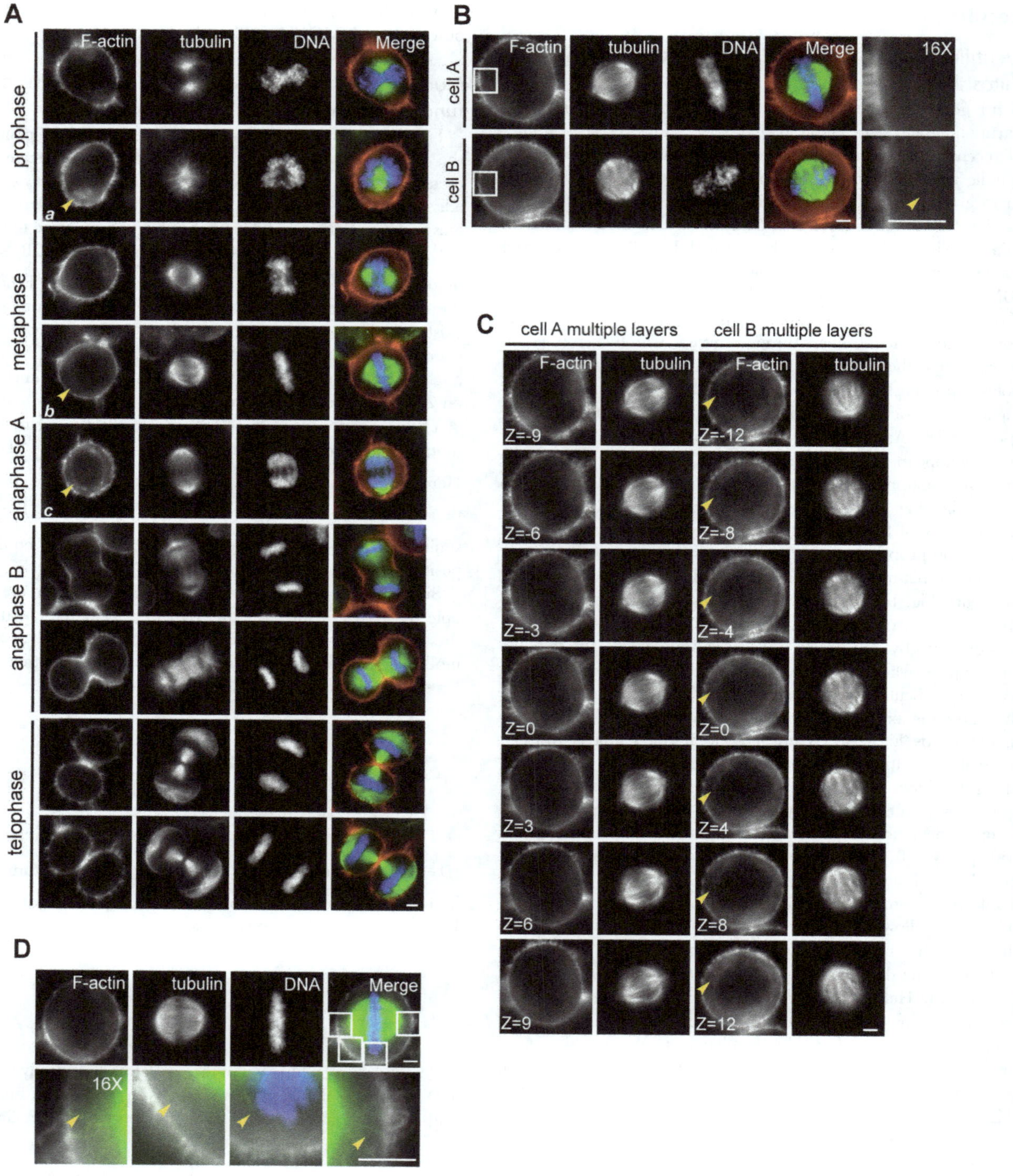

Figure 1. Identification of a ring-like F-actin structure during mitosis. (A) The distribution of F-actin in different phases of mitosis in HeLa cells. Asynchronized cells were fixed and co-stained for F-actin (red), microtubule (green) and DNA (blue). A ring-like F-actin structure appears during metaphase and anaphase and was indicated by the arrows (***a, b, c***). Scale bar, 5 μm. (B) The representative immunofluorescence images of two cells with cytoplasmic F-actin. Cell A represents the cells with slightly rotated spindles, and Cell B represents the cells with distinctly rotated spindle. The boxed areas are shown magnified in the right panels. Scale bar, 5 μm. (C) Multiple-layer images of Cell A and Cell B. The plane passing through the midpoint of spindle poles and parellel to substrate is chosen as Z = 0, and the images in Fig. 1B is taken at the plane Z = 0. The distance between layer Z and layer Z+1 is 0.2 μm. Scale bar, 5 μm. (D) Astral microtubules and cytoplasmic F-actin structure cross and distribute differently in cytoplasm. The yellow arrows indicate the detailed distribution of astral microtubules. The cytoplasmic F-actin structure distributes around the spindle continuously. The boxed areas are shown magnified 16 times in the bottom panels. Scale bar, 5 μm.

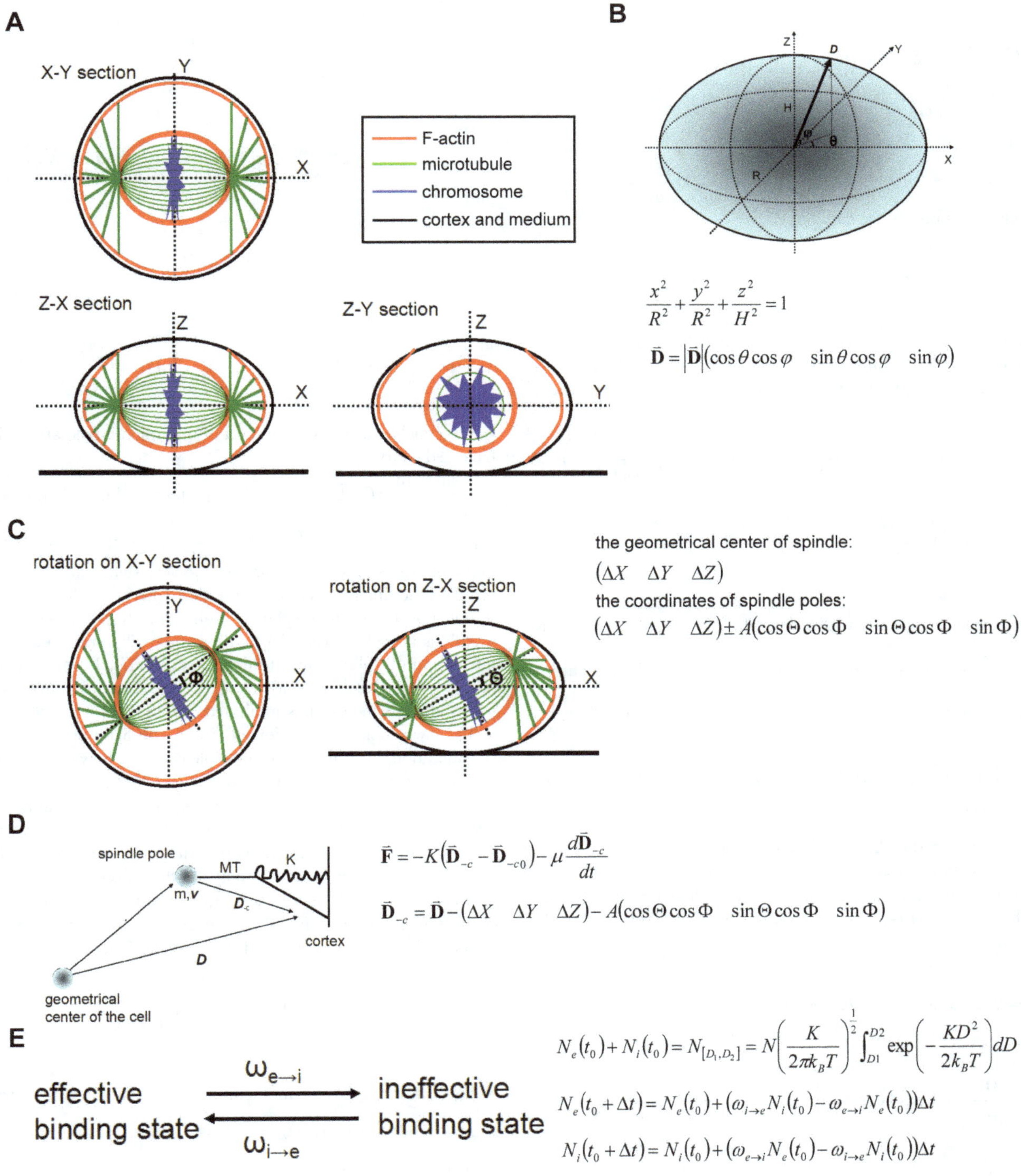

$$\frac{x^2}{R^2}+\frac{y^2}{R^2}+\frac{z^2}{H^2}=1$$

$$\vec{\mathbf{D}}=\left|\vec{\mathbf{D}}\right|(\cos\theta\cos\varphi \quad \sin\theta\cos\varphi \quad \sin\varphi)$$

the geometrical center of spindle:

$$(\Delta X \quad \Delta Y \quad \Delta Z)$$

the coordinates of spindle poles:

$$(\Delta X \quad \Delta Y \quad \Delta Z)\pm A(\cos\Theta\cos\Phi \quad \sin\Theta\cos\Phi \quad \sin\Phi)$$

$$\vec{\mathbf{F}}=-K\left(\vec{\mathbf{D}}_{-c}-\vec{\mathbf{D}}_{-c0}\right)-\mu\frac{d\vec{\mathbf{D}}_{-c}}{dt}$$

$$\vec{\mathbf{D}}_{-c}=\vec{\mathbf{D}}-(\Delta X \quad \Delta Y \quad \Delta Z)-A(\cos\Theta\cos\Phi \quad \sin\Theta\cos\Phi \quad \sin\Phi)$$

$$N_e(t_0)+N_i(t_0)=N_{[D_1,D_2]}=N\left(\frac{K}{2\pi k_BT}\right)^{\frac{1}{2}}\int_{D1}^{D2}\exp\left(-\frac{KD^2}{2k_BT}\right)dD$$

$$N_e(t_0+\Delta t)=N_e(t_0)+(\omega_{i\to e}N_i(t_0)-\omega_{e\to i}N_e(t_0))\Delta t$$

$$N_i(t_0+\Delta t)=N_i(t_0)+(\omega_{e\to i}N_e(t_0)-\omega_{i\to e}N_i(t_0))\Delta t$$

Figure 2. Modeling of spindle positioning and hypothesis of the function of ring-like F-actin structure. (A) The overview of a mitotic cell from three dimensions. X-axis links two spindle poles when the spindle is in its equilibrium position, and Z-axis is vertical to the substrate and passes through the midpoint of spindle poles, and Y-axis is simultaneously vertical to X-axis and Z-axis. Different regions are colored for F-actin (red), microtubule (green), chromosomes (blue), cortex and medium (black). (B) The geometrical hypothesis of cell. A mitotic HeLa cell is supposed to be an ellipsoid with its height H and radius R. Then, the geometry can be described with a formula, and the point on the surface can be positioned with an alterable vector ***D*** and two parameters θ, φ. (C) The schematic diagram of spindle rotation in two sections, X-Y and Z-X. The geometrical center of spindle is supposed to be translated from the geometrical center of cell, and the coordinate of two spindle poles can be expressed with **A**, the distance from spindle pole to equate plate. The rotation in X-Y and Z-X sections can be described with the parameters, **Θ, Φ**. (D) The hypothesis of oscillation. The microtubule-motor complex is simplified as an oscillator, and the oscillation follows Hooke's Law of Elasticity and is influenced by the obstruction from cytoplasm. Here, D_{-c} represents the vector from spindle pole to cell cortex, which can be decomposed into a regular vector ***D*** and the position of one spindle pole. (E) The dynamic transition between effective and ineffective connections or binding state. $\omega_{i\to e}$ and $\omega_{e\to i}$ were supposed to be two rate constant for this transition. We also supposed that only the oscillators with its |***D***| in the interval [D_1, D_2] and a positive momentum make effective connections. Then the number of effective or ineffective connections can be expressed as displayed in the figure.

$$N_e(t)=\frac{\omega_{i\to e}}{\omega_{i\to e}+\omega_{e\to i}}N_{[D_1,D_2]}-\left(\frac{\omega_{i\to e}}{\omega_{i\to e}+\omega_{e\to i}}N_{[D_1,D_2]}-N_e(t_0)\right)\exp(-(\omega_{i\to e}+\omega_{e\to i})(t-t_0)) \tag{4}$$

If we chose $N_e(\infty)=\lim_{t\to+\infty}N_e(t)=\frac{\omega_{i\to e}}{\omega_{i\to e}+\omega_{e\to i}}N_{[D_1,D_2]}$ to simplify equation (4), we can get:

$$N_e(t)=N_e(\infty)-(N_e(\infty)-N_e(t_0))\exp(-(\omega_{i\to e}+\omega_{e\to i})(t-t_0)) \tag{5}$$

In conclusion, in a very tiny area on the cell cortex, the approximate total momentum produced by the oscillators is as following, and the pushing force is not considered in this equation:

$$p(\theta,\varphi)=\sum_j p_j=\frac{N_e(t)}{(2\pi mk_BT)^{\frac{1}{2}}}\int_0^{+\infty}\left(p\bullet\exp\left(-\frac{p^2}{2mk_BT}\right)dp\right)=N_e(t)\left(\frac{mk_BT}{2\pi}\right)^{\frac{1}{2}} \tag{6}$$

Supposing the unit vector on the direction of $\vec{\mathbf{D}}_{-c}$ is $\vec{\mathbf{e}}_{-c}=\frac{\vec{\mathbf{D}}_{-c}}{|\vec{\mathbf{D}}_{-c}|}=\vec{\mathbf{e}}_{-c}(\theta,\varphi,\Theta,\Phi,\Delta X,\Delta Y,\Delta Z)$, the total momentum produced by all oscillators on the cortex is calculated as following:

$$\iint_{cortex} p(\theta,\varphi)\vec{\mathbf{e}}_{-c}d\theta d\varphi,\theta\in[-\alpha,\alpha],\varphi\in[-\beta,\beta],\alpha,\beta\in[0,\pi] \tag{7}$$

α,β relate to the distribution of all oscillators.

Then we simplified the calculation of the asymmetric motion. Supposing the coordination of one spindle pole is $(x\quad y\quad z)$, the length of the vector is $|(x\quad y\quad z)|<<H<R$, and H is close to R. Then we can get these:

$$\vec{\mathbf{D}}_{-c}=D(\cos\theta\cos\varphi\quad \sin\theta\cos\varphi\quad \sin\varphi)-(x\quad y\quad z),D\in[H,R] \tag{8}$$

$$\vec{\mathbf{e}}_{-c}=\frac{\vec{\mathbf{D}}_{-c}}{|\vec{\mathbf{D}}_{-c}|}\approx\left(\cos\theta\cos\varphi-\frac{x}{R}\quad \sin\theta\cos\varphi-\frac{y}{R}\quad \sin\varphi-\frac{z}{R}\right) \tag{9}$$

$$\iint_{\substack{\theta\in[-\alpha,\alpha]\\ \varphi\in[-\beta,\beta]}} p(\theta,\varphi)\vec{\mathbf{e}}_{-c}d\theta d\varphi=N_e(t)\left(\frac{mk_BT}{2\pi}\right)^{\frac{1}{2}}(-4\alpha\beta)\left(-\frac{\sin\alpha\sin\beta}{\alpha\beta}+\frac{x}{R}\quad \frac{y}{R}\quad \frac{z}{R}\right)=M\left(\frac{dx}{dt}\quad \frac{dy}{dt}\quad \frac{dz}{dt}\right) \tag{10}$$

We concluded that the minute translation of spindle pole will lead to the 3D-oscillation. First, the pattern of the oscillation is based on the components, while **M** is the equivalent mass of the spindle pole. We use a factor Q_t to simplify the presentation of part of the solution:

$$Q_t=\exp\left\{\left(-\frac{4\alpha\beta}{M}\left(\frac{mk_BT}{2\pi}\right)^{\frac{1}{2}}\right)\left[N_e(\infty)(t-t_0)+\frac{N_e(\infty)-N_e(t_0)}{\omega_{i\to e}+\omega_{e\to i}}\left(e^{-(\omega_{i\to e}+\omega_{e\to i})(t-t_0)}-1\right)\right]\right\} \tag{11}$$

So

$$(x_t\quad y_t\quad z_t)=\left(\frac{\sin\alpha\sin\beta}{\alpha\beta}R(1-Q_t)+Q_tx_0\quad Q_ty_0\quad Q_tz_0\right)$$

and

$$\lim_{t\to+\infty}Q_t=0 \tag{12}$$

$$\frac{d(x_t\quad y_t\quad z_t)}{dt}=\left(-\frac{4\alpha\beta}{M}\left(\frac{mk_BT}{2\pi}\right)^{\frac{1}{2}}\right)Q_tN_e(t_0)\left(x_0-\frac{\sin\alpha\sin\beta}{\alpha\beta}R\quad y_0\quad z_0\right) \tag{13}$$

We concluded that the position of one spindle pole at the final balanced state is $\left(\frac{\sin\alpha\sin\beta}{\alpha\beta}R\quad 0\quad 0\right)$, and the pattern of the oscillation is an exponential decay style. If we choose $\alpha=\frac{\pi}{2},\beta=\frac{\pi}{2}$ according to the previous works [27,34], we can get the very significant result: the spindle pole finally stays at the position where the distance from spindle pole to the equate plate is about 0.4 radius of the cell, while spindle is in its balanced place with some oscillation produced by fluctuation of pulling and pushing force [36,37]. Low concentration of Nocodazole mainly changes the distribution of astral microtubule, which results in altered α,β and $N_e(\infty)$.

Then we took the function of ring-like F-actin structure into consideration. We raised three possible manners how the structure performs on the spindle dynamics:

(1) It increases the potential energy of the oscillators. We assumed that the ring-like F-actin structure produces a conserved force field that increases the potential energy of the oscillators. The potential energy is proportional to the momentum of the oscillation and the offset to the equilibrium position. Here the coefficient of proportionality k_1 and k_2 are constants and I_{ring} refers to the relative intensity of the ring-like F-actin structure:

$$E_j=\frac{p^2}{2m}+\frac{1}{2}KD^2+I_{ring}(k_1p+k_2D)$$

The most probable momentum and offset change from $(p,D)_p=(0,0)$ to $(p,D)_p=-I_{ring}\left(k_1m,\frac{k_2}{K}\right)$ according to $\frac{\partial f(D,p)}{\partial p}=0$ and $\frac{\partial f(D,p)}{\partial D}=0$. The shortened astral microtubule in metaphase is observed in previous work [29]. Eventually, $N_{[D_1,D_2]}$ and $N_e(\infty)$ decrease regardless of the metaphase-anaphase transition. $N_e(\infty)$, mostly contributing to the factor Q_t, decreases mathematically and results in a decelerated velocity of spindle pole moving from the start point to the equilibrium position. This possibility does not affect the final position.

(2) It decreases the transition rate $\omega_{i\to e}$ and increases the transition rate $\omega_{e\to i}$. Some works have discovered the phenomenon that the number of astral microtubules raises from metaphase to anaphase (Fig. 1A; [28]). The ring-like F-actin structure is probably a mechanism to control the orchestrated

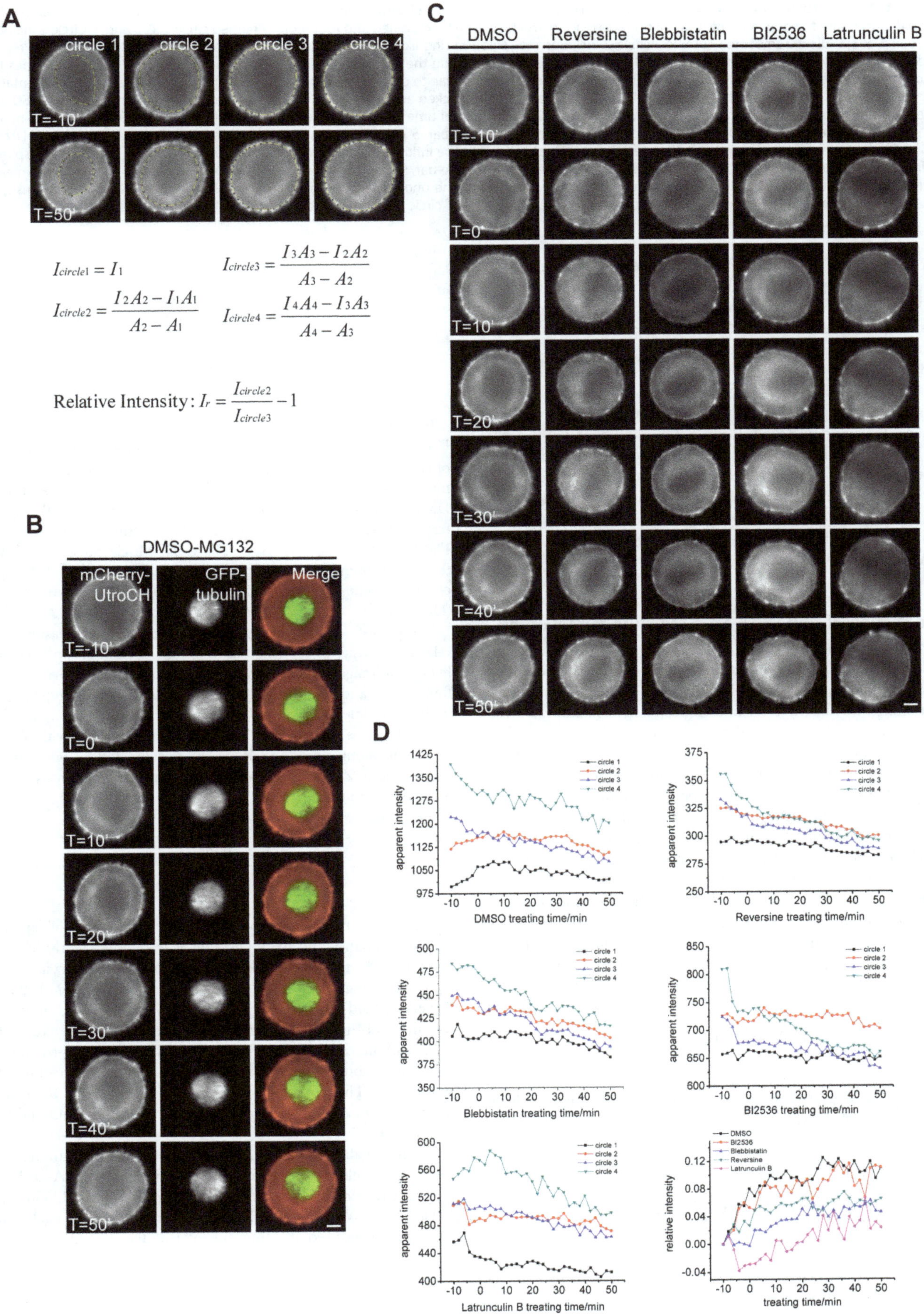
A
circle 1
circle 2
circle 3
circle 4
T=-10'
T=50'
$I_{circle1} = I_1$
$I_{circle2} = \frac{I_2A_2 - I_1A_1}{A_2 - A_1}$
$I_{circle3} = \frac{I_3A_3 - I_2A_2}{A_3 - A_2}$
$I_{circle4} = \frac{I_4A_4 - I_3A_3}{A_4 - A_3}$
Relative Intensity: $I_r = \frac{I_{circle2}}{I_{circle3}} - 1$
B
DMSO-MG132
mCherry-UtroCH
GFP-tubulin
Merge
T=-10'
T=0'
T=10'
T=20'
T=30'
T=40'
T=50'
C
DMSO
Reversine
Blebbistatin
BI2536
Latrunculin B
T=-10'
T=0'
T=10'
T=20'
T=30'
T=40'
T=50'
D
apparent intensity
DMSO treating time/min
Reversine treating time/min
Blebbistatin treating time/min
BI2536 treating time/min
Latrunculin B treating time/min
relative intensity
treating time/min

Figure 3. The perturbation of ring-like F-actin structure formation by chemical inhibitors and real-time imaging analyses. (A) The method to measure the apparent intensity of ring-like F-actin structure. A cell is classified into four regions named circle 1, 2, 3 and 4. Circle 1 includes the region of spindle-chromosome complex; circle 2 includes the region of ring-like F-actin structure just around the spindle, excluding the region inside circle 1; circle 3 includes the region of all cytoplasmic F-actin just inside the cortex, excluding the region inside circle 2; circle 4 includes the region of the whole cell body, excluding the region inside circle 3. The formulae to calculate apparent intensity are displayed here. (B) Representative images of a HeLa cell treated with DMSO and MG132. Cells were double blocked and released. MG132 was added at time point -5′, and DMSO was added at 0′. We acquired each image every 1 minute since -10′, and the total time was 1 hour. Cells were transfected with GFP-tubulin (green) and mCherry-UtroCH (red) to label microtubules and F-actin, respectively. Scale bar, 5 μm. (C) Representative images of HeLa cells treated with DMSO, BI2536, Blebbistatin, Reversine and Lat B. We used the same method as (B). The influence of chemical treatment on the ring-like structure and spindle position can be observed and measured from the supplemental movies. Scale bar, 5 μm. (D) The apparent intensity of the ring-like structure in each cell measured from the living cell imaging. The curve of circle 3 represents the photo-bleaching along the time. We chose the apparent intensity of circle 3 as the normalization factor. We also chose the apparent intensity of circle 2 as the apprent intensity of ring-like F-actin structure.

process to reduce the efficient connections between motor protein and cortex. This possibility will also result in a decreased $N_e(\infty)$.

On the other hand, relevant phenomenon is observed in the cells treated with Lat B. Lat B destroys cortical F-actin more or less and reduces the efficient connections [4].

(3) It increases the viscous force that the cytoplasm performs on the spindle to decelerate the rate of the translation and rotation of the spindle. This possibility is apparently related to the former two reasons. It slows down the velocity of the spindle motion directly, and finally prolongs the time needed to get to the equilibrium position for the cell, which can be analogized to the dynamic process of KT-MT connection. It is also possibly orchestrated by SAC. Moreover, the viscous force generated by the ring-like F-actin structure of proper intensity may significantly reduce the influence by the fluctuation of momentum and precisely position the spindle eventually.

Perturbation of ring-like F-actin structure formation by chemical inhibitors

Having established a mathematical model to elaborate the probable functions of ring-like F-actin structure in spindle positioning, we sought to define some possible factors involved in its formation. We proposed the following method to calculate the relative intensity of this ring-like F-actin structure in each cell (Fig. 3A). A cell is classified into four regions named circle 1, 2, 3 and 4. Circle 1 includes the region of spindle-chromosome complex; circle 2 includes the region of ring-like F-actin structure just around the spindle, excluding the region inside circle 1; circle 3 includes the region of all cytoplasmic F-actin just inside the cortex, excluding the region inside circle 2; circle 4 includes the region of the whole cell body, excluding the region inside circle 3.

We measured the apparent intensity of F-actin by using ImageJ to draw a polygon along the edge of the circles (Fig. 3A). Then we measured the mean gray-scale value and area inside the circles which are symbolized as following:

$$I_1, A_1, I_2, A_2, I_3, A_3, I_4, A_4$$

The mean apparent intensity of F-actin within each circle is calculated as following:

$$I_{circle1} = I_1$$

$$I_{circle2} = \frac{I_2A_2 - I_1A_1}{A_2 - A_1}$$

$$I_{circle3} = \frac{I_3A_3 - I_2A_2}{A_3 - A_2}$$

$$I_{circle4} = \frac{I_4A_4 - I_3A_3}{A_4 - A_3}$$

To discover the influence of those drugs on the mCherry-UtroCH labeled F-actin structure, we examined living cell images of each drug-treated group and measured the intensity. To enrich metaphase arrested cells, we added MG132 at -5' and add DMSO, Reversine, Blebbistatin, BI2536 and Lat B at 0', respectively. We found that the ring-like structure formed (Fig. 3B, Fig. S1A, Fig. S1B, Fig. S1C, Fig. S1D, Movie S3–S7). We also found that the intensity of ring-like F-actin structure of all groups, except for the Lat B group, was enhanced to various degrees (Fig. 3C).

To quantify differences between these groups, we measured the relative intensity of the ring-like structure of each group from the living cell images. Then we plotted the time-intensity curves of the four circles and found the slope $\Delta I_{circle3}/\Delta t$ relatively unchanged in the experiments (Fig. 3D, Table for Fig. 3D in Table S1), which means $I_{circle3}$ is a reasonable control that changes only with photo-bleaching along time, and it is dynamically stable and changes slightly along Z-axis. So we calculated the relative intensity of the actin structure in the cell as following:

$$I_r = \frac{I_{circle2}}{I_{circle3}} - 1$$

The curve of $I_{circle2}$ represents the formation process of ring-like F-actin structure, and we found that it decreases slightly in each drug-treated group. $I_{circle1}$ keeps nearly a constant deviation to $I_{circle2}$ in each group, while $I_{circle4}$ changes considerably in BI2536, Reversine and Latrunculin B groups. We concluded that the treatment of these drugs affects the cell cortex to some extent. In addition, curves of the relative intensity for each drug-treatment group are plotted together based on the same relative intensity start point. The groups of Blebbistatin, BI2536 and Reversine have curves of $\Delta I_r/\Delta t$ lying between the groups of DMSO and Lat B (Fig. 3D).

We next validated the aforementioned results by immunofluorescence of cells taken from given time points (Fig. 4A-DMSO, Fig. S2A-Reversine, Fig. S2B-Blebbistatin, Fig. S2C-BI2536, Fig. S2D-Lat B). We examined images of 30~50 cells for each time point and measured the intensity of ring-like F-actin structure.

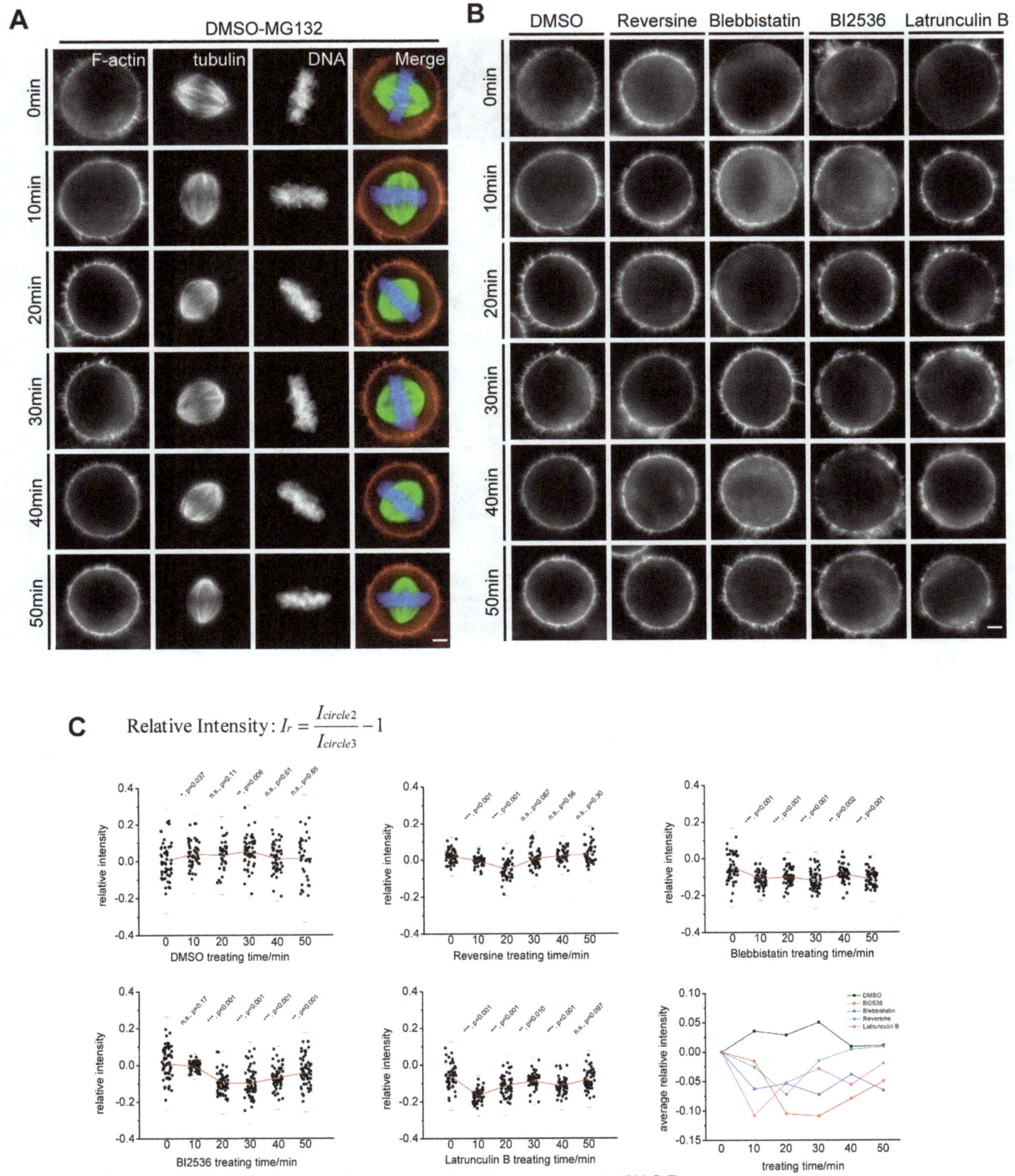

Figure 4. The perturbation of ring-like F-actin structure formation by chemical inhibitors and immunofluorescence analyses. (A) The immunofluorescence images of DMSO treated cells. Drug treatment was performed as mentioned in materials and methods, and cells were collected and fixed after drug treatment, respectively. Cells were immuno-stained for F-actin (red), microtubule (green) and DNA (blue). Scale bar, 5 μm. (B) Presentative immunofluorescence images of HeLa cells treated with DMSO, BI2536, Blebbistatin, Reversine and Lat B. Here we used the same method as (A). Scale bar, 5 μm. (C) The results of the treatment with DMSO, BI2536, Blebbistatin, Reversine and Lat B. MG132 was added at T = −10′. The start points are normalized in the last chart. The last chart suggests that Lat B, BI2536, Blebbistatin and Reversine inhibit the enhancement of the relative intensity. The significances displayed here demonstrate the differences between subsequent time points and T = 0′ by t-test. Red curves represent the mean value of the relative intensity of different time points, and red small bars represent the ±3×SD for a 95% confidence interval. Small black points represent the values of relative intensity of each cell. The formula to calculate relative intensity is displayed here.

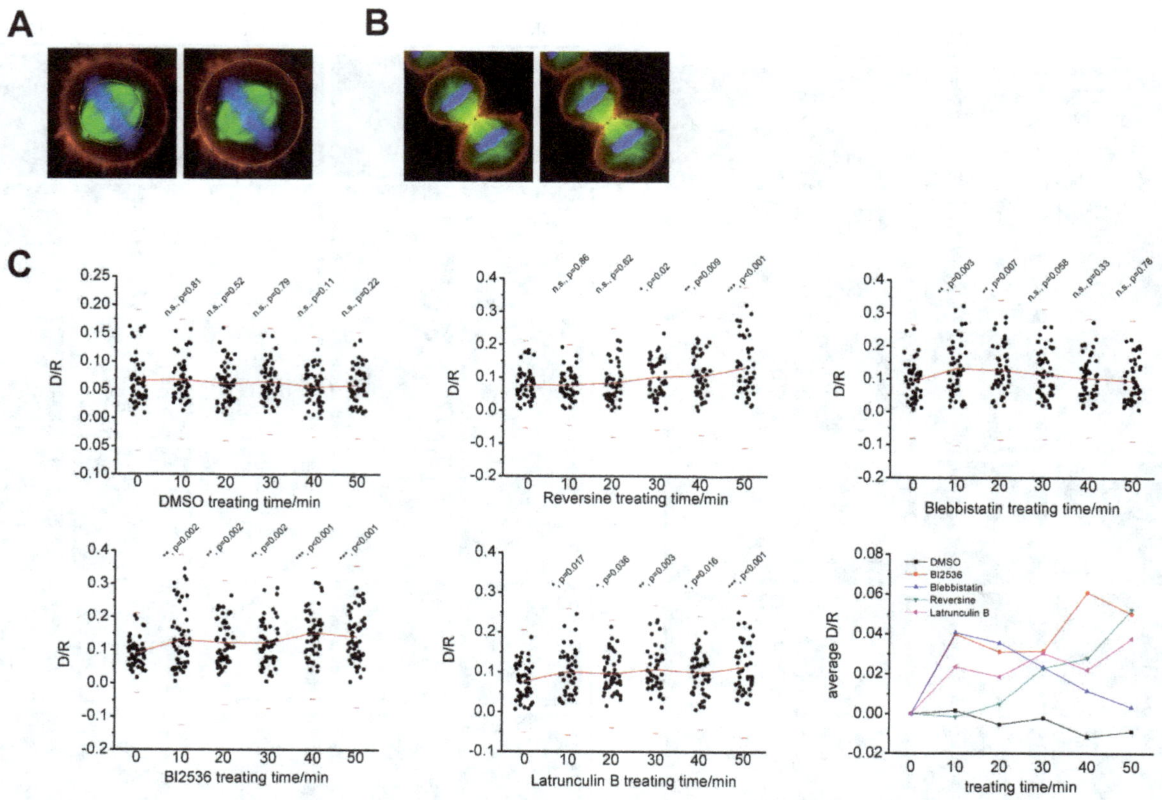

Red curves represent mean value, and small red bars represent ±3X S.D. .

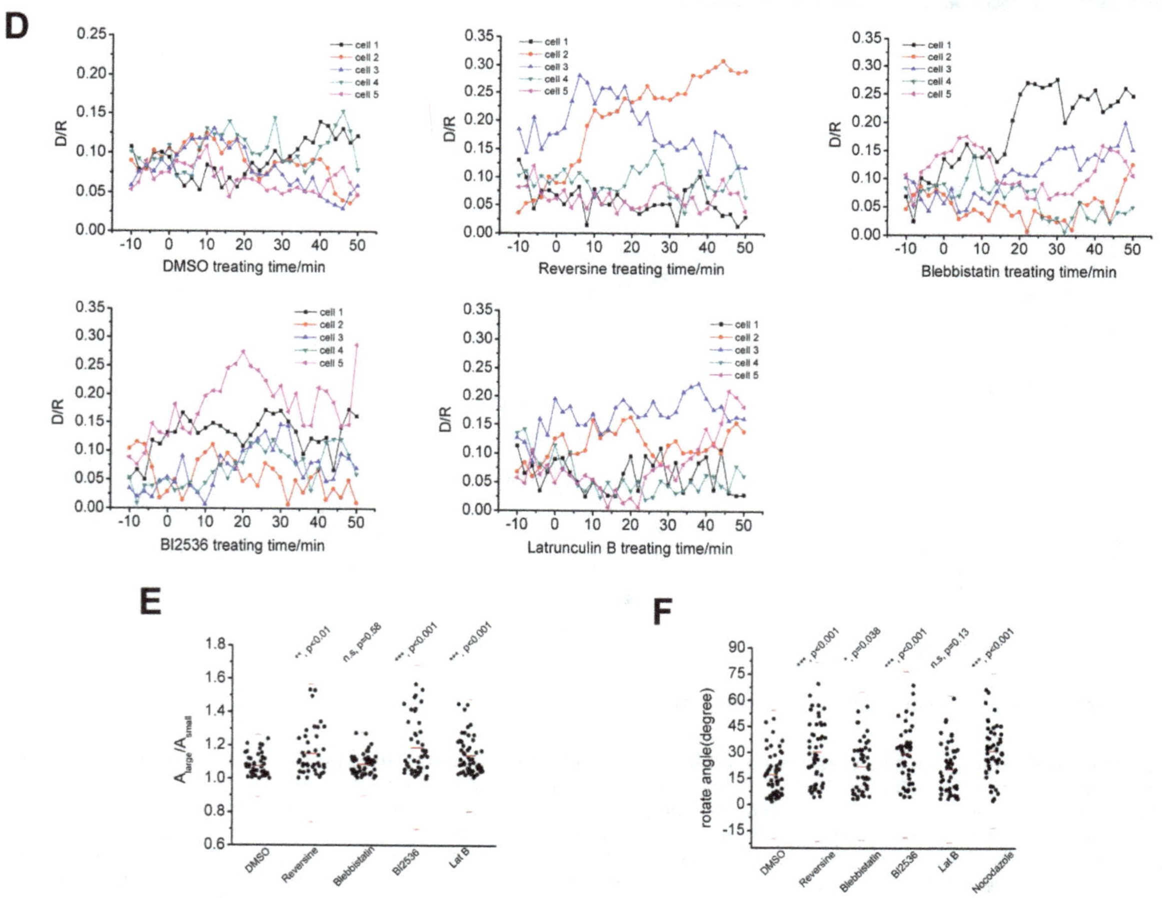

Large red bars represent mean value, and small red bars represent ±3X S.D

Figure 5. Treatment of chemical compounds alters spindle position and symmetric division. (A) Measurements for the relative translation of the spindle from the cell centroid (D/R). We draw two circles to determine the centroids of spindle and cell on the Z = 0 plane. The first circle highlights the spindle while the other one outlines the cell. Coordinates of the centroids of the circles were used to calculate the offset distance between them. Dividing the distance by the radius of the cell gives the relative distance which is expressed as D/R ratio. (B)Measurements for the area ratio of the daughter cells. The two polygons go around each daughter cell. Then the area ration equals the larger area divided by the smaller area. (C) The D/R changes along time with the treatment of drugs. The method is mentioned in materials and methods. The spindle moved away from the cell centroid in BI2536, Reversine and Lat B groups. However, the shift was finally recovered in Blebbistatin group. The significances displayed here demonstrate the differences between subsequent time points and T = 0′ by t-test. Red curves represent the mean value of D/R, and small red bars represent the ±3xSD for a 95% confidence interval. Small black points represent the values of D/R of each cell. (D) The curves presenting D/R along time by living cell imaging. The variation of D/R is enhanced in experimental groups comparing to the DMSO group. (E) The area ratio of daughter cells. BI2536 ($p<0.001$), Reversine ($p<0.01$) and Latruculin B ($p<0.001$) groups are significantly different from DMSO group, which means that the daughter cells of these groups intend to divide asymmetrically, but the Blebbistatin group is not (t-test $p = 0.58$ and F-test $p = 0.94$). Large red bars represent the mean values, and short red bars represent ±3xSD for a 95% confidence interval. Small black points represent the values of area ratio of each cell. (F)The rotating angle of spindles in cells treated with drugs. Reversine, BI2536 and Nocodazole groups are significantly different from DMSO group by t-test, which suggests that Mps1 and Plk1 play a role in spindle orientation. The cells were treated with MG132 for 2 hours and then the drugs for 1 hour, respectively.

DMSO group displays the largest variance in the relative intensity, but the mean is almost at the same level (Fig. 4C, Table for Fig. 4C in Table S1). Except for Blebbistatin group, the other groups have a decline of relative intensity after addition of drugs, but the decline is gradually recovered in a time-dependent manner. The cells do not recover from the treatment of Blebbistatin. These results indicated that the inhibition of Plk1, Mps1 or non-muscular Myosin delays the formation of the F-actin structure, which is consistent with previous works [13,34], and suggested that some factors link mitotic kinase machinery to the formation of ring-like F-actin structure in mitosis.

The cells arrested in metaphase for 2 hours form this ring-like structure (Fig. S3B). By the way, the ring-like structure still exists in the cells not treated with MG132 (Fig. 1A). Lat B significantly decreases the relative intensity of the ring-like F-actin structure, compared with DMSO group (Fig. S3D, Tables for Fig. S3D and S3F in Table S1). The relative intensity of the ring-like F-actin structures in other groups, except for Lat B and Reversine groups, is significantly enhanced after the metaphase arrest. Treatment with Reversine induces anaphase entry, suggesting that the formation of the ring-like structure is associated with SAC or metaphase-anaphase transition, while Plk1 also participates in the transition. On the other hand, deconstruction of astral microtubule or loss of motion power of Myosin can lead to a more apparent ring-like structure, suggesting potential relations between microtubule, actin filaments and Myosin in the formation of the ring-like structure.

Treatment of chemical compounds alters spindle position and symmetric division

The reported participation of F-actin structure in the regulation of spindle positioning is the precondition of contractile ring formation and symmetric division [10,32]. To explore the consequence of attenuated formation of the ring-like structure by the treatment of drugs, we measured the spindle position with the same groups of cells in Fig. 3 and Fig. 4 and cell area ratio of daughter cells in anaphase (Fig. 5A and 5B).

To measure the spindle position (Fig. 5A), we drew two circles to determine the centroid of spindle or cell on the Z = 0 plane. The first circle highlights the spindle while the other one outlines the cell. Coordinates of the centroids of the circles are used to calculate the offset distance between them. Dividing the distance by the radius of the cell gives the relative distance which is expressed as D/R ratio. From the viewpoint of the model, the curves of D/R along time represent the average motion of two spindle poles regardless of the dynamics in midzone. To measure the cell area ratio of daughter cells in anaphase (Fig. 5B), we drew two polygons to measure the area of each cell and the ratio equals the larger area divided by the smaller area. The image is projected on Z axis according to the maximum intensity.

We measured the groups treated with these drugs and made time course curves of spindle position (Fig. 5C, Tables for Fig. 5C and 5D in Table S1). Comparing with relative intensity of ring-like F-actin structure of each group displayed in Fig. 3D, the spindle position of the DMSO group is stable along time, while the spindles of the groups treated with BI2536, Reversine and Lat B are getting further away from the center of cell over time. The spindle position of the Blebbistatin group shows a slight recovery over the same period. Considering the relative intensity, the delay in the formation of ring-like F-actin structure is correlated with the perturbation of spindle position, which is probably due to less obstruction in cytoplasm. The inhibition of Myosin by Blebbistatin delays accurate spindle positioning, suggesting another pathway regulating spindle positioning. Together, these results indicated that the mitotic kinases such as Plk1 and Mps1 and motile Myosin are essential for accurate spindle positioning, which is coupled with the formation of the ring-like F-actin structure.

To assess how the drug treatment influences spindle position in a single cell over time, we examined the spindle position by living cell images of each group (Fig. 5D, Tables for Fig. 5C and 5D in Table S1). We found that the spindle positions in the cells treated with drugs except for DMSO have higher variance than the spindle position in DMSO group.

Both the formation of ring-like F-actin structure and the spindle position in Lat B group are perturbed. However, we should not attribute the perturbed positioning totally to the perturbed formation of ring-like F-actin structure, because the cortical F-actin is also influenced by the drug. Low concentration of Latrunculin A, a similar drug as Latrunculin B, is able to destroy cytoplasmic F-actin, but the completeness of cortical F-actin is conserved [31]. Thus we concluded that the formation of ring-like F-actin structure and spindle positioning are two parallel events under the regulation of mitotic signals and Myosin.

To discover the influence of the drugs on symmetric division, we measured the cell area ratio of daughter cells in anaphase (Fig. 5E, Tables for Fig. 5E and 5F in Table S1). Compared with DMSO group, the area ratios of BI2536, Reversine and Latrunculin B groups are significantly different. However, Blebbistatin group has no significant difference. This may due to the stable spindle position of the cells treated with Blebbistatin (e.g., Fig. S3A). Although there are much more factors involved in the positioning of contractile ring, this ratio also suggests potential relations between the formation of ring-like structure and symmetric division. But the detailed pathway remains unclear.

To address how the ring-like actin structure influences the spindle orientation, we measured the spindle angle and length of

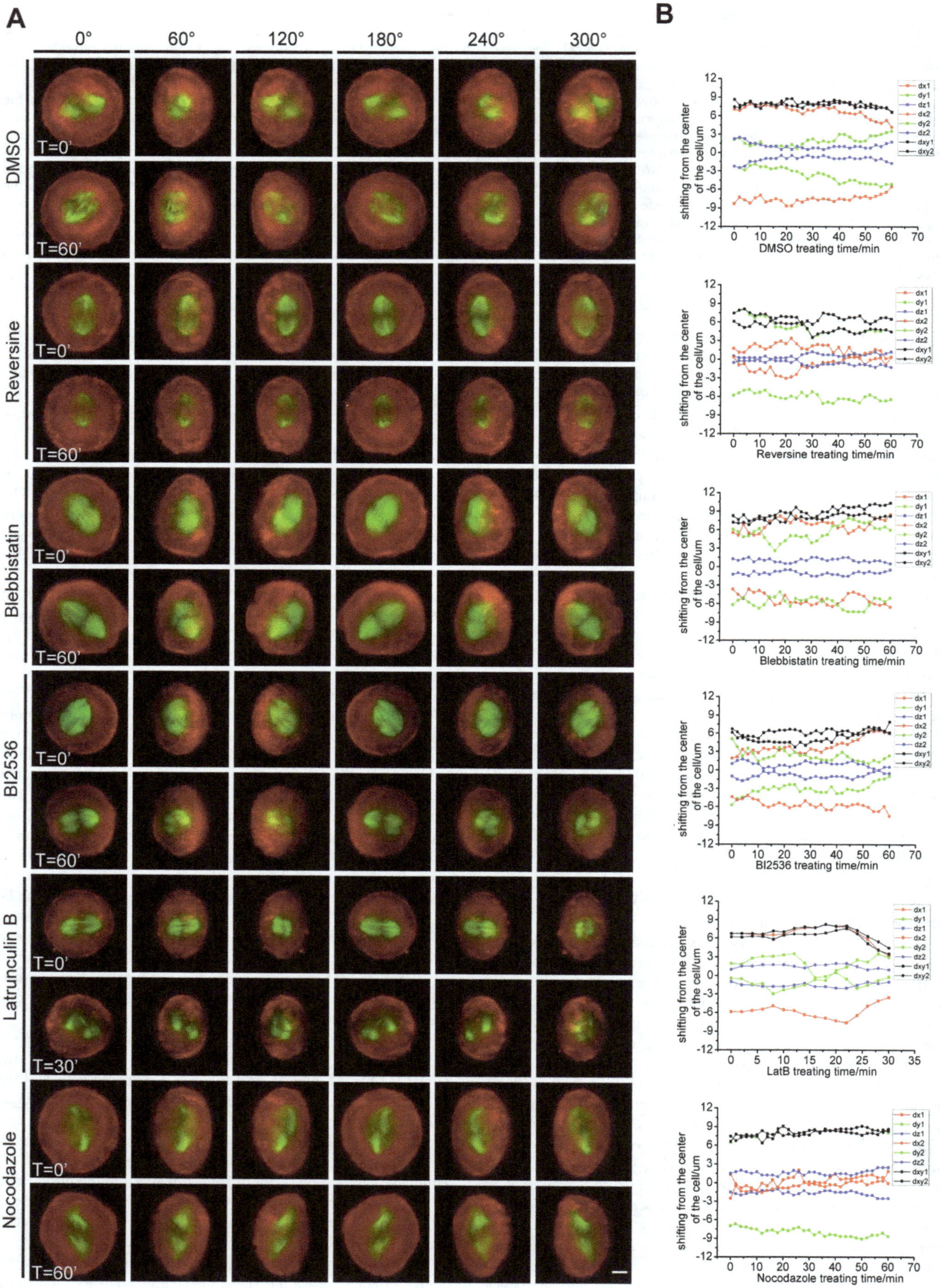
A
B
0°
60°
120°
180°
240°
300°
DMSO
Reversine
Blebbistatin
BI2536
Latrunculin B
Nocodazole
T=0'
T=60'
T=30'
dx1
dy1
dz1
dx2
dy2
dz2
dxy1
dxy2
shifting from the center of the cell/um
DMSO treating time/min
Reversine treating time/min
Blebbistatin treating time/min
BI2536 treating time/min
LatB treating time/min
Nocodazole treating time/min

Figure 6. 3D projected images of a single HeLa cell and 3D spindle positioning analysis. (A) 3D projected images of cells treated with DMSO, Reversine, Blebbistatin, BI2536, Lat B and Nocodazole. Cells were transfected with mCHerry-UtroCH (red) and GFP-tubulin (green) to label F-actin and microtubule. We added the drugs at time point T = 0′ and we ended up taking images at T = 60′, respectively. The spindle of cell treated with Lat B deformed critically after T = 30′. The cells are displayed in different rotating angles, 0°, 60°, 120°, 180°, 240° and 300°. Scale bar is 5 μm. (B) The spindle positioning plotting of the 3D projected images along time, and dx, dy and dz represent the coordinate value of spindle pole on X-axis, Y-axis and Z-axis, respectively. Numbers 1 and 2 represent the two spindle poles in each cell (Table S2). Then $(dx_1+dx_2)/2$, $(dy_1+dy_2)/2$ can be used to indicate the position of spindle. Red line represents the shifting on X-axis, green line represents the shifting on Y-axis, blue line represents the shifting on Z axis, and black line stands for the shifting on X-Y section. The rotation of spindle can be calculated between the red and green curves of each spindle pole. Spindle oscillation can be inferred from the vibrating amplitude and frequency of each red or green curve.

metaphase arrested cells (Fig. 5F, Tables for Fig. 5E and 5F in Table S1, Fig. S3B, Fig. S3D, Fig. S3F are same groups of cells). Lat B and Blebbistatin groups do not have significant difference with DMSO group at the level of $p<0.01$, but Reversine, BI2536 and Nocodazole groups do. Spindles in BI2536 and Nocodazole groups are significantly shorter than control (Fig. S3F, Tables for Fig. S3D and S3F in Table S1), while the spindle length in Reversine, Blebbistatin and Lat B groups has no significant difference from the control. These results suggest that spindle orientation is not significantly influenced by inhibiting Myosin motility or depolymerization of actin filament. The experimental concentration of Lat B may have very limited influence on cortical F-actin to alter spindle orientation in most cells we measured, which is consistent with previous publication [31]. However, altered spindle orientation partially reflects the situation of cortical F-actin. Thus these are not crucial evidences to correlate ring-like structure formation with spindle position.

Taken together, it remains unclear how these drugs influence the cortical stabilization. It is accepted that cortical complex influence spindle oscillation and positioning [10,11]. On the other hand, spindle orientation is influenced by microtubule-cortex interaction. Thus, both the situations are related to the completeness of cortical complex. Lat B and Blebbistatin mainly affect cytoplasmic F-actin and more or less influence the function of cortical complex. The treatment of Blebbistatin and Lat B have major influence on the formation of the ring-like F-actin structure but have minor influence on cortical complex. On the contrary, Reversine and BI2536 treatment have major influence on cortical complex.

3D projected images of a single HeLa cell and 3D spindle positioning analysis

To assess the influence that the drugs act on the ring-like F-actin structure and spindle, we acquired multiple-layer living cell images and made 3D projection (Fig. 6A and Movie S8–S19). We expressed mCherry-UtroCH to label F-actin and GFP-tubulin to label spindle. Before imaging, cells were treated with MG132 for 1 hour. Then we added drugs into the medium and labeled this time point as T = 0′. We took each image every 2 minutes, and the overall time was 1 hour. The images were 3D projected and displayed with an interval of 60° from 0° to 300°. We measured the positions of both spindle poles in each cell, and we plotted their shifting from the center of the cell along time (Fig. 6B, Table S2).

Green and red curves represent the position of spindle poles, and the distance between them reflects the length, orientation and position of spindle. Except for the Lat B treated cell, a distinct ring-like F-actin structure can be observed in the projected images. The spindle of DMSO treated cell rotates partially and oscillates with low frequency, and its length changes little along time (Fig. 6B-DMSO). The spindle of Reversine treated cell barely rotates and oscillates (Fig. 6B-Reversine). The spindle of Blebbistatin treated cell rotates slightly but oscillates with high frequency, and it elongates considerably (Fig. 6B-Blebbistatin). The spindle of BI2536 treated cell rotates to some extent and oscillates slightly (Fig. 6B-BI2536). The spindle of Lat B treated cell deforms significantly (Fig. 6B-Lat B). In Nocodazole treated cell, the spindle elongates and deforms, and it oscillates frequently (Fig. 6B-Nocodazole).

We had the 3D overview of the ring-like F-actin structure here. The result of Lat B treatment suggests that the perturbation of the ring-like F-actin structure is coupled with the altered configuration of spindle. The destruction of the structure may lead to uncontrolled spindle geometry rather than spindle length (Fig. S3F). The result of Blebbistatin treatment suggests that Myosin also functions in reducing the frequency of spindle oscillation.

Discussion

Accurate chromosome segregation in mitosis requires precise coordination of the microtubule-based spindle and the actin-based cell cortex. Thus, the major function of mitotic cytoplasmic actin filament is possible to enable spindle geometry to effectively prevent chromosome instability [38]. Recent studies have suggested a more direct role for the actin cytoskeleton in spindle formation [22], based on observed defects in spindle morphogenesis and orientation following perturbations on mitotic actin cytoskeleton [39,40,41,42] and actin-based hubs such as Myosin 10 and Ezrin-Radixin-Moesin (ERM) family protein [13,43,44]. These interactions possibly contribute to centrosome separation and spindle position through Myosin-driven cortical flow. It has been showed that loss of cortical F-actin in mitotic HeLa cells had little impact on overall period of mitosis or spindle bipolarity in isolated culture, even though the cortical F-actin was critically required in mitotic entry [37]. It would be interesting to ascertain the role of cytoplasmic F-actin, especially the ring-like F-actin structure, in mitotic processes such as mitotic entry and spindle bipolarity.

In this study, we analyzed the formation of ring-like F-actin structure using cell biological and computational approaches. The formation of this structure is parallel to spindle positioning and is regulated by Myosin and mitotic kinases, in consistence with the recent literature [13,29]. To elaborate spindle positioning in a quantitative manner, we formulated a mathematical model to simulate spindle positioning and orientation. According to previous works, we inferred that the cooperation of astral microtubule and cytoplasmic actin filament orchestrates the process of spindle positioning and orientation [2,3,10,36,37]. Thus, we raised an oscillator model based on previous work and got an approximate solution [35]. We predicted the final spindle pole position with $P_{final} = \frac{\sin\alpha \sin\beta}{\alpha\beta} R$. We also speculated the role of ring-like F-actin structure in spindle positioning with three hypotheses. All three hypotheses result in the decrease of effective connections between astral microtubule and cell cortex. In the model, we neglected the dynamics of kinetochore-microtubule and supposed the spindle is perfect and rigid, regardless of the alteration of spindle plasticity after the addition of these drugs.

However, the utility of our model is limited due to its hypotheses, as the species and inner properties of cells vary. Recent works have focused on how these oscillators act on spindle with pushing and pulling force [35,36]. In fact, the model we raised has calculated the influence of pulling force produced by the oscillators with D in an interval $[D_1, D_2]$ and a positive momentum. However, if we introduce the pushing force produced by the oscillators with D in another interval $[D_3, D_4]$ and a negative momentum, the calculation will result in partial neutralization due to the overlapped intervals. Here, $[D_3, D_4]$ refers to the situation that the growth of microtubule is more rapid than the velocity that motors walk on microtubule.

We have also raised questions on the formation, the structural property and the physical meanings of the ring-like F-actin structure. We used living cell imaging and immunofluorescence to observe the metaphase arrested HeLa cells treated with different drugs. We found that the inhibitors delay the formation of the ring-like F-actin structure to different extents. Interfering the formation of the ring-like F-actin structure by these inhibitors is accompanied with altered spindle positioning and asymmetric cell division simultaneously. The 3D projection has also suggested possible links between the ring-like F-actin structure and spindle positioning. Further experiments are needed to clarify the molecular mechanism.

It is important to study cytoplasmic F-actin network and screen the molecules participating in the interactions between cytoplasmic actin filament and spindle microtubule. Cytoplasmic F-actin network may function as a potential interactive hub to orchestrate spindle positioning, and some factors such as ERM members will likely come into play [45,46]. In a word, mechanical analysis and cytoplasmic factors are the center of the following study as well as molecular mechanism and cortical complex. The most intuitive meaning of studying the interaction between cytoplasmic actin filament and spindle microtubules is its contribution to artificially induce the growth of a group of cells. On the other hand, the study on cytoplasmic actin filament provides a method to study proteins involved in mitotic spindle geometry.

Supporting Information

Figure S1 The perturbation of ring-like F-actin structure formation by chemical inhibitors and real-time imaging analyses. Representative images of HeLa cells treated with MG132 plus Reversine(A), Blebbistatin(B), BI2536(C), Lat B(D). MG132 was added at $T = -5'$, and the other drugs were added at $0'$, respectively. We acquired each image every 1 minute, and the overall time was 1 hour. In (A), (B), (C) and (D) cells were transfected with GFP-tubulin (green) and mCherry-UtroCH (red) to label microtubules and F-actin, respectively. Scale bar, 5 μm.

Figure S2 The perturbation of ring-like F-actin structure formation by chemical inhibitors and immunofluorescence analyses. Representative immunofluorescence images of HeLa cells treated with MG132 and (A)Reversine, (B)Blebbistatin, (C)BI2536, (D)Lat B. Drug treatment was performed as mentioned in materials and methods, and cells were collected and fixed after drug treatment, respectively. In (A), (B), (C) and (D) cells were fixed and stained with Rhodamine-phalloidin (red), DM1A (green) and DAPI (blue). Scale Bar, 5 μm. The cells in the figures are only examples of each group.

Figure S3 Treatment of chemical compounds alters symmetric division and related properties of spindle and ring-like F-actin structure. (A) and (B) Representative immunofluorescence images of the groups on symmetric division(A), spindle orientation and relative intensity of ring-like structure in HeLa cells arrested in metaphase for 2 hours(B). Cells were released after double blocked by Thymidine and arrested in metaphase by MG132. Drug treatment were performed simultaneously and lasted for 2 hours. Except for Lat B group, a clear ring-like F-actin structure forms with the treatment of these drugs. This ring-like F-actin staining was mainly observed in metaphase or anaphase of asynchronized cells, and it was observed in all MG132-synchronized cells. In (A) and (B) cells were stained for F-actin (red), microtubule (green) and DNA (blue). Scale bar, 5 μm. (C) The ring-like F-actin structure is isotropic. We chose the planes parallel to the $Z = 0$ plane (Fig. 1C) with the interval of 1 μm between each plane, and the maximum interval is 5 μm. We equally divided each plane into 16 sectors and measured the apparent intensity of F-actin in each part of the circle 2, 3, 4 mentioned in Fig. 3. They are labeled as intracellular maximum, intracellular minimum and cell membrane. Then we got 16 values of each sectors on each plane. We compare the difference between $Z = 0$ plane and the others using t-test and F-test. Most of the p-value indicate that there is no significant difference between the planes, which means that the $Z = 0$ plane is sufficient for measurement. (D) Relative intensity of the ring-like F-actin structure in metaphase arrested cells (the same cells as displayed in Fig. S3B) treated with MG132 for 2 hours. The p-value of t-test between groups and control are marked. Except for Lat B group (significantly decrease) and Reversine group (no significance), the other groups have a significantly enhanced ring-like F-actin structure. Long red bars represent the mean value, and the short red bars represent the mean value ±3xSD. (E) The kymograph presenting the motion pattern of the ring-like F-actin structure. We select the first image of the movies (Movies B). Scale bar, 5 μm. Then we make kymographs by using a segment parallel (0°) or vertical (90°) to equate plate. Irregular teeth sequence is observed just inside the cortex, and it is different to previously reported [30,44]. Scale bar, 2.5 μm (horizontal, the length of the segment is 30 μm, relative to cellular scale) and 10 minutes (vertical, the total time of the movie is 40 minutes). Cells were transfected with GFP-H2B and mCherry-UTRO to label chromosomes and F-actin. (F) Spindle lengths in metaphase arrested cells (the same cells as displayed in Fig. S3B) treated with MG132 for 2 hours. The p-value of t-test between groups and control are marked. The spindle length in BI2536 and Nocodazole groups is significantly shorter than the control, and other groups have no significant difference. Long red bars represent the mean value, and the short red bars represent the mean value ±3xSD.

Table S1 The numerical values of results in figures. The worksheets titled "Fig. 3D", "Fig. 4C", "Fig. 5C and 5D", "Fig. 5E and 5F" and "Fig. S3D and S3F" present the raw data of values, average, standard deviation or significance in the corresponding figures as additional remarks, respectively. The worksheet titled "isotropic analysis-Fig. S3C" presents the significance between the planes along Z-axis. The quantitative method is illustrated in the legend of Fig. S3C.

Table S2 The coordinate values of spindle poles in 3D projection. This table additionally explains the numerical values in Fig. 6B. The worksheets titled "DMSO-MG132", "BI2536-MG132", "Reversine-MG132", "Blebbistatin-MG132", "Lat B-MG132" and "Nocodazole-MG132" present the directly measured coordinates of spindle poles (X1, X2, Y1, Y2, Z1, Z2) at each time point with corresponding drug treatments. Additionally, the converted coordinates according to the spindle coordinate instructed in Fig. 2B are presented (dx1, dx2, dy1, dy2, dz1, dz2).

Movie S1 The motion pattern of the ring-like F-actin structure in metaphase arrested Cell A. We took each image every 1 minute, and the total time was 40 minutes. Scale bar, 10 μm.

Movie S2 The motion pattern of the ring-like F-actin structure in metaphase arrested Cell B. We took each image every 1 minute, and the total time was 40 minutes. Scale bar, 10 μm.

Movie S3 The real time images on the plane Z = 0 of the DMSO-MG132 treated cell. We took each image every 1 minute, and the total time was 1 hour. Scale bar, 10 μm.

Movie S4 The real time images on the plane Z = 0 of the Reversine-MG132 treated cell. We took each image every 1 minute, and the total time was 1 hour. Scale bar, 10 μm.

Movie S5 The real time images on the plane Z = 0 of the Blebbistatin-MG132 treated cell. We took each image every 1 minute, and the total time was 1 hour. Scale bar, 10 μm.

Movie S6 The real time images on the plane Z = 0 of the BI2536-MG132 treated cell. We took each image every 1 minute, and the total time was 1 hour. Scale bar, 10 μm.

Movie S7 The real time images on the plane Z = 0 of the Lat B-MG132 treated cell. We took each image every 1 minute, and the total time was 1 hour. Scale bar, 10 μm.

Movie S8 The 3D projected images of DMSO treated cell at time point T = 0′. The structure is observed every 60° from 0° to 360°. We took images every 2 minutes, and the total time was 1 hour. Scale bar, 10 μm.

Movie S9 The 3D projected images of DMSO treated cell at time point T = 60′. The structure is observed every 60° from 0° to 360°. We took images every 2 minutes, and the total time was 1 hour. Scale bar, 10 μm.

Movie S10 The 3D projected images of Reversine treated cell at time point T = 0′. The structure is observed every 60° from 0° to 360°. We took images every 2 minutes, and the total time was 1 hour. Scale bar, 10 μm.

Movie S11 The 3D projected images of Reversine treated cell at time point T = 60′. The structure is observed every 60° from 0° to 360°. We took images every 2 minutes, and the total time was 1 hour. Scale bar, 10 μm.

Movie S12 The 3D projected images of Blebbistatin treated cell at time point T = 0′. The structure is observed every 60° from 0° to 360°. We took images every 2 minutes, and the total time was 1 hour. Scale bar, 10 μm.

Movie S13 The 3D projected images of Blebbistatin treated cell at time point T = 60′. The structure is observed every 60° from 0° to 360°. We took images every 2 minutes, and the total time was 1 hour. Scale bar, 10 μm.

Movie S14 The 3D projected images of BI2536 treated cell at time point T = 0′. The structure is observed every 60° from 0° to 360°. We took images every 2 minutes, and the total time was 1 hour. Scale bar, 10 μm.

Movie S15 The 3D projected images of BI2536 treated cell at time point T = 60′. The structure is observed every 60° from 0° to 360°. We took images every 2 minutes, and the total time was 1 hour. Scale bar, 10 μm.

Movie S16 The 3D projected images of Lat B treated cell at time point T = 0′. The structure is observed every 60° from 0° to 360°. We took images every 2 minutes, and the total time was 1 hour. Scale bar, 10 μm.

Movie S17 The 3D projected images of Lat B treated cell at time point T = 30′. After 30 minutes, the cell was unshaped for measuring. The structure is observed every 60° from 0° to 360°. We took images every 2 minutes, and the total time was 1 hour. Scale bar, 10 μm.

Movie S18 The 3D projected images of Nocodazole treated cell at time point T = 0′. The structure is observed every 60° from 0° to 360°. We took images every 2 minutes, and the total time was 1 hour. Scale bar, 10 μm.

Movie S19 The 3D projected images of Nocodazole treated cell at time point T = 60′. The structure is observed every 60° from 0° to 360°. We took images every 2 minutes, and the total time was 1 hour. Scale bar, 10 μm; In all movies, cells were transfected with mCherry-UtroCH (red), GFP-tubulin (green) or GFP-H2B (green) to label F-actin, microtubules and chromosomes, respectively.

Acknowledgments

We would like to thank members of our laboratory for insightful discussions.

Author Contributions

Conceived and designed the experiments: HL QZ XY. Performed the experiments: HL QZ HJ TZ PX. Analyzed the data: HL QZ DW XY. Contributed reagents/materials/analysis tools: WS. Wrote the paper: HL QZ WS DW FA ZD XY.

References

1. Brinkley BR, Stubblefield E, Hsu TC (1967) The effects of colcemid inhibition and reversal on the fine structure of the mitotic apparatus of Chinese hamster cells in vitro. J Ultrastruct Res 19: 1–18.
2. Théry M, Jiménez-Dalmaroni A, Racine V, Bornens M, Jülicher F (2007) Experimental and theoretical study of mitotic spindle orientation. Nature 447: 493–96.
3. Théry M, Racine V, Pepin A, Piel M, Chen Y, et al. (2005) The extracellular matrix guides the orientation of the cell division axis. Nat Cell Biol 7: 947–53.
4. Toyoshima F, Nishida E (2007) Intergrin-mediated adhesion orients the spindle parallel to the substratum in an EB1- and Myosin X-dependent manner. EMBO J 26: 1487–98.
5. Toyoshima F, Nishida E (2007) Spindle orientation in animal cell mitosis: roles of integrin in the control of spindle axis. J Cell Physiol 213: 407–11.
6. Grill SW, Howard J, Schaffer E, Stelzer EH, Hyman AA (2003) The distribution of active force generators controls mitotic spindle position. Science 301: 518–21.
7. Kozlowski C, Srayko M, Nedelec F (2007) Cortical microtubule contacts position the spindle in C. elegens embryos. Cell 129: 499–510.
8. Dunsch AK, Hammond D, Lloyd J, Schermelleh L, Gruneberg U, et al. (2012) Dynein light chain 1 and a spindle-associated adaptor promote dynein asymmetry and spindle orientation. J Cell Biol 198: 1039–54.
9. Zheng Z, Wan Q, Liu J, Zhu H, Chu X, et al. (2013) Evidence for dynein and astral microtubule-mediated cortical release and transport of Galphai/LGN/NuMA complex in mitotic cells. Mol Biol Cell 24: 901–13.
10. Kiyomitsu T, Cheeseman IM (2012) Chromosome-and spindle-pole-derived signals generate an intrinsic code for spindle position and orientation. Nat Cell Biol 14: 311–17.
11. Kiyomitsu T, Cheeseman IM (2013) Cortical dynein and asymmetric membrane elongation coordinately position the spindle in anaphase. Cell 154: 391–402.
12. Rosenblatt J, Cramer LP, Baum B, McGee KM (2004) Myosin II-dependent cortical movement is required for centrosome separation and positioning during mitotic spindle assembly. Cell 117: 361–372.
13. Woolner S, O'Brien LL, Wiese C, Bement WM (2008) Myosin-10 and actin filaments are essential for mitotic spindle function. J Cell Biol 182: 77–88.
14. Yao X, Anderson KL, Cleveland DW (1997) The microtubule-dependent motor centromere-associated protein E (CENP-E) is an integral component of kinetochore corona fibers that link centromeres to spindle microtubules. J Cell Biol 139: 435–47.
15. Lan W, Zhang X, Kline-Smith KL, Rosasco SE, Barrett-Wilt GA, et al. (2004) Aurora B phosphorylates centromeric MCAK and regulates its localozation and microtubule depolymerization activity. Curr Biol 14: 273–86.
16. Cimini D, Wan X, Hirel CB, Salmon ED (2006) Aurora kinase promotes turnover of kinetochore microtubules to reduce chromosome segregation errors. Curr Biol 16: 1711–18.
17. Yang Z, Tulu US, Wadsworth P, Rieder CL (2007) Kinetochore dynein is required for chromosome motion and congression independent of the spindle checkpoint. Curr Biol 17: 973–980.
18. Rieder CL, Cole RW, Khodjakov A, Sluder G (1995) The checkpoint delaying anaphase in response to chromosome monoorientation is mediated by an inhibition signal produced by unattached kinetochores. J Cell Biol 130: 941–48.
19. Sudakin V, Chan GK, Yen TJ (2001) Checkpoint inhibition of the APC/C in HeLa cells is mediated by a complex of BUBR1, BUB3, CDC20, and MAD2. J Cell Biol 154: 925–36.
20. Santaguida S, Tighe A, D'Alise AM, Taylor SS, Musacchio A (2010) Dissecting the role of MPS1 in chromosome biorientaion and the spindle checkpoint through the small molecular inhibitor Reversine. J Cell Biol 190: 73–87.
21. Rodriguez OC, Schaefer AW, Mandato CA., Forscher P, Bement WM, et al. (2003) Conserved microtubule-actin interactions in cell movement and morphogenesis. Nat Cell Biol 5: 599–609.
22. Sandquist JC, Kita AM, Bement WM (2011) And the dead shall rise: actin and Myosin return to the spindle. Dev Cell 21: 410–19.
23. Gundersen GG, Bretscher A (2003) Cell biology. Microtubule asymmetry. Science 300: 2040–41.
24. Gundersen GG, Gomes ER, Wen Y (2004) Cortical control of microtubulestability and polarization. Curr Opin Cell Biol 16: 106–12.
25. Perez-Moreno M, Jamora C, Fuchs E (2003) Sticky business: orchestrating cellular signals at adherens junctions. Cell 112: 535–48.
26. Gönczy P, Pichler S, Kirkham M, Hyman AA (1999) Cytoplasmic dynein is required foe distinct aspects of MTOC positioning, including centrosome separation, in the one cell stage Caenorhabditis elegans embryo. J Cell Biol 147: 135–50.
27. Maier B, Kirsch M, Anderhub S, Zentgraf H, Kramer A (2013) The novel actin/focal adhesion-associated protein MISP is involved in mitotic spindle positioning in human cells. Cell Cycle 12: 1457–71.
28. Zhu M, Settele F, Kotak S, Sanchez-Pulido L, Ehret L, et al. (2013) MISP is a novel Plk1 substrate required for proper spindle orientation and mitotic progression. J Cell Biol 200: 773–87.
29. Thaiparambil JT, Eggers CM, Marcus AI (2012) AMPK regulates mitotic spindle orientation through phosphorylation of Myosin regulatory light chain. Mol Cell Biol 32: 3203–17.
30. Mitsushima M, Aoki K, Ebisuya M, Matsumura S, Yamamoto T, et al. (2010) Revolving movement of a dynamic cluster of actin filaments during mitosis. J Cell Biol 191: 453–62.
31. Chew TG, Lorthongpanich C, Ang WX, Knowles BB, Solter D (2012) Symmetric cell division of the mouse zygote requires an actin network. Cytoskeleton (Hoboken) 69: 1040–46.
32. Laan L, Pavin N, Husson J, Romet-Lemonne G, van Duijn M, et al. (2012) cortical dynein controls microtubule dynamics to generate pulling force that position microtubule asters. Cell 148: 502–14.
33. Johnson VL, Scott MI, Holt SV, Hussein D, Taylor SS (2004) Bub1 is required for kinetochore localization of BubR1, Cenp-E, Cenp-F and Mad2, and chromosome congression. J Cell Sci 117: 1577–89.
34. Field CM, Lénárt P (2011) Bulk cytoplasmic actin and its functions in meiosis and mitosis. Curr Biol 21: R825–30.
35. Grill SW, Kruse K, Jülicher F (2005) Theory of mitotic spindle oscillations. Phys Rev Lett 94: 108104.
36. Pavin N, Laan L, Ma R, Dogterom M, Jülicher F (2012) Positioning of microtubule organizing centers by cortical pushing and pulling force. New Journal of Physics 14: 105025.
37. Ma R, Laan L, Dogterom M, Pavin N, Jülicher F (2014) General theory for the mechanics of confined microtubule asters. New Journal of Physics 16: 013018.
38. Lancaster SM, Berre ML, Dimitracopoulos A, Bonazzi D, Ziotekiewicz E, et al. (2013) Mitotic rounding alters cell geometry to ensure efficient bioplolar spindle formation. Dev Cell 25: 270–83.
39. Moulding DA, Blundell MP, Spiller DG, White MR, Cory GO, et al. (2007) Unregulated actin polymerization by WASP causes defects of mitosis and cytokinesis in X-linked neutropenia. J Exp Med 204: 2213–24.
40. Kaji N, Muramoto A, Mizuno K (2008) LIM kinase-mediated cofilin phosphorylation during mitosis is required for precise spindle positioning. J Biol Chem 283: 4983–92.
41. Kunda P, Pelling AE, Liu T, Baum B (2008) Moesin controls cortical rigidity, cell rounding, and spindle morphogenesis during mitosis. Curr Biol 18: 91–101.
42. Carreno S, Kouranti I, Glusman ES, Fuller MT, Echard A. et al. (2008) Moesin and its activating kinase Slik are required for cortical stability and microtubule organization in mitotic cells. J Cell Biol 180: 739–46.
43. Vilmos P, Jankovics F, Szathmári M, Lukácsovich T, Henn L, et al. (2009) Live imaging reveals that the Drosophila actin-binding ERM protein, moesin, co-localizes with the mitotic spindle. Eur J Cell Biol 88: 609–19.
44. Fink J, Carpi N, Betz T, Bétard A, Chebah M, et al. (2011) External forces control mitotic spindle positioning. Nat Cell Biol 13: 771–78.
45. Solinet S, Mahmud K, Stewman SF, Ben El, Kadhi K, et al. (2013) The actin-binding ERM protein Moesin binds to and stabilizes microtubules at the cell cortex. J Cell Biol 202: 251–60.
46. Okada S, Leda M, Hanna J, Savage NS, Bi E, et al. (2013) Dughter cell identity emerges from the interplay of Cdc42, septins, and exocytosis. Dev Cell 26: 148–61.

18

Alarming Levels of Drug-Resistant Tuberculosis in HIV-Infected Patients in Metropolitan Mumbai, India

Petros Isaakidis[1]*, Mrinalini Das[1], Ajay M V Kumar[2], Christopher Peskett[1], Minni Khetarpal[3], Arun Bamne[4], Balkrishna Adsul[5], Mamta Manglani[6], Kuldeep Singh Sachdeva[7], Malik Parmar[8], Avinash Kanchar[9], B.B. Rewari[9], Alaka Deshpande[10], Camilla Rodrigues[11], Anjali Shetty[11], Lorraine Rebello[1], Peter Saranchuk[12]

1 Médecins Sans Frontières, Mumbai, India, **2** International Union Against Tuberculosis and Lung Disease (The Union), South-East Asia Regional Office, New Delhi, India, **3** City TB Office, Bawala Wadi, Chinckpokli, Mumbai, India, **4** Brihanmumbai Municipal Corporation, Mumbai, India, **5** Mumbai District AIDS Control Society (MDACS), Mumbai, India, **6** Pediatric Centre of Excellence for HIV Care, L.T.M. Medical College & General Hospital, Sion, Mumbai, India, **7** Central TB Division, Directorate General of Health Services, Ministry of Health and Family Welfare, New Delhi, India, **8** World Health Organisation - Country Office for India, New Delhi, India, **9** Department of AIDS Control, National AIDS Control Organisation, New Delhi, India, **10** MGM Institute of Health Sciences, Navi Mumbai, India, **11** P.D. Hinduja National Hospital and Medical Research Centre, Mumbai, India, **12** Southern Africa Medical Unit (SAMU), Médecins Sans Frontières, Cape Town, South Africa

Abstract

Background: Drug-resistant tuberculosis (DR-TB) is a looming threat to tuberculosis control in India. However, no countrywide prevalence data are available. The burden of DR-TB in HIV-co-infected patients is likewise unknown. Undiagnosed and untreated DR-TB among HIV-infected patients is a major cause of mortality and morbidity. We aimed to assess the prevalence of DR-TB (defined as resistance to any anti-TB drug) in patients attending public antiretroviral treatment (ART) centers in greater metropolitan Mumbai, India.

Methods: A cross-sectional survey was conducted among adults and children ART-center attendees. Smear microscopy, culture and drug-susceptibility-testing (DST) against all first and second-line TB-drugs using phenotypic liquid culture (MGIT) were conducted on all presumptive tuberculosis patients. Analyses were performed to determine DR-TB prevalence and resistance patterns separately for new and previously treated, culture-positive TB-cases.

Results: Between March 2013 and January 2014, ART-center attendees were screened during 14135 visits, of whom 1724 had presumptive TB. Of 1724 attendees, 72 (4%) were smear-positive and 202 (12%) had a positive culture for *Mycobacterium tuberculosis*. Overall DR-TB was diagnosed in 68 (34%, 95% CI: 27%–40%) TB-patients. The proportions of DR-TB were 25% (29/114) and 44% (39/88) among new and previously treated cases respectively. The patterns of DR-TB were: 21% mono-resistant, 12% poly-resistant, 38% multidrug-resistant (MDR-TB), 21% pre-extensively-drug-resistant (MDR-TB plus resistance to either a fluoroquinolone or second-line injectable), 6% extensively drug-resistant (XDR-TB) and 2% extremely drug-resistant TB (XDR-TB plus resistance to any group-IV/V drug). Only previous history of TB was significantly associated with the diagnosis of DR-TB in multivariate models.

Conclusion: The burden of DR-TB among HIV-infected patients attending public ART-centers in Mumbai was alarmingly high, likely representing ongoing transmission in the community and health facilities. These data highlight the need to promptly diagnose drug-resistance among all HIV-infected patients by systematically offering access to first and second-line DST to all patients with 'presumptive TB' rather than 'presumptive DR-TB' and tailor the treatment regimen based on the resistance patterns.

Editor: Anil K. Tyagi, University of Delhi, India

Funding: This study was funded by Médecins Sans Frontières, Belgium. The funder was involved in study design, data collection and analysis. However, final preparation of the manuscript and the decision to publish rests with the first author.

Competing Interests: The authors have declared that no competing interests exist.

* Email: msfocb-asia-epidemio@brussels.msf.org

Introduction

India is a high burden country for tuberculosis (TB) and multidrug-resistant TB (MDR-TB). The World Health Organization has estimated that India accounted for 26% of the total number of TB cases worldwide in 2012, with 2.2% and 15% of the new and retreatment cases respectively being caused by multidrug-resistant strains [1]. Further, India is home to approximately 2.4 million people living with HIV [2] and considered to have a high burden on account of the large absolute numbers of people living with HIV in the country.

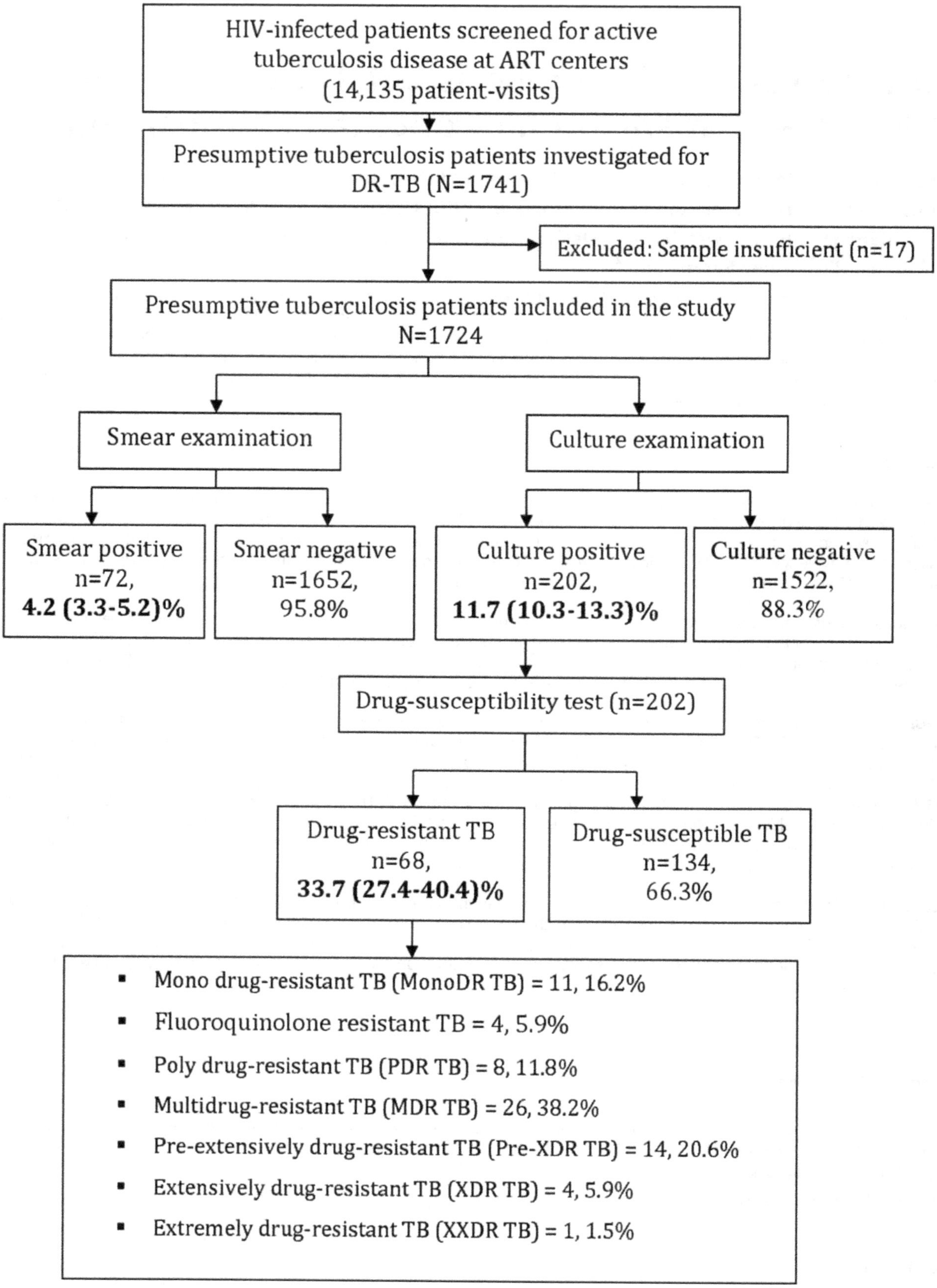

Figure 1. Drug-resistant tuberculosis among HIV-infected patients with presumptive tuberculosis, Mumbai, India.

The dual burden of HIV and TB/DR-TB in India is significantly high with a combined rate of 5.2%, ranging from 0.4% to 28.8% in various studies, with increasing trends noted in states having a higher burden of HIV infection [3–7]. However, nation-wide studies do not exist and previous studies have occurred mainly in hospitals and tertiary care centres [2,6–11]. A crude estimate from these studies suggests that 2500–3000 HIV-infected persons develop MDR-TB annually in India.

Country-wide or state-wide drug resistance surveys (DRS) aim to estimate the DR-TB burden at the country or state level. While this approach is scientifically and operationally acceptable, it may mask significant and important variance in the magnitude of the epidemic in different localities, communities or specific populations. For India, a vast country with an enormous burden of TB and a relatively large burden of HIV in absolute numbers, this statement seems to hold true; from an overcrowded impoverished slum in Mumbai to a small isolated village in the Northern Eastern Provinces of the country, one can assume that several different epidemics may exist. A description of such local epidemics is necessary so as to complement the country-wide prevalence estimate. While there is an urgent need for a nationally representative, country-wide DRS in India, specific studies to identify pockets of extremely high DR-TB prevalence or extensive drug resistance patterns are equally needed in order to advocate for and implement effective control strategies.

The overall aim of this study was to assess the burden of drug-susceptible and drug-resistant tuberculosis among HIV-infected patients attending antiretroviral treatment (ART) centers in the metropolitan area of Mumbai. The specific objectives were a) to determine the proportion of HIV-infected patients with DR-TB among those attending public ART centers, b) to describe drug susceptibility patterns among *Mycobacterium tuberculosis* isolates from this population, and c) to identify factors associated with TB and drug-resistant TB among HIV patients. We aimed to contribute to the evidence base that informs policies and practices and help to estimate the resources needed to control the epidemic in this specific group, as well as the community.

Methods

Ethics

The study was approved by the Institutional Ethics Committee of Grant Medical College and Sir J.J. Group of Hospitals (Mumbai, India), the Ethics Review Board of Médecins Sans Frontières (Geneva, Switzerland) and the Ethics Advisory Group of the International Union Against Tuberculosis and Lung Disease (Paris, France). The study protocol was approved by the Indian

Table 1. Demographic and clinical characteristics of HIV-infected patients with presumptive TB, Mumbai, India.

Characteristics	HIV-infected patients with presumptive TB (N = 1724)
	n (%)
Age [years, median (IQR)]	35.0 (24.3–44.0)
Sex of patients	
Male	1042 (60.4)
Female	671 (38.9)
Transgender	11 (0.6)
Family income per month (in Rupees)	
Less than 3500	88 (5.1)
3500–6999	910 (52.8)
7000 and above	454 (26.3)
Patient did not disclose	272 (15.6)
TB site	
Pulmonary	1688 (97.9)
Extra-pulmonary	36 (2.1)
ART status	
On ART	1386 (80.4)
Pre-ART	338 (19.6)
CD4 count, last visit (in cells/μl)	
Less than 200	258 (15.0)
200–349	351 (20.4)
350–499	289 (16.8)
500 and above	684 (39.7)
No information	142 (8.2)
ART duration* [months, median (IQR)]	26.0 (10.7–47.5)
Previous episode of TB	
Yes	933 (54.1)
No	791 (45.9)

ART: Antiretroviral treatment* Patients on ART with available information about ART initiation date, N = 1370.

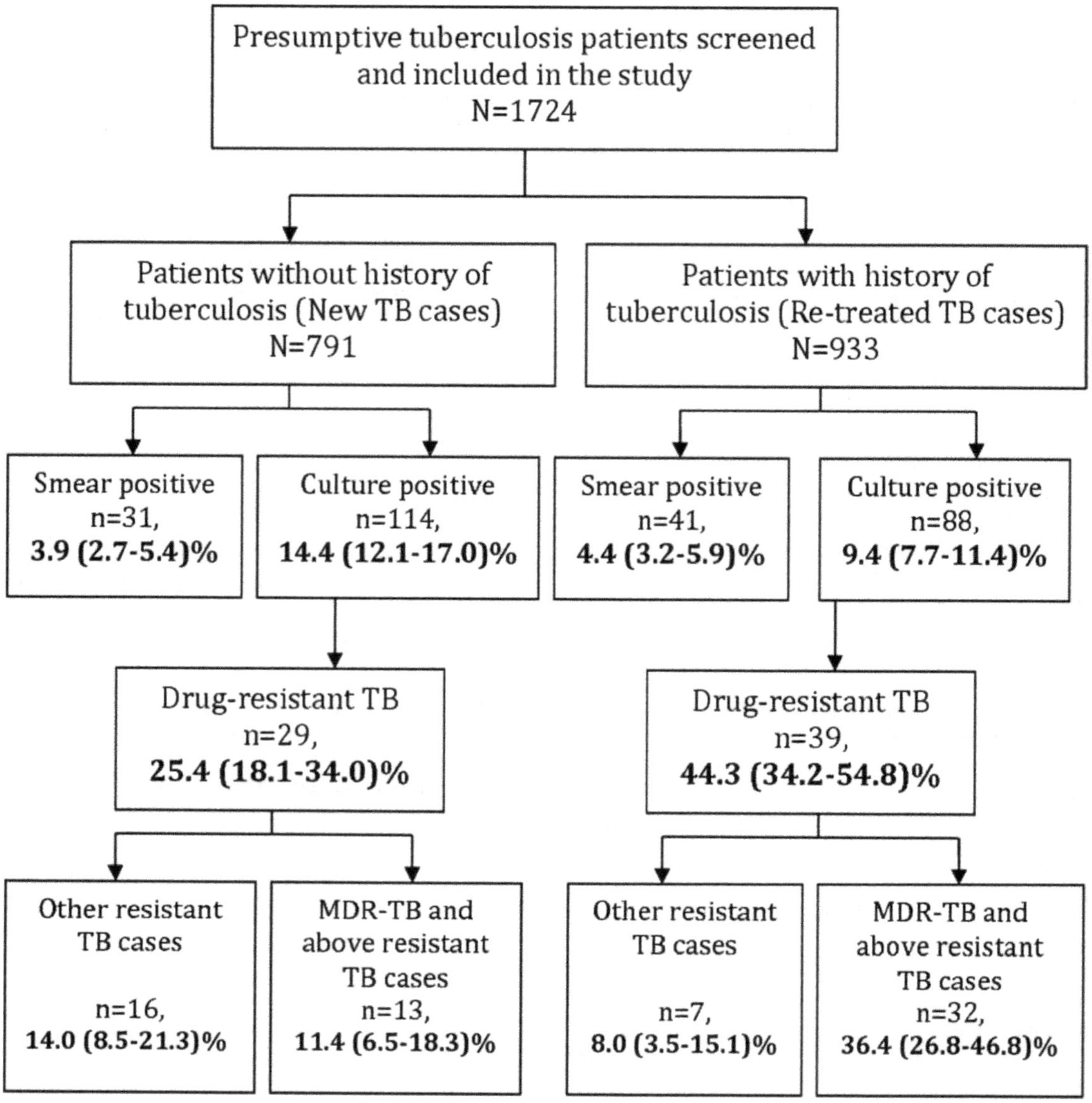

Figure 2. Distribution of Drug-resistant tuberculosis among HIV-infected (new and previously treated) with presumptive tuberculosis patients, Mumbai, India.

Council of Medical Research (ICMR), New Delhi, India. Informed consent was obtained from all study participants.

Study design

This was a cross-sectional survey among HIV-infected adult and paediatric patients attending public and public-private ART clinics in the greater metropolitan Mumbai area. All patients with presumptive pulmonary or extra-pulmonary TB were assessed with smear microscopy and conventional liquid culture. All M. tuberculosis isolates underwent drug susceptibility testing (DST) for first- and second-line anti-TB drugs.

Sample size

The desired sample size was determined separately for new and previously treated culture positive TB cases. Previous tuberculosis treatment was defined as any anti-tuberculosis treatment reported by the patient. Assuming a prevalence of MDR-TB of 3% among new cases and 17% among retreated cases, based on a DST survey conducted in Gujarat [12], a sample size of 123 confirmed new cases and 110 confirmed retreatment cases was sought in order to estimate the prevalence of MDR-TB, with 95% confidence intervals having a margin of error of 3% for new cases and 7% for retreated cases respectively.

Study setting and study population

The study was carried out in five Mumbai District AIDS Control Society (MDACS) ART Centres [1) KEM Hospital, 2) SION Hospital, 3) SION Centre of Excellence in Paediatric HIV Care, 4) Godrej Hospital, Vikhroli and 5) Larsen & Toubro Hospital, Andheri] as well as in two Maharashtra State AIDS Control Society (MSACS) ART Centres [1) Thane Civil Hospital and 2) Navi Mumbai (Vashi) Municipal Corporation Hospital].

All HIV-infected adult and paediatric patients enrolled in the ART centres were potentially eligible to be enrolled in the study, if they had presumptive pulmonary or extra-pulmonary TB based on symptom screening, regardless of the time they were enrolled in the centres or whether they were on ART or not at the time of the

Table 2. Resistance profile (first and second-line) for all drug-resistant tuberculosis patients, Mumbai, India.

Resistance profile (culture-based DST)	Total TB Patients (N=68), n (%)	New TB patients (N=29), n (%)	Previously treated TB patients (N=39), n (%)
H-mono	11 (16.2)	7 (24.1)	4 (10.3)
R-mono	-	-	-
Ofx-mono	1 (1.5)	1 (3.4)	-
Ofx Mfx	3 (4.4)	2 (6.9)	1 (2.6)
HE	7 (10.3)	6 (20.7)	1 (2.6)
HE Eto Ofx Mfx	1 (1.5)	-	1 (2.6)
HR	10 (14.7)	4 (13.8)	6 (15.4)
HRE	6 (8.8)	2 (6.9)	4 (10.3)
HR Eto	5 (7.4)	-	5 (12.8)
HR E Eto	5 (7.4)	2 (6.9)	3 (7.7)
HR Ofx Mfx E	2 (2.9)	2 (6.9)	-
HR Ofx Mfx Eto	1 (1.5)	1 (3.4)	-
HR Ofx Mfx E Lin	1 (1.5)	-	1 (2.6)
HR Ofx Mfx E Eto	8 (11.8)	1 (3.4)	7 (17.9)
HR Ofx Mfx E Eto PAS	2 (2.9)	-	2 (5.1)
HR Ofx Mfx Km Eto	1 (1.5)	-	1 (2.6)
HR Ofx Mfx Km E Eto	2 (2.9)	1 (3.4)	1 (2.6)
HR Ofx Mfx Km Cm E Eto	1 (1.5)	-	1 (2.6)
HR Ofx Mfx Km Cm E Eto PAS	1 (1.5)	-	1 (2.6)

H-isoniazid, R-rifampicin, E-ethambutol, Eto-ethionamide, Km-kanamycin, Cm-capreomycin, Ofx-ofloxacin, Mfx-Moxifloxacin, Lin- Linezolid, PAS- para-aminosalicylic acid.

study. Patients on TB treatment at the time of the study were excluded.

Recruitment and sampling procedure

All HIV-infected ART center attendees were screened by an MSF-employed nurse during the study period. Patients with presumptive TB were investigated using a standard diagnostic algorithm recommended by the World Health Organization [13] that included TB culture and DST. The nurse explained in detail the objectives of the study to the patient and/or caregiver and obtained the signature or thumbprint of the patient if consent was given to participate. When pulmonary TB was presumed, two sputum specimens were collected on the same day, one hour apart, at each study site/hospital laboratory. When extra-pulmonary TB (EPTB) was presumed, biological specimens (fine needle aspirates, pleural fluid, cerebrospinal fluid, etc) were obtained from extra-pulmonary sites. All specimens were transferred to Hinduja Hospital Microbiology Laboratory in Mumbai for culture and first- and second-line DST.

Conventional microscopy with Ziehl-Neelsen (ZN) staining for acid-fast bacilli and further sputum decontamination was performed using the N-acetyl-L-cysteine and sodium hydroxide method. Concentrated sediment was inoculated in one liquid culture tube for testing using the Mycobacterial growth indicator tube (MGIT 960) method. Positive cultures underwent microscopy with ZN staining to confirm cord formation, and speciation with MPT 64 antigen detection by Immunochromatography was carried out to confirm *M. tuberculosis* complex. Specimens fulfilling the above criteria underwent further testing with phenotypic DST using the MGIT System for the following drugs: isoniazid, rifampicin, ethambutol, ofloxacin, moxifloxacin, kanamycin, capreomycin, PAS, ethionamide, clofazimine and linezolid. Non-tuberculous Mycobacteria (NTM) speciation was done by molecular methods using Reverse Line Blot Hybridisation. Hinduja laboratory is quality controlled and has been accredited for first-line DST by the WHO Supranational Reference Laboratory in Bangalore and the College of American Pathologists. The laboratory was also accredited by the TB programme for second-line DST in December 2013; prior to this date, if a strain was suspected to have resistance to one or more second-line anti-TB drugs, it was sent to the National Tuberculosis Institute Laboratory in Bangalore for confirmation.

Multidrug-resistant tuberculosis (MDR-TB) was defined as resistance to both isoniazid and rifampicin; pre-XDR-TB was defined as MDR-TB with additional resistance to either a fluoroquinolone or a second-line injectable agent; and extensively drug-resistant tuberculosis (XDR-TB) was defined as MDR-TB with additional resistance to both a fluoroquinolone and an injectable agent. Extremely drug-resistant tuberculosis (XXDR-TB) was defined as XDR-TB with additional resistance to any group IV and/or group V TB drugs (PAS, ethionamide, clofazimine, linezolid) [13].

Management of those diagnosed with DR-TB

All patients diagnosed with MDR- or XDR-TB were managed in accordance with the national DR-TB treatment guidelines [14], while those with pre-XDR-TB were offered individualized treatment with 4 drugs likely to be effective.

Data collection and analysis

Demographics, clinical and laboratory data, antiretroviral treatment (yes/no) and duration on ART, as well as data on

Table 3. Demographic and clinical factors associated with culture-positive tuberculosis in HIV-infected patients, Mumbai, India.

Explanatory Variable	Patients with tuberculosis (N = 202), n (%)	Patients without tuberculosis (N = 1522), n (%)	Chi-square/t-test (p-value)	aPR[a] (95% CI)
Age [years, median (IQR)]	38.0 (32.0–43.3)	35.0 (22.0–44.0)	8.9 (<0.01)	0.99 (0.99–1.00)
Sex of patients				
Male	138 (13.1)	915 (86.9)	5.0 (0.02)	1.01 (0.99–1.03)
Female	64 (9.5)	607 (90.5)		
Family income per month⁺ (in Rupees)				
Less than 5000	96 (10.9)	788 (89.1)	0.2 (0.65)	
5000 and above	66 (11.6)	502 (88.4)		
ART status				
Pre-ART	72 (21.3)	266 (78.7)	37.3 (<0.01)	1.07 (1.04–1.10)
On ART	130 (9.4)	1256 (90.6)		
CD4 count, last visit* (in cells/μl)				
Less than 200	58 (22.5)	200 (77.5)	34.7 (<0.01)	1.08 (1.05–1.11)
200 and above	127 (9.6)	1197 (90.4)		
ART duration** [months, median (IQR)]	19.3 (5.2–35.7)	27.1 (11.3–47.9)	9.9 (<0.01)	
Previous episode of TB				
Yes	88 (9.4)	845 (90.6)	10.3 (<0.01)	1.01 (0.99–1.03)
No	114 (14.4)	677 (85.6)		

ART: Antiretroviral treatment, IQR: Inter-quartile range, CI; Confidence Intervals ⁺Patients with recorded family income, N = 1452* Patients with available information on CD4, last visit, N = 1582** Patients on ART with available information about ART initiation date, N = 1370[a] aPR; adjusted Prevalence Ratios (calculated by Poisson regression using multiple imputation for CD4 missing data).

previous TB treatment were doubly-entered into an EpiData database (Version 3.1, EpiData Association, Odense, Denmark), validated and analyzed.

To identify factors associated with TB and DR-TB, univariate and multivariate analyses were performed using Poisson and binary logistic regression models. Factors significant ($p = 0.05$) on univariate analysis were entered into the multivariate logistic regression models. Factors were coded as categorical variables and missing values for CD4 cell counts were imputed using a multiple imputation method. Transgender individuals (all were male to female) were grouped with biological males in the models. All factors were entered as a block into multivariate logistic regression models. Data analysis, including multivariate logistic regression models, was conducted with SPSS Version 20.0. Armonk, NY: IBM Corp. Released 2011).

Results

Screening for presumptive TB was carried-out during 14,135 patient visits at seven ART centers in metropolitan Mumbai between March 2013 and January 2014 (Figure 1). Individual patients might have been screened more than once during the study period. A total of 1741 HIV-infected patients with presumptive tuberculosis (TB) were identified. All of them consented to participate in the study and were investigated for drug-resistant TB. The sputum specimens of 17 patients were found insufficient for laboratory investigations and had to be excluded. Thus, 1724 (99%) of the eligible patients were included in the study.

Patient characteristics

The median age of the 1724 patients was 35 (Inter-quartile range, IQR: 24–44) years (Table 1) and the majority (60%) were male. A large proportion (53%) of patients had an average family income between 3500 and 7000 Indian National Rupees (equivalent to 60–120 USD) per month. Most of the patients (98%) had pulmonary TB. Among the entire study cohort, 80% were on ART during the study period and the majority (52%) had CD4 cell counts lower than 500 cells/μL at their last visit to an ART center. The median duration of exposure to ART prior to enrollment in the study was 26 months (IQR: 10.7–47.5). More than half (933/1724) of the presumptive TB patients had had at least one episode of active TB disease in the past.

Culture-positive and drug-resistant tuberculosis

All of the 1724 patients with presumptive TB included in the study (Figure 1) underwent smear, culture and drug susceptibility testing (DST). Of these, 72 (4.2%; 95% Confidence Intervals (CI): 3.3–5.2) patients had smear-positive TB while 202 (11.7%; 95% CI: 10.3–13.3) patients had culture-positive TB. Eleven TB

Table 4. Demographic and clinical factors associated with drug-resistant tuberculosis in HIV-infected tuberculosis patients, Mumbai, India.

Explanatory Variable	Patients with drug-resistant tuberculosis (N = 68), n (%)	Patients without drug-resistant tuberculosis (N = 134), n (%)	Chi-square/t-test (p-value)	aOR[a] (95% CI)
Age [years, median (IQR)]	35.5 (28.5–42.8)	38.0 (33.8–44.0)	2.15 (0.14)	0.98 (0.96–1.01)
Sex of patients				
Male	46 (33.3)	92 (66.7)	0.02 (0.88)	0.95 (0.49–1.82)
Female	22 (34.4)	42 (65.6)		
Family income per month⁺ (in Rupees)				
Less than 5000	36 (37.5)	60 (62.5)	1.8 (0.17)	
5000 and above	18 (27.3)	48 (72.7)		
ART status				
Pre-ART	22 (30.6)	50 (69.4)	0.48 (0.49)	0.96 (0.49–1.90)
On ART	46 (35.4)	84 (64.6)		
CD4 count, last visit* (in cells/µl)				
Less than 200	19 (32.8)	39 (67.2)	0.22 (0.88)	0.96 (0.48–1.93)
200 and above	43 (33.9)	84 (66.1)		
ART duration** [months, median (IQR)]	19.3 (5.7–31.3)	19.2 (3.2–43.7)		
Previous episode of TB				
Yes	39 (44.3)	49 (55.7)	7.93 (<0.01)	2.31 (1.24–4.30)
No	29 (25.4)	85 (74.6)		

ART: Antiretroviral treatment, CI; Confidence Intervals ⁺Patients with recorded family income, N = 162* Patients with available information about CD4 count, last visit N = 185** Patients on ART with available information about ART initiation date, N = 126[a] aOR; adjusted Odds ratios (calculated by binary logistic regression using multiple imputation for CD4 missing data).

patients were smear-positive but culture negative and 141 patients were culture-positive but smear-negative. Those patients having a history of TB had a higher rate of smear-positivity (4.4% versus 3.9%), but lower culture-positivity rate (9.4% versus 14.4%) as compared to patients without TB history (Figure 2).

Among all culture-positive TB patients, 68 or 33.7% (95% CI: 27.4–40.4) had some form of drug-resistant TB. A high proportion of MDR-TB and pre-XDR-TB, 38% (26/68) and 21% (14/68) respectively, was observed amongst drug-resistant TB patients. Table 2 shows the detailed resistance patterns of all patients with DR-TB.

Of the newly diagnosed (114/791) and previously treated (88/933) culture-positive TB patients, 25.4% (95% CI: 18.1–34.0) and 44.3% (95% CI: 34.2–54.8) patients had drug-resistant TB. The proportion of patients with multidrug-resistant TB and more advanced TB resistance profiles was higher (36% versus 11%) in previously treated patients compared to newly diagnosed TB patients.

Children and extra-pulmonary tuberculosis patients

In the study, 283 children aged less than 15 years were investigated. The median (IQR) age of these children was 11 (8–13) years, just over half of them were male (56%), and sixty-eight percent were on ART. Of the 283 children investigated, 5% (15/283) had culture-positive TB, of whom seven (46.7%, 7/15) had drug-resistant TB; one had polydrug-resistant TB, two had MDR-TB and four had pre-XDR-TB.

Among 1724 HIV-infected patients investigated during the study period, 36 patients had presumptive extra-pulmonary TB (EPTB). The median (IQR) age of these patients was 45 (40–47) years and three-quarters of them were male (27/36, 75%). Among the 36 investigated presumptive EPTB patients, 14% (5/36) patients had culture-positive TB. Of these, 40% (2/5) patients had DR-TB: one had INH mono-resistant TB while another had pre-XDR-TB.

Factors associated with culture-confirmed TB, DR-TB and MDR-TB

The demographic and clinical factors were assessed for association with culture-confirmed TB, DR-TB and MDR-TB. The univariate and bivariate analyses found age, ART status, CD4 count at last visit and previous episode of TB significantly related to culture-positive TB (Table 3). A multivariate Poisson regression model showed that older age, pre-ART status (i.e. not yet on ART), CD4 count less than 200 cells/µL at the last visit and a previous episode of TB were associated with culture-positive TB. None of the factors other than previous history of TB were associated with drug-resistant TB (Table 4) and multi-drug resistant TB (Table 5) in bivariate and multivariate binary logistic regression models.

Table 5. Demographic and clinical factors associated with multidrug-resistant tuberculosis in HIV-infected tuberculosis patients, Mumbai, India.

Explanatory Variable	Patients with multidrug-resistant tuberculosis (N = 45), n (%)	Patients with drug-susceptible tuberculosis (N = 134), n (%)	Chi-square/t-test (p-value)	aOR[a] (95% CI)
Age [years, median (IQR)]	38.0 (30.0–42.5)	38.0 (33.8–44.0)	1.85 (0.18)	0.98 (0.95–1.01)
Sex of patients				
Male	30 (24.6)	92 (75.4)	0.06 (0.80)	0.83 (3.8–1.83)
Female	15 (26.3)	42 (73.7)		
Family income per month⁺ (in Rupees)				
Less than 5000	21 (25.9)	60 (74.1)	1.03 (0.31)	
5000 and above	11 (18.6)	48 (81.4)		
ART status				
Pre-ART	12 (19.4)	50 (80.6)	1.69 (0.19)	0.85 (0.37–1.96)
On ART	33 (28.2)	84 (71.8)		
CD4 count, last visit* (in cells/µl)				
Less than 200	13 (25.0)	39 (75.0)	0.00 (1.00)	1.02 (0.43–2.41)
200 and above	28 (25.0)	84 (75.0)		
ART duration** [months, median (IQR)]	19.7 (5.7–34.8)	19.2 (3.2–43.7)	0.02 (0.88)	
Previous episode of TB				
Yes	32 (39.5)	49 (60.5)	16.2 (<0.01)	4.16 (1.93–8.95)
No	13 (13.2)	85 (86.7)		

ART: Antiretroviral treatment, CI; Confidence Intervals ⁺Patients with recorded family income, N = 140* Patients with available information about CD4 count, last visit N = 164** Patients on ART with available information about ART initiation date, N = 126[a]aOR; adjusted Odds ratios (calculated by binary logistic regression using multiple imputation for CD4 missing data).

Discussion

To our knowledge this is the first DR-TB survey carried out among HIV clinic attendees in India. This study shows that, among HIV-infected children and adults in Mumbai, the burden of drug-resistant tuberculosis is extremely high: almost one in four new TB cases and one in two of those previously treated for TB have a drug-resistant strain. Of just as great concern, a large proportion of these strains was resistant to one or more second-line tuberculosis drugs, especially fluoroquinolones.

The overall rate of culture positivity amongst presumptive TB cases was surprisingly low (11.7%). We hypothesize that this was due neither to limitations in laboratory techniques nor the presence of NTM disease, but instead to the broad inclusion criteria that required a person attending a study site to have just one of four possible TB symptoms as recommended by WHO [13]; a person with 'current cough', for example, who was otherwise stable was eligible for enrolment. Another possible contributor to the low rate of TB culture positivity was the relatively large number of poor quality specimens (e.g. consisting of saliva) despite active instruction being given by a dedicated study nurse at each site. In any case, this finding warrants further investigation.

Even though the overall yield of TB was small in the pediatric cohort as well, it remains significant that almost half of the children with TB were infected with drug-resistant strains, most commonly pre-XDR-TB. Since bacteriological confirmation of DR-TB is more challenging in young children than in adults, as they cannot expectorate sputum and are more likely to have paucibacillary and extra-pulmonary TB, we hypothesize that the burden of TB and DR-TB is likely to be underestimated among children in this study, similar to what has been found in a recent meta-analysis [15]. With less than 2% of all study participants having specimens taken from extrapulmonary sites, it is almost certain that EPTB is being underdiagnosed as well in this cohort. A separate analysis found no significant association between EPTB and DR-TB in children or adults.

Our statistical models revealed no significant associations between most demographic and clinical factors and the risk of DR-TB and MDR-TB. We believe that these findings are important for their lack of associations; it seems that most TB/HIV co-infected patients attending ART centers in Mumbai are at risk for DR-TB. Although the relatively small sample size limits the power of our analyses and calls for cautious interpretation, the lack of associations suggests that all those infected with HIV and presumed to have active TB be tested for drug-resistant strains.

Given the high population density in Mumbai, in which a large proportion of the population lives in slums under extreme poverty, the very high TB prevalence and the relatively high HIV burden reported in greater metropolitan Mumbai, these data are unlikely to be representative of a country as vast and diverse as India. Nevertheless the living conditions in Mumbai and common practices in the public and private health sectors (as for example the prescribing of inappropriate regimens and over-the-counter availability of fluoroquinolones and other drugs with anti-TB properties) are similar to those of other large metropolitan centres in the country, so these data could very well represent the DR-TB situation in such cities as New Delhi, Kolkata and Chennai.

While it may not be possible to generalise our estimates for the entire country or even for HIV-uninfected populations, they serve to highlight the overall magnitude of the DR-TB epidemic in Mumbai, which is not unknown [16,17]. A high prevalence of MDR-TB strains (11–68%) was reported in tertiary health facilities as early as 1991, followed by further documentation in 2006 [18–20], including information on the magnitude of the epidemic in children [21]. A study by D'Souza et al in 2009 [18] documented high levels of multiple drug resistance (both MDR and poly-drug resistance) amongst previously untreated cases in urban parts of Mumbai. In 2011 Udwadia et al reported a cases-series of totally-drug resistant TB (a term that has not officially been endorsed by WHO) in Mumbai, which captured the attention of local and international media [22,23]. However to-date such findings are often overlooked and their importance minimized as representing only selected populations, laboratory or tertiary care settings and small case-series. Our study confirms that there is more than one epidemic ongoing in Mumbai and reinforces the urgent need to accurately measure the overall prevalence and incidence of DR-TB around the country in order to define appropriate interventions. Studies in selected populations such as this complement the overall estimates and can help in directing resources and prioritizing interventions targeted at the most vulnerable groups.

This survey is subject to the usual limitations in survey design and data collection. There is likely to be a tendency for patients to not report previous treatment either because they do not remember (recall limitation) or, on purpose, to avoid going through a long course of treatment that includes daily injectable medication and is known among patients for debilitating side effects [24]. Such bias could have led to an overestimate of DR-TB among new cases and an underestimate among retreatment cases. However, most HIV-infected patients attending ART clinics are usually aware of tuberculosis and have been counseled and screened for TB on several occasions, so recall limitation is rather unlikely.

The majority of HIV-infected patients attending public and public-private ART centers in the city are likely to access the public national TB programme for TB diagnosis and treatment. However many still seek care from private practitioners or may switch between the public and private sectors. The contribution to DR-TB levels from suboptimal treatment regimens prescribed in the unregulated Indian private health sector has been well documented [25–27]. Cox et al in 2007 have shown that even under well-established DOTS programmes in areas with high levels of drug resistance, high levels of amplification of drug resistance are to be expected [28].

The high level of resistance to three or more first-line anti-TB drugs and to fluoroquinolones has been previously described by others [29]. The proportion of previously untreated cases in our study that were resistant to more than three drugs, especially isoniazid, rifampicin and a fluoroquinolone, was particularly alarming and highlights two major issues in the management of TB in the setting of HIV/ART clinics. Firstly, it points to the scenario of nosocomial transmission of TB and DR-TB. Those attending an ART clinic at least once a month are more likely to be exposed to susceptible and resistant strains of *M. tuberculosis* than the general population. Given that the ART centers in Mumbai are usually extremely busy, constantly crowded and that they often lack adequate TB infection control interventions, this scenario is not unlikely. Instead of hypothesizing that most cases of DR-TB are due to non-adherence among patients on treatment, exogenous infection or re-infection should first be considered [30,31]. Secondly, considering the high levels of resistance to second-line TB drugs and especially fluoroquinolones in this population, it is reasonable to assume that patients with presumptive TB may actually have pre-XDR-TB or even XDR-TB. This statement implies a huge investment in laboratory capacity in an already constrained public sector in Mumbai in order to screen all TB patients at the outset for strains that are resistant to fluoroquinolones and anti-TB injectables Nevertheless, we believe that it is a reasonable investment to make if the epidemic of DR-TB is to be controlled in the city in the future. Conversely, if DST is only offered afterward to those failing their TB treatment regimen, a large proportion of DR-TB cases will be missed due to the high risk of mortality among HIV-positive patients with untreated DR-TB [32].

There is an ongoing plan to systematically offer molecular TB diagnosis (mainly using Xpert MTB/RIF, also known as GeneXpert) to all HIV-infected patients in Mumbai and elsewhere in the country. While this is a giant leap forward, since GeneXpert can rapidly detect MTB and rifampicin resistance within 2 hours, we are concerned that 'scale up' of DR-TB diagnosis using this particular diagnostic may lead to suboptimal practices, since a diagnosis of rifampicin resistance alone and/or assumption that it represents a diagnosis of MDR-TB, may mask a diagnosis of pre-XDR or XDR-TB (or worse); the risks then associated with giving a suboptimal treatment regimen are significant both in terms of morbidity and mortality for the patient, as well as amplification of resistance and subsequent community transmission of resistant strains. While GeneXpert is an excellent and efficient diagnostic tool for MTB and screening test for DR-TB, in settings like Mumbai it is essential that it be complemented by culture and DST involving first- and second-line anti-TB drugs. The national programme has recently changed the policy to account for this risk, starting with HIV-infected patients in Mumbai and Maharashtra.

Our initial study protocol included fingerprinting studies using spoligotyping, which we had to abandon due to the high cost. Cox et al have in the past found a strong association between the Beijing genotype and amplification in situations of preexisting resistance in a central Asian setting [33]. Similarly, the proportion of the Beijing genotype was reported to be 35% in the urban Mumbai population studied by Almeida et al [34]. We need fingerprinting studies to establish how often nosocomial transmission occurs and to guide TB infection control interventions. Another area of research that is urgently needed relates to chemoprophylaxis for child contacts of DR-TB cases in Mumbai; preventative regimens that have shown to be effective in other settings are unlikely to prevent development of active disease in many children in Mumbai due to the high baseline rate of fluoroquinolone resistance [35].

Conclusion

Our findings strongly suggest that there is an ongoing DR-TB epidemic among people living with HIV and attending ART centers in Mumbai, which requires urgent, innovative and feasible models of care that allow for rapid and accurate detection and treatment of as many DR-TB patients as possible. Ideally all patients with presumptive TB attending any ART center in Mumbai, or settings with similar drug resistance patterns, should be screened with a rapid molecular diagnostic followed by DST to first- and second-line anti-TB drugs, including for fluoroquinolones, so that the correct diagnosis is made as early as possible and followed by prompt treatment initiation with an appropriate individualized regimen. The high rate of DR-TB amongst new TB patients also highlights the need for better TB infection control measures in order to prevent ongoing transmission of DR-TB in the community and health facilities, especially those attended by vulnerable populations, such as those living with HIV.

Acknowledgments

The authors wish to acknowledge the strong collaboration of hospital responsibles, heads of medical departments and ART centres and all staff from the seven ART Centers involved in this study. We thank the MSF nurses working within the 7 ART centres: Ujwala Pongurlekar, Prachi Salunke, Sonakshi Jadhav, Mansi Kulkarni, Jobin Joseph, Albert Thomas, and Louis Fernandes. We also thank Meenakshi Iyer for laboratory analyses and data entry. Finally, we acknowledge the participation within this study of the patients suffering from HIV and tuberculosis in Mumbai.

Author Contributions

Conceived and designed the experiments: PI. Performed the experiments: CP CR MM AS. Analyzed the data: PI MD. Contributed reagents/materials/analysis tools: AMVK MK AB BA MM MP AK BBR AD LR PS KSS. Contributed to the writing of the manuscript: PI MD PS. Critically reviewed several versions of the manuscript: AMVK MK AB BA MM MP AK BBR AD LR PS KSS CP AS.

References

1. World Health Organization (WHO) (2013), Global tuberculosis report 2013. WHO Press, Geneva, WHO/HTM/TB/2013.11.
2. Department of AIDS Control (2013), National AIDS Control Organization, Annual Report 2012–2013, Ministry of Health & Family Welfare, Government of India.
3. Paramasivan CN, Venkataraman P (2004) Drug resistance in tuberculosis in India. Indian J Med Res; 120: 377–386.
4. Deivanayagam CN, Rajasekaran S, Venkatesan R, Mahilmaran A, Ahmed PR, et al. (2002) Prevalence of acquired MDR TB and HIV co-infection. Indian J Chest Dis Allied Sci 44: 237–242.
5. Williams BG, Granich R, Chauhan LS, Dharmshaktu NS, Dye C (2005) The impact of HIV/AIDS on the control of tuberculosis in India. Proc Natl Acad Sci U S A 102: 9619–9624.
6. Swaminathan S, Paramasivan CN, Ponnuraja C, Iliayas S, Rajasekeran S (2005) Anti-tuberculosis drug resistance in patients with HIV and tuberculosis in South India. Int J Tuberc Lung Dis 9: 896–900.
7. Maniar JK, Kanuth RR, Mandalia S, Shah K, Maniar A (2006) HIV and tuberculosis: partners in crime. Indian J Dermatol Venereol Leprol 72: 276–82.
8. Pereira M, Tripathy S, Inamdar V, Ramesh K, Bhavsar M, et al. (2005) Drug resistance pattern of Mycobacterium tuberculosis in seropositive and seronegative HIV-TB patients in Pune, India. Indian J Med Res 121: 235–239.
9. Sethi S, Mewara A, Dhatwalia SK, Singh H, Yadav R, et al. (2013) Prevalence of multidrug resistance in *Mycobacterium tuberculosis* isolates from HIV seropositive and seronegative patients with pulmonary tuberculosis in north India. BMC Infect Dis 1471–2334/13/137.
10. Menon S, Dharmshale S, Chande C, Gohil A, Lilani S, et al. (2012) Drug resistance profiles of *Mycobacterium tuberculosis* isolates to first line anti-tuberculous drugs: a five years study. Lung India 29: 227–231.
11. Kumar P, Balooni V, Sharma BK, Kapil V, Sachdeva KS, et al. (2014) High degree of multi-drug resistance and hetero-resistance in pulmonary TB patients from Punjab state of India. Tuberculosis (Edinb) 94(1): 73–80.
12. Ramachandran R, Nalini S, Chandrasekar V, Dave PV, Sanghvi AS, et al. (2009) Surveillance of drug-resistant tuberculosis in the state of Gujarat, India Int J Tuberc Lung Dis 13(9): 1154–1160.
13. World Health Organization (2011) Guidelines for the programmatic management of drug-resistant tuberculosis. 2011 update. Geneva, Switzerland: WHO.
14. Central TB Division (2012) Programmatic Management for Drug-resistant Tuberculosis guidelines-May version, Directorate General of Heath Services, Ministry of Health and Family Welfare. Available: http://www.tbcindia.nic.in/pdfs/Guidelines%20for%20PMDT%20in%20India%20-%20May%202012.pdf. Accessed 2014 May 5.
15. Jenkins HE, Tolman AW, Yuen CM, Parr JB, Keshavjee S, et al. (2014) Incidence of multidrug-resistant tuberculosis disease in children: systematic review and global estimates. Lancet 383(9928): 1572–1579.
16. Almeida D, Rodrigues C, Udwadia ZF, Lalvani A, Gothi GD, et al. (2003) Incidence of multidrug-resistant tuberculosis in urban and rural India and implications for prevention. Clin Infect Dis 36: e152–4.
17. Singh S, Sankar MM, Gopinath K (2007) High rate of extensively drug-resistant tuberculosis in Indian AIDS patients. AIDS 21(17): 2345–7.
18. D'souza DT, Mistry NF, Vira TS, Dholakia Y, Hoffner S, et al. (2009) High levels of multidrug resistant tuberculosis in new and treatment-failure patients from the Revised National Tuberculosis Control Programme in an urban metropolis (Mumbai) in Western India. BMC Public Health 29: 9–211.
19. Rodrigues C, Shenai S, Sadani M, Thakkar P, Sodha A, et al. (2006) Multi drug-resistant tuberculosis in Mumbai: it's only getting worse. Int J Tuberc Lung Dis 10(12): 1421–1422.
20. Chowgule RV, D Lina (1998) Pattern of secondary acquired drug resistance to antituberculosis drugs in Mumbai, India 1991–1995. Ind J Chest Dis Allied Sciences 40: 23–31.
21. Karande S, Bavdekar SB (2002) Children and multidrug-resistant tuberculosis in Mumbai (Bombay), India. Emerg Infect Dis 8(11): 1360–1361.
22. Udwadia ZF, Amale RA, Ajbani KK, Rodrigues C (2011) Totally Drug-Resistant Tuberculosis in India. Clin Infect Dis. doi:10.1093/cid/cir889.
23. TIME Magazine (2013). Contagion; Why drug-resistant tuberculosis threatens us all. March 4, 2013.
24. Isaakidis P, Rangan S, Pradhan A, Ladomirska J, Reid T, et al. (2013) 'I cry every day': experiences of patients co-infected with HIV and multidrug-resistant tuberculosis. Trop Med & Int Health 18(9): 1128–1133.
25. Uplekar M, Juvekar S, Morankar S, Rangan S, Nunn P (1998) Tuberculosis patients and practitioners in private clinics in India. Int J Tuberc Lung Dis 2(4): 324–329.
26. Bhargava A, Pinto L, Pai M (2011) Mismanagement of tuberculosis in India: Causes, consequences, and the way forward. Hypothesis 9(1): e7.
27. Udwadia ZF, Pinto LM, Uplekar MW (2010) Tuberculosis management by private practitioners in Mumbai, India: has anything changed in two decades? PLoS One 5: e12023.
28. Cox HS, Niemann S, Ismailov G, Doshetov D, Orozco JD, et al. (2007) Risk of acquired drug resistance during short-course directly observed treatment of tuberculosis in an area with high levels of drug resistance. Clin Infect Dis 441421–1427.
29. Agrawal D, Udwadia ZF, Rodriguez C, Mehta A (2009) Increasing incidence of fluoroquinolone-resistant Mycobacterium tuberculosis in Mumbai, India. Int J Tuberc Lung Dis 13(1): 79–83.
30. Andrews JR, Gandhi NR, Moodley P, Shah NS, Bohlken L, et al. (2008) Exogenous reinfection as a cause of multidrug-resistant and extensively drug-resistant tuberculosis in rural South Africa. JID 198: 1582–1589.
31. March F, Garriga X, Rodriguez P, Moreno C, Garrigo M, et al. (1997) Acquired drug resistance in Mycobacterium tuberculosis isolates recovered from compliant patients with human immunodeficiency virus-associated tuberculosis. Clin Infect Dis 25: 1044–1047.
32. Gandhi NR, Shah NS, Andrews JR, Vella V, Moll AP, et al. (2010) HIV coinfection in multidrug- and extensively drug-resistant tuberculosis results in high early mortality. Am J Respir Crit Care Med 181: 80–86.
33. Cox HS, Kubica T, Doshetov D, Kebede Y, Rüsch-Gerdess S, et al. (2005). The Beijing genotype and drug resistant tuberculosis in the Aral Sea region of Central Asia. Respiratory research, 6(1): 134.
34. Almeida D, Rodrigues C, Ashavaid TF, Lalvani A, Udwadia ZF, et al. (2005). High incidence of the Beijing genotype among multidrug-resistant isolates of Mycobacterium tuberculosis in a tertiary care center in Mumbai, India. CID, 40(6): 881–886.
35. Seddon JA, Hesseling AC, Finlayson H, Fielding K, Cox H, et al. (2013) Preventive therapy for child contacts of multidrug-resistant tuberculosis: a prospective cohort study. CIDcit655.

19

Another "String to the Bow" of PJ34, a Potent Poly(ADP-Ribose)Polymerase Inhibitor: An Antiplatelet Effect through $P2Y_{12}$ Antagonism?

Marie Lechaftois[1], Elise Dreano[2,3], Bruno Palmier[1], Isabelle Margaill[1], Catherine Marchand-Leroux[1], Christilla Bachelot-Loza[2,3], Dominique Lerouet[1]*

1 EA4475-"Pharmacologie de la Circulation Cérébrale", Faculté des Sciences Pharmaceutiques et Biologiques, Université Paris Descartes, Comue Sorbonne Paris Cité, Paris, France, **2** Inserm UMR S1140, Paris, France, **3** Faculté des Sciences Pharmaceutiques et Biologiques, Université Paris Descartes, Comue Sorbonne Paris Cité, Paris, France

Abstract

Background: Neuro- and vasoprotective effects of poly(ADP-ribose)polymerase (PARP) inhibition have been largely documented in models of cerebral ischemia, particularly with the potent PARP inhibitor PJ34. Furthermore, after ischemic stroke, physicians are faced with incomplete tissue reperfusion and reocclusion, in which platelet activation/aggregation plays a key role. Data suggest that certain PARP inhibitors could act as antiplatelet agents. In that context, the present *in vitro* study investigated on human blood the potential antiplatelet effect of PJ34 and two structurally different PARP inhibitors, DPQ and INO-1001.

Methods and results: ADP concentrations were chosen to induce a biphasic aggregation curve resulting from the successive activation of both its receptors $P2Y_1$ and $P2Y_{12}$. In these experimental conditions, PJ34 inhibited the second phase of aggregation; this effect was reduced by incremental ADP concentrations. In addition, in line with a $P2Y_{12}$ pathway inhibitory effect, PJ34 inhibited the dephosphorylation of the vasodilator stimulated phosphoprotein (VASP) in a concentration-dependent manner. Besides, PJ34 had no effect on platelet aggregation induced by collagen or PAR1 activating peptide, used at concentrations inducing a strong activation independent on secreted ADP. By contrast, DPQ and INO-1001 were devoid of any effect whatever the platelet agonist used.

Conclusions: We showed that, in addition to its already demonstrated beneficial effects in *in vivo* models of cerebral ischemia, the potent PARP inhibitor PJ34 exerts *in vitro* an antiplatelet effect. Moreover, this is the first study to report that PJ34 could act *via* a competitive $P2Y_{12}$ antagonism. Thus, this antiplatelet effect could improve post-stroke reperfusion and/or prevent reocclusion, which reinforces the interest of this drug for stroke treatment.

Editor: Ferenc Gallyas, Jr, University of Pecs Medical School, Hungary

Funding: This work was supported by "Université Paris Descartes" and the following Societies: "Groupe de Réflexion sur la Recherche Cardiovasculaire," "Société Française de Pharmacologie et de Thérapeutique," "Fédération Française de Cardiologie" and "Société Française de Cardiologie." The funders had no role in study design, data collection and analysis, decision to publish, or preparation of the manuscript.

Competing Interests: The authors have declared that no competing interests exist.

* Email: dominique.lerouet@parisdescartes.fr

Introduction

Platelet adhesion, activation and aggregation are crucial in arterial thrombosis, and therefore, in the pathophysiology of ischemic stroke [1–4], a leading cause of death worldwide. Today, the only approved treatment for stroke is thrombolysis with the recombinant tissue plasminogen activator (rt-PA) that improves outcomes in acute ischemic stroke patients by restoring cerebral blood flow. Nevertheless, its use remains limited to less than 5% patients due to its narrow therapeutic window of 4.5 hours [5] and the related risk of hemorrhagic transformations [6]. Moreover, rt-PA induces recanalization in only half of the treated patients [7] and early arterial reocclusion also occurs after successful thrombolysis in about 20 to 30% of recanalized patients [8–11]. Another major health concern in survival patients is the high risk of recurrent strokes within the following few weeks after the first event [12]. In addition to lifestyle changes and to the control of risk factors (e.g. hypertension, diabetes, dyslipidemia), current guidelines recommend antiplatelet agents (mostly aspirin and clopidogrel) as the fundamental strategy of secondary stroke prevention in patients with noncardioembolic disease [13]. However the modest benefit of these agents and the potential risk of bleedings point out the need for novel strategies [14–16].

Almost 10 years ago, Alexy and collaborators [17] demonstrated *in vitro* that three poly(ADP-ribose)polymerase (PARP) inhibitors (4-hydroxyquinazoline; 2-mercapto-4(3H)-quinazolinone; HO-3089) were able to reduce aggregation induced by adenosine diphosphate (ADP). PARP is an ubiquitous nuclear enzyme catalyzing the synthesis of poly(ADP-ribose) from nicotinamide adenine dinucleotide (NAD) and physiologically involved in DNA repair. As platelets are small anucleate cells, they theoretically cannot contain this enzyme. To our knowledge, there is no data reporting PARP presence in platelets, but we confirmed its absence by measuring the protein expression and enzyme activity in human platelets (data not shown). Therefore, the potential antiplatelet effect of PARP inhibitors would be PARP-independent as suggested in Alexy's study [17]. Indeed, the authors attributed this effect to a potential competition between these inhibitors and ADP to bind to their platelet receptors, which might be due to a molecular structure resembling that of the adenine moiety of NAD and common with ADP. Such an inhibition of ADP-induced aggregation was not observed by Tóth and collaborators with INO-1001, another potent PARP inhibitor with a different structure [18]. Consequently, these data suggest that certain PARP inhibitors might exert antiplatelet effect and thus might prevent reocclusion after thrombolysis in ischemic stroke patients and/or be useful for secondary stroke prevention.

In pathophysiological conditions, such as stroke, the over-activation of PARP exerts deleterious effects, as demonstrated in several experimental models of cerebral ischemia [19,20]. In rodent models of cerebral ischemia, we and others have shown that PJ34 (N-(6-oxo-5,6-dihydro-phenanthridin-2-yl)-N,N-dimethylacetamide), a potent PARP inhibitor (IC50 = 17 nM), reduces infarct volume, blood-brain barrier permeability, brain edema, spontaneous and rt-PA-induced hemorrhagic transformations, inflammatory response, motor deficit, and enhances long-term neuronal survival and neurogenesis [21–28].

In that context, the aim of our study was to evaluate *in vitro* on human blood whether PJ34 exerts antiplatelet effect and the potential mechanism involved. Such an effect, in addition to the protective effects mentioned above, would reinforce the interest of PJ34 in stroke treatment. The effect of two other PARP inhibitors, that have also demonstrated beneficial effects in experimental models of cerebral ischemia [29–31], but with different chemical structures, was also studied (Figure 1): a dihydroisoquinolinone (3,4-dihydro-5-[4-(1-piperidinyl)butoxy]-1(2H)-isoquinolinone or DPQ; IC50~40 nM) and an isoindolinone derivative (INO-1001; IC50<15 nM). To our knowledge, this is the first work to report that PJ34 inhibits ADP-induced platelet aggregation in human platelet-rich plasma (PRP), probably acting *via* a $P2Y_{12}$ pathway inhibition.

Materials and Methods

Chemicals and reagents

ADP was obtained from Roche (Boulogne-Billancourt, France) and PAR1ap (activating peptide of protease-activated receptor 1), used as a thrombin receptor activator, from Bachem (Bubendorf, Switzerland). Collagen was purchased from Nycomed (kit SKF Solution, Austria Takeda Pharmaceuticals International, Zurich, Switzerland).

PJ34 was purchased from Sigma-Aldrich (Saint Quentin Fallavier, France), DPQ from Santa Cruz Biotechnology (Clin-iSciences, Nanterre, France) and INO-1001 from Seleck Chemicals (Euromedex, Souffelweyersheim, France).

All reagents were dissolved and diluted in distilled water, except DPQ that was dissolved in 100% DMSO and diluted in distilled water.

Human platelet aggregation studies

Venous blood from informed healthy donors was obtained from the French blood bank institute (EFS) according to the agreement between Paris Descartes University and EFS (C CPSL UNT No. 12/EFS/064).

PJ34

DPQ

INO-1001

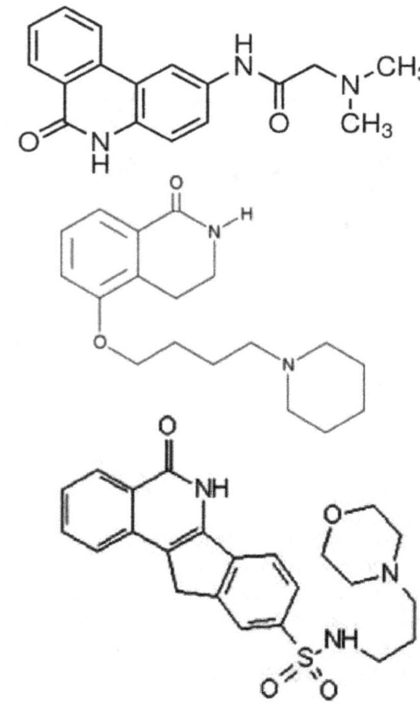

Figure 1. Chemical structure of the three PARP inhibitors: PJ34, DPQ and INO-1001.

Whole blood samples were collected from 35 volunteers into Vacutainer tubes containing 3.8% trisodium citrate (BD Vacutainer, Becton Dickinson, Le Pont de Claix, France) and centrifuged at 133 g for 20 minutes at 25°C (OrtoAlresa Digtor 21 R, Madrid, Spain) to obtain PRP. After carefully removing PRP, the pellet was centrifuged at 2630 g for 20 minutes at 25°C to obtain platelet-poor plasma (PPP). The final platelet count in PRP samples was adjusted to 2.5×10^{8} platelets/ml with autologous PPP.

Platelet aggregation was quantified in PRP by optical aggregometry using a PAP-8E Aggregometer (Bio/Data Corporation, Horsham, PA, USA) with a constant stirring rate of 1000 rpm at 37°C.

Ten microliters of PARP inhibitors (PJ34, DPQ or INO-1001) or vehicle (distilled water or 0.3% DMSO) were added to 230 µl of PRP in glass cuvettes. Samples were pre-incubated at 37°C for 10 minutes. After baseline adjustment, 10 µl of platelet agonist (ADP, collagen or PAR1ap) were added and aggregation was recorded for 8 minutes. A glass cuvette containing 20 µl of vehicle (distilled water or 0.3% DMSO) and 230 µl of PPP served as a control of "100% light transmission".

Agonist concentrations were adjusted for each donor to induce a maximum aggregation of about 65–70%: collagen (1−1.5 or 2 µg/ml) and PAR1ap (1−1.5 or 2 µM). Moreover, ADP concentration has to be determined for each donor to induce a biphasic aggregation curve (1.5−2–2.5−3–4 or 5 µM).

PJ34 was used at 1, 10, 25, 50 or 100 µM and the other PARP inhibitors (DPQ and INO-1001) at 50 µM.

References (=platelet agonists alone) were normalized to 100%. The maximal aggregation (%) measured in the presence of PARP inhibitor was compared to that of the corresponding reference, except for ADP-induced aggregation where maximal aggregation was distinguished for each phase.

To evaluate the antiaggregant effect of PJ34 on platelets stimulated with increasing ADP concentrations (1.5 to 10 µM),

PRP was pre-incubated with fixed concentrations of PJ34 (50, 100 or 500 μM). In this experiment, since the ADP concentration used did not always induce a biphasic aggregation curve, the maximum aggregation (%) in the presence of PJ34 was compared to the corresponding reference.

The concentrations of PARP inhibitors, platelet agonist or DMSO mentioned above correspond to the final concentration in 250 μl.

VASP phosphorylation

Vasodilator stimulated phosphoprotein (VASP) phosphorylation was measured using a modified commercial kit (PLT VASP/$P2Y_{12}$ assay, Biocytex, Marseille, France) on a FACS Calibur flow cytometer (Becton Dickinson, Franklin Lakes, USA). VASP is an intracellular platelet protein which phosphorylation is regulated by cyclic adenosine monophosphate (cAMP) and activation of a protein kinase pathway. Prostaglandin E1 (PGE1) activates this pathway resulting in VASP phosphorylation, whereas ADP inhibits this cascade through $P2Y_{12}$ receptors and thus reduces VASP phosphorylation.

Briefly, citrated whole blood from 4 healthy volunteers was pre-incubated for 10 minutes with PJ34 (final concentrations: 100, 250, 500 or 1000 μM) or its vehicle (distilled water). The results were expressed as the platelet reactivity index (PRI).

PRI is calculated using corrected mean fluorescence intensities (MFI) in the presence of (1) PGE1 alone (MFI PGE1) or (2) PGE1+ADP associated with PJ34 or its vehicle (MFI (PGE1+ADP±PJ34)), as follows:

PRI = [(MFI PGE1− MFI (PGE1+ADP±PJ34))/MFI PGE1] × 100.

One has to know that a low PRI is associated with a high VASP phosphorylation state, and therefore to an inhibition of ADP-induced platelet response.

Statistical analysis

Data are expressed as mean ± SD.

For PJ34, samples were compared with the vehicle group (=platelet agonist alone) using a one-way analysis of variance (ANOVA) followed by Dunnett's test.

For DPQ and INO-1001, comparisons with the vehicle group were evaluated by one-way ANOVA followed by Student t test.

Pearson correlation test was used to evaluate the relationship between PJ34 concentrations and ADP-induced platelet aggregation, and between PJ34 concentrations and PRI.

Statistical significance was assigned at $P<0.05$, after Bonferroni corrections for multiple comparisons when necessary.

All tests were performed with GraphPad Prism 5 (GraphPad Software, Inc., La Jolla, USA).

Results

Effect of PJ34 on ADP-induced platelet aggregation

The antiplatelet effect of PJ34 was first tested on ADP-induced PRP aggregation. ADP concentration has to be determined for each donor in order to induce a biphasic aggregation curve resulting from the activation of ADP receptors, $P2Y_1$ and $P2Y_{12}$, successively. Before normalization, basal maximal aggregation was about 64±9.8% with the first phase at 40±10.6% and the second one at 24±11.9%, as shown on the representative curve (Figure 2A).

PJ34 had no effect on the first phase of ADP-induced platelet aggregation, but inhibited the second one in a concentration-

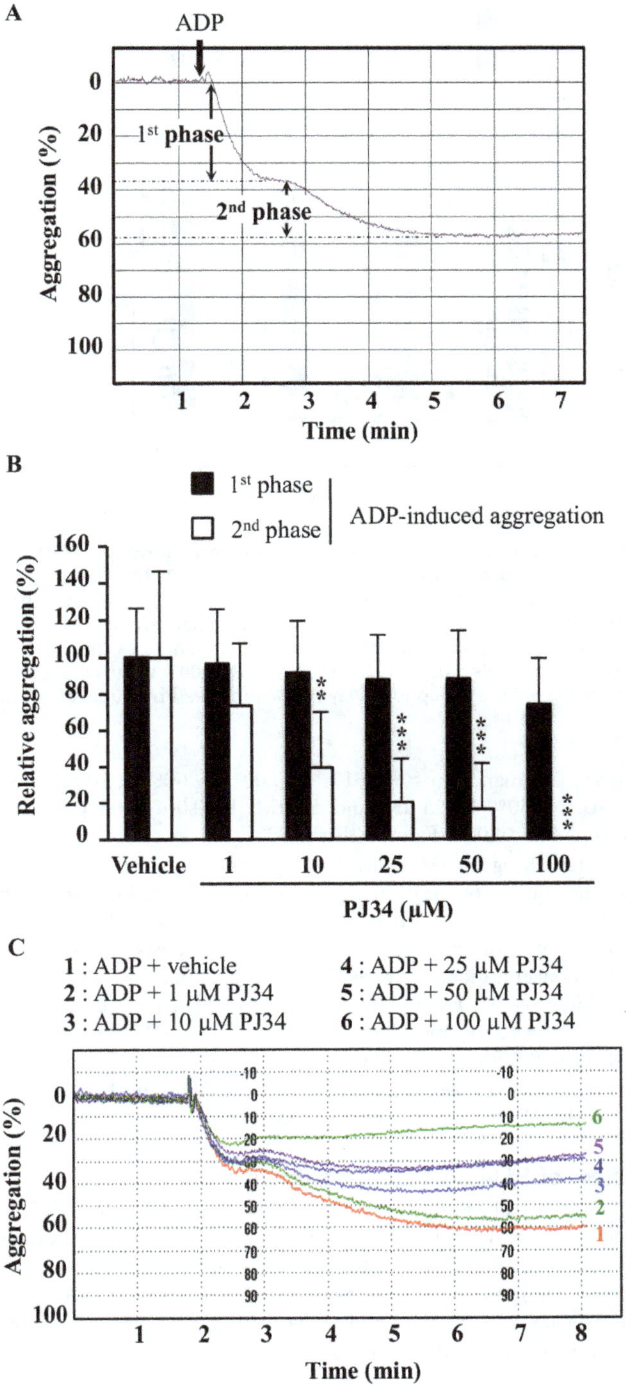

Figure 2. Effect of PJ34 on both phases of ADP-induced platelet aggregation. (A) ADP concentration (1.5 to 5 μM) was determined for each donor to produce a biphasic aggregation curve. (B) Human PRP samples were pre-incubated with PJ34 (1–100 μM) or its vehicle and then stimulated with ADP. Results are expressed relatively to ADP alone (=vehicle group; normalized to 100%) and presented as the mean ± SD (n=6–7). **$P<0.01$ and ***$P<0.001$ *versus* the corresponding vehicle group (one-way ANOVA followed by Dunnett's test). (C) Representative curves showing the effect of PJ34 or its vehicle on platelet aggregation induced by 2 μM ADP.

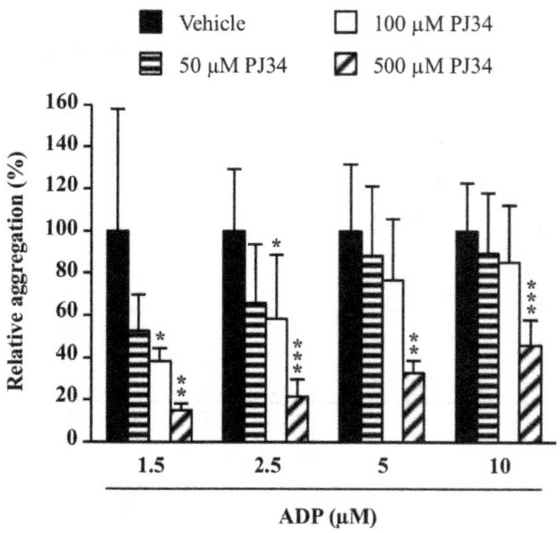

Figure 3. Effect of incremental concentrations of ADP on platelet aggregation in the presence of PJ34. Human PRP samples were pre-incubated with PJ34 or its vehicle and then stimulated with ADP. Results are expressed relatively to ADP alone (= vehicle group; normalized to 100%) and presented as the mean ± SD (n = 4–7). *P<0.05, **P<0.01 and ***P<0.001 *versus* the corresponding vehicle group (one-way ANOVA followed by Dunnett's test).

dependent manner (r = −0.617; P<0.001) by 60% at 10 μM (P<0.01), by 80% at 25 μM and 50 μM (P<0.001) and totally at 100 μM (P<0.001; Figures 2B and C).

Considering the concentration-dependent effect of PJ34 on the second phase of ADP-induced platelet aggregation, we then evaluated the potential competition between ADP and PJ34 using incremental concentrations of ADP. Figure 3 shows that the more ADP concentrations increased (up to 10 μM) the less PJ34 had an inhibitory effect. For instance, 100 μM of PJ34 reduced by 60% the platelet aggregation induced by 1.5 μM of ADP (P<0.05), by 40% the 2.5 μM ADP-induced platelet aggregation (P<0.05), by 25% the platelet aggregation induced by 5 μM and by 15% the 10 μM ADP-induced platelet aggregation.

Effect of PJ34 on VASP phosphorylation

Because the second aggregation phase induced by ADP is mainly dependent on the engagement of $P2Y_{12}$ receptor, leading to the inhibition of VASP phosphorylation, we used flow cytometry quantification of phosphorylated VASP (P-VASP) to investigate the interaction of PJ34 with $P2Y_{12}$ signaling. This method is one of the most valuable to evaluate the efficacy of $P2Y_{12}$ antagonists, such as clopidogrel [32]. In the test, a low PRI is associated with a high VASP phosphorylation state.

The PRI of ADP alone was 70±4.6%. PJ34 reduced the PRI in a concentration-dependent manner (r = −0.951; P<0.001) by 30% at 250 μM (P<0.01), 60% at 500 μM (P<0.001) and totally at 1000 μM (P<0.001; Figure 4).

Effect of PJ34 on collagen- and PAR1ap-induced platelet aggregation

In order to determine the specificity of PJ34 towards ADP-induced platelet aggregation, we next investigated the inhibitory effect of PJ34 on two other platelet agonists (collagen and PAR1ap). Since it is well known that secreted ADP constitutes a second feedback amplification signal in the setting of platelet aggregation, we used agonist concentrations inducing a strong

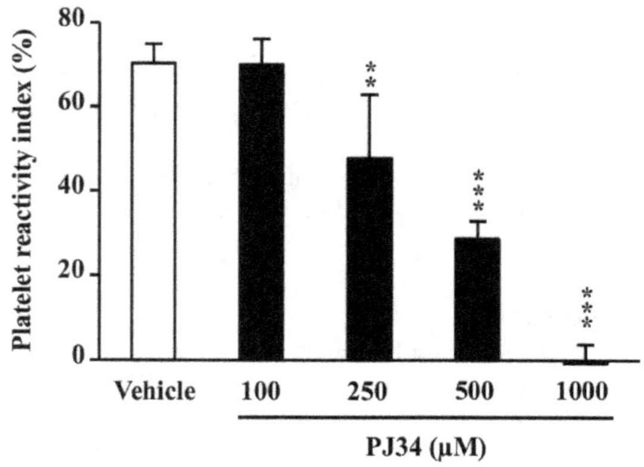

Figure 4. Effect of PJ34 on VASP phosphorylation. Human whole blood was pre-incubated with PJ34 or its vehicle and then stimulated with ADP. A low platelet reactivity index (PRI) is associated with a high VASP phosphorylation state and thus reflects $P2Y_{12}$ inhibition. Results are expressed relatively to ADP alone (= vehicle group) and presented as the mean ± SD (n = 3–4). **P<0.01 and ***P<0.001 *versus* vehicle (one-way ANOVA followed by Dunnett's test).

activation less dependent, or independent, on secreted ADP. We thus checked that the aggregation induced by these concentrations was not inhibited (or very slightly) by the selective $P2Y_{12}$ receptor antagonist 2MesAMP (2-methylthioadenosine 5′-monophosphate triethylammonium salt; data not shown) [33]. In these conditions, whatever the PJ34 concentration, no inhibitory effect was observed on either collagen- or PAR1ap-induced platelet aggregation (Figure 5).

Effect of two PARP inhibitors with different chemical structures on ADP-, collagen- and PAR1ap-induced platelet aggregation

To evaluate whether the inhibitory effect on ADP-induced platelet aggregation was specific to PJ34, we evaluated the effect of

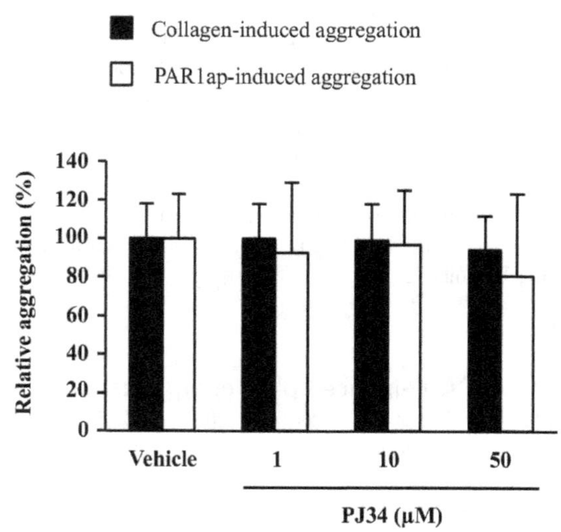

Figure 5. Effect of PJ34 on collagen- and PAR1ap-induced platelet aggregation. Human PRP samples were pre-incubated with PJ34 or its vehicle and then stimulated with either collagen (1 to 2 μg/ml) or PAR1ap (1 to 2 μM). Results are expressed relatively to platelet agonist alone (= vehicle group; normalized to 100%) and presented as the mean ± SD (n = 7–8).

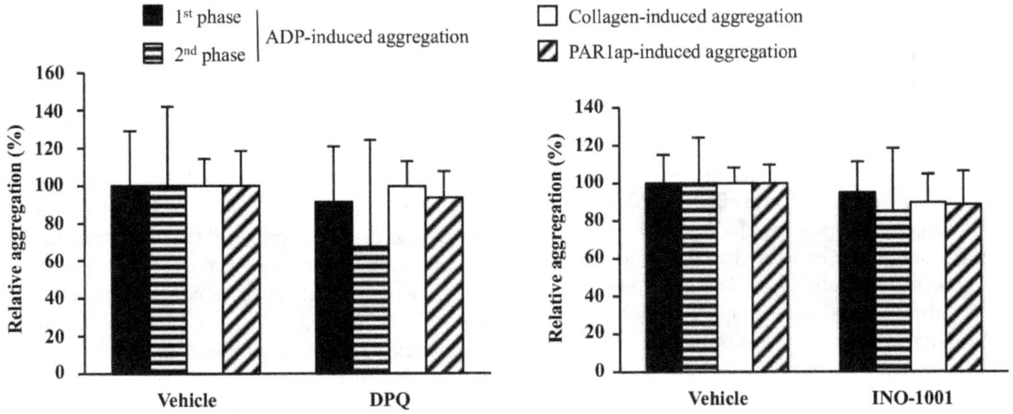

Figure 6. Effect of DPQ and INO-1001 on ADP-, collagen- or PAR1ap-induced platelet aggregation. Human PRP samples were pre-incubated with PARP inhibitor (50 μM) or its vehicle and then stimulated with ADP (1.5 to 5 μM; to produce a biphasic aggregation curve), collagen (1 to 2 μg/ml) or PAR1ap (1 to 2 μM). Results are expressed relatively to platelet agonist alone (=vehicle group; normalized to 100%) and presented as the mean ± SD (n=5–6).

two structural different PARP inhibitors, DPQ and INO-1001, at 50 μM. No significant effect of these inhibitors could be observed, although the second phase of ADP-induced platelet aggregation tended to be reduced by DPQ (Figure 6). DPQ and INO-1001 were devoid of effect on collagen- and PAR1ap-induced platelet aggregation in our experimental conditions (as explained above).

Discussion

Beside their physiological role in maintaining hemostasis, platelets are also involved in the formation of pathogenic thrombi. Platelet activation is triggered by a variety of agonists, such as sub-endothelial collagen, thromboxane A2 and ADP released from activated platelets or thrombin generated by the coagulation cascade [34]. These agonists act on different platelet receptors, but they all trigger signaling pathways leading to intracellular calcium concentration increase [35]. ADP, which is a weak agonist compared to collagen or thrombin, is however considered as the main amplifier of initial aggregation.

In this study, we showed that PJ34 inhibits ADP-induced platelet aggregation. This antiplatelet effect seems specific to ADP receptors since PJ34 does not inhibit collagen- or PAR1ap-induced platelet aggregation; both these agonists were used at concentrations inducing a strong activation less dependent, or independent, on secreted ADP. Our results are in accordance with those of Alexy and collaborators [17] who investigated the effects of three other PARP inhibitors (4-hydroxyquinazoline; 2-mercapto-4(3H)-quinazolinone; HO-3089) and found that they reduced ADP-, but not epinephrine- or collagen-induced platelet aggregation, presumably due to a competition between these PARP inhibitors and ADP for binding to its receptors.

To go further in this hypothetical mechanism, we examined which ADP receptor(s), i.e. $P2Y_1$ and/or $P2Y_{12}$, might be implicated. Indeed, the mechanism of ADP-induced platelet aggregation is complex, since the co-activation of both G protein-coupled receptors $P2Y_1$ and $P2Y_{12}$ is necessary to produce a complete aggregation response [36,37]. The Gq coupled-$P2Y_1$ receptor is essential in the initiation of ADP-induced platelet activation; it mediates calcium mobilization from internal stores, which results in platelet shape change, and weak and transient aggregation. The Gi coupled-$P2Y_{12}$ receptor activation, *via* lowering cAMP levels induces the amplification of platelet aggregation and secretion; this receptor plays a pivotal role in sustaining platelet aggregation. For that purpose, ADP concentrations were determined to produce a biphasic aggregation curve. In these conditions, PJ34 (10 to 100 μM) only inhibited the second phase of ADP-induced platelet aggregation without modifying the first one, suggesting that its antiaggregant effect is specifically linked to $P2Y_{12}$.

Moreover, we observed that incremental ADP concentrations (1.5 to 10 μM) reduced the inhibitory effect of PJ34 (50, 100 and 500 μM), and that the antiaggregant effect of 100 μM PJ34 even disappears when applying ADP at 10 μM, suggesting a competitive effect of PJ34 with ADP for $P2Y_{12}$. In order to test this hypothesis, we assessed by flow cytometry the phosphorylation state of the intracellular platelet protein VASP. This assay is commonly used in clinical practice to evaluate the efficiency of $P2Y_{12}$ antagonism in patients treated with clopidogrel [32]. Therefore, any specific $P2Y_{12}$ antagonist impedes VASP dephosphorylation, and consequently, promotes the phosphorylated form. This assay had to be performed with higher concentrations of PJ34 (100 to 1000 μM) than in aggregation studies. On one hand, these experimental conditions were partly attributed to the fact that whole blood has to be used with the commercial kit (PLT VASP/$P2Y_{12}$ assay) that does not work on PRP. It is important to note that, in both blood and plasma, ADP can be converted to adenosine, an inhibitor of platelet aggregation. However, adenosine is readily removed from blood through uptake into red blood cells, which makes it unavailable to inhibit platelet aggregation. Therefore, adenosine can exert more efficiently its inhibitor effect on platelet aggregation in PRP where red blood cells are absent [38]. This could explain that lower PJ34 concentrations are necessary to inhibit ADP-induced platelet aggregation in PRP. On the other hand, as the concentration of ADP provided in the kit is not specified, this concentration may be higher than those we used before. Whatever the reason, our results show that PJ34 increased the amount of P-VASP in a concentration-dependent manner, suggesting that PJ34 may act like a $P2Y_{12}$ antagonist.

Since our original hypothesis relied on a "PARP-independent" mechanism, we then examined whether two other PARP inhibitors with different chemical structure exert similar antiplatelet effect. We opted for DPQ and INO-1001 that also demonstrated beneficial effects in experimental models of cerebral ischemia [29–31]. The concentration of these PARP inhibitors (50 μM) was chosen based on the PJ34 concentration inducing an important antiaggregant effect, without referring to their IC50 for PARP accordingly to our hypothesis.

Neither DPQ nor INO-1001 modified platelet aggregation whatever the agonist used, although we noticed that the second phase of ADP-induced platelet aggregation tended to be inhibited by DPQ. However, due to the important variability between donors, this inhibition was not significant. Results with INO-1001 are consistent with previous data showing no effect of INO-1001 at 10 or 100 μM [18]. The authors suggested that this lack of antiplatelet effect might simply be explained by its structure, but they also suspected the concentrations used. Indeed, in Toth's study, INO-1001 concentrations are consistent with those preventing PARP activation in a cardiomyocyte oxidative challenge model or even with plasma concentrations measured in *in vivo* models, whereas Alexy and collaborators [17] showed that inhibition of ADP-induced platelet aggregation with their PARP inhibitors occurred at higher concentrations than those inhibiting PARP activity in similar cell culture.

In our study, PJ34 significantly inhibited the second phase of ADP-induced platelet aggregation by 60% at 10 μM, with a tendency at 1 μM (25%). Although these concentrations are higher than the IC50 for PARP inhibition (17 nM), they are similar to those used by Tóth and collaborators with the equipotent PARP inhibitor, INO-1001 (IC50<15 nM). Moreover, PJ34 concentrations are consistent with those commonly used in *in vitro* studies. So, for example, pre-treatment with 30–1000 nM PJ34 significantly protected neurons from cell death induced by oxygen and glucose deprivation in a dose-dependent manner [21]. PJ34 (10 or 100 μM) also protected cardiomyoblast cells against H_2O_2-induced injury [39]. In human umbilical vein endothelial cell culture, Mathews and Berk [40] showed that PJ34 at 10 μM reduced H_2O_2-induced cell death.

Other authors have already pointed out that PJ34 possessed PARP-independent properties [41–43]. Our results hereby highlight another specific facet of this PARP inhibitor that reinforces its superiority *versus* the others.

In conclusion, our study is the first one demonstrating that the PARP inhibitor PJ34 inhibits ADP-induced platelet aggregation *via* a potential competitive $P2Y_{12}$ antagonism. Moreover, since it is well established that pharmacological blockade of $P2Y_{12}$, either with thienopyridines such as clopidogrel or prasugrel or with the direct inhibitor ticagrelor, is a powerful antiplatelet strategy, this antiplatelet effect strengthens the interest of PJ34 in stroke treatment. Indeed, our results suggest that, in addition to its already demonstrated neuro- and vasoprotective effects in cerebral ischemia, PJ34 might also improve spontaneous or rt-PA-induced recanalization and/or prevent from early reocclusion.

Acknowledgments

The authors would like to thank Pr Pascale Gaussem for critically reviewing this manuscript.

Author Contributions

Conceived and designed the experiments: ML ED BP IM CML CBL DL. Performed the experiments: ML ED BP CBL. Analyzed the data: ML BP IM CBL DL. Contributed reagents/materials/analysis tools: ML ED BP CBL. Contributed to the writing of the manuscript: ML ED BP IM CML CBL DL.

References

1. del Zoppo GJ (1998) The role of platelets in ischemic stroke. Neurology 51 (3 Suppl 3): S9–14.
2. Yip HK, Liou CW, Chang HW, Lan MY, Liu JS, et al. (2005) Link between platelet activity and outcomes after an ischemic stroke. Cerebrovasc Dis 20: 120–128.
3. Stoll G, Kleinschnitz C, Nieswandt B (2008) Molecular mechanisms of thrombus formation in ischemic stroke: novel insights and targets for treatment. Blood 112: 3555–3562.
4. Franks ZG, Campbell RA, Weyrich AS, Rondina MT (2010) Platelet-leukocyte interactions link inflammatory and thromboembolic events in ischemic stroke. Ann N Y Acad Sci 1207: 11–17.
5. Hacke W, Kaste M, Bluhmki E, Brozman M, ECASS Investigators, et al. (2008) Thrombolysis with alteplase 3 to 4.5 hours after acute ischemic stroke. N Engl J Med 359: 1317–1329.
6. The National Institute of Neurological Disorders and Stroke rt-PA Stroke Study Group (1995) Tissue plasminogen activator for acute ischemic stroke. N Engl J Med 333: 1581–1587.
7. Rha JH, Saver JL (2007) The impact of recanalization on ischemic stroke outcome: a meta-analysis. Stroke 38: 967–973.
8. Alexandrov AV, Grotta JC (2002) Arterial reocclusion in stroke patients treated with intravenous tissue plasminogen activator. Neurology 59: 862–867.
9. Rubiera M, Alvarez-Sabín J, Ribo M, Montaner J, Santamarina E, et al. (2005) Predictors of early arterial reocclusion after tissue plasminogen activator-induced recanalization in acute ischemic stroke. Stroke 36: 1452–1456.
10. Saqqur M, Molina CA, Salam A, Siddiqui M, CLOTBUST Investigators, et al. (2007) Clinical deterioration after intravenous recombinant tissue plasminogen activator treatment: a multicenter transcranial Doppler study. Stroke 38: 69–74.
11. Balami JS, Sutherland BA, Buchan AM (2013) Complications associated with recombinant tissue plasminogen activator therapy for acute ischaemic stroke. CNS Neurol Disord Drug Targets 12: 155–169.
12. Mohan KM, Wolfe CD, Rudd AG, Heuschmann PU, Kolominsky-Rabas PL, et al. (2011) Risk and cumulative risk of stroke recurrence: a systematic review and meta-analysis. Stroke 42: 1489–1494.
13. Kirshner HS (2012) Antiplatelet and anticoagulation strategies in the prevention and treatment of ischemic stroke. Curr Pharm Des 18: 5261–5272.
14. Fabre JE, Gurney ME (2010) Limitations of current therapies to prevent thrombosis: a need for novel strategies. Mol Biosyst 6: 305–315.
15. Di Minno MN, Russolillo A, Camera M, Brambilla M, De Gregorio A, et al. (2011) New anti-thrombotic drugs for stroke prevention. Curr Vasc Pharmacol 9: 723–732.
16. Weber R, Brenck J, Diener HC (2012) Antiplatelet therapy in cerebrovascular disorders. Handb Exp Pharmacol 210: 519–546.
17. Alexy T, Toth A, Marton Z, Horvath B, Koltai K, et al. (2004) Inhibition of ADP-evoked platelet aggregation by selected poly(ADP-ribose) polymerase inhibitors. J Cardiovasc Pharmacol 43: 423–431.
18. Tóth O, Szabó C, Kecskés M, Pótó L, Nagy A, et al. (2006) In vitro effect of the potent poly(ADP-ribose) polymerase (PARP) inhibitor INO-1001 alone and in combination with aspirin, eptifibatide, tirofiban, enoxaparin or alteplase on haemostatic parameters. Life Sci 79: 317–323.
19. Komjáti K, Besson VC, Szabó C (2005) Poly (adp-ribose) polymerase inhibitors as potential therapeutic agents in stroke and neurotrauma. Curr Drug Targets CNS Neurol Disord 4: 179–194.
20. Curtin NJ, Szabo C (2013) Therapeutic applications of PARP inhibitors: Anticancer therapy and beyond. Mol Aspects Med 34: 1217–1256.
21. Abdelkarim GE, Gertz K, Harms C, Katchanov J, Dirnagl U, et al. (2001) Protective effects of PJ34, a novel, potent inhibitor of poly(ADP-ribose) polymerase (PARP) in in vitro and in vivo models of stroke. Int J Mol Med 7: 255–260.
22. Park EM, Cho S, Frys K, Racchumi G, Zhou P, et al. (2004) Interaction between inducible nitric oxide synthase and poly(ADP-ribose) polymerase in focal ischemic brain injury. Stroke 35: 2896–2901.
23. Haddad M, Rhinn H, Bloquel C, Coqueran B, Szabó C, et al. (2006) Anti-inflammatory effects of PJ34, a poly(ADP-ribose) polymerase inhibitor, in transient focal cerebral ischemia in mice. Br J Pharmacol 149: 23–30.
24. Haddad M, Beray-Berthat V, Coqueran B, Palmier B, Szabo C, et al. (2008) Reduction of hemorrhagic transformation by PJ34, a poly(ADP-ribose)polymerase inhibitor, after permanent focal cerebral ischemia in mice. Eur J Pharmacol 588: 52–57.
25. Haddad M, Beray-Berthat V, Coqueran B, Plotkine M, Marchand-Leroux C, et al. (2013) Combined therapy with PJ34, a poly(ADP-ribose)polymerase inhibitor, reduces tissue plasminogen activator-induced hemorrhagic transformations in cerebral ischemia in mice. Fundam Clin Pharmacol 27: 393–401.
26. Lenzsér G, Kis B, Snipes JA, Gáspár T, Sándor P, et al. (2007) Contribution of poly(ADP-ribose) polymerase to postischemic blood-brain barrier damage in rats. J Cereb Blood Flow Metab 27: 1318–1326.
27. Kauppinen TM, Suh SW, Berman AE, Hamby AM, Swanson RA (2009) Inhibition of poly(ADP-ribose) polymerase suppresses inflammation and promotes recovery after ischemic injury. J Cereb Blood Flow Metab 29: 820–829.
28. Teng F, Beray-Berthat V, Coqueran B, Lesbats C, Kuntz M, et al. (2013) Prevention of rt-PA induced blood-brain barrier component degradation by the

poly(ADP-ribose)polymerase inhibitor PJ34 after ischemic stroke in mice. Exp Neurol 248: 416–428.
29. Takahashi K, Pieper AA, Croul SE, Zhang J, Snyder SH, et al. (1999) Post-treatment with an inhibitor of poly(ADP-ribose) polymerase attenuates cerebral damage in focal ischemia. Brain Res 829: 46–54.
30. Giovannelli L, Cozzi A, Guarnieri I, Dolara P, Moroni F (2002) Comet assay as a novel approach for studying DNA damage in focal cerebral ischemia: differential effects of NMDA receptor antagonists and poly(ADP-ribose) polymerase inhibitors. J Cereb Blood Flow Metab 22: 697–704.
31. Komjáti K, Mabley JG, Virág L, Southan GJ, Salzman AL, et al. (2004) Poly(ADP-ribose) polymerase inhibition protect neurons and the white matter and regulates the translocation of apoptosis-inducing factor in stroke. Int J Mol Med 13: 373–382.
32. Aleil B, Ravanat C, Cazenave JP, Rochoux G, Heitz A, et al. (2005) Flow cytometric analysis of intraplatelet VASP phosphorylation for the detection of clopidogrel resistance in patients with ischemic cardiovascular diseases. J Thromb Haemost 3: 85–92.
33. Xiang B, Zhang G, Ren H, Sunkara M, Morris AJ, et al. (2012) The P2Y(12) antagonists, 2MeSAMP and cangrelor, inhibit platelet activation through P2Y(12)/G(i)-dependent mechanism. PLoS One 7: e51037.
34. Broos K, Feys HB, De Meyer SF, Vanhoorelbeke K, Deckmyn H (2011) Platelets at work in primary hemostasis. Blood Rev 25: 155–167.
35. Varga-Szabo D, Braun A, Nieswandt B (2009) Calcium signaling in platelets. J Thromb Haemost 7: 1057–1066.
36. Dorsam RT, Kunapuli SP (2004) Central role of the $P2Y_{12}$ receptor in platelet activation. J Clin Invest 113: 340–345.
37. Gachet C (2008) P2 receptors, platelet function and pharmacological implications. Thromb Haemost 99: 466–472.
38. Iyú D, Glenn JR, White AE, Fox SC, Heptinstall S (2011) Adenosine derived from ADP can contribute to inhibition of platelet aggregation in the presence of a $P2Y_{12}$ antagonist. Arterioscler Thromb Vasc Biol 31: 416–422.
39. Szepes M, Janicsek Z, Benkő Z, Cselenyák A, Kiss L (2013) Pretreatment of therapeutic cells with poly(ADP-ribose) polymerase inhibitor enhances their efficacy in an in vitro model of cell-based therapy in myocardial infarct. Int J Mol Med 31: 26–32.
40. Mathews MT, Berk BC (2008) PARP-1 inhibition prevents oxidative and nitrosative stress-induced endothelial cell death via transactivation of the VEGF receptor 2. Arterioscler Thromb Vasc Biol 28: 711–717.
41. Madison DL, Stauffer D, Lundblad JR (2011) The PARP inhibitor PJ34 causes a PARP1-independent, p21 dependent mitotic arrest. DNA Repair (Amst) 10: 1003–1013.
42. Antolín AA, Jalencas X, Yélamos J, Mestres J (2012) Identification of pim kinases as novel targets for PJ34 with confounding effects in PARP biology. ACS Chem Biol 7: 1962–1967.
43. Nasrabady SE, Kuzhandaivel A, Akrami A, Bianchetti E, Milanese M, et al. (2012) Unusual increase in lumbar network excitability of the rat spinal cord evoked by the PARP-1 inhibitor PJ-34 through inhibition of glutamate uptake. Neuropharmacology 63: 415–426.

20

Clinical Practice Guidelines and Consensus Statements in Oncology – An Assessment of Their Methodological Quality

Carmel Jacobs[1]*, Ian D. Graham[2,3], Julie Makarski[4], Michaël Chassé[2], Dean Fergusson[2,3], Brian Hutton[2], Mark Clemons[1,3]

1 Division of Medical Oncology, The Ottawa Hospital Cancer Centre and Department of Medicine, University of Ottawa, Ottawa, Ontario, Canada, 2 Department of Epidemiology and Community Medicine, University of Ottawa, Ottawa, Ontario, Canada, 3 Ottawa Hospital Research Institute and University of Ottawa, Department of Medicine, Ottawa, Ontario, Canada, 4 Independent Consultant, Hamilton, Ontario, Canada

Abstract

Background: Consensus statements and clinical practice guidelines are widely available for enhancing the care of cancer patients. Despite subtle differences in their definition and purpose, these terms are often used interchangeably. We systematically assessed the methodological quality of consensus statements and clinical practice guidelines published in three commonly read, geographically diverse, cancer-specific journals. Methods Consensus statements and clinical practice guidelines published between January 2005 and September 2013 in Current Oncology, European Journal of Cancer and Journal of Clinical Oncology were evaluated. Each publication was assessed using the Appraisal of Guidelines for Research and Evaluation II (AGREE II) rigour of development and editorial independence domains. For assessment of transparency of document development, 7 additional items were taken from the Institute of Medicine's standards for practice guidelines and the Journal of Clinical Oncology guidelines for authors of guidance documents.

Methods: Consensus statements and clinical practice guidelines published between January 2005 and September 2013 in Current Oncology, European Journal of Cancer and Journal of Clinical Oncology were evaluated. Each publication was assessed using the Appraisal of Guidelines for Research and Evaluation II (AGREE II) rigour of development and editorial independence domains. For assessment of transparency of document development, 7 additional items were taken from the Institute of Medicine's standards for practice guidelines and the Journal of Clinical Oncology guidelines for authors of guidance documents.

Findings: Thirty-four consensus statements and 67 clinical practice guidelines were evaluated. The rigour of development score for consensus statements over the three journals was 32% lower than that of clinical practice guidelines. The editorial independence score was 15% lower for consensus statements than clinical practice guidelines. One journal scored consistently lower than the others over both domains. No journals adhered to all the items related to the transparency of document development. One journal's consensus statements endorsed a product made by the sponsoring pharmaceutical company in 64% of cases.

Conclusion: Guidance documents are an essential part of oncology care and should be subjected to a rigorous and validated development process. Consensus statements had lower methodological quality than clinical practice guidelines using AGREE II. At a minimum, journals should ensure that that all consensus statements and clinical practice guidelines adhere to AGREE II criteria. Journals should consider explicitly requiring guidelines to declare pharmaceutical company sponsorship and to identify the sponsor's product to enhance transparency.

Editor: Eugenio Paci, ISPO, Italy

Funding: IG received funding from the Canadian Institutes of Health Research (CHIR) number; FRN:IOP 123548 (http://www.cihr-irsc.gc.ca/e/193.html). The funders had no role in study design, data collection and analysis, decision to publish, or preparation of the manuscript.

Competing Interests: Ian Graham was a member of the team that developed the AGREE II instrument. He has also been an author on practice guidelines from Cancer Care Ontario (CCO). He was not an author on any of the guidelines analysed in this manuscript. Brian Hutton has previously received funds for providing methodological advice to Amgen Canada for systematic reviews. Mark Clemons has previously been involved in the creation of practice guidelines for Cancer Care Ontario (CCO) and consensus statements for Roche; he was not an author on any of the guidelines analysed. No other authors have competing interests t o declare.

* Email: cjacobs@toh.on.ca

Table 1. Items from AGREE II (Domains 3 and 6) and additional items collected to assess Transparency of Document Development.

Criteria collected	Source
Rigour of development	
Systematic methods were used to search for evidence.	
The criteria for selecting the evidence are clearly described	
The strengths and limitations of the body of evidence are clearly described.	
The methods for formulating the recommendations are clearly described.	Domain 3 of AGREE II [5]
The health benefits, side effects, and risks have been considered in formulating the recommendations.	
There is an explicit link between the recommendations and the supporting evidence.	
The guideline has been externally reviewed by experts prior to its publication.	
A procedure for updating the guideline is provided.	
Editorial independence	
The views of the funding body have not influenced the content of the guideline.	Domain 6 of AGREE II [5]
Competing interests of guideline development group members have been recorded and addressed.	
Additional items to assess transparency of document development	
Was a systematic review performed? (yes – systematic review performed and documented, no – systematic review not performed or not documented)	IOM [3] JCO [10]
How was the guideline group established? (invited, not disclosed, other),	IOM [3]
Was the group privately funded? (yes, no, not disclosed)	JCO [10].
Was the group multidisciplinary? (yes, no, not disclosed)	JCO [10].
Consensus sponsor	
For guidelines where a pharmaceutical product was evaluated was a specific product endorsed in the statement? (yes- name of product, no)	
Name and manufacturer of product endorsed	

IOM = Institute of medicine,
JCO = Journal of clinical oncology.

Introduction

Consensus statements and clinical practice guidelines are widely used in oncology to improve the quality of patient care [1,2]. While both consensus statements and clinical practice guidelines are intended to provide guidance to clinicians, there are important differences between them. A *clinical practice guideline* (also called a medical guideline or clinical protocol) produces statements that are informed by a systematic review of the evidence and an assessment of the benefits and harms of alternative options [3]. A *consensus statement* is developed by an independent panel of experts, usually multidisciplinary, convened to review the research literature in an evidence-based manner for the purpose of advancing the understanding of an issue, procedure or method

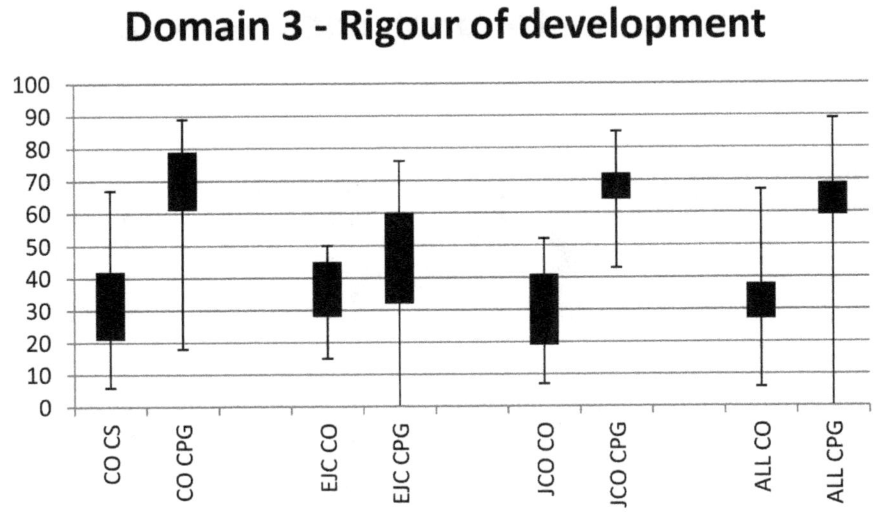

Figure 1. Range and 95% confidence intervals for Rigour of development scores. CO = Current Oncology. EJC = European Journal of Cancer. CS = Consensus statements. JCO = Journal of Clinical Oncology. CPG = Clinical practice guidelines.

Table 2. AGREE II: Rigour of development and Editorial Independence.

	CO	EJC	JCO	Overall	p-value, difference between means
AGREE II: Rigour of development (Domain 3)					
Consensus Statement (n = 34)					
Mean (95% Confidence Interval)	31 (21, 42)	36 (28, 45)	30 (19, 41)	32 (27, 38)	0.6400
Clinical Practice Guideline (n = 67)					
Mean (95% Confidence Interval)	70 (61, 79)	46 (32, 60)	68 (64, 72)	64 (59, 69)	0.0006
Mean difference Consensus Statement vs Clinical Practice Guideline					32 (24, 40)
Overall p-value Consensus Statement vs Clinical Practice Guideline					<0.0001
AGREE II: Editorial Independence (Domain 6)					
Consensus Statement (n = 34)					
Mean (95% Confidence Interval)	50 (38, 62)	44 (34, 54)	63 (56, 70)	53 (47, 59)	0.0305
Clinical Practice Guideline (n = 67)					
Mean (95% Confidence Interval)	75 (63, 86)	59 (52, 67)	66 (61, 70)	68 (63, 73)	0.0564
Mean difference Consensus Statement vs Clinical Practice Guideline					15 (7, 23)
Overall p-value Consensus Statement vs Clinical Practice Guideline					0.0003

[4]. Both documents provide recommendations for optimizing patient care [3].

Although consensus statements address topics in which the evidence base is less extensive compared to clinical practice guidelines, their development should still be methodologically rigorous and transparent [4]. To assist with maintaining methodological rigor, organizations such as Appraisal of Guidelines for Research and Evaluation (AGREE) [5], Institute of Medicine (IOM) [3] and Guidelines International Network (GIN) [6] have developed criteria to ensure objective, scientifically valid, and consistent standards for the development and reporting of high quality guidance documents.

Given their widespread availability and importance for both clinical practice and funding decisions [7], we sought to evaluate the methodological quality of both consensus statements and clinical practice guidelines published in three commonly accessed oncology-specific journals through the domains of rigor of development and editorial independence Information around the transparency of document development was also collected to assess whether or not pharmaceutical company sponsored guidelines were more likely to endorse a product manufactured by the sponsoring company.

Methods

Three oncology specific journals were searched for consensus statements and clinical practice guidelines published from January 2005–September 2013. Current Oncology (CO), the European Journal of Cancer (EJC) and the Journal of Clinical Oncology (JCO) were chosen as they have editorial offices in different

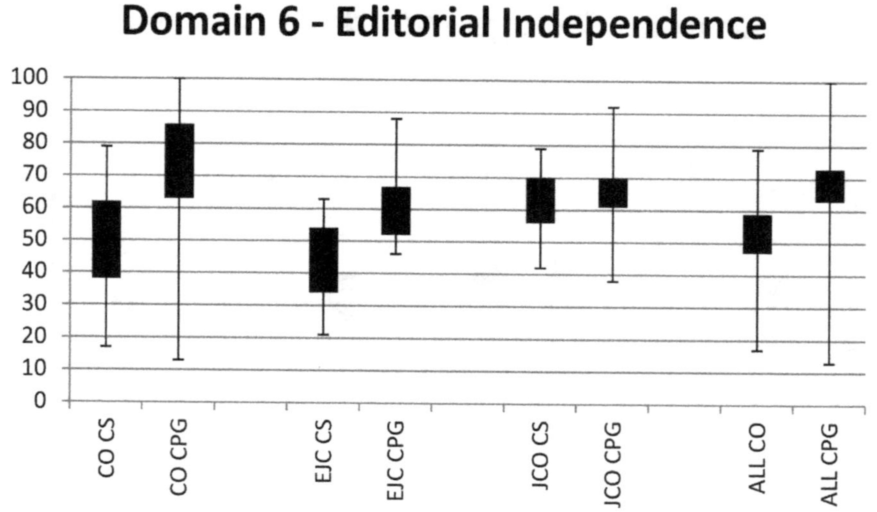

Figure 2. Range and 95% confidence intervals for Editorial independence scores. CO = Current Oncology. EJC = European Journal of Cancer. CS = Consensus statements. JCO = Journal of Clinical Oncology. CPG = Clinical practice guidelines.

Table 3. Additional items addressing Transparency of Document Development.

	CO n (%)	EJC n (%)	JCO n (%)	Overall n (%)	p-value
Systematic review performed					
Consensus Statement yes (n = 34)	3 (21)	3 (33)	0	6 (18)	0.1350
Clinical Practice Guideline yes (n = 67)	21 (88)	7 (54)	28 (93)	56 (84)	0.0082
Overall Consensus Statement vs Clinical Practice Guideline difference					<0.0001
How groups were established					
Consensus Statement (n = 34)					
Invited	6 (43)	5 (56)	1 (9)	12 (35)	0.1440
Not reported	6 (43)	4 (44)	7 (64)	17 (50)	
Other	2 (14)	0	3 (27)	5 (15)	
Clinical Practice Guideline (n = 67)					
Invited	4 (17)	5 (39)	5 (17)	14 (21)	0.0378
Not reported	7 (29)	7 (54)	9 (30)	23 (34)	
Other	13 (54)	1 (8)	16 (53)	30 (45)	
Overall Consensus Statement vs Clinical Practice Guideline difference					0.0106
Multidisciplinary					
Consensus Statement (n = 34)					
Yes	8 (57)	7 (78)	6 (55)	21 (62)	0.7182
No	1 (7)	0	0	1 (3)	
Not reported	5 (36)	2 (22)	5 (46)	12 (35)	
Clinical Practice Guideline (n = 67)					
Yes	19 (79)	8 (62)	23 (77)	50 (75)	0.4716
No	0	0	0	0	
Not reported	5 (21)	5 (39)	7 (23)	17 (25)	
Overall Consensus Statement vs Clinical Practice Guideline difference					0.1857
Privately funded meeting					
Consensus Statement (n = 34)					
Yes	9 (64)	2 (22)	0	11 (32)	<0.0001
No	1 (7)	0	0	1 (3)	
Not reported	4 (29)	7 (78)	11 (100)	22 (65)	
Clinical Practice Guideline (n = 67)					
Yes	1 (4)	5 (39)	0	6 (9)	<0.0001
No	15 (63)	0	16 (53)	31 (47)	
Not reported	8 (33)	8 (62)	14 (47)	30 (45)	
Overall Consensus Statement vs Clinical Practice Guideline difference					<0.0001
Consensus sponsors' product endorsed					
Consensus Statement (n = 34)					
Yes	9 (64)	1 (11)	0	10 (24.4)	<0.0001
Clinical Practice Guideline (n = 67)					
Yes	1 (4)	1 (8)	0	2 (3)	0.3012
Overall Consensus Statement vs Clinical Practice Guideline difference					<0.0001

countries and for their perceived prominence in North America and Europe. January 2005 was chosen as the starting date for eligibility, as this was the date by which all three journals had accessible electronic archives. Each journal's online search tool was used to search for the terms "consensus", "consensus guideline", "consensus statement", "clinical practice guideline", "practice guideline" or "medical guideline" in the title. Two reviewers (CJ, MC) reviewed each document retrieved to ensure they were consensus statements or practice guidelines, using the IOM criteria "statements that include recommendations intended to optimize patient care" [3].

As our primary focus related to evaluating the methodological quality, we opted to use Domain 3 of the AGREE II tool (Rigour of Development) and Domain 6 (Editorial Independence) to assess the documents. The rigour of development domain consists of 8 items, while the editorial independence domain consists of 2 items (items are shown in Table 1). AGREE II items are scored on a 7-point Likert scale ranging from 1 (strongly disagree) to 7 (strongly

Table 4. Current Oncology Consensus Statements and Clinical Practice Guidelines.

Current Oncology

Consensus Statements

Paper	Year published	Pharma sponsored	AGREE Domain 3 (%)	AGREE Domain 6 (%)	Sponsors product endorsed
Recommendations of the Canadian Consensus Group on the Management of Chronic Myeloid Leukemia [12]	2006	✓	50	50	✓
Updated recommendations from the Canadian National consensus meeting on HER2/neu testing in breast cancer [13]	2007	✓	7	17	✓
Colorectal Cancer Association of Canada Consensus Meeting on Practice Guidelines - Raising the Standard of Care in Canada for Early Stage Rectal Cancer [14]	2009	✓	22	64	✓
The role of the Epidermal Growth Factor Receptor Tyrosine Kinase Inhibitors as Therapy for Advanced, Metastatic and Recurrent Non-Small Cell Lung Cancer: A Canadian National Consensus Statement [15]	2009	✓	67	46	✓
Consensus recommendations for the use of anti-EGFR therapies in metastatic colorectal cancer [16]	2010		6	54	
Eastern Canadian Colorectal Cancer Consensus Conference: setting the limits of resectable disease [17]	2010	✓	32	21	✓
Consensus recommendations for the diagnosis and management of well-differentiated gastroenterohepatic neuroendocrine tumours: a revised statement from a Canadian national expert group [18]	2010	✓	23	79	✓
Diagnosis and management of hepatocellular carcinoma: results of a consensus meeting of The Ottawa Hospital Cancer Centre [19]	2010	✓	33	25	✓
Consensus Statements pre IOM 2011 (n = 8), Mean (95% Confidence Interval)	**30 (16, 44)**	**45 (29, 60)**			
Multidisciplinary Canadian consensus recommendations for the management and treatment of hepatocellular carcinoma [20]	2011	✓	56	75	✓
Canadian Expert Group consensus recommendations: KRAS testing in colorectal cancer [21]	2011		19	58	
Report from the 13th Annual Western Canadian Gastrointestinal Cancer Consensus Conference [22]	2012		43	46	
Consensus recommendations for cancer rehabilitation: research and education priorities [23]	2013		14	79	
Endocrine therapy for postmenopausal women with hormone receptor–positive her2–negative advanced breast cancer after progression or recurrence on nonsteroidal aromatase inhibitor therapy: a Canadian consensus statement [24]	2013	✓	40	63	✓
Eastern Canadian Colorectal Cancer Consensus Conference: standards of care for the treatment of patients with rectal, pancreatic, and gastrointestinal stromal tumours and pancreatic neuroendocrine tumours [25]	2013		29	33	
Consensus Statements post IOM 2011 (n = 6), Mean (95% Confidence Interval)			**34 (21, 46)**	**59 (45, 73)**	

Table 4. Cont.

Current Oncology					
Consensus Statements					
Paper	**Year published**	**Pharma sponsored**	**AGREE Domain 3 (%)**	**AGREE Domain 6 (%)**	**Sponsors product endorsed**
Clinical Practice Guidelines					
Bortezomib in Multiple Myeloma and Lymphoma: A systematic review and clinical practice guideline [26]	2006		82	88	
Guidelines for the diagnosis and management of carcinoid tumours, part 1: the gastrointestinal tract. A statement from a Canadian National Carcinoid Expert Group [27]	2006		20	13	
The role of oxaliplatin combined with 5-fluorouracil and folinic acid in the first- and second-line treatment of advanced colorectal cancer: a systematic review and clinical practice guideline [28]	2006		74	21	
Canadian Recommendations for the Treatment of Glioblastoma Multiforme [29]	2007	✓	19	17	✓
Melanoma Disease Site Group of Cancer Care Ontario's Program in Evidence-Based Care Mot. Temozolomide for the Treatment of Metastatic Melanoma: A Practice Guideline [30]	2007		80	92	
Ifosfamide-based combination chemotherapy in advanced soft tissue sarcoma: a systematic review and clinical practice guideline [31]	2007		61	96	
Management of Single Brain Metastases: A Practice Guideline [32]	2007		79	92	
Alemtuzumab in Chronic Lymphocytic Leukemia: A Systematic Review and Clinical Practice Guideline [33]	2007		81	100	
Single-Agent Interleukin-2 in the Treatment of Metastatic Melanoma: A Clinical Practice Guideline [34]	2007		78	100	
Biochemotherapy for the Treatment of Metastatic Malignant Melanoma: A Clinical Practice Guideline [35]	2008		43	75	
Dose-intensive Chemotherapy with Growth Factor or Autologous Bone Marrow/Stem Cell Transplant Support in First-line Treatment of Advanced or Metastatic Adult Soft Tissue Sarcoma – A Clinical Practice Guideline [36]	2008		89	100	
Epidermal growth factor receptor targeted therapy in stage III and IV head and neck cancer [37]	2010		85	79	
Follow-up for women after treatment for cervical cancer [38]	2010		78	79	
Clinical Practice Guidelines pre IOM 2011 (n = 13) Mean (95% Confidence Interval)			**67 (54, 80)**	**73 (55, 91)**	
Canadian College of Medical Geneticists guidelines for the indications, analysis, and reporting of cancer specimens [39]	2011		18	46	
Systemic therapy for advanced gastric cancer: a clinical practice guideline [40]	2011		84	83	

Table 4. Cont.

Paper	Year published	Pharma sponsored	AGREE Domain 3 (%)	AGREE Domain 6 (%)	Sponsors product endorsed
Current Oncology					
Consensus Statements					
Survivorship services for adult cancer populations: a pan-Canadian guideline [41]	2011		84	96	
Invasive mediastinal staging of non-small-cell lung cancer: a clinical practice guideline [42]	2011		75	83	
Management of a suspicious adnexal mass: a clinical practice guideline [43]	2012		80	63	
Lenalidomide in multiple myeloma – a practice guideline [44]	2013		75	83	
Chemotherapy (gemcitabine, docetaxel plus gemcitabine, doxorubicin, or trabectedin) in inoperable, locally advanced, recurrent, or metastatic uterine leiomyosarcoma: a clinical practice guideline [45]	2013		82	88	
Role of endolaryngeal surgery (with or without laser) compared with radiotherapy in the management of early (T1) glottic cancer: a clinical practice guideline [46]	2013		74	79	
Surgical margins and handling of soft-tissue sarcoma in extremities: a clinical practice guideline [47]	2013		77	100	
Liver resection for colorectal cancer metastases [48]	2013		80	83	
A pan-Canadian practice guideline and algorithm: screening, assessment, and supportive care of adults with cancer-related fatigue [49]	2013		75	38	
Clinical Practice Guidelines post IOM 2011 (n = 11) Mean (95% Confidence Interval)			**73 (62, 84)**	**77 (65, 88)**	

Table 5. European Journal of Cancer Consensus Statements and Clinical Practice Guidelines.

Paper	Year published	Pharma sponsored	AGREE Domain 3	AGREE Domain 6	Sponsors product endorsed
European Journal of Cancer					
Consensus Statements					
EORTC consensus recommendations for the treatment of mycosis fungoides/Sézary syndrome [50]	2006		43	50	
Towards a pan-European consensus on the treatment of patients with colorectal liver metastases. [51]	2006		41	38	
Consensus conference: Implementing treatment recommendations on yttrium-90 immunotherapy in clinical practice – Report of a European workshop [52]	2008	✓	27	42	✓
Diagnosis and treatment of melanoma: European consensus-based interdisciplinary guideline [53]	2010		39	38	
Breast cancer in pregnancy: Recommendations of an international consensus meeting. [54]	2010		49	21	
Consensus Statements pre IOM 2011 (n = 8), Mean (95% Confidence Interval)			**40 (33, 47)**	**38 (29, 47)**	
Consensus on Lung Cancer, new clinical recommendations and current status of biomarker assessment – First-line therapy. [55]	2011		15	38	
Highlights of the EORTC St. Gallen International Expert Consensus on the primary therapy of gastric, gastroesophageal and oesophageal cancer – Differential treatment strategies for subtypes of early gastroesophageal cancer. [56]	2012	✓	28	63	
Diagnosis and treatment of melanoma. European consensus-based interdisciplinary guideline – Update 2012 [57]	2012		35	63	
German, Austrian and Swiss consensus conference on the diagnosis and local treatment of the axilla in breast cancer [58]	2013		50	46	
Consensus Statements post IOM 2011 (n = 4), Mean (95% Confidence Interval)			**32 (18, 46)**	**53 (40, 65)**	
Clinical Practice Guidelines					
Guidelines for surgical treatment of hepatoblastoma in the modern era–recommendations from the Childhood Liver Tumour Strategy Group of the International Society of Paediatric Oncology (SIOPEL) [59]	2005		21	46	
Malignant ascites: systematic review and guideline for treatment. [60]	2006		63	46	
EORTC guidelines for the use of granulocyte-colony stimulating factor to reduce the incidence of chemotherapy-induced febrile neutropenia in adult patients with lymphomas and solid tumours. [61]	2006	✓	72	50	
EORTC guidelines for the use of erythropoietic proteins in anaemic patients with cancer: 2006 update [62]	2007	✓	60	88	
Tumour markers in colorectal cancer: European Group on Tumour Markers (EGTM) guidelines for clinical use [63]	2007		38	64	
Guidelines on the standards for the training of specialised health professionals dealing with breast cancer [64]	2007	✓	0	46	
Guidelines for the assessment of oral mucositis in adult chemotherapy, radiotherapy and haematopoietic stem cell transplant patients. European journal of cancer [65]	2008		69	58	
Diagnosis and antimicrobial therapy of lung infiltrates in febrile neutropenic patients: Guidelines of the infectious diseases working party of the German Society of Haematology and Oncology. [66]	2009		18	58	
The development of evidence-based guidelines on mouth care for children, teenagers and young adults treated for cancer [67]	2010		76	63	
2010 update of EORTC guidelines for the use of granulocyte-colony stimulating factor to reduce the incidence of chemotherapy-induced febrile neutropenia in adult patients with lymphoproliferative disorders and solid tumours [68]	2011	✓	63	50	✓
The development of evidence-based European guidelines on the management of depression in palliative cancer care [69]	2011		41	71	

Table 5. Cont.

European Journal of Cancer					
Consensus Statements					
Paper	**Year published**	**Pharma sponsored**	**AGREE Domain 3**	**AGREE Domain 6**	**Sponsors product endorsed**
Clinical Practice Guidelines pre IOM 2011 (n = 11) Mean (95% Confidence Interval)			**47 (32, 62)**	**58 (51, 66)**	
Paediatric intestinal cancer and polyposis due to bi-allelic PMS2 mutations: case series, review and follow-up guidelines. European journal of cancer [70]	2011		28	75	
EASL-EORTC clinical practice guidelines: management of hepatocellular carcinoma [71]	2012		49	58	
Clinical Practice Guidelines post IOM 2011 (n = 2) Mean (95% Confidence Interval)			**39 (18, 59)**	**67 (50, 83)**	

agree). Each domain score was calculated as per the AGREE II instructions included in the user's manual [5]. Domain score = [score obtained – minimum possible score]/[maximum possible score – minimum possible score × 100], giving a percentage score between 0 and 100. As the Standards and Guidelines Evidence (SAGE) directory has used AGREE II to evaluate English language cancer guidelines released since 2003 [8], if a document had been included in the SAGE database, this appraisal was used and a primary assessment of our own was not performed. The SAGE assessment utilises two trained evaluators to assess each document, discrepancies of a certain magnitude are resolved by a third and if required, fourth evaluator [9].

As we also wanted to assess issues surrounding the transparency of document development, and specific to whether or not pharmaceutical company sponsorship of the guideline development process was associated with product endorsement, each document was assess using an additional 7 items. These additional items were derived from the IOM standards for trustworthy clinical practice guidelines [3] and the JCO criteria for publishing consensus statements and clinical practice guidelines [10] (Table 1). These items included a statement on "Was a systematic review conducted?" Additional items related to transparency included, "How was the group established?", "Was the group multidisciplinary?", "Was the group privately funded?" and "What was the name of the funding body?" In order to assess any relationship between the sponsor of the group and recommendations, for pharmaceutical-related guidelines we also collected data on "Was a specific product endorsed in statement?", and if so, "Who was the manufacturer of product?".

Six reviewers appraised the documents, with each document appraised by two independent reviewers (see Acknowledgements). Discrepancy scores between reviewers for AGREE II were calculated using the concordance calculator for the SAGE database calculations [8]. We planned to resolve discrepancies in assessments as per SAGE, by third and if necessary fourth evaluators. For the additional items assessed, any discrepancies between the two reviewers were resolved by consensus.

Statistical analysis

For the two AGREE II domains of interests, we reported overall means with their 95% confidence intervals for each journal, stratified into separate categories of consensus statement and clinical practice guideline. We also stratified by year of document publication. We used the publication date of the IOM 'Clinical practice guidelines we can trust', March 2011 [3], as a time point in which to assess document quality over time. We compared overall differences between journals and between consensus statement or clinical practice guideline using analysis of variance (ANOVA). We also calculated the mean difference in scores between consensus statement and clinical practice guidelines with their corresponding 95% confidence intervals.

For the additional items collected addressing transparency of document development, we calculated the proportion of responses categorized as "Yes", "No", and "Not Reported". We assessed for differences in the journals' assessments using a chi-square test (or Fisher's Exact test when dealing with small cell counts in summary contingency tables) at a significance level of 5% while stratifying analyses into categories of consensus statement and clinical practice guideline. Finally, we compared overall items responses according to their consensus statement or clinical practice guideline category.

Agreement between reviewers was assessed by a concordance calculator, determining the number of standard deviations between reviewers, over each domain. A 'high' discrepancy score occurred when greater than 2 standard deviations were present between reviewers, 'medium' if >1.5 but <2 standard deviations and 'low' if <1.5 standard deviations.

Results

Identified Literature

The search identified a total of 104 documents for review. Three were excluded as one was a physician survey, one was a review of guidelines, and one was a letter to the editor. Therefore, 34 consensus statements and 67 practice guidelines were retained for assessment. The numbers and types of documents for each journal were; CO-14 consensus statements, 24 clinical practice guidelines, EJC -9 consensus statements, 13 clinical practice guidelines and JCO-11 consensus statements, 30 clinical practice guidelines.

AGREE II Rigour of development scores

When assessed across all three journals (Figure 1, Table 2), the mean scores for consensus statements were 32% (95% CI 27–38%) and for clinical practice guidelines 64% (95% CI 59–69%). The mean difference between guidelines was 32% ($p<0.0001$), indicating that clinical practice guidelines were scored significantly higher than consensus statements in terms of rigour of development. Analyses stratified by journal showed that rigour of development scores were significantly lower for consensus

Table 6. Journal of Clinical Oncology Consensus Statements and Clinical Practice Guidelines.

Paper	Year published	Pharma sponsored	AGREE Domain 3	AGREE Domain 6	Sponsors product endorsed
Journal of Clinical Oncology					
Consensus Statements					
Use of Positron Emission Tomography for Response Assessment of Lymphoma: Consensus of the Imaging Subcommittee of International Harmonization Project in Lymphoma. [72]	2007		49	63	
Definition, diagnosis, and management of intravascular large B-cell lymphoma: proposals and perspectives from an international consensus meeting. [73]	2007		9	67	
Consensus Report of the National Cancer Institute Clinical Trials Planning Meeting on Pancreas Cancer Treatment [74]	2009		7	67	
Venous Thromboembolism Prophylaxis and Treatment in Cancer: A Consensus Statement of Major Guidelines Panels and Call to Action [11]	2009		52	71	
Definition, Prognostic Factors, Treatment, and Response Criteria of Adult T-Cell Leukemia-Lymphoma: A Proposal From an International Consensus Meeting. [75]	2009		38	67	
International Myeloma Working Group Consensus Statement Regarding the Current Status of Allogeneic Stem-Cell Transplantation for Multiple Myeloma [76]	2010		23	46	
Renal Impairment in Patients With Multiple Myeloma: A Consensus Statement on Behalf of the International Myeloma Working Group [77]	2010		29	42	
Hepatocellular Carcinoma: Consensus Recommendations of the National Cancer Institute Clinical Trials Planning Meeting [78]	2010		35	67	
Future Directions in the Treatment of Neuroendocrine Tumors: Consensus Report of the National Cancer Institute Neuroendocrine Tumor Clinical Trials Planning Meeting. [79]	2011		30	67	
Consensus Statements pre IOM 2011 (n = 9), Mean (95% Confidence Interval)			**30 (20,40)**	**62 (55,69)**	
Clinical End Points and Response Criteria in Mycosis Fungoides and Sézary Syndrome: A Consensus Statement of the International Society for Cutaneous Lymphomas, the United States Cutaneous Lymphoma Consortium, and the Cutaneous Lymphoma Task Force of the European Organisation for Research and Treatment of Cancer. [80]	2011		8	63	
Platinum-Induced Ototoxicity in Children: A Consensus Review on Mechanisms, Predisposition, and Protection, Including a New International Society of Pediatric Oncology Boston Ototoxicity Scale. [81]	2012		45	79	
Consensus Statements post IOM 2011 (n = 29), Mean (95% Confidence Interval)			**27 (0,63)**	**71 (55,87)**	
Clinical Practice Guidelines					
American Society of Clinical Oncology Guideline Recommendations for Sentinel Lymph Node Biopsy in Early-Stage Breast Cancer. [82]	2005		75	73	
Colorectal Cancer Surveillance: 2005 Update of an American Society of Clinical Oncology Practice Guideline [83]	2005		65	79	
American Society of Clinical Oncology/College of American Pathologists Guideline Recommendations for Human Epidermal Growth Factor Receptor 2 Testing in Breast Cancer. [84]	2006		82	65	
2006 Update of Recommendations for the Use of White Blood Cell Growth Factors: An Evidence-Based Clinical Practice Guideline. [85]	2006		57	77	
American Society of Clinical Oncology Clinical Practice Guideline for the Use of Larynx-Preservation Strategies in the Treatment of Laryngeal Cancer. [86]	2006		65	54	
American Society of Clinical Oncology Guideline for Antiemetics in Oncology: Update 2006. [87]	2006		65	64	
American Society of Clinical Oncology Guideline: Recommendations for Venous Thromboembolism Prophylaxis and Treatment in Patients With Cancer. [88]	2007		81	63	

Table 6. Cont.

Journal of Clinical Oncology					
Consensus Statements					
Paper	**Year published**	**Pharma sponsored**	**AGREE Domain 3**	**AGREE Domain 6**	**Sponsors product endorsed**
Cancer Care Ontario and American Society of Clinical Oncology Adjuvant Chemotherapy and Adjuvant Radiation Therapy for Stages I-IIIA Resectable Non–Small-Cell Lung Cancer Guideline [89].	2007		79	88	
American Society of Clinical Oncology Endorsement of the Cancer Care Ontario Practice Guideline on Nonhormonal Therapy for Men With Metastatic Hormone-Refractory (castration-resistant) Prostate Cancer. [90]	2007		69	92	
American Society of Clinical Oncology 2007 Clinical Practice Guideline Update on the Role of Bisphosphonates in Multiple Myeloma. [91]	2007		60	75	
Initial Hormonal Management of Androgen-Sensitive Metastatic, Recurrent, or Progressive Prostate Cancer: 2007 Update of an American Society of Clinical Oncology Practice Guideline. [92]	2007		75	38	
American Society of Clinical Oncology 2008 Clinical Practice Guideline Update: Use of Chemotherapy and Radiation Therapy Protectants. [93]	2009		70	58	
Use of 5-alpha-reductase inhibitors for prostate cancer chemoprevention: American Society of Clinical Oncology/American Urological Association 2008 Clinical Practice Guideline. [94]	2009		76	71	
American Society of Clinical Oncology Clinical Practice Guideline Update on Chemotherapy for Stage IV Non–Small-Cell Lung Cancer [95].	2009		71	71	
American Society of Clinical Oncology Clinical Practice Guideline Update on the Use of Pharmacologic Interventions Including Tamoxifen, Raloxifene, and Aromatase Inhibition for Breast Cancer Risk Reduction [96].	2009		74	63	
American Society of Clinical Oncology/American Society of Hematology Clinical Practice Guideline Update on the Use of Epoetin and Darbepoetin in Adult Patients With Cancer [97].	2010		57	54	
American Society of Clinical Oncology Clinical Practice Guideline: Update on Adjuvant Endocrine Therapy for Women With Hormone Receptor–Positive Breast Cancer [98].	2010		54	54	
American Society of Clinical Oncology Clinical Practice Guideline on Uses of Serum Tumor Markers in Adult Males With Germ Cell Tumors [99].	2010		58	63	
American Society of Clinical Oncology/College of American Pathologists Guideline Recommendations for Immunohistochemical Testing of Estrogen and Progesterone Receptors in Breast Cancer [100].	2010		65	47	
Clinical Practice Guidelines pre IOM 2011 (n = 19) Mean (95% Confidence Interval)			**69 (64,72)**	**66 (60,72)**	
Antiemetics: American Society of Clinical Oncology Clinical Practice Guideline Update [101].	2011		72	67	
American Society of Clinical Oncology Endorsement of the Cancer Care Ontario Practice Guideline on Adjuvant Ovarian Ablation in the Treatment of Premenopausal Women With Early-Stage Invasive Breast Cancer [102].	2011		85	79	
2011 Focused Update of 2009 American Society of Clinica Oncology Clinical Practice Guideline Update on Chemotherapy for Stage IV Non–Small-Cell Lung Cancer [103].	2011		43	58	
American Society of Clinical Oncology Clinical Practice Guideline Update on the Use of Chemotherapy Sensitivity and Resistance Assays [104].	2011		54	58	
Sentinel Lymph Node Biopsy for Melanoma: American Society of Clinical Oncology and Society of Surgical Oncology Joint Clinical Practice Guideline [105].	2012		63	75	

Table 6. Cont.

Paper	Year published	Pharma sponsored	AGREE Domain 3	AGREE Domain 6	Sponsors product endorsed
Journal of Clinical Oncology					
Consensus Statements					
Appropriate Chemotherapy Dosing for Obese Adult Patients With Cancer: American Society of Clinical Oncology Clinical Practice Guideline [106].	2012		67	54	
Use of Pharmacologic Interventions for Breast Cancer Risk Reduction: American Society of Clinical Oncology Clinical Practice Guideline [107].	2013		82	63	
Fertility Preservation for Patients With Cancer: American Society of Clinical Oncology Clinical Practice Guideline Update [108].	2013		65	71	
Central Venous Catheter Care for the Patient With Cancer: American Society of Clinical Oncology Clinical Practice Guideline [109].	2013		80	58	
Breast Cancer Follow-Up and Management After Primary Treatment: American Society of Clinical Oncology Clinical Practice Guideline Update [110].	2013		48	71	
Antimicrobial Prophylaxis and Outpatient Management of Fever and Neutropenia in Adults Treated for Malignancy: American Society of Clinical Oncology Clinical Practice Guideline [111].	2013		81	71	
Clinical Practice Guidelines post IOM 2011 (n = 11) Mean (95% Confidence Interval)			**67 (59, 76)**	**66 (61, 71)**	

statements than clinical practice guidelines for manuscripts published in CO (31% [95% CI 21–40%] consensus statements, 70% [95% CI 61–79%] clinical practice guidelines) and JCO (30% [95% CI 19–41%] consensus statements, 68% [95% CI 64–72%] clinical practice guidelines). There was no significant difference between manuscripts published in EJC (36% [95% CI 28–45%] consensus statements, 46% [95% CI 32–60%] clinical practice guidelines). When comparing each journal with the others, all three had similar scores for consensus statements; however EJC clinical practice guidelines scored lower than Current Oncology (EJC 46% [95% CI 32–60%], CO 70% [95% CI 61–79%]) and JCO (68% [95% CI 64–72%]). Discrepancy levels between the reviewers were low with the exception of one consensus statement published in the Journal of Clinical Oncology [11] which had a high discrepancy score.

AGREE II Editorial independence scores

When assessed across all three journals (Figure 2, Table 2), the mean score for consensus statements was 53% (95% CI 47–59%) and for clinical practice guidelines was 68% (95% CI 63–73%). The mean difference between consensus statement and clinical practice guideline scores was 15% ($p = 0.0003$), indicating that clinical practice guidelines were scored significantly higher than consensus statements with respect to editorial independence. Editorial independence scores were significantly lower for consensus statements than clinical practice guidelines in documents published in CO (50% [95% CI 38–62%] consensus statements, 75% [95% CI 63–86%] clinical practice guidelines). This difference seen to a lesser extent in EJC (44% [95% CI 34–54%] consensus statements, 59% [95% CI 52–67%] clinical practice guidelines) and no difference was seen in JCO (63% [95% CI 56–70%] consensus statements, 66% [95% CI 61–70%] clinical practice guidelines). EJC (44% [95% CI 35–54%]) scored lower than JCO (63% [95% CI 56–70%]) on consensus statements, but similarly to CO. No journal appeared to perform better or worse than the other journals with regard to clinical practice guidelines. Discrepancy levels between the reviewers were low for all documents.

Additional transparency of document development item scores

Consensus statements infrequently referenced or conducted a systematic review on the topic of the guideline (6/34 = 18%), a step which was much more common with clinical practice guidelines (56/67 = 83%) ($p = 0.018$) (Table 3). The largest discrepancy was seen in JCO where 0/11 (0%) of consensus statements documented a systematic review compared to 28/30 (93%) of clinical practice guidelines. Neither consensus statements (50%) nor clinical practice guidelines (34%) consistently declared how their development group was established. Consensus statements were more likely than clinical practice guidelines to state that participants were "invited" (12/34 = 35% vs 14/67 = 21%; $p = 0.01$). Guideline groups were multidisciplinary in 21 out of 34 (62%) consensus statements and 50 out of 67 (75%) clinical practice guidelines groups. Group member roles were not declared in 35% (12/34) of the consensus statements nor in 25% (17/67) of clinical practice guidelines ($p = 0.19$).

While consensus statements were more likely to declare private funding (11/34 = 32%) than clinical practice guidelines (6/67 = 9%) ($p<0.0001$), many documents did not declare their source of funding (22/34 = 65% of consensus statements versus 31/67 = 46% of clinical practice guidelines). If a source of funding was declared, the funding body was recorded (Table 3).

With respect to whether or not a document endorsed a product made by the sponsoring company (Table 3), this occurred less frequently in clinical practice guidelines (2/67 = 3%) than in consensus statements (10/34 = 29%) ($p<0.0001$). In CO, consensus statements endorsed the product of the sponsoring company in

9/14 (64%) of cases. All of these documents declared financial support from the sponsoring company, but none explicitly declared the link between the sponsoring company and the product endorsed. Four percent of clinical practice guidelines published in CO endorsed the sponsor's product. This trend was seen to a lesser extent in EJC with 11% of consensus statements endorsing sponsors products and 8% of clinical practice guidelines. No document published by JCO documented a relationship between pharmaceutical company funding and product endorsement in the guideline.

Have consensus statements and clinical practice guidelines improved over time?

When assessed chronologically, there is no association with document quality over time, using the date of publication of the IOM 'Clinical practice guidelines we can trust', March 2011 as a reference point (Tables 4,5 and 6). There may be a trend of declining pharmaceutical sponsorship of documents in recent years.

Discussion

As the terms consensus statement and clinical practice guidelines are often used interchangeably and both are used to improve clinical care, their methodological rigour and transparency of development is essential. Here we report the results of a review of the methodological quality of consensus statements and clinical practice guidelines in a limited sample of the oncology literature. While others have published on quality assessment of clinical guidelines in oncology using either the AGREE or AGREE II tool [112–117], to our knowledge this is the first such comprehensive review of both consensus statement and practice guidelines in oncology.

As literature assessing the quality of consensus statements is limited [118], we used tools developed for clinical practice guidelines and collected additional information that would help assess the transparency of guideline development. AGREE II is a validated appraisal tool for assessing the methodological development quality and reporting of practice guidelines; it does not assess the actual content of clinical recommendations [5]. AGREE II assesses how well a guideline performs on each of the 6 domains (scope and purpose, stakeholder involvement, rigour of development, clarity of presentation, applicability and editorial independence). We felt the rigour of development (an assessment of the evidentiary base and methods used to formulate recommendations) and editorial independence (an assessment of bias and competing interests influencing recommendation formulation [5]) were the most appropriate for our evaluation.

For both the rigour of development and editorial independence domains, consensus statements scored consistently less well than did practice guidelines. In the only publication we found evaluating practice guidelines in comparison to consensus statements, although not specific to oncology [118], similar differences were seen, with consensus statements scoring significantly lower than clinical practice guidelines across 4 of the 6 AGREE II domains (stakeholder involvement, rigour of development, clarity, and presentation and applicability). We could show no improvement in document quality over time.

Performing a systematic review is an essential element of guideline development [119]. Both IOM [120] and JCO [10] state that "clinical practice guideline developers should use systematic reviews" and that "guidelines/recommendations should be driven by a high level of evidence" respectively. We felt it was necessary to specifically ask 'was a systematic review performed?' We asked this question even though AGREE II domain 3.1 assess if 'systematic methods were used to search for evidence' (scored on a continuum of whether a guideline reports what databases were searched, the search terms used, the search time periods and the inclusion of a full search strategy). In the current study systematic reviews were performed more frequently by clinical practice guidelines than consensus statements across all three journals. With respect to the processes by which a clinical practice guideline group was established and the role of individual members, this was inconsistently reported. There were however significant differences between these items in consensus statements and clinical practice guidelines.

Of particular interest was the role of the funding body for the development of the guidance document. While no information can be gleaned for whether this association is real or implied, several observations can be made. Overall, consensus statements and clinical practice guidelines published in the three journals studied either did not declare or were not explicit about the funding source for the document (funding source not declared in 65% consensus statements, 45% clinical practice guidelines). For documents with topics related to pharmaceutical products, when the document was sponsored by a pharmaceutical company, documents endorsed the sponsor's product in both consensus statements (29%) and to a lesser degree in clinical practice guidelines (3%). However, in the CO journal, 64% of consensus statements published endorsed the sponsors product, whereas only 4% of clinical practice guidelines endorsed the sponsors product. Further, this association was not reported in the conflict of interest statement. This absence of reporting contravenes standards published by medical societies [121,122] and could question the integrity and quality of published guidance documents [123,124].

We acknowledge a number of study limitations. Although we feel that consensus statements should be subjected to the same rigorous criteria for their development as practice guidelines, the AGREE II tool has not been validated for evaluation of consensus statements [5,118]. The additional items we included for assessment from the IOM guideline standards and JCO authorship guidance on consensus statements and clinical practice guidelines also have not been validated. Consensus statements and clinical practice guidelines analyzed here may not be representative of all oncology consensus statements and clinical practice guidelines released between January 2005 and September 2013, nor representative of all oncology journals. A brief PubMed search suggests over 900 oncology guidance documents were published in peer-reviewed journals over the same time period, translating to a sample of 11% of these documents. Finally, we chose only three journals from which to sample. Our rational for selecting them was that they commonly publish both consensus statements and clinical practice guidelines, are prominent journals in their locale of origin and are geographically diverse. We appreciate that these journals may not be representative of all oncology journals.

Conclusions

While consensus statements and clinical practice guidelines are developed with slightly different approaches and methods, both are used to inform clinical and policy decisions. As such both documents should be developed using equally rigorous and transparent methods and subjected to high quality standards. Here we have shown that consensus statements score lower than clinical practice guidelines for scores of rigour of development and editorial independence. Consensus statements are also less likely to include a systematic review of the literature and were more likely to be sponsored by a pharmaceutical company and to endorse a specific pharmaceutical product. Unfortunately transparency of document development was generally poor in both types of documents and there was infrequent documentation of sources of funding, how guideline groups were established and who comprised their guideline development groups.

Given the important role of guidance we feel that both consensus statements and clinical practice guidelines should be subject to the same rigorous and high quality development criteria. We suggest that journals encourage authors of guidance documents to use the AGREE II and IOM criteria when developing their documents and require journal reviewers to use these same criteria when undertaking their peer-review of these documents. While there are quality differences between each of the journals sampled in our study, this was most pronounced around the issues of private funding and product endorsement. Readers of guidance documents published within these journals should be made aware of the presence of private funding and sponsorship should be made transparent through their reporting so that readers can acknowledge such conflicts and potential bias.

Acknowledgments

We would like to acknowledge Chika Agbassi, Fulvia Baldassarre, Judy Brown, Nadia Coakley, Karen Spithoff, and Caroline Zwaal for their assistance in data collection.

Author Contributions

Conceived and designed the experiments: CJ IG DF M. Clemons BH. Performed the experiments: CJ JM M. Chasse M. Clemons. Analyzed the data: CJ IG JM M. Chasse BH M. Clemons. Contributed reagents/ materials/analysis tools: CJ JM M. Chasse M. Clemons. Contributed to the writing of the manuscript: CJ IG JM M. Chasse DF BH M. Clemons.

References

1. Woolf SH, Grol R, Hutchinson A, Eccles M, Grimshaw J (1999) Potential benefits, limitations, and harms of clinical guidelines. BMJ 318: 527–530.
2. Grimshaw JM, Russell IT (1993) Effect of clinical guidelines on medical practice: a systematic review of rigorous evaluations. Lancet 342: 1317–1322.
3. Graham RMM, Miller Wolman D, Greenfield S, Steinberg E, Editors, Committee on Standards for Developing Trustworthy Clinical Practice Guidelines Clinical Practice Guidelines We Can Trust.: Institute of Medicine.
4. (2009) Mosby's Medical Dictionary. 8th Edition ed: Elsevier.
5. Brouwers MC, Kho ME, Browman GP, Burgers JS, Cluzeau F, et al. (2010) AGREE II: advancing guideline development, reporting and evaluation in health care. Cmaj 182: E839–842.
6. Guidelines International Network. Available: http://www.g-i-n.net/. Accessed 26 May 2014.
7. Canadian partnership against cancer and pCODR. (2013) How cancer drug funding decisions are made Available: http://www.pcodr.ca/idc/groups/ pcodr/documents/pcodrdocument/pcodr-funding-tutorial.pdf. Accessed 28 April 2014.
8. Brouwers (2010) Standards and Guidelines Evidence (SAGE) Directory of Cancer Guidelines. Available: http://www.cancerview.ca/cv/portal/Home/ TreatmentAndSupport/TSProfessionals/ClinicalGuidelines/GRCMain/ GRCSAGE?_afrLoop=176960541903000&lang=en&_afrWindowMode=0&_ adf.ctrl-state=n8sm6f4dx_85. Accessed 28 September 2013.
9. Brouwers MC, Rawski E, Spithoff K, Oliver TK (2011) Inventory of Cancer Guidelines: a tool to advance the guideline enterprise and improve the uptake of evidence. Expert Rev Pharmacoecon Outcomes Res 11: 151–161.
10. Oncology JoC Information for Contributors.
11. Khorana AA, Streiff MB, Farge D, Mandala M, Debourdeau P, et al. (2009) Venous Thromboembolism Prophylaxis and Treatment in Cancer: A Consensus Statement of Major Guidelines Panels and Call to Action. Journal of Clinical Oncology 27: 4919–4926.
12. Laneuville P, Barnett MJ, Belanger R, Couban S, Forrest DL, et al. (2006) Recommendations of the canadian consensus group on the management of chronic myeloid leukemia. Curr Oncol 13: 201–221.
13. Hanna W, O'Malley F P, Barnes P, Berendt R, Gaboury L, et al. (2007) Updated recommendations from the Canadian National Consensus Meeting on HER2/neu testing in breast cancer. Curr Oncol 14: 149–153.
14. Colorectal Cancer Association of Canada consensus meeting: raising the standards of care for early-stage rectal cancer (2009) Curr Oncol 16: 50–56.
15. Ellis PM, Morzycki W, Melosky B, Butts C, Hirsh V, et al. (2009) The role of the epidermal growth factor receptor tyrosine kinase inhibitors as therapy for advanced, metastatic, and recurrent non-small-cell lung cancer: a Canadian national consensus statement. Curr Oncol 16: 27–48.
16. Cripps C, Gill S, Ahmed S, Colwell B, Dowden S, et al. (2010) Consensus recommendations for the use of anti-egfr therapies in metastatic colorectal cancer. Curr Oncol 17: 39–45.
17. Vickers M, Samson B, Colwell B, Cripps C, Jalink D, et al. (2010) Eastern Canadian Colorectal Cancer Consensus Conference: setting the limits of resectable disease. Curr Oncol 17: 70–77.
18. Kocha W, Maroun J, Kennecke H, Law C, Metrakos P, et al. (2010) Consensus recommendations for the diagnosis and management of well-differentiated gastroenterohepatic neuroendocrine tumours: a revised statement from a Canadian National Expert Group. Curr Oncol 17: 49–64.
19. Asmis T, Balaa F, Scully L, Papadatos D, Marginean C, et al. (2010) Diagnosis and management of hepatocellular carcinoma: results of a consensus meeting of The Ottawa Hospital Cancer Centre. Curr Oncol 17: 6–12.
20. Sherman M, Burak K, Maroun J, Metrakos P, Knox JJ, et al. (2011) Multidisciplinary Canadian consensus recommendations for the management and treatment of hepatocellular carcinoma. Curr Oncol 18: 228–240.
21. Aubin F, Gill S, Burkes R, Colwell B, Kamel-Reid S, et al. (2011) Canadian Expert Group consensus recommendations: KRAS testing in colorectal cancer. Curr Oncol 18: e180–184.
22. Vickers MM, Pasieka J, Dixon E, McEwan S, McKay A, et al. (2012) Report from the 13th annual Western canadian gastrointestinal cancer consensus conference; calgary, alberta; september 8–10, 2011. Curr Oncol 19: e468–477.
23. McEwen S, Egan M, Chasen M, Fitch M (2013) Consensus recommendations for cancer rehabilitation: research and education priorities. Curr Oncol 20: 64–69.
24. Pritchard KI, Gelmon KA, Rayson D, Provencher L, Webster M, et al. (2013) Endocrine therapy for postmenopausal women with hormone receptor-positive her2-negative advanced breast cancer after progression or recurrence on nonsteroidal aromatase inhibitor therapy: a Canadian consensus statement. Curr Oncol 20: 48–61.
25. Di Valentin T, Biagi J, Bourque S, Butt R, Champion P, et al. (2013) Eastern Canadian Colorectal Cancer Consensus Conference: standards of care for the treatment of patients with rectal, pancreatic, and gastrointestinal stromal tumours and pancreatic neuroendocrine tumours. Curr Oncol 20: e455–464.
26. Reece D, Imrie K, Stevens A, Smith CA (2006) Bortezomib in multiple myeloma and lymphoma: a systematic review and clinical practice guideline. Curr Oncol 13: 160–172.
27. Maroun J, Kocha W, Kvols L, Bjarnason G, Chen E, et al. (2006) Guidelines for the diagnosis and management of carcinoid tumours. Part 1: the gastrointestinal tract. A statement from a Canadian National Carcinoid Expert Group. Curr Oncol 13: 67–76.
28. Jonker D, Rumble RB, Maroun J (2006) Role of oxaliplatin combined with 5-fluorouracil and folinic acid in the first- and second-line treatment of advanced colorectal cancer. Curr Oncol 13: 173–184.
29. Mason WP, Maestro RD, Eisenstat D, Forsyth P, Fulton D, et al. (2007) Canadian recommendations for the treatment of glioblastoma multiforme. Curr Oncol 14: 110–117.
30. Quirt I, Verma S, Petrella T, Bak K, Charette M, et al. (2007) Temozolomide for the Treatment of Metastatic Melanoma: A Practice Guideline. Current Oncology, {S1}14.
31. Verma S, Younus J, Stys-Norman D, Haynes AE, Blackstein M (2007) Ifosfamide-based combination chemotherapy in advanced soft-tissue sarcoma: a practice guideline. Curr Oncol 14: 144–148.
32. Mintz A, Perry J, Spithoff K, Chambers A, Laperriere N (2007) Management of single brain metastasis: a practice guideline. Curr Oncol 14: 131–143.
33. Fraser G SC, Imrie K, Meyer R (2007) Alemtuzumab in Chronic Lymphocytic Leukemia: A Systematic Review and Clinical Practice Guideline. Current Oncology, {S1}14.
34. Petrella T, Quirt I, Verma S, Haynes AE, Charette M, et al. (2007) Single-Agent Interleukin-2 in the Treatment of Metastatic Melanoma: A Clinical Practice Guideline. Curr Oncol 14: 21–26.
35. Verma S, Petrella T, Hamm C, Bak K, Charette M (2008) Biochemotherapy for the treatment of metastatic malignant melanoma: a clinical practice guideline. Curr Oncol 15: 85–89.
36. Verma S, Younus J, Haynes AE, Stys-Norman D, Blackstein M (2008) Dose-intensive chemotherapy with growth factor or autologous bone marrow or stem-cell transplant support in first-line treatment of advanced or metastatic adult soft tissue sarcoma: a clinical practice guideline. Curr Oncol 15: 80–84.
37. Cripps C, Winquist E, Devries MC, Stys-Norman D, Gilbert R (2010) Epidermal growth factor receptor targeted therapy in stages III and IV head and neck cancer. Curr Oncol 17: 37–48.
38. Elit L, Fyles AW, Oliver TK, Devries-Aboud MC, Fung-Kee-Fung M (2010) Follow-up for women after treatment for cervical cancer. Curr Oncol 17: 65–69.

39. Dawson AJ, McGowan-Jordan J, Chernos J, Xu J, Lavoie J, et al. (2011) Canadian College of Medical Geneticists guidelines for the indications, analysis, and reporting of cancer specimens. Curr Oncol 18: e250–255.
40. Mackenzie M, Spithoff K, Jonker D (2011) Systemic therapy for advanced gastric cancer: a clinical practice guideline. Curr Oncol 18: e202–209.
41. Howell D, Hack TF, Oliver TK, Chulak T, Mayo S, et al. (2011) Survivorship services for adult cancer populations: a pan-Canadian guideline. Curr Oncol 18: e265–281.
42. Darling GE, Dickie AJ, Malthaner RA, Kennedy EB, Tey R (2011) Invasive mediastinal staging of non-small-cell lung cancer: a clinical practice guideline. Curr Oncol 18: e304–310.
43. Dodge JE, Covens AL, Lacchetti C, Elit LM, Le T, et al. (2012) Management of a suspicious adnexal mass: a clinical practice guideline. Curr Oncol 19: e244–257.
44. Chen C, Baldassarre F, Kanjeekal S, Herst J, Hicks L, et al. (2013) Lenalidomide in multiple myeloma-a practice guideline. Curr Oncol 20: e136–149.
45. Gupta AA, Yao X, Verma S, Mackay H, Hopkins L (2013) Chemotherapy (gemcitabine, docetaxel plus gemcitabine, doxorubicin, or trabectedin) in inoperable, locally advanced, recurrent, or metastatic uterine leiomyosarcoma: a clinical practice guideline. Curr Oncol 20: e448–454.
46. Yoo J, Lacchetti C, Hammond JA, Gilbert RW (2013) Role of endolaryngeal surgery (with or without laser) compared with radiotherapy in the management of early (T1) glottic cancer: a clinical practice guideline. Curr Oncol 20: e132–135.
47. Kandel R, Coakley N, Werier J, Engel J, Ghert M, et al. (2013) Surgical margins and handling of soft-tissue sarcoma in extremities: a clinical practice guideline. Curr Oncol 20: e247–254.
48. Gallinger S, Biagi JJ, Fletcher GG, Nhan C, Ruo L, et al. (2013) Liver resection for colorectal cancer metastases. Curr Oncol 20: e255–265.
49. Howell D, Keller-Olaman S, Oliver TK, Hack TF, Broadfield L, et al. (2013) A pan-Canadian practice guideline and algorithm: screening, assessment, and supportive care of adults with cancer-related fatigue. Curr Oncol 20: e233–246.
50. Trautinger F, Knobler R, Willemze R, Peris K, Stadler R, et al. (2006) EORTC consensus recommendations for the treatment of mycosis fungoides/Sézary syndrome. European journal of cancer (Oxford, England: 1990) 42: 1014–1030.
51. Van Cutsem E, Nordlinger B, Adam R, Köhne C-H, Pozzo C, et al. (2006) Towards a pan-European consensus on the treatment of patients with colorectal liver metastases. European journal of cancer (Oxford, England: 1990) 42: 2212–2221.
52. Zinzani PL, d'Amore F, Bombardieri E, Brammer C, Codina JG, et al. (2008) Consensus conference: Implementing treatment recommendations on yttrium-90 immunotherapy in clinical practice – Report of a European workshop. European journal of cancer (Oxford, England: 1990) 44: 366–373.
53. Garbe C, Peris K, Hauschild A, Saiag P, Middleton M, et al. (2010) Diagnosis and treatment of melanoma: European consensus-based interdisciplinary guideline. European journal of cancer (Oxford, England: 1990) 46: 270–283.
54. Amant F, Deckers S, Van Calsteren K, Loibl S, Halaska M, et al. (2010) Breast cancer in pregnancy: Recommendations of an international consensus meeting. European journal of cancer (Oxford, England: 1990) 46: 3158–3168.
55. Gridelli C, Rossi A, Maione P (2011) 2010 Consensus on Lung Cancer, new clinical recommendations and current status of biomarker assessment – First-line therapy. European journal of cancer (Oxford, England : 1990) 47: S248-S257.
56. Lutz MP, Zalcberg JR, Ducreux M, Ajani JA, Allum W, et al. (2012) Highlights of the EORTC St. Gallen International Expert Consensus on the primary therapy of gastric, gastroesophageal and oesophageal cancer – Differential treatment strategies for subtypes of early gastroesophageal cancer. European journal of cancer (Oxford, England: 1990) 48: 2941–2953.
57. Garbe C, Peris K, Hauschild A, Saiag P, Middleton M, et al. (2012) Diagnosis and treatment of melanoma. European consensus-based interdisciplinary guideline – Update 2012. European journal of cancer (Oxford, England: 1990) 48: 2375–2390.
58. German Austrian and Swiss consensus conference on the diagnosis and local treatment of the axilla in breast cancer (2103) European journal of cancer (Oxford, England: 1990) 49: 2277–2283.
59. Czauderna P, Otte JB, Aronson DC, Gauthier F, Mackinlay G, et al. (2005) Guidelines for surgical treatment of hepatoblastoma in the modern era– recommendations from the Childhood Liver Tumour Strategy Group of the International Society of Paediatric Oncology (SIOPEL). Eur J Cancer 41: 1031–1036.
60. Becker G, Galandi D, Blum HE (2006) Malignant ascites: systematic review and guideline for treatment. Eur J Cancer 42: 589–597.
61. Aapro MS, Cameron DA, Pettengell R, Bohlius J, Crawford J, et al. (2006) EORTC guidelines for the use of granulocyte-colony stimulating factor to reduce the incidence of chemotherapy-induced febrile neutropenia in adult patients with lymphomas and solid tumours. Eur J Cancer 42: 2433–2453.
62. Bokemeyer C, Aapro MS, Courdi A, Foubert J, Link H, et al. (2007) EORTC guidelines for the use of erythropoietic proteins in anaemic patients with cancer: 2006 update. Eur J Cancer 43: 258–270.
63. Duffy MJ, van Dalen A, Haglund C, Hansson L, Holinski-Feder E, et al. (2007) Tumour markers in colorectal cancer: European Group on Tumour Markers (EGTM) guidelines for clinical use. Eur J Cancer 43: 1348–1360.
64. Cataliotti L, De Wolf C, Holland R, Marotti L, Perry N, et al. (2007) Guidelines on the standards for the training of specialised health professionals dealing with breast cancer. Eur J Cancer 43: 660–675.
65. Quinn B, Potting CM, Stone R, Blijlevens NM, Fliedner M, et al. (2008) Guidelines for the assessment of oral mucositis in adult chemotherapy, radiotherapy and haematopoietic stem cell transplant patients. Eur J Cancer 44: 61–72.
66. Maschmeyer G, Beinert T, Buchheidt D, Cornely OA, Einsele H, et al. (2009) Diagnosis and antimicrobial therapy of lung infiltrates in febrile neutropenic patients: Guidelines of the infectious diseases working party of the German Society of Haematology and Oncology. Eur J Cancer 45: 2462–2472.
67. Glenny AM, Gibson F, Auld E, Coulson S, Clarkson JE, et al. The development of evidence-based guidelines on mouth care for children, teenagers and young adults treated for cancer. European Journal of Cancer 46: 1399–1412.
68. Aapro MS, Bohlius J, Cameron DA, Dal Lago L, Donnelly JP, et al. (2011) 2010 update of EORTC guidelines for the use of granulocyte-colony stimulating factor to reduce the incidence of chemotherapy-induced febrile neutropenia in adult patients with lymphoproliferative disorders and solid tumours. Eur J Cancer 47: 8–32.
69. Rayner L, Price A, Hotopf M, Higginson IJ (2011) The development of evidence-based European guidelines on the management of depression in palliative cancer care. Eur J Cancer 47: 702–712.
70. Herkert JC, Niessen RC, Olderode-Berends MJ, Veenstra-Knol HE, Vos YJ, et al. (2011) Paediatric intestinal cancer and polyposis due to bi-allelic PMS2 mutations: case series, review and follow-up guidelines. Eur J Cancer 47: 965–982.
71. (2012) EASL-EORTC clinical practice guidelines: management of hepatocellular carcinoma. Eur J Cancer 48: 599–641.
72. Juweid ME, Stroobants S, Hoekstra OS, Mottaghy FM, Dietlein M, et al. (2007) Use of Positron Emission Tomography for Response Assessment of Lymphoma: Consensus of the Imaging Subcommittee of International Harmonization Project in Lymphoma. Journal of Clinical Oncology 25: 571–578.
73. Ponzoni M, Ferreri AJM, Campo E, Facchetti F, Mazzucchelli L, et al. (2007) Definition, Diagnosis, and Management of Intravascular Large B-Cell Lymphoma: Proposals and Perspectives From an International Consensus Meeting. Journal of Clinical Oncology 25: 3168–3173.
74. Philip PA, Mooney M, Jaffe D, Eckhardt G, Moore M, et al. (2009) Consensus Report of the National Cancer Institute Clinical Trials Planning Meeting on Pancreas Cancer Treatment. Journal of Clinical Oncology 27: 5660–5669.
75. Tsukasaki K, Hermine O, Bazarbachi A, Ratner L, Ramos JC, et al. (2009) Definition, Prognostic Factors, Treatment, and Response Criteria of Adult T-Cell Leukemia-Lymphoma: A Proposal From an International Consensus Meeting. Journal of Clinical Oncology 27: 453–459.
76. Lokhorst H, Einsele H, Vesole D, Bruno B, Miguel JS, et al. (2010) International Myeloma Working Group Consensus Statement Regarding the Current Status of Allogeneic Stem-Cell Transplantation for Multiple Myeloma. Journal of Clinical Oncology 28: 4521–4530.
77. Dimopoulos MA, Terpos E, Chanan-Khan A, Leung N, Ludwig H, et al. (2010) Renal Impairment in Patients With Multiple Myeloma: A Consensus Statement on Behalf of the International Myeloma Working Group. Journal of Clinical Oncology 28: 4976–4984.
78. Thomas MB, Jaffe D, Choti MM, Belghiti J, Curley S, et al. (2010) Hepatocellular Carcinoma: Consensus Recommendations of the National Cancer Institute Clinical Trials Planning Meeting. Journal of Clinical Oncology 28: 3994–4005.
79. Kulke MH, Siu LL, Tepper JE, Fisher G, Jaffe D, et al. (2011) Future Directions in the Treatment of Neuroendocrine Tumors: Consensus Report of the National Cancer Institute Neuroendocrine Tumor Clinical Trials Planning Meeting. Journal of Clinical Oncology 29: 934–943.
80. Olsen EA, Whittaker S, Kim YH, Duvic M, Prince HM, et al. (2011) Clinical End Points and Response Criteria in Mycosis Fungoides and Sézary Syndrome: A Consensus Statement of the International Society for Cutaneous Lymphomas, the United States Cutaneous Lymphoma Consortium, and the Cutaneous Lymphoma Task Force of the European Organisation for Research and Treatment of Cancer. Journal of Clinical Oncology 29: 2598–2607.
81. Brock PR, Knight KR, Freyer DR, Campbell KCM, Steyger PS, et al. (2012) Platinum-Induced Ototoxicity in Children: A Consensus Review on Mechanisms, Predisposition, and Protection, Including a New International Society of Pediatric Oncology Boston Ototoxicity Scale. Journal of Clinical Oncology 30: 2408–2417.
82. Lyman GH, Giuliano AE, Somerfield MR, Benson AB, 3rd, Bodurka DC, et al. (2005) American Society of Clinical Oncology guideline recommendations for sentinel lymph node biopsy in early-stage breast cancer. J Clin Oncol 23: 7703–7720.
83. Desch CE, Benson AB, Somerfield MR, Flynn PJ, Krause C, et al. (2005) Colorectal Cancer Surveillance: 2005 Update of an American Society of Clinical Oncology Practice Guideline. Journal of Clinical Oncology 23: 8512–8519.
84. Wolff AC, Hammond MEH, Schwartz JN, Hagerty KL, Allred DC, et al. (2006) American Society of Clinical Oncology/College of American Pathologists Guideline Recommendations for Human Epidermal Growth Factor

Receptor 2 Testing in Breast Cancer. Journal of Clinical Oncology 25: 118–145.

85. Smith TJ, Khatcheressian J, Lyman GH, Ozer H, Armitage JO, et al. (2006) 2006 Update of Recommendations for the Use of White Blood Cell Growth Factors: An Evidence-Based Clinical Practice Guideline. Journal of Clinical Oncology 24: 3187–3205.
86. Pfister DG, Laurie SA, Weinstein GS, Mendenhall WM, Adelstein DJ, et al. (2006) American Society of Clinical Oncology Clinical Practice Guideline for the Use of Larynx-Preservation Strategies in the Treatment of Laryngeal Cancer. Journal of Clinical Oncology 24: 3693–3704.
87. Kris MG, Hesketh PJ, Somerfield MR, Feyer P, Clark-Snow R, et al. (2006) American Society of Clinical Oncology Guideline for Antiemetics in Oncology: Update 2006. Journal of Clinical Oncology 24: 2932–2947.
88. Lyman GH, Khorana AA, Falanga A, Clarke-Pearson D, Flowers C, et al. (2007) American Society of Clinical Oncology Guideline: Recommendations for Venous Thromboembolism Prophylaxis and Treatment in Patients With Cancer. Journal of Clinical Oncology 25: 5490–5505.
89. Pisters KMW, Evans WK, Azzoli CG, Kris MG, Smith CA, et al. (2007) Cancer Care Ontario and American Society of Clinical Oncology Adjuvant Chemotherapy and Adjuvant Radiation Therapy for Stages I-IIIA Resectable Non–Small-Cell Lung Cancer Guideline. Journal of Clinical Oncology 25: 5506–5518.
90. Basch EM, Somerfield MR, Beer TM, Carducci MA, Higano CS, et al. (2007) American Society of Clinical Oncology Endorsement of the Cancer Care Ontario Practice Guideline on Nonhormonal Therapy for Men With Metastatic Hormone-Refractory (castration-resistant) Prostate Cancer. Journal of Clinical Oncology 25: 5313–5318.
91. Kyle RA, Yee GC, Somerfield MR, Flynn PJ, Halabi S, et al. (2007) American Society of Clinical Oncology 2007 Clinical Practice Guideline Update on the Role of Bisphosphonates in Multiple Myeloma. Journal of Clinical Oncology 25: 2464–2472.
92. Loblaw DA, Virgo KS, Nam R, Somerfield MR, Ben-Josef E, et al. (2007) Initial Hormonal Management of Androgen-Sensitive Metastatic, Recurrent, or Progressive Prostate Cancer: 2007 Update of an American Society of Clinical Oncology Practice Guideline. Journal of Clinical Oncology 25: 1596–1605.
93. Hensley ML, Hagerty KL, Kewalramani T, Green DM, Meropol NJ, et al. (2009) American Society of Clinical Oncology 2008 Clinical Practice Guideline Update: Use of Chemotherapy and Radiation Therapy Protectants. Journal of Clinical Oncology 27: 127–145.
94. Kramer BS, Hagerty KL, Justman S, Somerfield MR, Albertsen PC, et al. (2009) Use of 5-alpha-reductase inhibitors for prostate cancer chemoprevention: American Society of Clinical Oncology/American Urological Association 2008 Clinical Practice Guideline. J Clin Oncol 27: 1502–1516.
95. Azzoli CG, Baker S, Temin S, Pao W, Aliff T, et al. (2009) American Society of Clinical Oncology Clinical Practice Guideline Update on Chemotherapy for Stage IV Non–Small-Cell Lung Cancer. Journal of Clinical Oncology 27: 6251–6266.
96. Visvanathan K, Chlebowski RT, Hurley P, Col NF, Ropka M, et al. (2009) American Society of Clinical Oncology Clinical Practice Guideline Update on the Use of Pharmacologic Interventions Including Tamoxifen, Raloxifene, and Aromatase Inhibition for Breast Cancer Risk Reduction. Journal of Clinical Oncology 27: 3235–3258.
97. Rizzo JD, Brouwers M, Hurley P, Seidenfeld J, Arcasoy MO, et al. (2010) American Society of Clinical Oncology/American Society of Hematology Clinical Practice Guideline Update on the Use of Epoetin and Darbepoetin in Adult Patients With Cancer. Journal of Clinical Oncology 28: 4996–5010.
98. Burstein HJ, Prestrud AA, Seidenfeld J, Anderson H, Buchholz TA, et al. (2010) American Society of Clinical Oncology Clinical Practice Guideline: Update on Adjuvant Endocrine Therapy for Women With Hormone Receptor–Positive Breast Cancer. Journal of Clinical Oncology 28: 3784–3796.
99. Gilligan TD, Seidenfeld J, Basch EM, Einhorn LH, Fancher T, et al. (2010) American Society of Clinical Oncology Clinical Practice Guideline on Uses of Serum Tumor Markers in Adult Males With Germ Cell Tumors. Journal of Clinical Oncology 28: 3388–3404.
100. Hammond MEH, Hayes DF, Dowsett M, Allred DC, Hagerty KL, et al. (2010) American Society of Clinical Oncology/College of American Pathologists Guideline Recommendations for Immunohistochemical Testing of Estrogen and Progesterone Receptors in Breast Cancer. Journal of Clinical Oncology 28: 2784–2795.
101. Basch E, Prestrud AA, Hesketh PJ, Kris MG, Feyer PC, et al. (2011) Antiemetics: American Society of Clinical Oncology Clinical Practice Guideline Update. Journal of Clinical Oncology 29: 4189–4198.
102. Griggs JJ, Somerfield MR, Anderson H, Henry NL, Hudis CA, et al. (2011) American Society of Clinical Oncology Endorsement of the Cancer Care Ontario Practice Guideline on Adjuvant Ovarian Ablation in the Treatment of Premenopausal Women With Early-Stage Invasive Breast Cancer. Journal of Clinical Oncology 29: 3939–3942.
103. Azzoli CG, Temin S, Aliff T, Baker S, Brahmer J, et al. (2011) 2011 Focused Update of 2009 American Society of Clinical Oncology Clinical Practice Guideline Update on Chemotherapy for Stage IV Non–Small-Cell Lung Cancer. Journal of Clinical Oncology 29: 3825–3831.
104. Burstein HJ, Mangu PB, Somerfield MR, Schrag D, Samson D, et al. (2011) American Society of Clinical Oncology Clinical Practice Guideline Update on the Use of Chemotherapy Sensitivity and Resistance Assays. Journal of Clinical Oncology 29: 3328–3330.
105. Wong SL, Balch CM, Hurley P, Agarwala SS, Akhurst TJ, et al. (2012) Sentinel Lymph Node Biopsy for Melanoma: American Society of Clinical Oncology and Society of Surgical Oncology Joint Clinical Practice Guideline. Journal of Clinical Oncology 30: 2912–2918.
106. Griggs JJ, Mangu PB, Anderson H, Balaban EP, Dignam JJ, et al. (2012) Appropriate Chemotherapy Dosing for Obese Adult Patients With Cancer: American Society of Clinical Oncology Clinical Practice Guideline. Journal of Clinical Oncology 30: 1553–1561.
107. Visvanathan K, Hurley P, Bantug E, Brown P, Col NF, et al. (2013) Use of Pharmacologic Interventions for Breast Cancer Risk Reduction: American Society of Clinical Oncology Clinical Practice Guideline. Journal of Clinical Oncology 31: 2942–2962.
108. Loren AW, Mangu PB, Beck LN, Brennan L, Magdalinski AJ, et al. (2013) Fertility Preservation for Patients With Cancer: American Society of Clinical Oncology Clinical Practice Guideline Update. Journal of Clinical Oncology 31: 2500–2510.
109. Schiffer CA, Mangu PB, Wade JC, Camp-Sorrell D, Cope DG, et al. (2013) Central venous catheter care for the patient with cancer: American Society of Clinical Oncology clinical practice guideline. J Clin Oncol 31: 1357–1370.
110. Khatcheressian JL, Hurley P, Bantug E, Esserman LJ, Grunfeld E, et al. (2013) Breast Cancer Follow-Up and Management After Primary Treatment: American Society of Clinical Oncology Clinical Practice Guideline Update. Journal of Clinical Oncology 31: 961–965.
111. Flowers CR, Seidenfeld J, Bow EJ, Karten C, Gleason C, et al. (2013) Antimicrobial Prophylaxis and Outpatient Management of Fever and Neutropenia in Adults Treated for Malignancy: American Society of Clinical Oncology Clinical Practice Guideline. Journal of Clinical Oncology 31: 794–810.
112. Fervers B, Burgers JS, Haugh MC, Brouwers M, Browman G, et al. (2005) Predictors of high quality clinical practice guidelines: examples in oncology. Int J Qual Health Care 17: 123–132.
113. Burgers JS, Fervers B, Haugh M, Brouwers M, Browman G, et al. (2004) International assessment of the quality of clinical practice guidelines in oncology using the Appraisal of Guidelines and Research and Evaluation Instrument. J Clin Oncol 22: 2000–2007.
114. de Haas ER, de Vijlder HC, van Reesema WS, van Everdingen JJ, Neumann HA (2007) Quality of clinical practice guidelines in dermatological oncology. J Eur Acad Dermatol Venereol 21: 1193–1198.
115. Shimbo T, Fukui T, Ishioka C, Okamoto K, Okamoto T, et al. (2010) Quality of guideline development assessed by the Evaluation Committee of the Japan Society of Clinical Oncology. Int J Clin Oncol 15: 227–233.
116. Langton JM, Drew AK, Mellish L, Olivier J, Ward RL, et al. (2011) The quality of web-based oncology guidelines and protocols: how do international sites stack up? Br J Cancer 105: 1166–1172.
117. Hogeveen SE, Han D, Trudeau-Tavara S, Buck J, Brezden-Masley CB, et al. (2012) Comparison of international breast cancer guidelines: are we globally consistent? cancer guideline AGREEment. Curr Oncol 19: e184–190.
118. Lopez-Olivo MA, Kallen MA, Ortiz Z, Skidmore B, Suarez-Almazor ME (2008) Quality appraisal of clinical practice guidelines and consensus statements on the use of biologic agents in rheumatoid arthritis: a systematic review. Arthritis Rheum 59: 1625–1638.
119. Collaboration TC (2014) Understanding Searching Techniques to Inform HTA, Systematic Reviews and Guideline Development.
120. Graham R, Mancher M, Wolman DM, Greenfield S, Steinberg E (2011) Clinical Practice Guidelines We Can Trust. The National Academies Press.
121. Mendelson TB, Meltzer M, Campbell EG, Caplan AL, Kirkpatrick JN (2011) COnflicts of interest in cardiovascular clinical practice guidelines. Archives of Internal Medicine 171: 577–584.
122. American Society of Clinical Oncology (2013) Conflict of Interest Policy Implementation for Clinical Practice Guidelines of American Society of Clinical Oncology. http://www.asco.org/sites/www.asco.org/files/conflict_of_interest_policy_implementation_for_clinical_practice_guidelines_8.8.2013_0.pdf [Accessed 28 May 2014].
123. Norris SL, Holmer HK, Ogden LA, Burda BU (2011) Conflict of interest in clinical practice guideline development: a systematic review. PLoS One 6: e25153.
124. Cosgrove L, Bursztajn HJ, Erlich DR, Wheeler EE, Shaughnessy AF (2013) Conflicts of interest and the quality of recommendations in clinical guidelines. Journal of Evaluation in Clinical Practice 19: 674–681.

Comparison of Long-Term Survival and Toxicity of Cisplatin Delivered Weekly versus Every Three Weeks Concurrently with Intensity-Modulated Radiotherapy in Nasopharyngeal Carcinoma

Chang-Juan Tao[1,2¶], Li Lin[1¶], Guan-Qun Zhou[1], Ling-Long Tang[1], Lei Chen[1], Yan-Ping Mao[1], Mu-Sheng Zeng[3], Tie-Bang Kang[3], Wei-Hua Jia[3], Jian-Yong Shao[4], Hai-Qiang Mai[5], Ai-Hua Lin[6], Jun Ma[1], Ying Sun[1]*

1 Department of Radiation Oncology, Sun Yat-sen University Cancer Center, State Key Laboratory of Oncology in South China, Collaborative Innovation Center for Cancer Medicine, Guangzhou, Guangdong Province, People's Republic of China, **2** Department of Radiation Oncology, Zhejiang Cancer Hospital, Hangzhou, Zhejiang Province, People's Republic of China, **3** Department of Experimental Research, Sun Yat-sen University Cancer Center, State Key Laboratory of Oncology in South China, Collaborative Innovation Center for Cancer Medicine, Guangzhou, Guangdong Province, People's Republic of China, **4** Department of Pathology, Sun Yat-sen University Cancer Center, State Key Laboratory of Oncology in South China, Collaborative Innovation Center for Cancer Medicine, Guangzhou, Guangdong Province, People's Republic of China, **5** Department of Nasopharyngeal Carcinoma, Sun Yat-sen University Cancer Center, State Key Laboratory of Oncology in South China, Collaborative Innovation Center for Cancer Medicine, Guangzhou, Guangdong Province, People's Republic of China, **6** Department of Medical Statistics and Epidemiology, School of Public Health, Sun Yat-sen University, Guangzhou, Guangdong Province, People's Republic of China

Abstract

Background: We aimed to compare the long-term survival outcomes and acute toxicity of cisplatin administered weekly versus every three weeks concurrently with intensity-modulated radiotherapy (IMRT) in patients with nasopharyngeal carcinoma (NPC).

Methods: This was a retrospective review of 154 patients with histologically proven, non-disseminated NPC who were treated using IMRT between January 2003 and December 2007. Seventy-three patients (47.4%) received 5–7 weeks of 30–40 mg/m^2 cisplatin weekly; 81 patients (52.6%) received two or three cycles of 80 mg/m^2 cisplatin every three weeks. IMRT was delivered at 68 Gy/30 fractions to the nasopharyngeal gross target volume and 60–66 Gy to the involved neck area.

Results: The clinical characteristics and treatment factors of the two groups were well-balanced. The median follow-up was 74 months (range, 6–123 months), and the 5-year overall survival, disease-free survival, locoregional relapse-free survival, and distant metastasis-free survival rates were 85.2% vs. 78.9% ($P=0.318$), 71.6% vs. 71.0% ($P=0.847$), 93.5% vs. 92.6% ($P=0.904$), and 80.9% vs. 80.1% ($P=0.925$) for the group treated every three weeks and weekly, respectively. Subgroup analyses indicated no significant differences in the survival rates of the two groups among patients with early- or advanced-stage disease. The incidence of acute toxicities was similar between groups.

Conclusion: IMRT with concurrent cisplatin administered weekly or every three weeks leads to similar long-term survival outcomes and acute toxicity in NPC regardless of whether patients have early- or advanced-stage disease.

Editor: Apar Kishor Ganti, University of Nebraska Medical Center, United States of America

Funding: This work was supported by grants from the National Natural Science Foundation of China (No. 8172409), the Sun Yat-Sen University Clinical Research 5010 Program (No. 2012011), the Natural Science Foundation of Guangdong Province (No. S2013010012220), the Science and Technology project of Guangzhou City, China (No. 132000507), the Health & Medical Collaborative Innovation Project of Guangzhou City, China (201400000001), and the National Science & Technology Pillar Program during the Twelfth Five-year Plan Period (2014BAI09B10). The funders had no role in study design, data collection and analysis, decision to publish, or preparation of the manuscript.

Competing Interests: The authors have declared that no competing interests exist.

* Email: sunying@sysucc.org.cn

¶ These authors contributed equally to this work.

Introduction

Nasopharyngeal carcinoma (NPC) is highly prevalent in southern China; incidence rates range between 15 and 50 per 100,000 individuals [1]. Due to the anatomical location and radiosensitivity of NPC, radiation therapy (RT) is the mainstay treatment. According to the 7th Edition of the American Joint Commission on Cancer (AJCC) staging system [2], 60–70% of patients present with stage III–IVB disease at diagnosis [3]. Several randomized clinical trials and meta-analyses have consistently demonstrated that concurrent chemoradiotherapy

(CCRT) confers survival benefit in locoregionally advanced NPC [4–11].

The National Comprehensive Cancer Network recommends that CCRT with cisplatin (CDDP) be delivered at an intermediate dose weekly or at a high dose at 3-week intervals for stage II–IVB NPC. The Intergroup 0099 trial (INT-0099) [3] and NPC-9901 trial [5] compared concurrent CDDP (100 mg/m^2) every three weeks with RT alone; compliance to the intensive regimen was poor, and CCRT was associated with a high incidence of acute toxicity. Two other phase III clinical trials [6–7] evaluated the efficiency of CCRT with weekly CDDP (40 mg/m^2) during RT; CCRT conferred survival benefit and weekly CDDP was well-tolerated. Therefore, it is of great importance to identify the optimal administration schedule for CDDP during CCRT in patients with NPC.

To the best of our knowledge, only one study [12] has compared the dose delivery and survival outcomes of weekly CDDP versus CDDP every three weeks delivered concurrently with RT in locally advanced NPC. However, in that study, the clinical characteristics and treatment factors were unevenly distributed, and the majority of patients were treated with 3-dimensional conformal RT. Radiation technology has evolved rapidly in recent years, especially with the introduction of intensity-modulated radiotherapy (IMRT). In NPC, this treatment modality has excellent local control and less late toxicities [13]. With the widespread application of IMRT, reevaluating the survival outcomes and toxicity of concurrent weekly CDDP versus CDDP every three weeks in patients with NPC undergoing CCRT would be worthwhile.

Therefore, we aimed to compare the long-term survival outcomes and acute toxicities of weekly CDDP versus CDDP every three weeks delivered concurrently with IMRT in patients with NPC. Our results will help guide clinical CCRT treatment strategies in NPC.

Materials and Methods

Patient characteristics

Between January 2003 and December 2007, we reviewed the records of 749 patients with newly diagnosed, untreated, non-disseminated NPC who were treated using IMRT at our center. We excluded 595 patients (79.4%): 214 (28.6%) who were treated with RT only, 274 (36.6%) who received neoadjuvant chemotherapy, 86 (11.5%) who received concurrent chemotherapy using a combination of CDDP and 5-fluorouracil, and 21 (2.8%) who received concurrent chemotherapy with taxol. We included the remaining 154 patients in our retrospective study; 115 were male and 39 were female (male:female ratio, 2.95:1) and the median age was 44.0 years (range, 13–73 years). One hundred and fifty patients (97.4%) had a pathological diagnosis of World Health Organization (WHO) type II or III NPC, only one patient (0.6%) had WHO type I NPC, and three patients (1.9%) had basaloid squamous cell carcinoma. The ethics committee of Sun Yat-sen University Cancer Center approved this study. Written consent was waived because this was a retrospective study; verbal consent was obtained from the patients via telephone and documented in the informed consent form if the patient agreed to participate in this study, as was consent on behalf of the children enrolled. The Institutional Review Board approved the use of verbal consent.

All patients underwent pre-treatment evaluation, which included complete patient history, physical and neurological examination, hematological and biochemical profiles, magnetic resonance imaging (MRI) scan of the neck and nasopharynx, chest radiography, abdominal sonography, and single-photon emission computed tomography whole-body bone scans. Positron emission tomography/computed tomography (CT) was performed on 41 patients (26.6%). All patients were restaged according to the 7th edition of the AJCC staging system. The stage distribution was as follows: stage II, 40/154 (26%); stage III, 66/154 (42.8%); stage IVA, 38/154 (24.7%); stage IVB, 10/154 (6.5%). Table 1 lists the characteristics of the patient cohort.

Radiotherapy

All patients were immobilized in the supine position with a head, neck, and shoulder thermoplastic mask. We obtained two sets of images, i.e., with and without contrast, from the CT simulator for treatment planning purposes. CT was performed after administering intravenous contrast medium, and we obtained 3-mm slices from the head to 2 cm below the sternoclavicular joint. The primary tumor and upper neck above the caudal edge of the cricoid cartilage were treated by IMRT. The target volumes were delineated using a previously described institutional treatment protocol [14] in accordance with the International Commission on Radiation Units and Measurements reports 50 and 62. The clinical target volumes (CTVs) were individually delineated based on the tumor invasion pattern [15]. The contoured images were transferred to a Corvus version 3.0 inverse IMRT planning system (Peacock; Nomos Corp., Deer Park, IL, USA). The prescribed radiation dose (as per the protocol) was total dose of 68 Gy in 30 fractions at 2.27 Gy/fraction to the planning target volume (PTV) of the primary gross tumor volume (GTV), 60–64 Gy to the nodal GTV PTV, 60 Gy to the CTV-1 PTV (i.e., high-risk regions), and 54 Gy to the CTV-2 PTV (i.e., low-risk regions) and CTV-N (i.e., neck nodal regions). Treatment was delivered by a dynamic, multileaf intensity-modulating collimator (MIMiC; Nomos Corp., Sewickley, PA, USA). A conventional anterior or anteroposterior opposing cervical technique was used for the lower neck. All patients were treated with one fraction daily over five days per week. All targets were treated simultaneously using the simultaneous integrated boost technique.

Concurrent chemotherapy

All patients were treated with CCRT; eight patients (5.2%) also received adjuvant chemotherapy using CDDP and 5-fluorouracil for two or three cycles. CCRT was initiated on the first day of RT and the choice of every three weeks or weekly CDDP was based on oncologists' opinions. Seventy-three patients (47.4%) received 30–40 mg/m^2 CDDP weekly for 5–7 planned weeks, and 81 patients (52.6%) received two or three cycles of 80 mg/m^2 CDDP every three weeks. In both groups, 5-hydroxytryptamine 3 antagonists and dexamethasone were administered as antiemetic prophylaxis.

Follow-up

The duration of follow-up was calculated from the first day of treatment to either the day of death or day of the last follow-up. Patients were examined at least every three months during the first two years, and every six months thereafter until death. At every follow-up, we assessed disease status with complete physical examination, nasopharyngoscopy, hematological and biochemical profiles, chest radiography, abdominal ultrasonography, and CT/MRI scans of the nasopharynx and cervical region. Acute toxicities were scored according to the Common Terminology Criteria for Adverse Events v3.0 (CTCAE v3.0).

Statistical analysis

We used Statistical Package for the Social Sciences version 16.0 (SPSS, Chicago, IL, USA) for statistical analysis. We compared

Table 1. Clinical characteristics of patients.

Characteristic	Weekly cisplatin (n = 73)	Cisplatin every three weeks (n = 81)	P*
Age (years)			.351
≤50	52	63	
>50	21	18	
≤18	0	3	.247
>18	73	78	
Sex			.581
Male	56	59	
Female	17	22	
Histology			.116
WHO I	1	0	
WHO II	7	3	
WHO III	65	75	
BSCC	0	3	
T classification†			.651
T1	7	13	
T2	17	17	
T3	31	30	
T4	18	21	
N classification†			.538
N0	14	13	
N1	42	55	
N2	12	8	
N3	5	5	
Staging†			.939
II	18	22	
III	33	33	
IVA	17	21	
IVB	5	5	
OTT (days)			.554
Median	43	44	
SD	4.3	4.0	
Response rate			.258
CR	60	61	
PR	11	19	

WHO: World Health Organization; BSCC: basaloid squamous cell carcinoma; CR: complete response; PR: partial response; SD: standard deviation; OTT: overall treatment time.

*P-values were calculated using the chi-square test (or Fisher's exact test) and Mann–Whitney U test.

†According to the 7th AJCC/International Union against Cancer staging system.

and analyzed the clinical characteristics and toxicity rates of the two treatment groups using the chi-square test (or Fisher's exact test, if indicated). Overall treatment time and cumulative CDDP dose were compared using the Mann–Whitney U test. All events were measured from the start of treatment. The following end points (time to the first defined event) were assessed: overall survival (OS), disease-free survival (DFS), locoregional relapse–free survival (LRRFS), distant metastasis–free survival (DMFS). Actuarial rates were calculated using the Kaplan–Meier method [16]. Multivariate analyses using the Cox proportional hazards model

Table 2. Acute toxicity according to CTCAE v3.0.

Toxicity	Weekly cisplatin (n = 73)					Every three week cisplatin (n = 81)					P*
	Grade0	Grade1	Grade2	Grade3	Grade4	Grade0	Grade1	Grade2	Grade3	Grade4	
Hematological											
Leucopenia	30	17	20	5	1	23	28	25	5	0	0.312
Anemia	58	9	4	2	0	61	17	3	0	0	0.233
Thrombocytopenia	62	4	2	3	2	74	2	2	2	1	0.583
Non-hematological											
Dermatitis	0	59	13	1	0	0	54	24	3	0	0.121
Mucositis	0	29	21	23	0	0	23	34	23	1	0.139
Dysphagia	29	33	8	3	0	31	32	13	5	0	0.715
Nausea/Vomiting	32	24	17	0	0	36	27	15	3	0	0.295
Xerostomia	15	27	31	0	0	11	31	39	0	0	0.498
Ototoxicity	52	19	2	0	0	57	23	1	0	0	0.767
Neurotoxicity	70	2	1	0	0	77	3	1	0	0	0.632

*P-values were calculated with the chi-square test (or Fisher's exact test, if indicated).

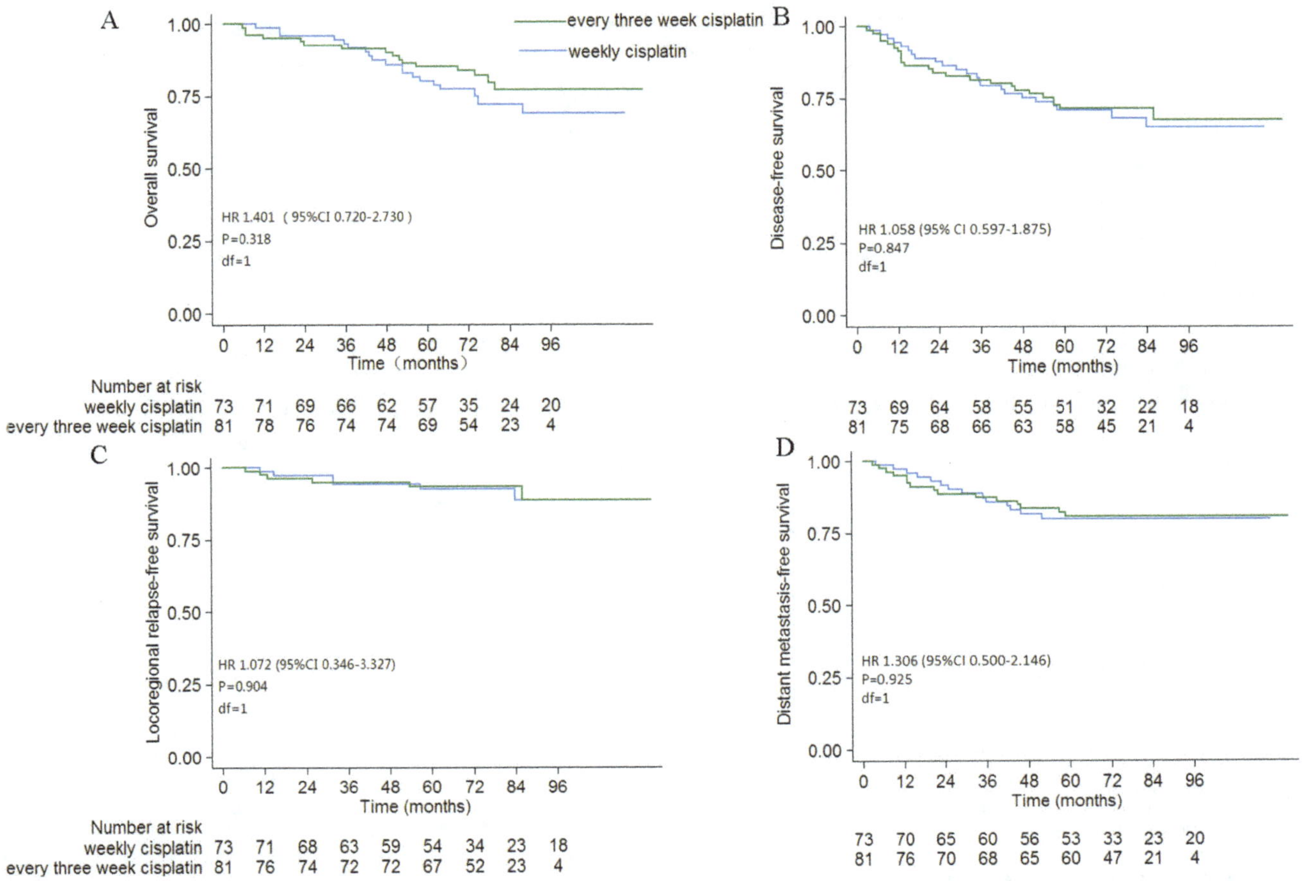

Figure 1. Survival curves for patients with NPC. (A) OS, (B) DFS, (C) LRRFS, and (D) DMFS. Hazard ratios (HRs) were calculated with an unadjusted Cox proportional hazards model; *P*-values were calculated with the unadjusted log-rank test.

were used to test for independent significance using backward elimination of insignificant explanatory variables of different parameters [17]. Host factors (age and sex) were included as covariates in all tests. The criterion for statistical significance was set at $a = 0.05$ and *P*-values were determined using 2-sided tests.

Results

Patient characteristics

Both groups were well-balanced in terms of baseline demographic and clinical characteristics and treatment factors (Table 1). Tumor response was evaluated via endoscopy and MRI scans of the neck and nasopharynx at three months after RT. The composite overall response rate for the primary site and neck region was 97.3% and 98.7% for the weekly and every three week CDDP group, respectively ($P = 0.258$).

Treatment compliance and acute toxicities

All 154 patients tolerated the treatment well and completed the prescribed dose of RT. The median overall treatment time was 43 days in the weekly group and 44 days in the every three weeks group ($P = 0.554$). In the weekly group, 66 patients (90.4%) received at least five weeks of CDDP and only four patients (5.5%) received seven weeks of CDDP. In the every three weeks group, 72 patients (88.9%) completed two cycles of CDDP and five patients (6.2%) received three cycles of CDDP. The median cumulative dose received during concurrent CCRT was 180 and 160 mg/m^2 CDDP for the weekly and every three weeks group, respectively ($P = 0.10$). Reductions in the number of chemotherapy cycles were mostly due to patient refusal, severe mucositis, or prolonged severe leucopenia.

Systemic toxicities were similar in both groups (Table 2). No treatment-related deaths were observed in either cohort. The most commonly recorded non-hematological adverse event was grade 3–4 mucositis in 23 patients (31.5%) in the weekly group and 24 patients (29.6%) in the every three weeks group ($P = 0.139$). The most common hematological adverse event was grade 3–4 leucopenia in six patients (8.2%) in the weekly group and five patients (6.2%) in the every three weeks group ($P = 0.312$).

Patterns of failure and survival rates

The overall median follow-up time was 74 months (range, 6–123 months). Twelve of the 154 patients (7.8%) developed locoregional relapse. There was distant metastasis in 29/154 patients (18.8%), and 35/154 patients (22.7%) died. The sites of relapse were local in 7/154 patients (4.5%), regional in 7/154 patients (4.5%), and both local and regional in 2/154 patients (1.3%). Three patients (1.9%) experienced both locoregional and distant failure.

The overall 5-year OS, DFS, LRRFS, and DMFS rates were 82.3%, 71.3%, 93.1%, and 80.5%, respectively. The 5-year OS, DFS, LRRFS, and DMFS rates were not significantly different between the two treatment groups (every three weeks vs. weekly: OS = 85.2% vs. 78.9%, $P = 0.318$; DFS = 71.6% vs. 71.0%, $P = 0.847$; LRRFS = 93.5% vs. 92.6%, $P = 0.904$; DMFS = 80.9%

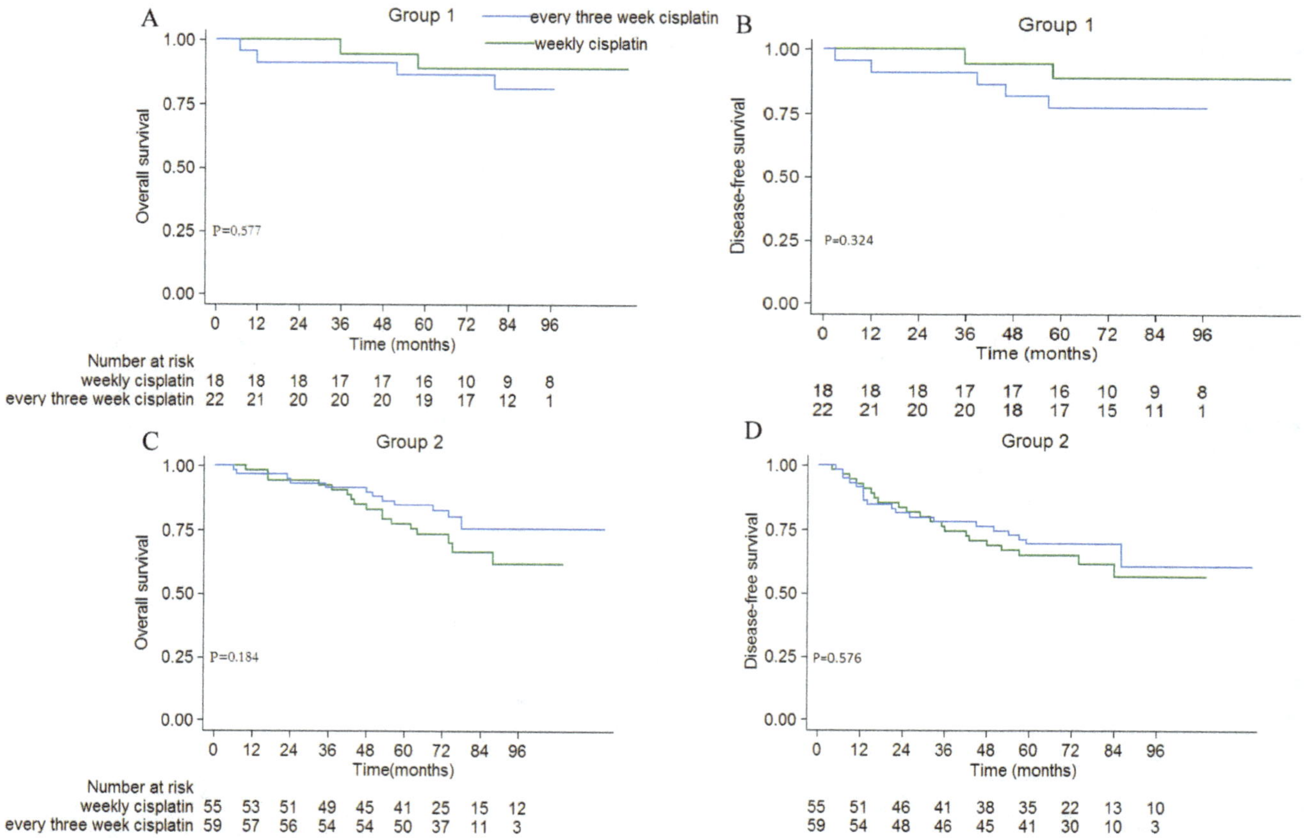

Figure 2. OS and DFS curves for NPC patients stratified by clinical stage. Group 1: patients with stage II disease; Group 2: patients with stage III–IVB disease. *P*-values were calculated with the unadjusted log-rank test.

vs. 80.1%, $P = 0.925$; Fig. 1). The 5-year OS and DFS rates for patients with early- or advanced-stage disease in the two treatment groups were not significantly different (Fig. 2).

Prognostic factors

Univariate analysis revealed that age and N classification were significant prognostic factors for OS ($P = 0.009$ and 0.011, respectively). The 5-year OS rate for patients who received

Table 3. Summary of multivariate analysis of prognostic factors in the 154 patients.

End point	HR (95% CI)	*P*-value†
OS		
Age, >50 years vs. ≤50 years	2.809 (1.404–5.620)	0.004
N classification (N0–1 vs. N2–3)	2.830 (1.388–5.767)	0.004
Chemotherapy regimen, weekly vs. every three weeks	0.862 (0.428–1.738)	0.679
DFS		
N classification (N0–1 vs. N2–3)	2.241 (1.213–4.141)	0.010
Chemotherapy regimen, weekly vs. every three weeks	1.099 (0.604–2.001)	0.757
DMFS		
N classification (N0–1 vs. N2–3)	2.752 (1.271–5.961)	0.010
Chemotherapy regimen, weekly vs. every three weeks	1.331 (0.607–2.917)	0.475
LRRFS		
Chemotherapy regimen, weekly vs. every three weeks	1.280 (0.382–4.288)	0.689

HR: hazard ratio; CI: confidence interval; OS: overall survival; DFS: disease-free survival; DMFS: distant metastasis-free survival; LRRFS: locoregional relapse-free survival.
†P-values were calculated using an adjusted Cox proportional hazards regression model adjusted for age (>50 years vs. ≤50 years), sex (male vs. female), T classification (T1–2 vs. T3–4), N classification (N0–1 vs. N2–3), chemotherapy regimen, (weekly vs. every three weeks) and cumulative cisplatin dose, (≥160 mg/m2 vs. <160 mg/m2). Only variables that were significantly associated with survival are presented except for the chemotherapy regimen.

cumulative CDDP≥160 mg/m^2 was 84.1% compared to 73.3% for patients who received cumulative CDDP<160 mg/m^2 ($P = 0.175$).

Multivariate analysis was performed to adjust for various prognostic factors. The following parameters were included in the Cox proportional hazards model by backward elimination of insignificant explanatory variables: age (>50 years vs. ≤50 years), sex, T classification (T1–2 vs. T3–4), N classification (N0–1 vs. N2–3), concurrent chemotherapy regimen (CDDP weekly vs. every three weeks), and cumulative CDDP dose (≥160 mg/m^2 vs. <160 mg/m^2). Multivariate analysis demonstrated that the CCRT regimen was not a significant prognostic factor for any end point. Age and N classification were significant predictive factors for OS; furthermore, N classification was the only significant prognostic factor for DFS and DMFS (Table 3).

Discussion

NPC is a highly chemosensitive tumor and CCRT has long been a standard treatment option for locoregionally advanced NPC. Treatment regimens delivering medium doses of CDDP weekly or high CDDP doses every three weeks have been evaluated. Weekly medium doses are efficient and simple to administer, especially for outpatients; high doses every three weeks are more effective for reducing distant metastasis, but may lead to more severe acute toxicities [4–7].

In this retrospective study, we observed that CDDP-based (both weekly and every three weeks) CCRT led to similar long-term survival outcomes and acute toxicities in patients with NPC receiving IMRT regardless of whether the patients had early- or advanced-stage disease. Our results are in agreement with that of Jagdis et al. [12], which showed that 40 mg/m^2 CDDP weekly and 100 mg/m^2 CDDP every three weeks had similar deliverability, toxicity profiles, and comparable survival outcomes in locally advanced NPC.

In our study, the overall 5-year OS, DFS, LRRFS, and DMFS rates were 82.3%, 71.3%, 93.1%, and 80.5%, respectively. CDDP delivered both weekly or every three weeks concurrently with IMRT achieved excellent OS. Distant metastasis was the predominant mode of failure. One approach to improving the strategy tested in this study would be changing the sequence to induction–concurrent, as substantially better tolerance and compliance rates have been reported for induction–concurrent regimens [18]. The meta-analysis by OuYang et al. in 2013 [19] also showed that neoadjuvant chemotherapy effectively enhances OS and reduces the rate of distant metastasis in NPC.

With respect to dose delivery, both treatment groups achieved similar cumulative dose intensities; however, a low proportion of patients completed seven weeks of weekly CDDP or three cycles of every three week CDDP. The compliance rates in the present study are lower than that of previously published trials [4–7]. This may be because the weekly CDDP regimen was mostly administered to outpatients and the regimen given every three weeks was mainly administered to inpatients at our center. Poor outpatient compliance and inadequate numbers of inpatient beds led to delays in administering chemotherapy, which often resulted in patients missing the final cycle of chemotherapy.

We adopted an every three week CDDP dose of 80 mg/m^2 in our study, which was effective with low toxicity. The INT-0099 regimen is widely used, where 100 mg/m^2 CDDP is administered on days 1, 22, and 43 with radical RT, given its impressive results compared to RT alone when treating NPC. Regrettably, only 63% of patients in the chemoradiation arm of INT-0099 completed all three cycles of concurrent chemotherapy as planned. Ho et al. [20] compared the dose intensity and toxicity of CDDP administered weekly and every three weeks concurrently to 52 patients with locally advanced squamous head and neck cancer. They found that 100 mg/m^2 CDDP every three weeks with RT was less well tolerated than 40 mg/m^2 CDDP weekly or 80 mg/m^2 CDDP every three weeks and resulted in fewer patients achieving a cumulative dose of >200 mg/m^2. Therefore, the optimal CDDP dose in CCRT regimes for NPC warrants further exploration.

The dose intensity of CDDP is an important prognostic factor in NPC patients receiving CCRT [21–22]. Using pooled data from three prospective trials (in which most patients were treated with conventional RT), Loong et al. [21] explored the prognostic significance of the total CDDP dose delivered during CCRT and reported that patients with stage II or III NPC who received more than five weeks of 40 mg/m^2 CDDP weekly had significantly better OS than patients who received less than five weeks. In our study, a cumulative dose of ≥160 mg/m^2 led to obviously better OS, although the difference was not significant (84.1% vs. 73.3%, $P = 0.175$); this may be related to the small number of patients who received a cumulative dose of <160 mg/m^2. Additionally, the use of IMRT has improved the long-term outcome for patients with NPC, which may render detection of the survival benefit of a higher total CDDP dose difficult.

The toxicity profiles of both groups were similar. However, there was a slightly higher incidence of grade 3–4 hematological toxicity and oropharyngeal mucositis in the weekly CDDP group, although the difference was not significant. The main reasons for this observation may be the inadequate monitoring of blood counts and poor oral care in outpatients in the weekly CDDP group. It is worth noting that there was a lower incidence of grade 3–4 dermatitis, dysphagia, and gastrointestinal reactions in patients who received CDDP weekly even though they received a relatively high median cumulative dose.

To our knowledge, this is the first single-institution study to review the difference between CDDP administered weekly and every three weeks concurrently with IMRT in NPC. The principal limitation of this study is its retrospective nature. However, the clinical characteristics of the patients in the two groups were well-balanced, which may reduce potential selection bias. To derive a definitive conclusion, a randomized phase II study of CCRT with CDDP administered every three weeks versus weekly in patients with locally advanced NPC is ongoing in Korea. The findings of this study will aid in the standardization of CCRT regimens for NPC.

Conclusions

IMRT in conjunction with concurrent CDDP chemotherapy administered weekly or every three weeks leads to similar long-term survival outcomes and acute toxicities in NPC regardless of whether the patient has early- or advanced-stage disease. The results of this study require further validation in prospective, multi-center controlled trials.

Author Contributions

Conceived and designed the experiments: C-JT LL YS. Performed the experiments: C-JT LL YS G-QZ L-LT LC Y-PM M-SZ T-BK W-HJ J-YS H-QM JM. Analyzed the data: C-JT LL YS A-HL. Contributed reagents/materials/analysis tools: H-QM A-HL JM. Wrote the paper: C-JT LL YS G-QZ.

References

1. Jemal A, Bray F, Center MM, Ferlay J, Ward E, et al. (2011) Global cancer statistics. CA Cancer J Clin 61: 69–90.
2. Edge SB, Byrd DR, Compton CC, Fritz AG, Greene FL, et al. (2009) American Joint Committee on Cancer Manual for Staging of Cancer [M]. 7th ed. Philadelphia: JB Lippincott. 649 p.
3. Chen L, Mao YP, Xie FY, Liu LZ, Sun Y, et al. (2012) The seventh edition of the UICC/AJCC staging system for nasopharyngeal carcinoma is prognostically useful for patients treated with intensity-modulated radiotherapy from an endemic area in China. Radiat Oncol Biol Phys 104: 331–337.
4. Al-Sarraf M, LeBlanc M, Giri PG, Fu KK, Cooper J, et al. (1998) Chemoradiotherapy versus radiotherapy in patients with advanced nasopharyngeal cancer: phase III randomized Intergroup Study 0099. J Clin Oncol 16: 1310–1317.
5. Lee AW, Lau WH, Tung SY, Chua DT, Chappell R, et al. (2005) Preliminary results of a randomized study on therapeutic gain by concurrent chemotherapy for regionally-advanced nasopharyngeal carcinoma: NPC-9901 trial by the Hong Kong Nasopharyngeal Cancer Study Group. J Clin Oncol 23: 6966–6975.
6. Lee AW, Tung SY, Chua DT, Ngan RK, Chappell R, et al. (2010) Randomized trial of radiotherapy plus concurrent-adjuvant chemotherapy vs. radiotherapy alone for regionally advanced nasopharyngeal carcinoma. J Natl Cancer Inst 102: 1188–1198.
7. Chen Y, Sun Y, Liang SB, Zong JF, Li WF, et al. (2013) Progress report of a randomized trial comparing long-term survival and late toxicity of concurrent chemoradiotherapy with adjuvant chemotherapy versus radiotherapy alone in patients with stage III to IVB nasopharyngeal carcinoma from endemic regions of China. Cancer 119: 2230–2238.
8. Chan AT, Leung SF, Ngan RK, Teo PM, Lau WH, et al. (2005) Overall survival after concurrent cisplatin-radiotherapy compared with radiotherapy alone in locoregionally advanced nasopharyngeal carcinoma. J Natl Cancer Inst 97: 536–539.
9. Lin JC, Jan JS, Hsu CY, Liang WM, Jiang RS, et al. (2003) Phase III study of concurrent chemoradiotherapy versus radiotherapy alone for advanced nasopharyngeal carcinoma: positive effect on overall and progression-free survival. J Clin Oncol 21: 631–637.
10. Chen L, Hu CS, Chen XZ, Hu GQ, Cheng ZB, et al. (2012) Concurrent chemoradiotherapy plus adjuvant chemotherapy versus concurrent chemoradiotherapy alone in patients with locoregionally advanced nasopharyngeal carcinoma: a phase 3 multicentre randomised controlled trial. Lancet Oncol 13: 163–171.
11. Baujat B, Audry H, Bourhis J, Chan AT, Onat H, et al. (2006) Chemotherapy in locally advanced nasopharyngeal carcinoma: an individual data meta-analysis of eight randomized trials and 1753 patients. Int J Radiat Oncol Biol Phys 64: 47–56.
12. Jagdis A, Laskin J, Hao D, Hay J, Wu J, et al. (2012) Dose delivery analysis of weekly versus 3-weekly cisplatin concurrent with radiation therapy for locally advanced nasopharyngeal carcinoma (NPC). Am J Clin Oncol Oct 29.
13. Peng G, Wang T, Yang KY, Zhang S, Zhang T, et al. (2012) A prospective, randomized study comparing outcomes and toxicities of intensity-modulated radiotherapy vs. conventional two-dimensional radiotherapy for the treatment of nasopharyngeal carcinoma. Radiother Oncol 104: 286–293.
14. Zhao C, Han F, Lu LX, Huang SM, Lin CG, et al. (2004) Intensity modulated radiotherapy for local-regional advanced nasopharyngeal carcinoma. Ai Zheng 23: 1532–1537.
15. Liang S, Sun Y, Liu L, Chen Y, Chen L, et al. (2009) Extension of local disease in nasopharyngeal carcinoma detected by magnetic resonance imaging: improvement of clinical target volume delineation. Int J Radiat Oncol Biol Phys 75: 742–750.
16. Kaplan EL, Meier P (1958) Nonparametric estimation from incomplete observation. J Am Stat Assoc 53: 457–481.
17. Cox DR (1972) Regression models and life tables. J R Stat Soc B 34: 187–220.
18. Lee AWM, Ng WT, Chan OSH, Sze HCK (2012) If concurrent-adjuvant chemoradiotherapy is beneficial for locoregionally advanced nasopharyngeal carcinoma, would changing the sequence to induction-concurrent achieve better outcome? J Radiat Oncol 1: 107–115.
19. OuYang PY, Xie C, Mao YP, Zhang Y, Liang XX, et al. (2013) Significant efficacies of neoadjuvant and adjuvant chemotherapy for nasopharyngeal carcinoma by meta-analysis of published literature-based randomized, controlled trials. Ann Oncol 24: 2136–2146.
20. Ho KF, Swindell R, Brammer CV (2008) Dose intensity comparison between weekly and 3-weekly Cisplatin delivered concurrently with radical radiotherapy for head and neck cancer: A retrospective comparison from New Cross Hospital, Wolverhampton, UK. Acta Oncol 47: 1513–1518.
21. Loong HH, Ma BB, Leung SF, Mo F, Hui EP, et al. (2012) Prognostic significance of the total dose of cisplatin administered during concurrent chemoradiotherapy in patients with locoregionally advanced nasopharyngeal carcinoma. Radiother Oncol 104: 300–304.
22. Chen QY, Wen YF, Guo L, Liu H, Huang PY, et al. (2011) Concurrent chemoradiotherapy vs radiotherapy alone in stage II nasopharyngeal carcinoma: phase III randomized trial. J Natl Cancer Inst 103: 1761–1770.

Permissions

All chapters in this book were first published in PLOS ONE, by The Public Library of Science; hereby published with permission under the Creative Commons Attribution License or equivalent. Every chapter published in this book has been scrutinized by our experts. Their significance has been extensively debated. The topics covered herein carry significant findings which will fuel the growth of the discipline. They may even be implemented as practical applications or may be referred to as a beginning point for another development.

The contributors of this book come from diverse backgrounds, making this book a truly international effort. This book will bring forth new frontiers with its revolutionizing research information and detailed analysis of the nascent developments around the world.

We would like to thank all the contributing authors for lending their expertise to make the book truly unique. They have played a crucial role in the development of this book. Without their invaluable contributions this book wouldn't have been possible. They have made vital efforts to compile up to date information on the varied aspects of this subject to make this book a valuable addition to the collection of many professionals and students.

This book was conceptualized with the vision of imparting up-to-date information and advanced data in this field. To ensure the same, a matchless editorial board was set up. Every individual on the board went through rigorous rounds of assessment to prove their worth. After which they invested a large part of their time researching and compiling the most relevant data for our readers.

The editorial board has been involved in producing this book since its inception. They have spent rigorous hours researching and exploring the diverse topics which have resulted in the successful publishing of this book. They have passed on their knowledge of decades through this book. To expedite this challenging task, the publisher supported the team at every step. A small team of assistant editors was also appointed to further simplify the editing procedure and attain best results for the readers.

Apart from the editorial board, the designing team has also invested a significant amount of their time in understanding the subject and creating the most relevant covers. They scrutinized every image to scout for the most suitable representation of the subject and create an appropriate cover for the book.

The publishing team has been an ardent support to the editorial, designing and production team. Their endless efforts to recruit the best for this project, has resulted in the accomplishment of this book. They are a veteran in the field of academics and their pool of knowledge is as vast as their experience in printing. Their expertise and guidance has proved useful at every step. Their uncompromising quality standards have made this book an exceptional effort. Their encouragement from time to time has been an inspiration for everyone.

The publisher and the editorial board hope that this book will prove to be a valuable piece of knowledge for researchers, students, practitioners and scholars across the globe.

List of Contributors

Jefferson W. Daniel and José C. E. Veiga
Division of Neurosurgery, Santa Casa de São Paulo - Faculty of Medical Sciences, São Paulo, Brazil

Teemu J. Murtola
University of Tampere, School of Medicine, Tampere, Finland
Tampere University Hospital, Department of Urology, Tampere, Finland

Kala Visvanathan
Johns Hopkins Bloomberg School of Public Health, Department of Epidemiology, Baltimore, Maryland, United States of America
Sidney Kimmel Comprehensive Cancer Center, Johns Hopkins School of Medicine, Baltimore Maryland, United States of America

Miia Artama
University of Helsinki, Helsinki, Finland,

Harri Vainio
Finnish Institute of Occupational Health, Helsinki, Finland

Eero Pukkala
University of Tampere, School of Health Sciences, Tampere, Finland
The Finnish Cancer Registry, Institute for Statistical and Epidemiological Cancer Research, Helsinki, Finland

Serene M. L. Lee, Natalja Fröse, Tobias S. Schiergens and Wolfgang E. Thasler
Department of General, Visceral, Transplantation, Vascular and Thoracic Surgery, Grosshadern Hospital, Ludwig Maximilians University, Munich, Germany

Celine Schelcher and Reinhard M. K. Thasler
Tissue Bank, Department of General, Visceral, Transplantation, Vascular and Thoracic Surgery, Grosshadern Hospital, Ludwig Maximilians University, Munich, Germany

Rüdiger P. Laubender and Ulrich Mansmann
Institute for Medical Information Processing, Biometry and Epidemiology, Grosshadern Hospital, Ludwig Maximilians University, Munich, Germany

Wenjun Zhao, Lirong Wei, Dongming Tan, Guangsong Su, Yanwen Zheng and Chao He
Cyrus Tang Hematology Center, Jiangsu Institute of Hematology, the First Affiliated Hospital, Soochow University, Suzhou, Jiangsu Province, PR China

Zhengwei J. Mao
Division of Hematopathology, Department of Laboratory Medicine and Pathology, University of Minnesota Medical Center-Fairview, Minneapolis, Minnesota, United States of America

Timothy P. Singleton
Department of Laboratory of Medicine and Pathology, University of Minnesota, Minneapolis, Minnesota, United States of America

Bin Yin
Cyrus Tang Hematology Center, Jiangsu Institute of Hematology, the First Affiliated Hospital, Soochow University, Suzhou, Jiangsu Province, PR China
Thrombosis and Hemostasis Key Lab of the Ministry of Health, Soochow University, Suzhou, Jiangsu Province, PR China
Collaborative Innovation Center of Hematology, Soochow University, Suzhou, Jiangsu Province, PR China

Nicola Magrini, Giulio Formoso, Emilio Maestri, Francesco Nonino, Barbara Paltrinieri, Claudio Voci, Lucia Magnano and Anna Maria Marata
Drug Evaluation Area, Emilia-Romagna Regional Agency for Health and Social Care, Bologna, Italy

Oreste Capelli and Lisa Daya
Local Health Authority, Modena, Italy

Cinzia Del Giovane
Department of Clinical and Diagnostic Medicine and Public Health, University of Modena and Reggio Emilia, Modena, Italy

Yuanming Shen, Jiansong Zhou, Yang Li, Feng Ye, Xiaoyun Wan, Weiguo Lu, Xing Xie and Xiaodong Cheng
Department of Gynecologic Oncology, Women's Hospital, School of Medicine, Zhejiang University, Hangzhou, China

Min Zhang, Mingquan Shang, Weiwei Yang, Junli Chen and Hong Shang
Key Laboratory of AIDS Immunology of National Health and Family Planning Commission, Department of Laboratory Medicine, The First Affiliated Hospital, China Medical University, Shenyang, China
Collaborative Innovation Center for Diagnosis and Treatment of Infectious Diseases, Hangzhou, China

Zhe Wang
Disease Prevention and Control Center of Henan Province, Zhengzhou, China

Angelo Gámez-Pozo, Rocío López-Vacas, Julia Berges-Soria and Juan A. Fresno Vara
Instituto de Genética Médica y Molecular (INGEMM) - IdiPAZ, Hospital La Paz, Madrid, Spain

Ramón M. Pérez Carrión
Medical Oncology Department, Hospital Quirón, Pozuelo de Alarcón, Madrid, Spain

Luis Manso, Cesar Mendiola and Eva M. Ciruelos
Medical Oncology Department, Hospital 12 de Octubre, Madrid, Spain

Carmen Crespo
Medical Oncology Department, Hospital Ramón y Cajal, Madrid, Spain

Isabel Álvarez López
Medical Oncology Department, Hospital de Donostia, San Sebastián, Pais Vasco, Spain

Mireia Margeli
Medical Oncology Department, Hospital Germans Trias i Pujol, Badalona, Barcelona, Spain

Juan L. Bayo Calero
Medical Oncology Department, Hospital Juan Ramón Jiménez, Huelva, Spain

Xavier González Farre
Medical Oncology Department, Hospital Clinic de Barcelona, Barcelona, Spain

Ana Santaballa
Medical Oncology Department, Hospital La Fe, Valencia, Spain

Ruth Afonso
Medical Oncology Department, Hospital Nuestra Señora de la Candelaria, Santa Cruz de Tenerife, Spain

Juan Lao
Medical Oncology Department, Hospital Miguel Servet, Zaragoza, Spain

Gustavo Catalán
Medical Oncology Department, Hospital Son Llàtzer, Palma de Mallorca, Spain

José V. Álvarez Gallego
Medical Oncology Department, Complejo Hospitalario de Zamora, Zamora, Spain

José Miramón López
Medical Oncology Department, Hospital Serranía de Ronda, Ronda, Málaga, Spain

Francisco J. Salvador Bofill
Medical Oncology Department, Hospital Virgen de Valme, Sevilla, Spain

Manuel Ruiz Borrego
Medical Oncology Department, Hospital Virgen del Rocío, Sevilla, Spain

Enrique Espinosa and Pilar Zamora
Medical Oncology Department, Hospital La Paz, Madrid, Spain

Jie Ge, Zihua Chen and Zhikang Chen
Department of Gastrointestinal Surgery, Xiangya Hospital, Central South University, Changsha, Hunan, P. R. China

Jin Huang, Jinxiang Chen and Weijie Yuan
Department of Oncology, Xiangya Hospital, Central South University, Changsha, Hunan, P. R. China

Zhenghao Deng
Department of Pathology, Xiangya Hospital, Central South University, Changsha, Hunan, P. R. China

Ling-Long Tang, Rui Guo, Guanqun Zhou, Ying Sun and Jun Ma
Department of Radiation oncology, Sun Yat-sen University Cancer Center; State Key Laboratory of Oncology in South China; Collaborative Innovation Center for Cancer Medicine, Guangzhou, Guangdong, People's Republic of China

Li-Zhi Liu and Li Li
Imaging Diagnosis and Interventional Center, State Key Laboratory of Oncology in South China, Sun Yatsen University Cancer Center, Collaborative Innovation Center for Cancer Medicine, Guangzhou, Guangdong, People's Republic of China

Ai-Hua Lin
Department of Medical Statistics and Epidemiology, School of Public Health, Sun Yat-sen University, Guangzhou, Guangdong, People's Republic of China

Haiqiang Mai
Department of Nasopharyngeal Carcinoma, Sun Yat-Sen University Cancer Center, Collaborative Innovation Center for Cancer Medicine, Guangzhou, Guangdong, People's Republic of China

Jianyong Shao
Department of Molecular Diagnostics, State Key Laboratory of Oncology in South China, Sun Yat-Sen University Cancer Center, Collaborative Innovation Center for Cancer Medicine, Guangzhou, Guangdong, People's Republic of China

Edward Yepes
IBSAL-CIETUS (Instituto de Investigación Biomédica de Salamanca-Centro de Investigación de Enfermedades Tropicales de la Universidad de Salamanca), Facultad de Farmacia, Universidad de Salamanca, Salamanca, Spain
Instituto de Biología Molecular y Celular del Cáncer, Centro de Investigación del Cáncer, CSIC-Universidad de Salamanca, Campus Miguel de Unamuno, Salamanca, Spain

Rubén E. Varela-M, E L Habib Dakir and Faustino Mollinedo
Instituto de Biología Molecular y Celular del Cáncer, Centro de Investigación del Cáncer, CSIC-Universidad de Salamanca, Campus Miguel de Unamuno, Salamanca, Spain

Julio López-Abán and Antonio Muro
IBSAL-CIETUS (Instituto de Investigación Biomédica de Salamanca-Centro de Investigación de Enfermedades Tropicales de la Universidad de Salamanca), Facultad de Farmacia, Universidad de Salamanca, Salamanca, Spain

Shahid Husain, Yasir Abdul, Sudha Singh, Anis Ahmad and Mahvash Husain
Hewitt Laboratory of the Ola B. Williams Glaucoma Center, Department of Ophthalmology, Storm Eye Institute, Medical University of South Carolina, Charleston, South Carolina, United States of America

Kristina Star and I. Ralph Edwards
Uppsala Monitoring Centre, WHO Collaborating Centre for International Drug Monitoring, Uppsala, Sweden

Imti Choonara
Academic Division of Child Health, University of Nottingham, Derbyshire Children's Hospital, Nottingham, United Kingdom

Mogens K. Boisen and Benny V. Jensen
Department of Oncology, Herlev University Hospital, Herlev, Denmark

Christian Dehlendorff
Statistics, Bioinformatics and Registry, Danish Cancer Society Research Center, Copenhagen, Denmark

Dorte Linnemann and Estrid V. S. Høgdall
Department of Pathology, Herlev University Hospital, Herlev, Denmark

Boye S. Nielsen
Bioneer, Hørsholm, Denmark

Jim S. Larsen
Department of Oncology, Roskilde Hospital, Roskilde, Denmark

Kell Østerlind
Department of Oncology, Rigshospitalet, Copenhagen, Denmark

Svend E. Nielsen
Department of Oncology and Palliation, Hillerød Hospital, Hillerød, Denmark

Line S. Tarpgaard, Camilla Qvortrup and Per Pfeiffer
Department of Oncology, Odense University Hospital, Odense, Denmark

Niels H. Holländer
Department of Oncology, Næstved Hospital, Næstved, Denmark

Nina Keldsen
Department of Oncology, Herning Hospital, Herning, Denmark

Torben F. Hansen
Department of Oncology, Vejle Hospital, Vejle, Denmark

Brita B. Jensen
Department of Medicine, Queen Ingrid Hospital, Nuuk, Greenland
Department of Oncology, Sydvestjysk Hospital, Esbjerg, Denmark

Julia S. Johansen
Department of Oncology, Herlev University Hospital, Herlev, Denmark
Department of Medicine, Herlev University Hospital, Herlev, Denmark

Daniel Purcaru
Department of Medical Ethics, Transilvania University, Brasov, Romania
Department of Clinical Research, Neomed Medical Center, Brasov, Romania

Adrian Preda
Department of Psychiatry and Human Behavior, University of California Irvine School of Medicine, Irvine, California, United States of America
University of California Irvine Neuropsychiatric Center, Orange, California, United States of America

Daniela Popa
Faculty of Psychology and Sciences of Education, Transilvania University, Brasov, Romania

Marius Alexandru Moga
Department of Medical and Surgical Specialties, Faculty of Medicine, Transilvania University, Brasov, Romania

Liliana Rogozea
Department of Fundamental Disciplines and Clinical Prevention, Faculty of Medicine, Transilvania University, Brasov, Romania

Huan Lu, Qun Zhao, Hao Jiang, Peng Xia, Dongmei Wang, Zhen Dou and Xuebiao Yao
Anhui Key Laboratory of Cellular Dynamics and Chemical Biology, University of Science and Technology of China, Hefei, Anhui, China

Tongge Zhu
Anhui Key Laboratory of Cellular Dynamics and Chemical Biology, University of Science and Technology of China, Hefei, Anhui, China
Department of Physiology, Morehouse School of Medicine, Atlanta, Georgia, United States of America

William Seffens and Felix Aikhionbare
Department of Physiology, Morehouse School of Medicine, Atlanta, Georgia, United States of America

Petros Isaakidis, Mrinalini Das, Christopher Peskett and Lorraine Rebello
Médecins Sans Frontières, Mumbai, India

Ajay M V Kumar
International Union Against Tuberculosis and Lung Disease (The Union), South-East Asia Regional Office, New Delhi, India

Minni Khetarpal
City TB Office, Bawala Wadi, Chinckpokli, Mumbai, India

Arun Bamne
Brihanmumbai Municipal Corporation, Mumbai, India

Balkrishna Adsul
Mumbai District AIDS Control Society (MDACS), Mumbai, India

Mamta Manglani
Pediatric Centre of Excellence for HIV Care, L.T.M. Medical College & General Hospital, Sion, Mumbai, India

Kuldeep Singh Sachdeva
Central TB Division, Directorate General of Health Services, Ministry of Health and Family Welfare, New Delhi, India,

Malik Parmar
World Health Organisation - Country Office for India, New Delhi, India,

Avinash Kanchar and B.B. Rewari
Department of AIDS Control, National AIDS Control Organisation, New Delhi, India,

Alaka Deshpande
MGM Institute of Health Sciences, Navi Mumbai, India,

Camilla Rodrigues and Anjali Shetty
P.D. Hinduja National Hospital and Medical Research Centre, Mumbai, India,

Peter Saranchuk
Southern Africa Medical Unit (SAMU), Médecins Sans Frontières, Cape Town, South Africa

Marie Lechaftois, Bruno Palmier, Isabelle Margaill, Catherine Marchand-Leroux and Dominique Lerouet
EA4475-"Pharmacologie de la Circulation Cérébrale", Faculté des Sciences harmaceutiques et Biologiques, Université Paris Descartes, Comue Sorbonne Paris Cité, Paris, France

Elise Dreano and Christilla Bachelot-Loza
Inserm UMR S1140, Paris, France
Faculté des Sciences Pharmaceutiques et Biologiques, Université Paris Descartes, Comue Sorbonne Paris Cité, Paris, France

Carmel Jacobs
Division of Medical Oncology, The Ottawa Hospital Cancer Centre and Department of Medicine, University of Ottawa, Ottawa, Ontario, Canada

Ian D. Grahamn and Dean Fergusson
Department of Epidemiology and Community Medicine, University of Ottawa, Ottawa, Ontario, Canada
Ottawa Hospital Research Institute and University of Ottawa, Department of Medicine, Ottawa, Ontario, Canada

Julie Makarsk
Independent Consultant, Hamilton, Ontario, Canada

Michaël Chassé and Brian Hutton
Department of Epidemiology and Community Medicine, University of Ottawa, Ottawa, Ontario, Canada

Mark Clemons
Division of Medical Oncology, The Ottawa Hospital Cancer Centre and Department of Medicine, University of Ottawa, Ottawa, Ontario, Canada
Ottawa Hospital Research Institute and University of Ottawa, Department of Medicine,
Ottawa, Ontario, Canada

Chang-Juan Tao
Department of Radiation Oncology, Sun Yat-sen University Cancer Center, State Key Laboratory of Oncology in South China, Collaborative Innovation Center for Cancer Medicine, Guangzhou, Guangdong Province, People's Republic of China
Department of Radiation Oncology, Zhejiang Cancer Hospital, Hangzhou, Zhejiang Province, People's Republic of China

Li Lin, Guan-Qun Zhou, Ling-Long Tang, Lei Chen, Yan-Ping Mao, Jun Ma and Ying Sun
Department of Radiation Oncology, Sun Yat-sen University Cancer Center, State Key Laboratory of Oncology in South China, Collaborative Innovation Center for Cancer
Medicine, Guangzhou, Guangdong Province, People's Republic of China

Mu-Sheng Zeng, Tie-Bang Kang and Wei-Hua Jia
Department of Experimental Research, Sun Yat-sen University Cancer Center, State Key Laboratory of Oncology in South China, Collaborative Innovation Center for Cancer Medicine, Guangzhou, Guangdong Province, People's Republic of China

Jian-Yong Shao
Department of Pathology, Sun Yat-sen University Cancer Center, State Key Laboratory of Oncology in South China, Collaborative Innovation Center for Cancer Medicine, Guangzhou, Guangdong Province, People's Republic of China

Hai-Qiang Mai
Department of Nasopharyngeal Carcinoma, Sun Yat-sen University Cancer Center, State Key Laboratory of Oncology in South China, Collaborative Innovation Center for Cancer Medicine, Guangzhou, Guangdong Province, People's Republic of China

Ai-Hua Lin
Department of Medical Statistics and Epidemiology, School of Public Health, Sun Yatsen
University, Guangzhou, Guangdong Province, People's Republic of China

Juan Carlos Q. Velez and John M. Arthur
Division of Nephrology, Department of Medicine, Medical University of South Carolina, Charleston, South Carolina, United States of America
Medical Service, Ralph H. Johnson Veterans Affairs Medical Center, Charleston, South Carolina, United States of America

Michael G. Janech, Megan P. Hicks, Thomas A. Morinelli, Jessalyn Rodgers and Wayne R. Fitzgibbon
Division of Nephrology, Department of Medicine, Medical University of South Carolina, Charleston, South Carolina, United States of America

Sally E. Self
Department of Pathology, Medical University of South Carolina, Charleston, South Carolina, United States of America

Index